An Eighteen-Hundred-Year-Old Chinese Medical Text on Miscellaneous Disease by Zhāng Jī (Zhāng Zhòng-Jǐng)

金匱要略

JĪN GUÌ YÀO LÜÈ

ESSENTIAL PRESCRIPTIONS OF THE GOLDEN CABINET

Translation and Commentaries

NIGEL WISEMAN
SABINE WILMS

PARADIGM PUBLICATIONS
TAOS, NEW MEXICO USA

An Eighteen-Hundred-Year-Old Chinese Medical Text on Miscellaneous Disease by Zhāng Jī (Zhāng Zhòng-Jǐng)

Jīn Guì Yào Lüè

Essential Prescriptions of the Golden Cabinet

‡ TRANSLATION AND COMMENTARIES ‡

Library of Congress Cataloging-in-Publication Data

Zhang, Zhongjing, fl. 168-196.
[Jin gui yao lüe. English]
Jin guì yào lüè : translation and commentaries = Essential prescriptions of the golden cabinet / Zhang Zhòng-Jing ; translated [and commented] by Nigel Wiseman and Sabine Wilms.
p. ; cm.
Parallel title: Essential prescriptions of the golden cabinet
Includes index.
In English; includes original text in Chinese.
ISBN 978-0-912111-91-9 (hardcover : alk. paper)
I. Wiseman, Nigel. II. Wilms, Sabine. III. Title. IV. Title: Essential prescriptions of the golden cabinet.
[DNLM: 1. Zhang, Zhongjing, fl. 168-196. Jin gui yao lue. English & Chinese. 2. Medicine, Chinese Traditional. WZ 294]
R733
615.8'8--dc23

2013003515

Published by Paradigm Publications, Taos, New Mexico USA
www paradigm-pubs.com
Distributed by Redwing Books, 202 Bendix St., Taos, NM 87571 USA
www.redwingbooks.com

Preface

This English translation of the *Jīn Guì Yào Lüè* ("Essential Prescriptions of the Golden Cabinet") complements that of the *Shāng Hán Lùn, Translation and Commentaries* by Mitchell, Féng, and Wiseman, published by Paradigm in 1999. Both the *Jīn Guì Yào Lüè* and *Shāng Hán Lùn* were pieced together from fragments of the no longer extant *Shāng Hán Zá Bìng Lùn* ("On Cold Damage and Miscellaneous Diseases") by Zhāng Jī of the Eastern Hàn Dynasty. The *Shāng Hán Lùn* represents the portion of it dealing with externally contracted disease, while the *Jīn Guì Yào Lüè* is the portion dealing with miscellaneous diseases, i.e., everything other than external contractions. The value of making these texts accessible to a Western audience requires no explanation, nor does the worth of their contribution. These two books together are among the earliest extant texts of Chinese medicine, making them a unique interface between the theories of the *Nèi Jīng* and the pragmatic approach of medicinal therapy that was fully recognized and widely adopted, only centuries later, in the Sòng Dynasty.

The continuous influence of these texts into modern times is easy to see. To this day, the *Shāng Hán Lùn* and *Jīn Guì Yào Lüè* are taught as subjects of their own in the Chinese medicine world, not merely for historical perspective but because they have contributed enormously to the shaping of Chinese medicine over its entire history. In any modern textbook of formulas, as many as 20% of the formulas are from Zhāng Jī's work. These formulas, now often used for conditions other than those for which they may have been prescribed originally, are valued today for the elegance with which so few ingredients treat so many aspects of a condition.

The *Jīn Guì Yào Lüè* is presented in 25 chapters, most of which deal with two or three closely related diseases. The final three chapters cover miscellaneous formulas and foodstuffs. Each chapter includes an introduction to the material, followed by the original lines of the text, which herein are rendered in simplified Chinese characters, Pīnyīn, and English translation. This is followed by notes to elucidate obscure phrases in the original text, a synopsis of the content of the line, and a detailed explanatory commentary.

Our translation strategy is the same as was used for our translation of the *Shāng Hán Lùn.* The translation of each line is as exact as possible. Substantial additions required in English to ensure grammatical sense are placed in brackets. We adopt a source-oriented approach to the translation of terms to preserve as far as possible the original concepts; e.g., "fox-creeper" for 狐惑 *hú huò*, rather than the superficially more explicit "throat-anus-genital pattern."

—Nigel Wiseman

Table of Contents

Introduction

Together with the *Shāng Hán Lùn* ("On Cold Damage"), the *Jīn Guì Yào Lüè* ("Essential Prescriptions of the Golden Cabinet") is widely studied and used by practitioners of Chinese medicine in both China and the West. As the earliest extant classics on medicinal formulas, these two texts together were originally rendered as a single text of sixteen scrolls called the *Shāng Hán Zá Bìng Lùn* ("On Cold Damage and Miscellaneous Diseases") by Zhāng Jī (Zhāng Zhòng-Jǐng) during the Eastern Hàn period, around the end of the second century CE. Unfortunately, this important text was lost soon after completion in the war-related upheavals that accompanied the collapse of the Hàn dynasty. In the following Western Jìn period, Wáng Shū-Hé (210-285 CE), who also left a mark in the history of Chinese medicine as the compiler of the *Mài Jīng* ("Pulse Canon"), collected the extant fragments of Zhāng Zhòng-Jǐng's work. He arranged them into two separate books: the *Shāng Hán Lùn* in ten scrolls, and another text on "miscellaneous diseases" in six scrolls, which in later centuries became known as the *Jīn Guì Yào Lüè*. It is in this form and under these titles that we most commonly access Zhāng Zhòng-Jǐng's clinical insights today.

The *Jīn Guì Yào Lüè,* and its sister volume the *Shāng Hán Lùn*, are treasures composed by arguably the most brilliant medical mind that China ever produced, the Hàn Dynasty physician Zhāng Jī. Exerting an influence on the development of Chinese medicine unmatched by any other medical scholar, Zhāng integrated the then relatively new theories of systematic correspondence laid down in the *Huáng Dì Nèi Jīng* and the *Nàn Jīng* with an already vast practical knowledge in the use of medicinals. His brilliance was not fully recognized by Chinese physicians until centuries later in the Sòng Dynasty, when Zhāng's combination of theory and practice became a mainstream feature of Chinese medicine that survived centuries of scrutiny from successive generations of medical scholars, and buttressed traditional medicine against the challenge of Western medicine in the 20th century. Combining theoretical etiologies with detailed diagnosis and skillfully devised treatments, Zhāng's work has had a profound influence on traditional medicine in China for nearly two thousand years.

The *Jīn Guì Yào Lüè* covers diseases other than external contractions (which are dealt with in the *Shāng Hán Lùn*), including lung diseases, water swelling, phlegm disease, dispersion-thirst, impediment (*bì*), summerheat stroke, mounting diseases, and gynecological disorders, to name just a few. The first chapter explains the etiology of disease and treatment principles, while the last discusses food prohibitions.

Textual History

As its title suggests, Zhāng Zhòng-Jǐng's *Shāng Hán Lùn* discusses the diagnosis and treatment of cold damage conditions, which are conditions related to external contraction, especially of wind and cold. His *Jīn Guì Yào Lüè* is thought to reflect that section of the original *Shāng Hán Zá Bìng Lùn* that was called "miscellaneous diseases" (杂病 *zá bìng*), basically a catch-all phrase for any conditions which could not be traced to externally contracted evils.

The full title of this present text is *Jīn Guì Yào Lüè Fāng Lùn*, "Essential Prescriptions and Discussions from the Golden Cabinet." This title tells us several things about the book. First, it is an indication of the value that the author (or more accurately, the person who named the text as such) placed on the book's content. "Golden Cabinet" refers to a cabinet-like storage box made of gold, hence a place where a person of great wealth would store his or her most valuable items. Second, the text is characterized as containing both "prescriptions" and "discussions," or in other words, clinical as well as theoretical information. This combination positions it at an interesting fulcrum in the textual history of Chinese medicine, namely the intersection between theoretical classics like the *Huáng Dì Nèi Jīng* ("Yellow Emperor's Inner Canon") and *Nàn Jīng* ("Classic of Difficult Issues"), which were mostly concerned with the flow of qì and blood through the vessels and the correlation of the human body to the macrocosm, and formulary collections like the *Qiān Jīn Fāng* ("Thousand Gold Pieces Prescriptions") by Sūn Sī-Miǎo, which primarily matched lists of symptoms to specific formulas without providing any diagnostic or etiological explanation for the rationale behind a treatment. By contrast, the *Jīn Guì Yào Lüè* includes detailed diagnostic guidelines and etiological reasoning in addition to instructions for treatment primarily with medicinal formulas (and some references to acupuncture, moxibustion, and other therapeutic modalities). Zhāng Zhòng-Jǐng thus created a medical classic with outstanding significance for both theory and practice, centuries before other medical authors attempted to follow in his footsteps during the Sòng period.

Due to the turbulence of its historical times, it is impossible to reconstruct the exact format, content, and organization of Zhāng Zhòng-Jǐng's work today. Nevertheless, its significance for the history of medicine and its applicability in modern clinical practice has inspired much research, especially in China, to approximate its original form as much as possible on the basis of later reprints, fragments that have been recovered in China and Japan in archaeological sites, and quotations in received texts.

By order of the Sòng Imperial court in the 11th century, both the *Shāng Hán Lùn* and the *Jīn Guì Yào Lüè* were included among a small selection of early Chinese medical classics to be collated, annotated, and reissued in woodblock print. This monumental effort was completed by a large editorial team from the Office for the Correction of Medical Texts, which had been established in 1057 CE. While these scholars had access to the ten scrolls of the *Shāng Hán Lùn* which had been edited by Wáng Shū-Hé, the part on "miscellaneous diseases" had not survived. Instead, they painstakingly had to recreate the *Jīn Guì Yào Lüè* on the basis of quotations found in other medical classics like the *Mài Jīng* ("Pulse Canon"), *Zhū Bìng Yuán Hòu Lùn* ("Origin and Indicators of Disease"), and *Qiān Jīn Fāng* ("Thousand Gold Pieces Prescriptions"), as well as a summary of Zhāng Zhòng-Jǐng's work in three scrolls entitled *Jīn Guì Yù Hán Yào Luè Fāng* ("Essential Prescriptions from the Golden Cabinet and Jade Sheath"). These Sòng editors matched the prescriptions with the descriptions of symptoms, arranged the text by disease categories into 25 chapters in three parts, and lastly added select outstanding prescriptions by other physicians of the times, all with the goal of making this text as clinically useful as possible. This Sòng revision has been the standard version of the text ever since, and also the version on which subsequent editions such as this one are based. It is thus important for the discerning reader to keep in mind that we are looking at a Hàn dynasty text that was lost for several centuries and reconstructed, rearranged, and supplemented by Sòng dynasty scholars approximately eight hundred years later.

The Author Zhāng Zhòng-Jǐng

As is true for most other authors of early Chinese texts, we know very few historically reliable facts about Zhāng Zhòng-Jǐng's life. The few details we have present the picture of a skilled physician deeply concerned with the terrible suffering he witnessed as a result of the collapse of the dynasty of the Hàn rulers which occurred in tandem with a series of natural disasters and particularly lethal epidemics.

Zhāng Jī, or Zhāng Zhòng-Jǐng (his more widely known courtesy name), lived during the Eastern Hàn dynasty from approximately 150 to 219 CE. He is said to have been born to a family of physicians in Niè-Yáng (涅阳) in present-day Nán-Yáng County (南阳) in Hé-Nán Province (河南). He received his medical training from the physician Zhāng Bó-Zǔ 张伯祖, and a number of historical texts mention his medical talents in diagnosis, prognosis, and treatment with medicinal prescriptions. As he himself explained in the preface to the *Shāng Hán Lùn* (c.f. Mitchell, Féng, and Wiseman, p. 29), losing two thirds of his family in less than ten years, most of them due to externally contracted diseases, motivated him to immerse himself in the medical literature available at the time and collect the most efficacious treatments he could find into the work he titled *Shāng Hán Zá Bìng Lùn*. While he knew that his book might not allow readers to cure every disease they encountered, his intention was to assist them in at least discerning the origins of disease. The success of his intention can be confirmed in light of the continued importance of this book for both the theory and practice of Chinese medicine to this day.

Description and Outline of the Text

In the version reconstructed by the Sòng editors, the *Jīn Guì Yào Lüè* consists of 25 chapters that deal mostly with various conditions of internal medicine, but also contains sections on gynecology, some external medicine, emergency treatments, and advice on the prevention and treatment of food poisoning. Here is a brief summary of the text:

The first chapter serves as a preface, presenting Zhāng Zhòng-Jǐng's general guidelines on diagnosis, treatment, and prevention. It emphasizes the cosmic interrelations between cycles inside and outside the human body in accordance with five-phase correspondences through the vehicle of qì. Accordingly, the *Jīn Guì Yào Lüè* defines health as the result of a free flow of internal qì in the five viscera, and disease as a state of disharmony or lack of flow, caused by an invasion of external evil qì, most notably abnormal climatic influences. In addition, Zhāng Zhòng-Jǐng recognizes other pathogenic factors like intemperate sexual intercourse, injuries from metal blades, and insect or animal bites. As a result, prevention is primarily the recommended course of action for a life free from disease: cultivating right qì on the one hand and taking precautions to avoid injury on the other hand. Next, the preface offers some basic diagnostic rules to predict the course of disease, related to the inspection of the face, quality of the voice and breath, and nature of the pulse, especially in relation to the prevailing seasonal qì. The chapter concludes by describing a number of disease patterns and pathomechanisms to demonstrate general rules in the progression of disease, related to yīn and yáng, the difference between internal and external and chronic and sudden conditions, the type of invading evil, and which viscera or bowel may be affected first.

The following chapters each discuss a disease or category of diseases in terms of causes, main signs and pulses, pattern identification, treatment principles, and prognosis, with occasional references to adverse or contraindicated treatments or transmuted patterns. In most cases, a number of medicinal prescriptions are given to treat specific variations or stages of the diseases covered in that chapter, sometimes with reference to acumoxa therapy, dietary prescriptions, or other treatments.

Specifically, Chapter 2 covers tetany, dampness, and thermoplegia, all of which are conditions caused by the contraction of external evils that manifest in greater yáng exterior patterns. Chapter 3 discusses the diagnosis and treatment of hundred union disease, fox-creeper, and yīn and yáng toxin, placed together because they are all caused by externally contracted heat. In both these chapters, we can see how Zhāng Zhòng-Jǐng's sophisticated understanding of the underlying roots of these various conditions allowed him to group them together, describe their diagnostic differences, offer precise methods of pattern identification, and give specific treatment recommendations. He not only arranged prescriptions and their accompanying lists of symptoms in chapters on the basis of the root etiology of diseases, but further explained this organizational scheme with references to underlying patterns of the causation and transformation of disease. Though composed at an earlier date, this exemplary approach was centuries ahead of any comparable texts. Prescription collections such as the *Bèi Jí Qiān Jīn Yào Fāng* ("A Thousand Gold Pieces Emergency Prescriptions") or the *Wài Tái Mì Yào*

("Secrets from the Wài Tái Library"), merely presented prescriptions and long lists of symptoms associated with each of them, but did not include any references to etiology, pattern identification, or treatment principles. The *Zhū Bìng Yuán Hòu Lùn* ("Origin and Indicators of Disease") listed all known diseases by etiology and symptoms but did not related them to each other, differentiate them, or give advice on treatment.

To continue this summary of the content of the *Jīn Guì Yào Lüè,* Chapter 4, on malaria, stands out for the diversity of recommended treatments, namely sweating, ejection, precipitation, warming, needling, moxibustion, and dietary therapy. As in Chapter 3, the conditions in Chapter 5 are grouped together because they are due to contraction of the same external evil: in this case wind-stroke and joint-running, both of which are due to contraction of wind evil in combination with depletion of right qì.

The importance Zhāng Zhòng-Jǐng accorded to the problem of vacuity taxation is reflected in the sophisticated differentiation of this disease category in Chapter 6. He identifies eight different patterns by pulses, signs, and pathomechanisms, offers six prescriptions, and additionally describes the pulses, signs, and treatment of blood impediment, including both a medicinal prescription and acumoxa therapy. Chapter 7 deals with lung disease in the closely related subcategories of lung wilting, pulmonary welling-abscess, and cough with qì ascent. In Chapter 8, which covers running piglet qì, three different treatments are given, depending on the affected viscus (liver or kidney) and whether the disease has already occurred or is about to occur. The diseases in the next two chapters are grouped together because of their location. Chapter 9 discusses chest impediment, shortness of breath, and heart pain, all of which are focused in the chest, and Chapter 10 covers abdominal fullness, cold mounting, and abiding food, which are all diseases that primarily affect the spleen, stomach, and intestines.

Each of the next handful of chapters discuss specific variations of disease categories. Chapter 11 deals with wind and cold striking the five viscera (conditions of internal wind and cold, as distinct from those of external wind and cold as discussed in the *Shāng Hán Lùn*), as well as with accumulations and gatherings. The discussion of phlegm-rheum and cough in Chapter 12 contains the first reference in Chinese medical literature to the concept of phlegm (*tán* 痰). Chapter 13 discusses dissipation-thirst, inhibited urination, and strangury, or in other words, conditions related to abnormal thirst and urination due to problems in the kidney and bladder. Chapter 14, "Water Qì," covers water swelling and qì distention due to debilitation of yáng qì, which is invariably linked to the lung, spleen, and kidney.

Chapter 15, focusing on jaundice, first explains the different causes of this disease (diet, alcohol, sexual taxation), and then differentiates a number of pathomechanisms with associated signs and treatments. Chapter 16 covers fright and palpitation and a variety of bleeding conditions, combined in one chapter because they are related to problems with the heart, blood, and vessels. Chapter 17 covers retching, vomiting, hiccup, and diarrhea, closely related and mutually conducive conditions that are related to stomach and intestinal disharmonies.

The following two chapters serve as catch-all for sundry conditions that are not prevalent or important enough to warrant their own separate chapters but may only be superficially related to each other. Chapter 18 covers sores (referring to incised wounds, that is, any injury from metal blades), welling-abscess and intestinal welling-abscess, and wet spreading sores, grouped together because they were all considered conditions of external medicine. Chapter 19 covers hobbled dorsum of the foot, swelling of the fingers and arms, cramping, yīn fox-like mounting, and roundworm.

Placed almost at the very end of the *Jīn Guì Yào Lüè,* Chapters 20 through 22 deal with conditions specific to the females, namely "Pregnancy," "Post-Partum," and "Miscellaneous [Female] Diseases." A medical historian searching for early traces of a gender-specific understanding of the female body would recognize that these three chapters did not yet reflect a clear conception of gynecological conditions beyond isolated statements. Most notably, Zhāng Zhòng-Jǐng states, "Women's diseases are caused by vacuity, accumulated cold, and bound qì, which cause the menstrual fluids to stop flowing." As the various entries show, Zhāng Zhòng-Jǐng saw female conditions of abnormal vaginal discharge (*dài xià* 带下, literally "below the girdle") as related primarily to a combination of vacuity with an invasion of wind and/or cold, and less frequently to "heat entering the blood chamber"). As these circumstances interrupted and disordered menstruation, they led to problems with fertility, and particularly occurred during and after pregnancy and childbirth.

Many scholars question whether the last three chapters of the *Jīn Guì Yào Lüè* were actually composed by Zhāng Zhòng-Jǐng himself or were added later by the Sòng dynasty editors. Regardless of their age and authorship, they contain valuable clinical information on miscellaneous formulas, mostly emergency treatments. The final two chapters, "Fowls, Beasts, Fish, and Insects: Contraindications and Treatments," and "Fruits, Vegetables, and Grains: Contraindications and Treatments," expound on dietary therapy and the prevention of food poisoning.

Weights and Measures

Weights and measures in Zhāng Zhòng-Jǐng's time followed a system that bears resemblance to the the those that are now labeled as "traditional," as opposed to the modern metric weights and measures now commonly used in the Chinese world. Some of the terms, such as 斤 *jīn* and 两 *liǎng* are the same, but the weights or measures they denote are different from those of today.

Weights and Measures		
Unit	**Traditional Equivalent**	**Metric Equivalent**
Weight		
dàn 石	120 jīn	300 kg
jīn 斤	16 liǎng	250 grams (roughly)
liǎng 两	1/16 of a jīn	15.6 grams (see below)
zhū 朱	1/12 of a liǎng	1.3 grams

Volume		
dǒu 斗 (also called "dipper")	10 shēng	2 liters
shēng 升	1/10 of a dǒu	200 milliliters
gě 合	1/10 of a shēng	20 milliliters
qián-spoonful 钱匕	see below	1.5–1.8 grams
square-inch-spoonful 方寸匕	see below	5 ml
Length		
chǐ 尺		23 cm

Liǎng 两 *liǎng*

There is disagreement regarding the weight of one *liǎng* during Zhāng Jī's time. Some estimates roughly equate one *liǎng* to 15.6 grams; however, other sources suggest that the weight of one *liǎng* during the Eastern Hàn dynasty was closer to 13.9 grams.

Confusion regarding the precise weight of the ancient *liǎng* has remained unresolved for centuries, and no definitive answer exists in the absence of new historical evidence. In the Ming dynasty, the famous author Lǐ Shí-Zhēn 李时珍 stated, "In ancient times, one *liǎng* was equivalent to one [contemporary] *qián*." Around the same time period, the Ming dynasty author Zhāng Jǐng-Yuè 张景岳 stated, "One ancient *liǎng* is equivalent to six *qián*." While it is known that one *qián* weighed about 3.7 grams during the Ming dynasty, precise answers about the weight of the ancient Hàn dynasty *liǎng* have remained elusive for centuries. Lǐ Shí-Zhēn's statement may have influenced other sources, as numerous contemporary Chinese textbooks assume an equivalent weight of 3 grams per ancient *liǎng* in Zhāng Jī's formulas; however, other contemporary textbooks cite the much higher equivalent dose of 15.6 grams.

Qián 钱匕 *qián bǐ* (spoonful)

There is disagreement as to whether the *qián* is a unit of volume or weight. According to definitions contained in premodern literature, it was used as a measure of volume for powdered substances. One *qián* was the amount of the substance that could be piled on a 铜钱 *tóng qián*, which was a copper coin with a square hole in the center. Modern textbooks indicate that a square-inch-spoonful is equivalent to 1.5–1.8 grams. Scholars have recently questioned this, suggesting that it was a unit of weight equal to the weight of such a copper coin, which in the Han Dynasty was about 13.175–15.625 grams.

In several places in the *Jīn Guì Yào Lüè*, the character 钱 *qián* appears alone as a measure. This is probably an abbreviation for 钱匕 *qián bǐ*, and should not be confused with the 钱 *qián* of later and modern times.

Since copper coins had characters, piling a substance on a coin so that only one character was covered would be one 字 *zì* ("one characterful"). Although *zì* appears in the *Shāng Hán Lùn,* it does not appear in the *Jīn Guì Yào Lüè.*

Square-inch-spoonful 方寸匕 *fāng cùn bǐ*

A square-inch spoon was a scooping utensil one inch (or one *cùn*) square. One *cùn* varied in length over history. According to present research, one *cùn* in the Hàn Dynasty was about 2.34 cm and one square-inch-spoonful was equivalent to roughly 5 ml. Some modern textbooks indicate that it is 6–9 grams.

Piece 枚 *méi*
The Chinese 枚 *méi* is a measure word for small, usually round items, used in Chinese medical texts to describe fruits, certain roots, egg yolks, and lumps of minerals. In English translation, it usually appears as "piece." Thus, "jujube (大枣 *dà zǎo*, Jujubae Fructus) 12 pieces" means 12 jujubes (jujube fruits); "unripe bitter orange (枳实 *zhǐ shí*, Aurantii Fructus Immaturus) 5 pieces" means 5 whole fruits; "peach kernel (桃仁 *táo rén*, Persicae Semen) 50 pieces" means 50 peach kernels; "aconite (附子 *fù zǐ*, Aconiti Radix Lateralis Praeparata) 1 piece" means one root; "gypsum (石膏 *shí gāo*, Gypsum Fibrosum) 12 pieces" means 12 lumps.

Conclusion

As the name suggests, the *Jīn Guì Yào Lüè* is truly worth being stored in a "golden cabinet." The preface to the Sòng dynasty reprint described its value this way: "This book can bring a person back to life" (此书可以活人)" because "the efficacy [of its treatments] is divine" (其效若神). Unique in the context of its time and for many centuries to come, unsurpassed in clinical value except by its companion the *Shāng Hán Lùn,* the *Jīn Guì Yào Lüè* applied the theoretical premises of the Hàn dynasty classics like the *Huáng Dì Nèi Jīng* and *Nàn Jīng* to the diagnosis and treatment of diseases, with particular attention paid to pulses and medicinal prescriptions. Disease was understood as the lack of harmony between external cycles in nature, most notably the cycle of the seasons, and the internal cycles inside the human body, as manifested in the movement of qì and blood via the channels and network vessels through the whole body, but especially in the viscera and bowels.

Much like the authors of the theoretical classics, Zhāng Zhòng-Jǐng adhered to and emphasized the medical ideal of prevention, or at least preemptive diagnosis and treatment, as articulated in the famous expression,上工治未病 ("The superior practitioner treats disease before it arises"). Zhāng Zhòng-Jǐng's professional training and practice as a physician and his witnessing of the suffering due to epidemics in the last years of the Hàn dynasty underscored his foremost concern—to help his fellow humans be as healthy as possible in the constraints of their circumstances. Thus for proponents of an historically-rooted practice of Chinese medicine, the *Jīn Guì Yào Lüè* is a prime example of the importance and clinical value of combining a concrete understanding of the diagnosis and treatment of disease with a deeper insight into the fundamental unity of the human microcosm and the macrocosm—"as above, so below." This unity is, after all, where the root of all illness and well-being is found in the true framework of Chinese traditional medicine.

SABINE WILMS

脏腑经络先后并脉证第一

CHAPTER 1

Bowels and Viscera, and Channels and Network Vessels

Disease Sequence, Pulses, and Signs

OVERVIEW

This first chapter describes the causes and pathomechanisms of disease of the bowels and viscera and of the channels and network vessels, the sequence in which they occur, and the pulses and signs by which they are recognized. It forms a general introduction to the *Jīn Guì Yào Lüè* as a whole. Short as it is, it covers and provides copious examples of a broad range of subjects including prevention of disease, causes of disease, pathomechanisms, diagnostics, principles of treatment, nursing, and prognosis.

Throughout the broad-ranging contents, emphasis is given to an holistic view of health and disease, stressing not only the relationship of the human body to the natural world outside the body, but as well to the unity within the body. Grasping the interdependence and interactions among the bowels and viscera and among the channels and network vessels leads to comprehending how an imbalance or disharmony manifests as disease. Thus disease in one bowel or viscus can affect another bowel or viscus. Disease in one channel can affect another. Disease evils contracted through the channels and network vessels can pass into the bowels and viscera. Disease evils of the bowels and viscera can manifest along the pathways of the channels and network vessels.

‡ Schematic Overview

Humankind and Nature

1. Changes in weather: There are [times when a given season] has not yet arrived, but [its qì] arrives; when [a given season] arrives, but [its qì] does not arrive; when [a given season] arrives, but the previous season's qì fails to leave; [and when a given season] arrives and [its qì is] excessive.

2. Mutual responsiveness of humankind and nature: Human beings are endowed with the five constants and rely on wind qì for birth and growth. If the original true [qì] of the five viscera flows freely, the person is calm and in harmony.

3. Non-responsiveness: When the visiting qì of evil wind strikes people, they often die.

Causes of Disease and Pathomechanisms

1. Internal causes: Channels and network vessels contracting evil and passing it to the bowels and viscera.

2. External causes: Strike through the skin, causing stopped passage through the limbs, nine orifices, and blood vessels.

3. Other injuries: sexual activity; incised wounds, insect and animal injuries, and disasters.

Characteristics of Evils

1. Mist: A clear evil that resides in the upper body, damaging the skin and interstices.
2. Dampness: A turbid evil that resides in the lower body, flowing into the joints.
3. Wind: A major evil striking the exterior; floating pulse.
4. Cold: A minor evil striking in the interior; tight pulse.
5. Food: When food evils strike, they damage the spleen and stomach.
6. Extreme cold damages the channels
7. Extreme heat damages the network vessels.
8. Prevalence of yīn and yáng: Yáng without yīn—reversing yáng.

Categorization of Disease Patterns

1. Channels and network vessels contracting disease:
   a) Eighteen yáng diseases: Headache, pulling pain in the nape, lumbus, spine, arm, and foot (3 × 6 = 18).
   b) Eighteen yīn diseases: Cough, qì ascent, panting, belching, dysphagia, rumbling intestines, distention and fullness, heart pain, and hypertonicity (3 × 6 = 18).
2. Bowels and viscera contracting the six excesses:
   a) Disease of qì.
   b) Disease of blood.
   c) Disease of both qì and blood. The five viscera each have 18 diseases, combing to make 90 diseases. The six bowels each have 18 diseases, combining to make 108 diseases.

3. Disease caused by diet, lifestyle, and affective disturbances: The five taxations, seven damages, and six extremes.
4. Women's diseases: Thirty-six women's diseases.

Prevention (Treating Disease Before it Arises)

1. Health cultivation: Maintaining a healthy body so that disease cannot enter the interstices.
   a) Avoid evil wind from disturbing the channels and network vessels.
   b) Avoid breaking the law.
   c) Avoid cuts, animal and insect injuries, and natural disasters.
   d) Avoid excesses of sexual activity.
   e) In clothing and diet, apply temperance in consumption of cold, hot, bitter, sour, acrid, and sweet things.

Measures after disease has arisen

1. Treat early: If by chance [wind evil] strikes the channels and network vessels, a physician must treat it immediately, before it flows into the bowels and viscera. As soon as the limbs feel heavy and stagnant, treat the patient with conduction (*dǎo yǐn*), exhalation and inhalation, acupuncture and moxibustion, or paste rubbing.
2. Prevent passage and mutations: If you see disease of the liver, you know that it will pass from the liver to the spleen, so you must first replenish the spleen.

Four Examinations

1. Inspection
   a) Tip of the nose
      Blue-green: Pain in the abdomen.
      Slightly black: Water qì.
   b) Facial complexion
      Yellow: Cold on the chest.
      White: Blood collapse.
   c) Face and eyes
      Blue-green: Pain.
      Black: Taxation.
      Red: Wind; slight redness at the wrong season means death.
      Yellow: Difficult defecation.
      Fresh and shiny: Lodged rheum.
      Eyes, straight and round: Untreatable.
2. Listening and Smelling:
   a) Voice

If the patient has a quiet voice and tends to cry when frightened, the disease is in the joints.

If the sound of the voice is dull and not clear, this is disease in the heart and diaphragm.

If the sound of the voice is wispy, fine, and long, the disease is in the head.

b) Breathing

Shaking shoulders: Hardness in the heart.

Qì ascent in the chest: Cough.

Open mouth and shortness of breath: Lung wilting with spitting of foam. (Repletion patterns can be treated by precipitation; vacuity patterns are difficult to treat).

Faint and rapid: Center burner (treat with precipitation).

Long inhalation: Lower burner (difficult to treat).

Hasty: Upper burner (difficult to treat).

Breathing with shaking and trembling: Impossible to treat.

3. Inquiry

a) Understanding likes and dislikes: When the five viscera are diseased and receive what they require, recovery ensues. If they are averse to what they receive, disease ensues.

b) History of disease: If patients suddenly crave to eat something they normally do not like, they will [suffer from] heat effusion.

4. Palpation

a) Correlation of complexion and pulse: The pulse at the inch opening moves in accord with the season during which each of the five viscera are in turn effulgent (correspondence of complexion and pulse): No disease.

b) Examples of pulses

Floating pulse: At the front (inch opening) means the disease is in the exterior; at the back (cubit) means the disease is in the interior.

Large sunken and slippery inch pulse: A sunken pulse indicates [blood] repletion. A slippery pulse indicates exuberant qì.

PRINCIPLES OF TREATMENT

1. Treatment Principles

a) Do not evacuate vacuity; do not replenish repletion; supplement insufficiency and reduce superabundance.

b) All diseases in the viscera, if they are to be attacked, should be attacked in accordance with what [evil] the patient has contracted.

2. Pattern identification as the basis for determining treatment

a) Dual disease of exterior and interior

In disease in which a physician has precipitated, and [the patient] subsequently has incessant clear-grain diarrhea and generalized pain, you must quickly rescue the interior.

Afterwards, [if there is still] generalized pain but the eliminations have returned to normal, then you must quickly rescue the exterior.

b) Simultaneous presence of chronic and acute diseases

First treat the sudden disease.

Then treat the intractable disease.

OUTCOME AND PROGNOSIS

1. Case Studies

a) Desertion of the pulse

When the disease enters the viscera, the patient dies.

When the disease enters the bowels, the patient recovers.

b) Sudden depression

Green blue lips and cold body means that the disease is entering the viscera, in which case the person dies.

Harmonious warmth of the body and spontaneous sweating means the patient will recover.

c) Wet spreading sores

When spreading from the mouth to limbs they can be treated.

When spreading from the limbs toward the mouth, they are difficult to cure.

2. Hundred diseases

a) Disease in the exterior can be treated. (Easy to treat.)

b) When the disease enters the interior, the patient dies. (Difficult to treat.)

Line 1.1

(1)问曰：上工治未病，何也？师曰：夫治未病者，见肝之病，知肝传脾，当先实脾，四季脾旺不受邪，即勿补之。中工不晓相传，见肝之病，不解实脾，惟治肝也。

(2)夫肝之病，补用酸，助用焦苦，益用甘味之药调之。酸入肝，焦苦入心，甘入脾。脾能伤肾，肾气微弱，则水不行；水不行，则心火气盛；心火气盛，则伤肺；肺被伤，则金气不行；金气不行，则肝气盛。故实脾，则肝自愈。此治肝补脾之要妙也。肝虚则用此法，实则不再用之。

(3)经曰：虚虚实实，补不足，损有余。是其义也。余藏准此。

(1) Wèn yuē: Shàng gōng zhì wèi bìng, hé yě? Shī yuē: Fū zhì wèi bìng zhě, jiàn gān zhī bìng, zhī gān chuán pí, dāng xiān shí pí, sì jì pí wàng bù shòu xié, jí wù bǔ zhī. Zhōng gōng bù xiǎo xiāng chuán, jiàn gān zhī bìng, bù jiě shí pí, wéi zhì gān yě.

(2) Fū gān zhī bìng, bǔ yòng suān, zhù yòng jiāo kǔ, yì yòng gān wèi zhī yào tiáo zhī. Suān rù gān, jiāo kǔ rù xīn, gān rù pí. Pí néng shāng shèn, shèn qì wēi ruò, zé shuǐ bù xíng; shuǐ bù xíng, zé xīn huǒ qì shèng; xīn huǒ qì shèng zé shāng fèi; fèi bèi shāng, zé jīn qì bù xíng; jīn qì bù xíng, zé gān qì shèng. Gù shí pí, zé gān zì yú. Cǐ zhì gān bǔ pí zhī yào miào yě. Gān xū zé yòng cǐ fǎ, shí zé bù zài yòng zhī.

(3) Jīng yuē: xū xū shí shí, bǔ bù zú, sǔn yǒu yú. Shì qí yì yě. Yú zàng zhǔn cǐ.

(1) Question: "The superior practitionēr[1] treats disease before it arises.[2] What does this mean?" The Master[3] says: "Treating disease before it arises means for example that if you see disease of the liver, you know that it will pass from the liver to the spleen, [thus you] must first replenish the spleen.[4] Supplementation is unnecessary [only if] the spleen is effulgent [throughout] the four seasons.[5] The practitioner of medium proficiency does not know about the passage of disease. Thus when he sees liver disease, he does not understand the need to replenish the spleen, and treats only the liver."

(2) In liver disease, supplement with sourness, assist with charred and bitter [flavors], and boost with medicinals of sweet flavor to harmonize. Sourness enters the liver, charred and bitter [flavors] enter the heart, and sweetness enters the spleen. The spleen can damage the kidney.[6] When kidney qì is weak, water fails to move; when water fails to move, heart fire becomes exuberant; when heart fire becomes exuberant, it damages the lung; when the lung is damaged, metal qì fails to move; and when metal qì fails to move, liver qì becomes exuberant. Therefore when you replenish the spleen, the liver recovers on its own. This is the main subtlety of treating the liver by supplementing the spleen. Use this method to treat liver vacuity, but not to treat repletion.

(3) The *Classic*[7] says, "To avoid evacuating vacuity and replenishing repletion,[8] supplement insufficiency and reduce superabundance." This is what is meant here. The other viscera follow this [scheme too].

TEXT NOTES, LINE 1.1

[1] Superior practitioner 上工 *shàng gōng*: In ancient China, a superior practitioner was one with a nine-out-of-ten success rate, a mediocre practitioner (中工 *zhōng gōng*) was one with a seven-out-of-ten success rate, and an inferior practitioner (下工 *xià gōng*) was one with a six-out-of-ten success rate.

[2] Treat disease before it arises 治未病 *zhì wèi bìng*: To prevent disease from arising. Here, it clearly means to treat bowels and viscera that are not yet affected by disease, so as to prevent the transmission and transmutation of disease. The term also means to prevent the advance of disease.

[3] The Master 师 *shī*: This is presumed to mean Zhāng Jī. If this is so, it may well be that the text, at least in part, was written down by students rather than by Zhāng himself. A considerable number of lines are formatted as a student's question followed by the Master's answer.

[4] Replenish the spleen 实脾 *shí pí*: Supplement the spleen.

[5] The spleen is effulgent [throughout] the four seasons 四季脾旺 *sì jì pí wàng*: The spleen belongs to earth, which is supposed to be effulgent through the four seasons. Here the meaning is that spleen qì is exuberant for the whole of the year.

[6] The spleen can damage the kidney 皮能伤肾 *pí néng shāng shèn*: The spleen can restrain the kidney, which is associated with water.

[7] The Classic 经 *jīng*: This is an almost literal quotation of two *Nèi Jīng* passages: *Líng Shū* 1, "The Nine Needles and Twelve Sources," and *Sù Wèn* 70, "Great Treatise on the Five Normal Rules."

[8] Evacuate vacuity and replenish repletion 虚虚实实 *xū xū shí shí*: To exacerbate vacuity by draining and exacerbate repletion by supplementation.

SYNOPSIS, LINE 1.1

This line describes the notion of treating disease before it arises. Through the example of liver disease giving rise to spleen disease, we can see that "treating disease before it arises" means preventing particular conditions from arising during the course of disease.

COMMENTARY, LINE 1.1

This line opens with the notion, central to Chinese medicine, of treating disease before it arises, which means identifying any pathological buildup and preventing it from spreading or developing further. Physicians can only do this when they fully understand the relationships between each of the internal organs and how diseases develop and spread from one locus to another.

For example, when there is liver repletion, the spleen is threatened. According to five-phase theory, wood restrains earth. When wood becomes too strong, it overwhelms earth. Hence, earth has to be fortified to prevent this. So in liver repletion, if the spleen is weak, it has to be regulated and supplemented to protect it from being damaged by the liver. This is treating spleen disease before it arises. The overwhelming cycle only applies in repletion, not in vacuity.

Vacuity and repletion must be carefully distinguished. Again this point is explained through the example of the liver. Sourness is the flavor that enters the liver. In liver vacuity, sourness is therefore appropriate for supplementation. Charred and bitter flavors are associated with the heart. Because wood engenders fire, the heart is the child of the liver. Supplementing the child can fortify the mother, so charred and bitter flavors can be used to complement sour. Lastly, sweetness is used to regulate center qì. This approach is appropriate for liver vacuity, but not for liver repletion.

The section from "sourness enters the liver" to "this is the main subtlety of treating the liver by supplementing the spleen" explains in detail the reasons for using sour, sweet, charred, and bitter flavors to treat liver vacuity. In terms of the five phases, liver-wood is normally restrained by lung-metal. When the liver becomes vacuous, the normal relationship is upset, and lung-metal is bound to rebel against it. Before lung-metal rebels against liver-wood, it is appropriate to use sourness to supplement the liver itself and use burnt-bitter flavors to assist heart-fire.

There are three reasons for assisting heart fire: When heart-fire is effulgent, (1) it can affect qì in the liver; (2) it can prevent the draining of liver qì, and (3) it can restrain the lung, preventing it from restraining the liver and allowing the liver to recover. Sweetness is used because it enters the spleen. Supplementing the spleen enhances the ability of spleen-earth to restrain kidney-water (supplementing earth to dam water). This is what is meant by "the spleen can damage the kidney." When the yīn-cold water qì of the kidney is kept in check, this prevents "water qì damaging the heart." When the lesser fire of the heart is exuberant, it can restrain lung metal, which in turn helps to prevent lung-metal from rebelling against liver-wood. Moreover, it is said that "earth can luxuriate wood" (土能荣木 *tǔ néng róng mù*): When spleen qì is exuberant, it can help to supplement the vacuity of the liver.

Finally, the last section explains that vacuity is normally treated by supplementation and repletion by drainage. If drainage is used to treat vacuity, or supplementation is used to treat repletion, this is to commit the error of "evacuating vacuity" or "replenishing repletion." In either case, the patient is harmed.

Line 1.2

(1)夫人禀五常，因风气而生长，风气虽能生万物，亦能害万物。如水能浮舟，亦能覆舟。若五藏元真通畅，人即安和，客气邪风，中人多死，千般疢难，不越三条：一者，经络受邪，入藏腑为内所因也；二者，四肢九窍，血脉相传，壅塞不通，为外皮肤所中也；三者，房室金刃，虫兽所伤。以此详之，病由都尽。

(2)若人能养慎，不令邪风干忤经络，适中经络，未流传脏腑，即医治之，四肢纔觉重滞，即导引吐纳，针灸膏摩，勿令九窍闭塞。更能无犯王法，禽兽灾伤，房室勿令竭乏，服食节其冷、热、苦、酸、辛、甘，不遗形体有衰，病则无由入其腠理。腠者，三焦通会元真之处，为血气所注；理者，是皮肤脏腑之文理也。

(1) Fū rén bǐng wǔ cháng, yīn fēng qì ér shēng zhǎng, fēng qì suī néng shēng wàn wù, yì néng hài wàn wù. Rú shuǐ néng fú zhōu, yì néng fù zhōu. Ruò wǔ zàng yuán zhēn tōng chàng, rén jí ān hé, kè qì xié fēng, zhōng rén duō sì, qiān bān chèn nàn, bù yuè sān tiáo: yī zhě, jīng luò shòu xié rù zàng fǔ wéi nèi suǒ yīn yě; èr zhě, sì zhī jiǔ qiào, xuè mài xiāng chuán, yōng sè bù tōng, wéi wài pí fū suǒ zhòng yě; sān zhě, fáng shì jīn rèn, chóng shòu suǒ shāng. Yǐ cǐ xiáng zhī, bìng yóu dōu jìn.

(2) Ruò rén néng yǎng shèn, bù lìng xié fēng gān wǔ jīng luò, shì zhōng jīng luò, wèi liú chuán fǔ zàng, jí yī zhì zhī, sì zhī cái jué zhòng zhì, jí dǎo yǐn tù nà, zhēn jiǔ gāo mó, wù lìng jiǔ qiào bì sè. Gèng néng wú fàn wáng fǎ, qín shòu zāi shāng, fáng shì wù lìng jié fá, fú shí jié qí lěng, rè, kǔ, suān, xīn, gān, bù yí xing tǐ yǒu shuāi, bìng zé wú yóu rù qí còu lǐ. Còu zhě, sān jiāo tōng huì yuán zhēn zhī chù, wéi xuè qì suǒ zhù; lǐ zhě, shì pí fū zàng fǔ zhī wén lǐ yě.

(1) Human beings are endowed with the qì of the five constants[1] and rely on wind qì[2] for birth and growth. Although wind qì can engender the myriad things, it can also damage them, just as water can float a boat and also capsize it. If the original true [qì][3] of the five viscera flows freely, the person is calm and in harmony; when the visiting qì of evil wind[4] strikes people, they often die. A thousand afflictions fall into no more than three categories. The first [category] is evil being contracted by the channels and network vessels and entering the bowels and viscera. This constitutes internal causation. The second is when passage through the limbs, the nine orifices, or the blood vessels becomes congested and stopped. This constitutes an external strike through the skin. The third is injury due to bedroom [activity],[5] metal blades, or insects and animals. Using these [three categories] to examine disease, the origins of all conditions can be thoroughly understood.

(2) If people can cultivate [right qì] and take precautions [against contraction of wind evil], they can prevent wind evil from disturbing the channels and network vessels. But if by chance [wind evil] strikes the channels and network vessels, a physician must treat it immediately, before it flows into the bowels and viscera. As soon as the limbs feel heavy and stagnant, treat the patient with conduction,[6] inhalation and exhalation,[7] acupuncture and moxibustion, or paste rubbing[8] to prevent the nine orifices from becoming blocked. Furthermore, avoid transgressing imperial law[9] and being injured by beast or fowl; in bedroom [activities], do not exhaust yourself; as regards clothing and diet, regulate heat and cold and the consumption of cold, hot, bitter, sour, acrid, and sweet flavors. Thus you prevent the body from becoming debilitated. As a result, disease has no place from which to enter the interstitial grain. The interstices are the site of the confluence of the original true [qì] of the triple burner, whereunto the blood and qì pour. Grain refers to the grain of the skin and of the bowels and viscera.

TEXT NOTES, LINE 1.2

[1] Five constants 五常 *wǔ cháng*: The constant laws of the five phases.

[2] Wind qì 风气 *fēng qì*: Climatic influences.

[3] Original and true [qì] 元真 *yuán zhēn*: Original qì (元气 *yuán qì*) or true qì (真气 *zhēn qì*).

[4] Visiting qì and evil wind 客气邪风 *kè qì xié fēng*: Abnormal climatic influences affecting the body.

[5] Bedroom [activity] 房室 *fáng shì*: A euphemism for sexual intercourse. Also 房事 *fáng shì*, literally, bedroom matters.

[6] Conduction 导引 *dǎo yǐn*: An ancient calisthenic method of health cultivation through exercising the sinews and bones and guiding qì throughout the body.

[7] Inhalation and exhalation 吐纳 *tù nà*: The body inhales clear qì and expels turbid qì. Inhalation and exhalation here refer to the art of regulating respiration for the cultivation of health and elimination of disease.

[8] Paste rubbing 膏摩 *gāo mó*: A method of treatment whereby medicinal paste is applied over a given area and rubbed into the skin.

[9] Avoid transgressing imperial law 无犯王法 *wú fàn wáng fǎ*: This warning against committing criminal acts refers to the fact that in traditional China, breaking the law endangered the body, because it was punished physically by torture and mutilation.

Synopsis, Line 1.2

This line arranges the causes of disease in three categories. It emphasizes the importance of preventing disease and treating it in its early stages.

Commentary, Line 1.2

This line describes the relationship between humankind and nature and the causes of disease, as well as its prevention and early treatment.

Human beings are subject to the five climatic influences associated with the five phases: wind (wood), summerheat (fire), dampness (earth), dryness (metal), and cold (water). Under normal circumstances, these nourish all life, but abnormal climatic influences are damaging. However, when people's original qì is exuberant, they remain healthy. This is the principle often expressed as "when right qì is conserved within, evil cannot interfere" (正气存内，邪气不可干 *zhèng qì cún nèi, xié qì bù kě gān*). It is only when right qì is insufficient that evil can exploit the vacuity and enter the body, causing damage and in some cases death.

There are many different diseases, but there are only three basic causes. The first cause is evil entering the channels and network vessels and then passing into the bowels and viscera. This is evil exploiting vacuity to enter the inner body. The second cause is congestion and stoppage in the passage between the limbs and orifices and the blood vessels. The third is a miscellaneous group of factors including excessive sexual activities, incised wounds, and insect and animal bites.

The second section states that if people take all precautions to prevent illness, evil qì will not invade the channels. If, through neglect, evil is allowed to enter the channels, action should promptly be taken to prevent it from passing into the viscera. If the limbs feel heavy and stagnant, techniques such as conduction (*dǎo yǐn*) exercises and qì cultivation, acupuncture and moxibustion, and paste rubbing can be applied to prevent blockage in the nine orifices. To keep in health, people must abide by the law so as to avoid physical repercussions. They must also avoid injuries sustained from fowl or beast and show temperance in sexual behavior and diet. If they thereby keep strong and healthy, disease will not enter through the interstices. The interstices are governed by the triple burner and are intimately related to the skin and bowels and viscera. They are the point of confluence of original true qì and a place through which blood and qì flow. When the ability to resist external evils is weakened, the interstices become their point of entry into the body.

Line 1.3

问曰：病人有气色见于面部，愿闻其说。师曰：鼻头色青，腹中痛，苦冷者死；鼻头色微黑者，有水气；色黄者，胸上有寒；色白者，亡血也。设微赤非时者死。其目正圆者痉，不治。又色青为痛，色黑为劳，色赤为风，色黄者便难，色鲜明者有留饮。

Wèn yuē: Bìng rén yǒu qì sè jiàn yú miàn bù, yuàn wén qí shuō. Shī yuē: Bí tóu sè qīng, fù zhōng tòng, kǔ lěng zhě sì. Bí tóu sè wēi hēi zhě, yǒu shuǐ qì; sè huáng zhě, xiōng shàng yǒu hán; sè bái zhě, wáng xuè yě. Shè wēi chì fēi shí zhě sǐ, qí mù zhèng yuán zhě jìng, bù zhì. Yòu sè qīng wéi tòng, sè hēi wéi láo, sè chì wéi fēng, sè huáng zhě biàn nán, sè xiān míng zhě yǒu liú yǐn.

Question: "Patients have [various different] qì colors[1] appearing on the face. I would like to hear the doctrine [concerning this]."

The Master says: "If the tip of the nose is green-blue in color and there is pain and coldness in the abdomen, the patient will die. If the tip of the nose is slightly black in color, there is water qì. If the complexion is yellow, there is cold on the chest; if white, blood has collapsed. If it is slightly reddened at the wrong time, [the patient] will die. If the eyes are straight and round,[2] this is tetany, which cannot be treated. Also, green-blue means pain; black means taxation, red means wind; yellow means difficult defecation; and a fresh shiny complexion means lodged rheum."[3]

TEXT NOTES, LINE 1.3

[1] Qì color 气色 *qì sè*: Complexion.

[2] Eyes are straight and round 正圆 *zhèng yuán*: The eyes are wide open and stare fixedly ahead.

[3] Lodged rheum 留饮 *liú yǐn*: See Chapter 12, "Phlegm-Rheum and Cough."

SYNOPSIS, LINE 1.3

This line describes the diagnostic and prognostic significance of the different complexions.

COMMENTARY, LINE 1.3

This line describes the inspection of the face. The tip of the nose is the "king of the face." It belongs to the spleen; hence its normal color is yellow. When other colors appear on the nose, they can be understood in terms of the relationships between the five phases.

A green-blue nose indicates liver-wood restraining spleen-earth. It is likely to be accompanied by pain in the abdomen. If there is also aversion to cold, this is caused by yáng qì debilitation and constitutes a life-threatening situation.

Black is the color associated with the water phase. A slightly black nose thus means kidney-water rebelling against spleen-earth and hence the presence of water qì.

Yellow is the color of spleen-earth; when the complexion of the whole face is yellow, this is disease of the spleen preventing the distribution of liquid and causing water to collect in the chest and diaphragm. Thus a yellow complexion indicates "cold on the chest," which is understood to mean cold rheum.

A white complexion means excessive loss of blood, referred to here as blood collapse. If in blood collapse the complexion is slightly red outside the hot season, this is due to damage to yīn and vacuous yáng floating upward.

If the eyes stare straight ahead and do not move, this is due to exuberant wind evil and expiration of the essential qì of the five viscera. This is a sign of tetanic disease, which is difficult to treat. It should be noted that when the text says "[the patient] dies" or "cannot be treated," this is meant to describe an extremely critical situation. It does not necessarily mean that the physician should give up all effort to save the patient. Zhāng Zhòng-Jǐng does not consider tetany to be inherently untreatable since in Chapter 2 he discusses methods of treating it.

The final sentence further discusses the significance of the various facial complexions.

Green-blue is the color that indicates stopped flow in the vessels and hence pain.

Black is the color of the kidney. Because taxation fatigue causes insufficiency of kidney essence, a black complexion is observed in patients suffering from taxation fatigue.

Red is the color of fire. Wind is a yáng evil that commonly arises from a transformation of fire; hence the text says that a red complexion means wind.

Yellow is the color of spleen-earth. Thus a bright yellow complexion reflects damp-heat brewing and stagnation of spleen qì, which usually manifests in difficult defecation.

A "fresh shiny complexion" is understood to refer to a puffy face with a glossy complexion, which arises when water-rheum collecting internally floods up into the face; hence a fresh shiny complexion indicates lodged rheum.

Line 1.4

师曰：病人语声寂然，喜惊呼者，骨节间病；语声喑喑然不彻者，心膈间病；语声啾啾然细而长者，头中病。

Shī yuē: Bìng rén yǔ shēng jì rán, xǐ jīng hū zhě, gǔ jié jiān bìng; yǔ shēng yīn yīn rán bù chè zhě, xīn gé jiān bìng; yǔ shēng jiū jiū rán xì ér cháng zhě, tóu zhōng bìng.

The Master says: "If the patient has a quiet voice[1] but exhibits a tendency to cry from fright, he has disease in the joints. If the sound of the voice is dull[2] and not clear, this is disease in the heart and diaphragm. If the sound of the voice is wispy,[3] fine and long, the disease is in the head."

Text Notes, Line 1.4

[1] Quiet 寂然 *jì rán*: Tending not to talk and not to talk loudly.

[2] Dull 喑喑然 *yīn yīn rán*: A low faint voice.

[3] Wispy 啾啾然 *jiū jiū rán*: Faint but clear.

Synopsis, Line 1.4

This line discusses the clinical significance of the patient's voice.

Commentary, Line 1.4

This line describes the significance of the voice in diagnosis. When a patient usually remains quiet, but cries out suddenly now and again, this is a sign of pain in the joints that makes physical movement difficult and painful. Such a patient will normally tend to keep still and quiet, but will cry out in pain when movement causes pain. When the voice is low, faint, and unclear, this may reflect disease in the heart and diaphragm, such as chest bind, heart glomus, and anguish. This is because in such conditions, the airways become obstructed. When the patient's voice is very faint, this is because of a severe headache that is exacerbated by the sound of his own voice. Because the airways are not obstructed, the voice is clear.

Line 1.5

师曰：息摇肩者，心中坚；息引胸中上气者咳；息张口短气者，肺痿唾沫。

Shī yuē: Xī yáo jiān zhě, xīn zhōng jiān; xī yǐn xiōng zhōng shàng qì zhě ké; xī zhāng kǒu duǎn qì zhě, fèi wěi tuò mò.

The Master says: "When breathing shakes the shoulders,[1] this indicates hardness in the heart;[2] when breathing causes qì ascent in the chest, this indicates cough; when breathing gives rise to open mouth and shortness of breath, this indicates lung wilting[3] with spitting of foam."

Text Notes, Line 1.5

[1] Breathing shakes the shoulders 息摇肩 *xī yáo jiān*: Raised shoulder breathing.

[2] Hardness in the heart 心中坚 *xīn zhōng jiān*: Hardness and fullness in the chest,

usually because of repletion evil causing obstruction and stagnation.

SYNOPSIS, LINE 1.5

This line discusses how to understand disease by the patient's respiration.

COMMENTARY, LINE 1.5

This line describes three kinds of respiratory problems. First is the condition in which a patient has difficulty in breathing and lifts his shoulders. Such a condition may be due to vacuity or repletion. "Hardness in the heart" is how the author describes the repletion condition in which evil qì is congesting the chest and causing difficulty in breathing, flaring of the nostrils, oppression in the chest, and cough and panting.

Second is a condition in which breathing causes qì ascent in the chest and cough. This arises because there is evil in the chest obstructing the airways, impairing the depurative downbearing of the lung qì, and causing qì to ascend counterflow; hence the cough.

Third is the condition in which a patient has to open his mouth to breathe but despite this has shortness of breath. This happens in lung wilting when the lung is weak and cannot perform its breathing function properly. This tends to be accompanied by ejection of foamy drool.

[3] Lung wilting 肺痿 *fèi wěi*: See Chapter 7, "Lung Wilting."

Line 1.6

师曰：吸而微数，其病在中焦，实也。当下之即愈。虚者不治。在上焦者，其吸促；在下焦者，其吸远，此皆难治。呼吸动摇振振者，不治。

Shī yuē: Xī ér wēi shuò, qí bìng zài zhōng jiāo, shí yě. Dāng xià zhī jí yù. Xū zhě bù zhì. Zài shàng jiāo zhě, qí xī cù; zài xià jiāo zhě, qí xī yuǎn, cǐ jiē nán zhì. Hū xī dòng yáo zhèn zhèn zhě, bù zhì.

The Master says: "If inhalation is faint and rapid, the disease is in the center burner, [which is a condition of] repletion. [This] must be cured by precipitation. Vacuity cannot be treated. [If the disease is in] the upper burner, inhalation is hasty;[1] if in the lower burner, breathing is long.[2] These [cases] are hard to treat. Breathing with shaking and trembling cannot be treated."

TEXT NOTES, LINE 1.6

[1] Inhalation is hasty 吸促 *xī cù*: Inhalation is short and shallow.

[2] Inhalation is long 吸远 *xī yuǎn*: Inhalation is slow, drawn out, and difficult.

[3] Shaking and trembling 动摇振振 *dòng yáo zhèn zhèn*: Tremor of the whole body.

SYNOPSIS, LINE 1.6

This line describes how to determine on the basis of respiration whether the disease is in the upper or lower body, whether it is vacuity or repletion, and whether it is treatable or not.

COMMENTARY, LINE 1.6

This line discusses different patterns of inhalation.

The first instance refers to faint and rapid inhalation, which indicates that the disease is in the center burner. In this case, the pathomechanism is evil qì congesting the center burner and affecting depurative downbearing of lung qì. This is treated by precipitation. As soon as the qì dynamic is freed, breathing will return to normal.

When there is vacuity, the condition is not so easily treated. If in spite of the repletion, right qì is vacuous, then the patient will not be able to withstand precipitation and so cannot be treated.

If the disease is in the upper burner, which here essentially refers to the lung, it manifests with hasty inhalation. This is caused by great vacuity of the lung.

If the disease is in the lower burner, which essentially refers to the kidney, the patient presents with long inhalation, which is due to debilitation of original kidney and the kidney failing to absorb qì.

If there is generalized tremor, the vacuity is even more severe. The line as a whole thus suggests that abnormalities of inhalation that form vacuity patterns are difficult to treat.

Line 1.7

师曰：寸口脉动者，因其旺时而动，假令肝旺色青，四时各随其色。肝色青而反色白，非其时色脉，皆当病。

Shī yuē: Cùn kǒu mài dòng zhě, yīn qí wàng shí ér dòng, jiǎ lìng gān wàng sè qīng, sì shí gè suí qí sè. Gān sè qīng ér fǎn sè bái, fēi qí shí sè mài, jiē dāng bìng.

The Master says: "The pulse at the inch opening moves in accord with the season during which each of the five viscera are effulgent. For example, in the spring it reflects an effulgent liver and is accompanied by a green-blue complexion, since each of the four seasons has its own color.[2] When the liver complexion [should be] green-blue but instead is white, the complexion and pulse are unsynchronized, so the patient must be ill."

TEXT NOTES, LINE 1.7

[1] Inch opening 寸口 *cùn kǒu*: The term has two meanings. On a more general level, it refers to the wrist pulse, which is divided into three sections: inch, bar, and cubit. The other meaning is the inch section of the wrist pulse. The *Jīn Guì Yào*

Lüè reflects two methods of pulse-taking. One is the three-sections method, which involves examining the inch opening (the stirring pulse of the hand greater yīn), the instep yáng pulse (at ST-42 *chōng yáng*) on the yáng brightness channel), and the lesser yīn pulse (at KI-3 *tài xī*) on the foot lesser yīn channel). The other method involves only examining the wrist pulse (and its three sections, the inch, the bar, and cubit). The meaning of the term has to be deduced from the context. Here, it refers in general to the pulse on all three sections of each wrist.

[2] Each of the four seasons having its own color 四时各随其色 *sì shí gè suí qí sè*: Green-blue in the spring; red in the summer; white in the autumn; black in the winter.

Synopsis, Line 1.7

This line explains the diagnostic significance of complexion and pulse in relation to the seasons.

Commentary, Line 1.7

The complexion and pulse vary according to the seasons. To determine whether a pulse is normal or not, one has to take account of the seasons. This principle is demonstrated in the present line by the example of the liver-pulse that is prevalent in spring. In the spring, the liver is effulgent. Thus, at this time the pulse is normally stringlike and the complexion green-blue. If the complexion is white and the pulse is downy (downy being the normal pulse of autumn), then both the pulse and complexion are abnormal.

Line 1.8

问曰：有未至而至，有至而不至，有至而不去，有至而太过，何谓也？师曰：冬至之后，甲子夜半少阳起，少阳之时阳始生，天得温和。以未得甲子，天因温和，此为未至而至也；以得甲子而天未温和，为至而不至也；以得甲子而天大寒不解，此为至而不去也；以得甲子而天温如盛夏五六月时，此为至而太过也。

Wèn yuē: Yǒu wèi zhì ér zhì, yǒu zhì ér bù zhì, yǒu zhì ér bù qù, yǒu zhì ér tài guò, hé wèi yě? Shī yuē: Dōng zhì zhī hòu, jiǎ zǐ yè bàn shào yáng qǐ, shào yáng zhī shí yáng shǐ shēng, tiān dé wēn hé. Yǐ wèi dé jiǎ zǐ, tiān yīn wēn hé, cǐ wéi wèi zhì ér zhì yě; Yǐ dé jiǎ zǐ ér tiān wèi wēn hé, wéi zhì ér bù zhì yě; yǐ dé jiǎ zǐ ér tiān dà hán bù jiě, cǐ wéi zhì ér bù qù yě; yǐ dé jiǎ zǐ ér tiān wēn rú shèng xià wǔ liù yuè shí, cǐ wéi zhì ér tài guò yě.

Question: "There are [times when a given season] has not yet arrived, but [its qì] arrives; when [a given season] arrives, but [its qì] does not arrive; when [a given season] arrives, but the previous season's qì fails to leave; [and when a given season] arrives and [its qì is] excessive. What does this mean?"

The Master says: "At midnight of the *jiǎ-zǐ* day[1] after the winter solstice,[2] lesser yáng rises.[3] At the time of lesser yáng, yáng begins to be engendered and the weather becomes warm and congenial. If the weather becomes warm and congenial before *jiǎ-zǐ*, this is a case of qì arriving before its season. If *jiǎ-zǐ* has already arrived, but the weather has not become warm and congenial, this is a case of qì failing to arrive in time for its season. If the time of *jiǎ-zǐ* has arrived but severely cold weather fails to resolve, this is a case of the season arriving and [the previous season's qì] not leaving. If the weather at the arrival of *jiǎ-zǐ* is warm as in the height of summer in the fifth and sixth months, this is a case of [the season] arriving and [the qì] being excessive."

TEXT NOTES, LINE 1.8

[1] Jiǎ-zǐ 甲子 *jiǎ zǐ*: In ancient times, the ten heavenly stems (S) and 12 earthly branches (B) were used to measure time in 60-day cycles. The ten heavenly stems are: 甲、乙、丙、丁、戊、已、更、辛、壬、癸 *jiǎ, yǐ, bǐng, dīng, wù, yǐ, gēng, xīn, rén, guǐ*. The twelve earthly branches are 子、丑、寅、卯、辰、巳、午、未、申、酉、戌、亥 *zǐ, chǒu, yín, mǎo, chén, sì, wǔ, wèi, shēn, yǒu, xū, hài*. These were combined starting with 甲子 *jiǎ zǐ* and ending with 癸亥 *guì hài*, making a total of 60 combinations. The 甲子 *jiǎ zǐ* referred to here is the first day of *jiǎ zǐ* occurring at midnight 60 days after the winter solstice.

[2] Winter solstice 冬至 *dōng zhì*: The 12th solar term in the lunar calendar.

[3] Lesser yáng rises 少阳起 *shào yáng qǐ*: An ancient representative method of classifying time, starting with *shào yang* and ending with *jué yīn*.

SYNOPSIS, LINE 1.8

This line describes the ways in which the weather can be inappropriate for the time of year.

COMMENTARY, LINE 1.8

Extremes—excesses and deficiencies—in weather conditions can cause illness.

This passage demonstrates the various types of unseasonable weather by using as an example the time of lesser yáng rising, which occurs 60 days after the winter solstice.

At this time, yáng qì is engendered and the weather should therefore gradually become warmer. If the weather becomes unseasonably warm before this time, this is an instance of the weather arriving before the season. If, however, the weather fails to turn warm, this is a case of the season arriving and the weather not changing accordingly. If the weather instead remains cold, this is the season arriving and the cold weather remaining longer than it should. If lastly the weather turns unseasonably warm as in summer, this is weather arriving excessively. All these situations are abnormal and can cause disease. Thus, people should adapt to them appropriately.

Line 1.9

师曰：病人脉浮者在前，其病在表；浮者在后，其病在里。腰痛背强不能行，必短气而极也。

Shī yuē: Bìng rén mài fú zhě zài qián, qí bìng zài biǎo; fú zhě zài hòu, qí bìng zài lǐ. Yāo tòng bèi qiáng bù néng xíng, bì duǎn qì ér jí yě.

The Master says: "When the patient has a floating pulse in front [of the bar],[1] the disease is in the exterior. When a floating pulse is behind [the bar],[2] the disease is in the interior. [In the latter case, there is] lumbar pain, rigidity of the back, inability to walk, and shortness of breath in the extreme."[3]

TEXT NOTES, LINE 1.9

[1] In front 前 *qián*: The inch position of the pulse, in front of the bar, closest to the hand.

[2] Behind 后 *hòu*: The cubit position of the pulse, behind the bar, furthest from the hand.

[3] In the extreme 极 *jí*: Critically severe.

SYNOPSIS, LINE 1.9

This line describes the significance of one and the same pulse condition appearing at different positions.

COMMENTARY, LINE 1.9

Normally, a floating pulse reflects disease in the exterior. However, this type of floating pulse must be present at the inch section, that is, in front of the bar. The inch section is yáng and governs the exterior, thus a floating pulse at the inch section means disease of the exterior and reflects right qì fighting the invading evil.

If the floating pulse appears at the cubit section, that is, behind the bar, the significance is different. The cubit section is yīn and governs the interior. A floating pulse at the cubit means disease of the interior, usually insufficiency of kidney yīn with vacuous yáng floating outward and yáng qì unable to keep itself concealed. It should also be pointed out that in an exterior repletion pattern, the floating pulse should be floating and forceful; in interior vacuity patterns, the floating pulse is floating and forceless.

The cubit postion belongs to the kidney, which stores essence and governs the bones. The lumbus is the house of the kidney and its vessels run along the spine. In kidney vacuity, essence and marrow are lacking and the lumbar spine is deprived of nourishment; hence there is lumbar pain and stiff back, wilting bones preventing the patient from walking, and in severe cases inability to absorb qì, causing shortness of breath and panting.

Line 1.10

问曰：经云厥阳独行何谓也？师曰：此为有阳无阴，故称厥阳。

Wèn yuē: jīng yún jué yáng dú xíng hé wèi yě? Shī yuē: Cǐ wéi yǒu yáng wú yīn, gù chēng jué yáng.

Question: The Classic[1] mentions "reversing yáng[2] going alone"; what does this mean? The Master says, "This is yáng without yīn; hence it is called reversing yáng."

TEXT NOTES, LINE 1.10

[1] The Classic 经 *jīng*: It is not known to what book this refers.

[2] Reversing yáng 厥阳 *jué yáng*: "Reversing" here means counterflow rising. Reversing yáng denotes solitary exuberant yáng qì rising counterflow.

SYNOPSIS, LINE 1.10

This line explains the pathomechanism of reversing yáng.

COMMENTARY, LINE 1.10

Normally, yīn and yáng maintain a coordinated balance in the body. If yīn qì is depleted, however, yáng qì loses its support, there is upbearing without downbearing, and yáng without yīn. This is what is called "reversing yáng going alone."

Line 1.11

问曰：寸脉沉大而滑，沉则为实，滑则为气。实气相搏，血气入脏即死，入腑即愈，此为卒厥。何谓也？师曰：唇口青，身冷，为入脏即死；如身和，汗自出，为入腑即愈。

Wèn yuē: cùn mài chén dà ér huá, chén zé wéi shí, huá zé wéi qì. Shí qì xiāng bó, xuè qì rù zàng jí sǐ, rù fǔ jí yù, cǐ wéi zú jué. Hé wèi yě? Shī yuē: Chún kǒu qīng, shēn lěng, wéi rù zàng jí sǐ; rú shēn hé, hàn zì chū, wéi rù fǔ jí yù.

Question: "In cases with a large sunken and slippery inch pulse, since a sunken pulse indicates [blood] repletion and a slippery pulse indicates qì [repletion],[1] the patient suffers from qì and blood contending with each other. If blood and qì enter the viscera, [the patient] will die; if they enter the bowels, the patient will recover. This is the condition of sudden reversal.[2] What does this mean?" The Master says: "Green-blue lips and a cold body mean that [evil] has entered the viscera and that the patient will die. A [warm and] harmonious body[3] and spontaneous sweating indicate that [evil] has entered the bowels and that the patient will recover."

TEXT NOTES, LINE 1.11

[1] Repletion and qì 实气 *shí qì*: "Replete" here means blood repletion, while "qì" means qì repletion. The entire phrase means that there is evil repletion in both qì and blood.

[2] Sudden reversal 卒厥 *cù jué*: Sudden loss of consciousness.

[3] Body is [warm and] in harmony 身和 *shēn hé*: The body is normal in temperature. "Harmony" is often used in the *Jīn Guì Yào Lüè* to mean health or normality.

SYNOPSIS, LINE 1.11

This line discusses the pathomechanism and prognosis of sudden reversal.

COMMENTARY, LINE 1.11

The first sentence explains sudden reversal in terms of the pulse. However, the sentence contains omissions. To make sense, it should read: "…sunken means blood repletion, while slippery means qì repletion. When blood repletion and qì repletion contend with each other…" The left inch position reflects the heart's function of governing blood, while the right inch position represents the lung's function of governing qì. Because sudden reversal is characterized by simultaneous blood repletion and qì repletion, it is reflected in the inch positions of both wrists.

"Repletion and qì contend with each other" means that blood [repletion] and qì [repletion] co-exist and exacerbate each other. When this happens, blood and qì can flow counter to their normal direction and ascend to the upper body, which is called "sudden reversal."

In the statement "… [if] blood and qì enter the viscera, the patient will die; [if they] enter the bowels, the patient will recover," blood and qì refer to pathological blood and qì.

When blood and qì are in a pathological state of repletion, they behave like disease evils. The distinction between entering the viscera and entering the bowels rests on the understanding that the viscera store, but do not discharge, while the bowels discharge, but do not store. When pathological qì and blood enter the viscera, there is no way out, so the patient dies. By contrast, when pathological qì and blood enter the bowels, they can escape. When qì and blood enter the viscera, the lips turn green-blue as a result of inhibited movement of blood. The body turns cold as a result of the debilitation of yáng qì. Original true qì cannot move, and the upward, downward, inward, and outward pathways are all blocked. This is why the text says, "if blood and qì enter the viscera, [the patient] dies."

By contrast, qì and blood can escape when they enter the bowels. Although there is sudden clouding and reversal cold of the extremities, the condition is only temporary. In a short time, qì and blood resume their normal flow, yáng qì reaches the exterior, and the evil qì can discharge from the body. The body becomes warm again, sweat flows, and the patient finally recovers. This is why it is said, "when qì and blood enter the bowels, the patient will recover. This is the condition of sudden reversal."

Line 1.12

问曰：脉脱入脏即死，入腑即愈，何谓也？师曰：非为一病，百病皆然。譬如浸淫疮，从口起流向四肢者，可治；从四肢流来入口者，不可治；病在外者，可治；入里者，即死。

Wèn yuē: mài tuō rù zàng jí sǐ, rù fǔ jí yù, hé wèi yě? Shī yuē: Fēi wéi yī bìng, bǎi bìng jiē rán. Pì rú jìn yín chuāng, cóng kǒu qǐ liú xiàng sì zhī zhě, kě zhì; cóng sì zhī liú lái rù kǒu zhě, bù kě zhì; bìng zài wài zhě, kě zhì; rù lǐ zhě, jí sǐ.

Question: "When the pulse deserts,[1] [if evil qì] has entered the viscera, [the patient] dies, [while if evil qì] has entered the bowels, [the patient] recovers. Why is this so?" The Master says: "This applies not just to a single disease, but to all the hundred diseases. Take wet spreading sores[2] as an example: If they begin at the mouth and spread to the four limbs, they can be treated, but if they begin in the limbs and spread to the mouth, they cannot be treated. When the disease is in the exterior, it can be treated; when it enters the interior, [the patient] dies."

TEXT NOTES, LINE 1.12

[1] The pulse deserts 脉脱 *mài tuō*: The pulse suddenly becomes undetectable, indicating that evil qì is obstructing right, so that there is temporary stoppage in the vessels.

[2] Wet spreading sores 浸淫疮 *jìn yín chuāng*: A type of sore that begins locally and spreads to other parts of the body. See Chapter 18, "Sores, Welling-Abscesses, Intestinal Welling-Abscesses and Wet Spreading Sores."

SYNOPSIS, LINE 1.12

This line discusses the difference between disease spreading from the outside in and from the inside out through the example of wet spreading sores.

COMMENTARY, LINE 1.12

This line continues the discussion on sudden reversal that started in line 1.11. In sudden reversal, the pulse may be large, sunken, and slippery, but it also suddenly may become hidden. When blood and qì enter the viscera, the patient dies; when they enter the bowels, the patient recovers.

The difference between the two pathomechanisms is relatively minor. The present line develops the notion that in general evils moving toward the inner body are difficult to treat, while those moving outward are easier to treat. The example given is that of wet spreading sores. Those that spread from the mouth outward to the limbs can be treated, while those that spread from the limbs into the mouth cannot be treated.

In contrast to this distinction between inward and outward movement of disease, the preceding line makes the distinction between entering the bowels and entering the viscera, and explains the difference in the outcome in terms of the storing and discharging actions of the viscera and bowels respectively. If the difference in outcome in line 1.11 were explained completely in terms of depth of penetration (the viscera being deeper than the bowels) instead, the principle discussed in the present line would also explain the phenomena described there.

Line 1.13

(1)问曰：阳病十八何谓也？师曰：头痛、项、腰、脊、臂、脚掣痛。阴病十八何谓也？师曰：咳、上气、喘、哕、咽、肠鸣、胀满、心痛、拘急。五脏病各有十八，合为九十病；人又有六微，微有十八病，合为一百八病，五劳、七伤、六极、妇人三十六病，不在其中。

(2)清邪居上，浊邪居下，大邪中表，小邪中里，槃饪之邪，从口入者，宿食也。五邪中人，各有法度，风中于前，寒中于暮，湿伤于下，雾伤于上，风令脉浮，寒令脉急，雾伤皮腠，湿流关节，食伤脾胃，极寒伤经，极热伤络。

(1) Wèn yuē: Yáng bìng shí bā hé wèi yě? Shī yuē: Tóu tòng, xiàng, yāo, jǐ, bèi, jiǎo chè tòng. Yīn bìng shí bā hé wèi yě? Shī yuē: Ké, shàng qì, chuǎn, yuē, yān, cháng míng zhàng mǎn, xīn tòng jū jí. Wǔ zàng bìng gè yǒu shí bā, hé wéi jiǔ shí bìng; rén yòu yǒu liù wēi, wēi yǒu shí bā bìng, hé wéi yī bǎi bā bìng, wǔ láo, qī shāng, liù jí, fù rén sān shí liù bìng, bù zài qí zhōng.

(2) Qīng xié jū shàng, zhuó xié jū xià, dà xié zhòng biǎo, xiǎo xié zhòng lǐ, gǔ rèn zhī xié, cóng kǒu rù zhě, sù shí yě. Wǔ xié zhòng rén, gè yǒu fǎ dù, fēng zhòng yú qián, hán zhōng yú mù, shī shāng yú xià, wù shāng yú shàng, fēng lìng mài fú, hán lìng mài jí, wù shāng pí còu, shī liú guān jié, shí shāng pí wèi, jí hán shāng jīng, jí rè shāng luò.

(1) Question: "There are eighteen yáng diseases.[1] What are they?" The Master says, "Headache, pulling pain in the nape, pulling pain in the lumbus, pulling pain in the spine, pulling pain in the arm, and pulling pain in the foot." "There are eighteen yīn diseases.[2] What are they?" The Master says: "Cough, qì ascent, panting, belching, dysphagia,[3] rumbling intestines, distention and fullness, heart pain, and hypertonicity. The five viscera each have eighteen diseases, combining to make ninety diseases. People also have six minor conditions[4] [of the bowels]", which each have eighteen diseases, combining to make one hundred and eight. The five taxations,[5] seven damages,[6] six extremes,[7] and the thirty-six women's diseases[8] are not among these."

(2) Clear evils dwell in the upper body; turbid evils dwell in the lower body. Major evils strike the exterior; minor evils strike the interior. Food evils[9] enter through the mouth, giving rise to abiding food. The five evils[10] strike people each in their own way. Wind strikes before [noon]; cold strikes in the evening. Dampness damages the lower body; mist damages the upper body. Wind makes the pulse floating; cold makes the pulse tense.[11] Mist damages the interstices of the skin; dampness flows into the joints. Food damages the spleen and stomach. Extreme cold damages the channels; extreme heat damages the network vessels.

Text Notes, Line 1.13

[1] Yáng disease 阳病 *yáng bìng*: Disease in the exterior and channels and network vessels.

[2] Yīn disease 阴病 *yīn bìng*: Disease in the interior, in the bowels and viscera.

[3] Dysphagia 咽 *yàn*: Blockage in the throat preventing swallowing.

[4] Six minor conditions 六微 *liù wēi*: Based on textual parallelism, commentators and scholars explain it as referring to diseases of the six bowels, which are considered minor in comparison with the diseases that affect the five viscera.

[5] Five taxations 五劳 *wǔ láo*: The *Nèi Jīng* ("The Inner Canon") explains damage by the five taxations in this way: "Prolonged vision damages the blood; prolonged lying damages qì; prolonged sitting damages the flesh; prolonged standing damages the bones; and prolonged walking damages the sinews (*Sù Wèn* ("Plain Questions") 23, "Treatise Explaining the Five Qì")."

[6] Seven damages 七伤 *qī shāng*: The *Zhū Bìng Yuán Hòu Lùn* ("Origin and Indicators of Disease") states that great satiety damages the spleen; great anger and qì counterflow damage the liver; straining, lifting heavy [weights], and prolonged sitting in damp places damage the kidney; coldness of the body and cold drinks damage the lung; anxiety and worry damage the heart; wind, rain, cold, and summerheat damage the physical body; and great fear damages the mind. In the chapter on "Vacuity Taxation" of the same text, the seven damages are alternatively defined as food damage, anxiety damage, drinking damage, bedroom taxation damage, hunger damage, taxation damage, and channel and network construction and defense qì damage.

[7] Six extremes 六极 *liù jí*: This expression refers to extreme taxation detriment in the six aspects of qì, blood, sinews, bones, flesh, and essence.

[8] Thirty-six women's diseases 妇人三十六病 *fù rén sān shí liù bìng*: This is a standard term for gynecological conditions that consists of the twelve concretions, nine pains, the seven harms, five damages, and three intractable diseases.

[9] Food evil 槃饪之邪 *gǔ rèn zhī xié*: Literally, "evil of grain and cooked food," it refers here more generally to food as a cause of illness.

[10] The five evils 五邪 *wǔ xié*: Wind, cold, dampness, fog, and food and drink.

[11] Tense 急 *jí*: Tight.

Synopsis, Line 1.13

This line classifies disease patterns, calculates their number, and describes the general laws by which evils strike people.

Commentary, Line 1.13

This line presents an ancient classification of disease and evils. First, there is a broad classification into yáng diseases and yīn diseases, yáng diseases being those that affect the exterior and the channels, yīn diseases being those that affect the viscera and bowels in the interior. The line tells us there are eighteen yáng diseases and that these are "headache, pulling pain in the nape, lumbus, spine, arm, and foot." These items amount only to six. The number eighteen derives from the threefold division of each disease into construction disease, defense disease, and construction-defense disease (6 × 3 = 18).

We are told that there are also eighteen yīn diseases: Cough, qì ascent, panting, belching, dysphagia, rumbling intestines, distention and fullness, heart pain, and hypertonicity. The figure eighteen derives from there being both vacuity and repletion forms of each of the nine diseases (9 × 2 = 18).

Each of the five viscera has eighteen diseases. These are contraction of the six excesses: wind, cold, summerheat, dampness, dryness, and fire. Each kind of contraction is further divided into three types: qì aspect disease, blood aspect disease, and dual disease of qì and blood. Thus in all there are eighteen diseases (6 × 3 = 18). Since the five viscera each have eighteen diseases, the viscera have a total of ninety diseases (18 × 5 = 90). The "six minor conditions" is generally understood to refer to diseases of the six bowels (the bowels being of lesser importance than the viscera). Alternatively, it may also refer to the diseases caused by the six excesses that strike the bowels, which are less severe than those caused by the six excesses striking the viscera. The ambiguity makes no difference as regards the meaning of the text, which is clear: the bowels also have diseases caused by the six excesses, each of which are subdivided into the three types of qì aspect disease, blood aspect disease, and dual disease of qì and blood, making a total of a hundred and eight (6 × 6 × 3 = 108).

The five taxations, seven damages, six extremes, and the thirty-six women's disease are not caused by the six excesses and hence are not included in the previously mentioned diseases.

The second section of the line describes the different ways in which evils strike the body. It rests on a fivefold classification of evils: wind, cold, dampness, mist, and food and drink. Clear evil, i.e., mist and dew, affect the upper part of the body; turbid evil, i.e., water and dampness, affect the lower part of the body. Major evil, i.e., wind, being diffuse, strikes the exterior; minor evil, i.e., cold, being tight and compact, strikes the channels in the interior. Food evil refers to abiding food, which affects the spleen and stomach.

The second part of the second section further elucidates the laws by which evils strike the body. Wind is a yáng evil. It strikes the body before noon and gives rise to a pulse that is floating and moderate. Cold is a yīn evil. It strikes the body after evening comes and gives rise to a pulse that is usually tight and urgent. Dampness is a heavy turbid evil. It damages the lower body and flows into people's joints. Mist is a clear evil. It damages the upper body and reaches into the interstices of the skin. The spleen governs movement and transformation, and intemperance in eating and drinking damages the spleen and stomach. The channels are in the interior and are yīn; the network vessels are in the outer body and are yáng. Cold qì homes to yīn, hence extreme cold damages the channels. Heat qì homes to yáng; hence extreme heat damages the network vessels.

Line 1.14

问曰：病有急当救里、救表者，何谓也？师曰：病，医下之，续得下利清谷不止，身体疼痛者，急当救里，后身体疼痛，清便自调者，急当救表也。

Wèn yuē: Bìng yǒu jí dāng jiù lǐ, jiù biǎo zhě, hé wèi yě? Shī yuē: Bìng, yī xià zhī, xù dé xià lì qīng gǔ bù zhǐ, shēn tǐ téng tòng zhě, jí dāng jiù lǐ, hòu shēn tǐ téng tòng, qīng biàn zì tiáo zhě, jí dāng jiù biǎo yě.

Question: "There are diseases where you must quickly rescue the interior and those where you must quickly rescue the exterior. What does this mean?" The Master says: "In conditions where a physician has precipitated and [the patient] continues to suffer from incessant clear-grain diarrhea[1] and generalized pain, you must quickly rescue the interior. Afterwards, [if there is still] generalized pain, but the eliminations have returned to normal,[2] then you must quickly rescue the exterior."

Text Notes, Line 1.14

[1] Clear-grain diarrhea 下利清谷 *xià lì qīng gǔ*: Diarrhea with stool containing undigested food.

[2] Eliminations have returned to normal 清便自调 *qīng biàn zì tiáo*: The stool has returned to normal.

Synopsis, Line 1.14

This line discusses the principles for deciding priorities in the treatment of dual disease of the exterior and interior.

Commentary, Line 1.14

When exterior and interior patterns appear together, it is important to determine which is the acute and which is the chronic. The acute pattern is treated first. When the disease is in the exterior, precipitation cannot be given. If precipitation is mistakenly given, this will damage the spleen and stomach and cause incessant clear-grain diarrhea without eliminating the generalized pain of the exterior pattern. Because the interior pattern is the more severe, it must be treated first. Owing to incessant clear-grain diarrhea, right qì is already weakened and not only unable to resist the evil, but if allowed to develop further, will give way to yáng collapse. If sweating were applied to address the exterior pattern at this point, it might exacerbate the yáng vacuity, giving rise to a critical condition of desertion in the upper and lower body. So the correct approach is rather to return the stool to normal and then to take swift action to rescue the exterior. If exterior signs are still present after the diarrhea has stopped, they must be treated quickly to prevent the evil from entering the interior and causing more complications.

Line 1.15

夫病痼疾，加以卒病，当先治其卒病，后乃治其痼疾也。

Fū bìng gù jí, jiā yǐ cù bìng, dāng xiān zhì qí zú bìng, hòu nǎi zhì qí gù jí yě.

When an intractable disease[1] is added to by a sudden disease,[2] you must first treat the sudden disease and afterwards treat the intractable disease.

TEXT NOTES, LINE 1.15

[1] Intractable disease 痼疾 *gù jí*: A chronic disease that resists treatment.

[2] Sudden disease 卒病 *cù bìng*: An acute disease of sudden onset.

SYNOPSIS, LINE 1.15

This line offers principles for deciding priorities in the treatment of intractable and sudden disease.

COMMENTARY, LINE 1.15

This line follows on from the previous line in that it is concerned with determining priorities when two disease patterns are present, this time an old disease pattern and a new one. The principle of coping with this is the same: treat the more acute problem first and the chronic problem afterwards. The old disease is chronic and cannot be treated quickly. The new disease is acute, and delay in coping with it will allow it to develop further.

Line 1.16

师曰：五脏病各有所得者愈；五脏病各有所恶，各随其所不喜者为病。病者素不应食，而反暴思之，必发热也。

Shī yuē: Wǔ zàng bìng gè yǒu suǒ dé zhě yù; wǔ zàng bìng gè yǒu suǒ wù, gè suí qí suǒ bù xǐ zhě wéi bìng. Bìng zhě sù bù yīng shí, ér fǎn bào sī zhī, bì fā rè yě.

The Master says: "In disease of the five viscera, if each gets what is appropriate [for it], recovery ensues. Since they each have things to which they are averse, if they get what they dislike, disease ensues as a consequence. If patients suddenly crave to eat something they normally do not like, they will [suffer from] heat effusion."

SYNOPSIS, LINE 1.16

This line discusses the importance of treatment and nursing in accordance with the likings and aversions of the five viscera.

COMMENTARY, LINE 1.16

In the treatment of disease, the five viscera each have their specific requirements in regards to diet and environment. If they are supplied with what they need, the patient will recover. By contrast, if a patient is given inappropriate diet and nursing care during recovery, the viscera will respond to their aversions and the disease will be exacerbated accordingly. Heart disease, for example, can result in blood heat, and the patient should therefore not be exposed to hot foods or clothing. If a patient suddenly experiences unusual food cravings, this is a sign that evil qì has affected visceral qì. If this pathogenic qì is fortified by inappropriate food, it can therefore result in heat effusion (fever).

Line 1.17

夫诸病在藏欲攻之，当随其所得而攻之，如渴者，与猪苓汤，余皆仿此。

Fū zhū bìng zài zàng yù gōng zhī, dāng suí qí suǒ dé ér gōng zhī, rú kě zhě, yǔ zhū líng tāng, yú jiē fǎng cǐ.

All diseases in the viscera,[1] if they are to be attacked,[2] should be attacked in accord with what [evil] the patient has contracted. For example, for thirst, I give *zhū líng tāng* (猪苓汤 Polyporus Decoction). [All] other diseases are like this too.

TEXT NOTES, LINE 1.17

[1] In the viscera 在脏 *zài zàng*: In the interior.

[2] Attack 攻 *gōng*: To treat.

SYNOPSIS, LINE 1.17

This line stresses the need to determine treatment of any disease on the basis of the evil the patient has contracted.

COMMENTARY, LINE 1.17

When treating the various internal diseases, the physician must prescribe treatment in accordance with the evil the patient has contracted. For example, in cases of thirst and inhibited urination, if it is caused by heat binding water and damaging yīn, Polyporus Decoction (*zhū líng tāng*) is appropriate because it fosters yīn and disinhibits water, thereby removing water and eliminating heat.

痉湿暍病脉证治第二

CHAPTER 2

Tetany, Dampness, and Thermoplegia

Pulses, Signs, Treatments

‡ Overview

This chapter deals with tetany, dampness, and thermoplegia. All three are caused by contraction of external evils and are characterized in the initial stage by greater yáng exterior patterns. For this reason, they are discussed together in one chapter.

Tetany

Tetany (痉 *jìng*) is a disease of the sinews that manifests in severe spasm such as rigidity in the neck, clenched jaw, convulsions of the limbs, and arched-back rigidity. It arises in external contraction or by internal damage by three pathomechanisms: cold causing contracture and tautness; the sinews being deprived of nourishment; and/or exuberant heat stirring wind. In the present chapter, the emphasis is on tetany due to external contraction of wind-cold, but tetany arising through inappropriate treatment is also discussed. While *Nèi Jīng* ("The Inner Canon") contains odd descriptions of tetany conditions and their causes here and there, it was Zhāng Jī who first gave the first complete description of the tetany due to externally contracted wind and its treatment.

Dampness

Dampness disease affects the flesh and joints and is characterized by heat effusion, generalized heaviness, and joint pain. It is called dampness disease because it it caused by dampness, which either can be contracted externally or can arise internally. The present chapter concentrates mainly on external dampness, which often combines with other evils like wind or cold to invade the fleshy exterior and spread to the joints. If there is concurrent internal dampness, there may also be inhibited urination. Treatment of dampness generally centers on protecting yáng qì, in combination with promotion of slight sweating for external dampness and disinhibiting urine for internal dampness. While the *Nèi Jīng* ("The Inner Canon") mentions the process and symptoms of disease caused by dampness in passing, the systematic identification and treatment of dampness disease originates in the *Jīn Guì*.

THERMOPLEGIA

Thermoplegia (中暍 *zhòng yè*) is commonly referred to in modern texts as summerheat damage (伤暑 *shāng shǔ*). The English term *thermoplegia*, literally meaning "heat stroke," has been chosen to represent this condition wherever it is called *zhòng yè* in the Chinese. Thermoplegia is the contraction of summerheat-heat in the summer months. It is characterized by heat effusion, spontaneous sweating, vexing thirst, reddish urine, shortage of qì, and a vacuous pulse. At onset, it is usually characterized by exterior signs. Often, it is complicated by cold or dampness. Furthermore, it invariably causes damage to both qì and yīn, creating a vacuity-repletion complex. The condition described in this chapter is basically identical to what *Sù Wèn* ("Plain Questions") 53, "Treatise on Points to Remember When Needling" describes as "qì vacuity generalized heat that is contracted through summerheat damage." However, this differs from the thermoplegia (or summerheat strike) described in the *Zhū Bìng Yuán Hòu Lùn* ("The Origin and Indicators of Disease") as arising "when [people] traveling far under a torrid sun suddenly cloud and collapse."

‡ SCHEMATIC OVERVIEW

TETANY

1. Causes: Pre-existing insufficiency of fluids, complicated by a contraction of external evils that obstruct the sinews.

2. Main signs: Generalized heat with cold lower extremities, stiffness of the neck and nape, aversion to cold and periodic head heat, red face, red eyes, shaking of the head only, sudden clenching of the jaw, arched-back rigidity.

3. Main pulse: tight and stringlike when pressed, from top to bottom.

4. Tetany caused by external contraction of wind evil

a) Pattern identification

Hard tetany: greater yáng disease with heat effusion, no sweating, and with aversion to cold.

Soft tetany: greater yáng disease with heat effusion, sweating, and absence of aversion to cold.

b) Treatment

Hard tetany: Pueraria Decoction (*gé gēn tāng*) for greater yáng disease with absence of sweating, scant urine, qì surging up into the chest, and clenched jaw with inability to speak.

Soft tetany: Trichosanthes and Cinnamon Twig Decoction (*guā lóu guì zhī tāng*) for greater yáng disease with generalized stiffness and stretching, but with a pulse that is sunken and slow.

Evil entering yáng brightness: Major Qì-Coordinating Decoction (*dà chéng qì tāng*) to treat fullness in the chest, clenched jaw, lying without [the back] touching the mat, and hypertonicity in the legs.

5. Tetany caused by damage to yīn from inappropriate treatment

a) Greater yáng disease: tetany arising from excessive promotion of sweating.

b) Wind disease: tetany arising from precipitation followed by promotion of sweating.

c) Sores: tetany arising from inappropriate use of sweating in patients with generalized pain.

6. Prognosis

a) Greater yáng disease with heat effusion and a sunken and fine pulse is called tetany.

b) Tetanic disease moxibustion sores: difficult to treat.

c) Fulminant abdominal distention.

d) If the pulse remains as before or turns hidden and stringlike, this means tetany.

DAMP DISEASE

1. Causes

a) External cause: "damage from exposure to wind during sweating, enduring damage from consumption of cold substances."

b) Internal cause: Impaired movement and transformation with water-damp collecting internally.

2. Main signs: heat effusion, generalized heaviness, pain in the joints.

3. Treatment principles

a) External dampness: promote slight sweating.

b) Internal dampness: disinhibit urine.

4. Pattern identification

a) Cold-damp

Mild pattern: generalized pain, heat effusion, yellow face, panting, headache, nasal congestion and vexation, a large pulse, ability to eat and drink naturally. Pathomechanism: disease in the head, cold-damp in the center, harmony in the abdomen. Method of treatment: insufflation of medicinals into the nose.

Exterior repletion: Vexing generalized pain. Treatment: Do not attack with fire. Use Ephedra Decoction Plus White Atractylodes (*má huáng jiā zhú tāng*) to disperse cold and dispel dampness.

b) Wind-damp

Exterior repletion: Generalized pain and heat effusion worsening in late afternoon. Formula: Ephedra, Apricot Kernel, Coix, and Licorice Decoction (*má xìng yì gān tāng*) to dispel wind and transform dampness.

Exterior vacuity: Floating pulse, generalized heaviness, sweating, and aversion to wind. Use Fangji and Astragalus Decoction (*fáng jǐ huáng qí tāng*) to boost qì and move impediment.

c) Yáng vacuity

Wind more pronounced: Vexing generalized pain with inability to turn sides. Use Cinnamon Twig and Aconite Decoction (*guì zhī fù zǐ tāng*) to dispel wind and transform dampness.

Dampness more pronounced: Hard stool, uninhibited urination. Use White Atractylodes and Aconite Decoction (*bái zhú fù zǐ tāng*) to warm the channels and dispel dampness.

Wind and damp equally pronounced: Vexing generalized pain, pulling pain preventing bending and stretching, sweating, shortness of breath, aversion to wind, inhibited urination, and in some cases light generalized sweating. Use Licorice and Aconite Decoction (*gān cǎo fù zǐ tāng*) to warm the channels and dispel dampness.

5. Treatment contraindications

a) Contraindication against precipitation

Transmuted pattern: "Dampness patients sweat only from the head, suffer from rigidity of the back, and desire to be covered with bedclothes and face the fire. If precipitation is performed early, the result is hiccup or fullness in the chest with inhibited urination, and a tongue that resembles [one that has] fur. This is because there is heat in the cinnabar field and cold on the chest. If there is thirst with a desire for water but inability to drink, the result is vexing dryness of the mouth."

Death pattern: "When dampness patients after precipitation treatment manifest with sweating on the forehead, slight panting, and uninhibited urination, they will die. If there is incessant diarrhea, they also die."

Beware to attack with fire.

Thermoplegia

1. Causes: Contraction of summerheat-heat qì or voracious consumption of cold drinks and entering water when sweating.

2. Pulse and Signs

a) Pulse: stringlike and fine; scallion-stalk and slow.

b) Signs: Heat effusion, aversion to cold, generalized heaviness and pain, shivering and body hair standing erect after urinating, reverse flow of the extremities, heat effusion at the slightest physical taxation, and dry front teeth.

3. Pattern Identification

a) Prevalence of summerheat-heat.

b) Prevalence of summerheat-damp.

4. Treatment contraindications

a) Sweating is contraindicated because it makes the aversion to cold more severe.

b) Warm needling is contraindicated because it makes the heat effusion more severe.

c) Repeated precipitation is contraindicated because it makes the strangury more severe.

Line 2.1

太阳病，发热无汗，反恶寒者，名曰刚痉。

Tài yáng bìng, fā rè wú hàn, fǎn wù hán zhě, míng yuē gāng jìng.

Greater yáng disease[1] with heat effusion and absence of sweating, but with aversion to cold is called "hard tetany."[2]

TEXT NOTES, LINE 2.1

[1] Greater yáng disease 太阳病 *tài yáng bìng*: Cold damage disease affecting greater yáng. See the discussion on greater yáng in the *Shāng Hán Lùn* ("On Cold Damage") (Féng, Mitchell, and Wiseman, pp. 33–295).

[2] Hard tetany 刚痉 *gāng jìng:* Tetany characterized by heat effusion, absence of sweating, aversion to cold, rigidity of the neck, shaking head, clenched jaw, hypertonicity or convulsions of the extremities (in severe cases, arched-back rigidity), and a tight stringlike pulse.

SYNOPSIS, LINE 2.1

This line discusses the signs of hard tetany.

COMMENTARY, LINE 2.1

According to a literal reading of the text, heat effusion without sweating and with aversion to cold constitutes hard tetany. Of course, it is known that these signs indicate patterns of greater yáng exterior repletion caused by an invasion of wind-cold. They only constitute hard tetany when they are accompanied by signs such as stiffness of the neck and nape, clenched jaw, or in severe cases arched-back rigidity. Hence, the original text contains an ellipsis.

When wind-cold assails the body and right qì resists it, the fight between right and evil gives rise to heat effusion. Cold causes contracture and tautness. When cold fetters the outer body, defensive yáng cannot reach the exterior, and the interstices close; hence there is aversion to cold without sweating. When cold evil affects the sinews of greater yáng, the distribution of fluids is affected. As a result, the sinews are deprived of nourishment and become hypertonic, hence there is stiffness of the neck and nape, clenched jaw, and arched-back rigidity.

"Hard tetany" is so called not due to any quality of the tetany signs themselves, but because the tetany occurs in a repletion pattern without sweating. See the following line, which discusses soft tetany.

Line 2.2

太阳病，发热汗出，而不恶寒，名曰柔痓。

Tài yáng bìng, fā rè hàn chū, ér bù wù hán, míng yuē róu jìng.

Greater yáng disease with heat effusion and sweating and without aversion to cold is called "soft tetany."[1]

TEXT NOTE, LINE 2.2

1. Soft tetany 柔痓 *róu jìng*: Tetany characterized by generalized heat [effusion], sweating, rigidity of the neck, shaking of the head, clenched jaw, hypertonicity of the extremities, arched-back rigidity, and a slow sunken pulse.

SYNOPSIS, LINE 2.2

This line discusses the signs of soft tetany.

COMMENTARY, LINE 2.2

When external evils cause tetany, the disease must begin in greater yáng; hence the greater yáng disease signs described in this line. When wind evil assails the exterior, right qì fights the evil, giving rise to heat effusion. Wind by nature causes opening and discharge; when it damages defense, defense qì fails to perform its securing action, so the interstices become loose. The result is sweating and aversion to cold. External evils can obstruct the greater yáng sinews and hamper the distribution of fluids. In patients suffering from pre-existing insufficiency of liquid, this can deprive the sinews of nourishment and make them tense; hence the stiffness of the nape and back, clenched jaw, and in severe cases arched-back rigidity.

The difference between the hard tetany discussed in the preceding line and the soft tetany discussed in the present line lies not in the nature of the tetany but in the nature of the pattern in which the tetany occurs. Hard tetany means tetany occurring in exterior repletion without sweating, while soft tetany occurs in exterior vacuity patterns with sweating.

Line 2.3

太阳病，发热脉沉而细者，名曰痓，为难治。

Tài yáng bìng, fā rè mài chén ér xì zhě, míng yuē jìng, wéi nán zhì.

Greater yáng disease with heat effusion and a sunken and fine pulse is called tetany. It is difficult to treat.

SYNOPSIS, LINE 2.3

This line explains the prognosis of tetany indicated by the pulse condition.

COMMENTARY, LINE 2.3

Heat effusion in greater yáng disease indicates that the disease in the exterior. In such patterns, the pulse ought to be floating. If there is tetany, the pulse is likely to be sunken and slow or else stringlike and tight. If the pulse is sunken and fine, this means that yīn humor is depleted internally and that right qì is insufficient and thus incapable of fighting the disease effectively. In a situation of exuberant evil and right vacuity, the prognosis is not good, since attack and supplementation are both difficult. This applies not only to tetanic disease, but is also true of any other form of disease in the exterior.

Line 2.4

太阳病，发汗太多，因致痉。

Tài yáng bìng, fā hàn tài duō, yīn zhì jìng.

In greater yáng disease, excessive promotion of sweating [can] cause tetany.

SYNOPSIS, LINE 2.4

This line discusses tetany due to excessive promotion of sweating in greater yáng disease.

COMMENTARY, LINE 2.4

Greater yáng disease of the exterior is normally treated by promoting sweating. Cinnamon Twig Decoction (*guì zhī tāng*) is used to promote sweating and resolve the fleshy exterior. However, as we are told in line 12 of the chapter on "Greater Yáng Disease" in the *Shāng Hán Lùn*, the aim is to give the formula "until the whole body is moist, as if sweating very lightly. You cannot [allow the sweat] to flow like water." Under Ephedra Decoction (má huáng tāng), which opens the exterior and promotes sweating, we are also told to "cover [the patient with bedclothes] to obtain light sweating." Because sweat is derived from the fluids of the body, excessive sweating can cause damage to fluids. By depriving the sinews of nourishment, it causes them to contract, thereby giving rise to tetanic disease.

Line 2.5

夫风病下之则痉，复发汗必拘急。

Fū fēng bìng xià zhī zé jìng, fù fā hàn bì jū jí.

In wind disease, precipitation results in tetany. If you additionally promote sweating, you will invariably cause hypertonicity.

Synopsis, Line 2.5

This line discusses tetany due to inappropriate precipitation of wind disease.

Commentary, Line 2.5

The meaning of "wind disease" in this line has long been the subject of disagreement among scholars. One view, held by Wèi Lì-Tōng 魏荔彤, Cáo Jiā-Dá 槽家达, and others, is that it refers to externally contracted wind in greater yáng wind-strike. Another view, held by Huáng Yuán-Yù 黄元御, is that it refers to internal wind. When we consider this issue in the context of Zhāng Jī's thoughts on greater yáng wind-strike and wind-stroke in miscellaneous diseases, here the interpretation as external wind makes greater sense.

Wind disease is treated by coursing and dispersing. If you apply offensive precipitation, you will damage the fluids and thereby deprive the sinews of moisture, giving rise to possible tetany. If you promote sweating after precipitating, before the wind evil is resolved, you will damage the fluids yet further. Hypertonicity and contracture of the limbs is thus even more likely to arise.

Line 2.6

疮家虽身疼痛，不可发汗，汗出则痉。

Chuāng jiā suī shēn téng tòng, bù kě fā hàn, hàn chū zé jìng.

Even if patients who suffer from sores[1] experience generalized pain, you must not promote sweating; sweating will result in tetany.

Text Note, Line 2.6

[1]Patients who suffer from sores 疮家 *chuāng jiā*: Patients with a history of sores on the body, typically over an extended period. In a wider sense the term includes patients suffering from incised wounds.

SYNOPSIS, LINE 2.6

This line discusses tetany due to inappropriate promotion of sweating in patients with enduring sores or incised wounds.

COMMENTARY, LINE 2.6

When a person has had sores for a long time, the continual purulence will cause depletion of liquid and blood. A person with incised wounds may have lost blood and hence may suffer from yīn-blood vacuity. Because liquid and blood are of the same origin, damage to liquid affects the blood and damage to the blood affects liquid. Even if such patients have exterior signs like generalized pain, they should therefore not be given sweating treatment, since this might cause further damage to liquid and blood, thereby depriving the sinews of nourishment and giving rise to tetany.

After Zhāng Jī's time, tetanic disease in patients with wounds came to be called 破伤风 *pò shāng fēng*, that is, lock-jaw.

Line 2.7

病者，身热足寒，颈项强急，恶寒，时头热，面赤目赤，独头动摇，卒口噤，背反张者，痉病也。若发其汗者，寒湿相得，其表益虚，即恶寒甚，发其汗已，其脉如蛇。

Bìng zhě, shēn rè zú hán, jǐng xiàng jiàng jí, wù hán, shí tóu rè, miàn chì mù chì, dú tóu dòng yáo, cù kǒu jìn, bèi fǎn zhāng zhě, jìng bìng yě. Ruò fā qí hàn zhě, hán shī xiāng dé, qí biǎo yì xū, jí wù hán shèn, fā qí hàn yǐ, qí mài rú shé.

If a patient [presents with] generalized heat [effusion], cold in the lower extremities, rigid neck and nape, aversion to cold, a periodically hot head, red face, red eyes, shaking of the head only, sudden clenching of the jaw, and arched-back rigidity, this is tetany. If you promote sweating in such a patient, cold and dampness will exacerbate each other, so that the exterior will be even more vacuous. This means that the aversion to cold will be aggravated. After sweating, the pulse becomes snake-like.[1]

TEXT NOTE, LINE 2.7

1. "The pulse becomes snake-like" 脉如蛇 *mài rú shé*: According to most commentators, this expression is understood to describe a pulse that is bending and turning in agitation like a snake, instead of stretched out straight. Alternatively, it could refer to the amorphous quality of a pulse that is difficult to grasp.

SYNOPSIS, LINE 2.7

This line discusses the signs of tetanic disease, specifically the pulse and signs in patients where sweating has been promoted inappropriately.

COMMENTARY, LINE 2.7

The first sentence depicts the pathomechanism of externally contracted wind-cold entering the interior, transforming into heat, and giving rise to tetany. When wind-cold assails the outer body and invades the greater yáng exterior, defense qì and right qì engage in a struggle that gives rise to generalized heat effusion and aversion to cold. If the exterior evil transforms into heat and enters yáng brightness before the exterior has been resolved, evil heat will fume upward, giving rise to head heat and red face and eyes. At the same time, the evil causes yáng qì to become depressed and thereby prevents it from reaching the lower body, hence cold lower extremities (feet or feet and legs). Exuberant heat stirs wind and when wind begins to stir, there is shaking of the head. When exuberant heat scorches liquid, the sinews are deprived of nourishment, hence stiffness of the neck, sudden clenching of the jaw, and arched-back rigidity.

The latter part of the present line has been the subject of disagreement. One interpretation, held by Zhào Yǐ-Dé 赵以德, Xú Zhōng-Kě 徐忠可, and others is that it describes the pulse signs after inappropriate use of sweating. In their opinion, the symptoms described in the earlier part of the line are manifestations of exterior evil entering the interior, transforming into heat, damaging liquid, and stirring wind. These should be treated by clearing heat and engendering liquid, as well as resolving the exterior, thereby treating the exterior and interior simultaneously. Inappropriately resolving the exterior with warmth and acridity in such a situation will not only fail to eliminate the exterior evil, but by promoting sweating it will also give rise to exterior vacuity and thereby cause the dampness of sweat to contend with the exterior cold evil. This will make the aversion to cold even more severe. After sweating, right qì is left vacuous, but the evil is still not eliminated. As a result, the pulse meanders like a snake—deep, hidden, and inhibited.

A second interpretation, held by Wú Qiān 吴谦, Cǎo Yǐng-Fǔ 曹颖甫, and others, is that the latter part of the line does not belong with the first part. This interpretation is one that is well worth considering. The pattern described here is one of tetany that results from external wind entering the interior and transforming into heat. It is likely to be related to a pre-existing surfeit of yáng or insufficiency of fluids. However, it is not entirely clear why inappropriate promotion of sweating with warmth and acridity should not have caused damage to yáng through excessive sweating rather than damage to liquid. Supporting this interpretation is the phrase "[so that] the exterior [will be] even more vacuous." This suggests that initially there had been exterior vacuity, a fact that would be hard to reconcile with the pathomechanism described in the first half of the line.

Line 2.8

暴腹胀大者，为欲解。脉如故，反伏弦者痉。

Bào fù zhàng dà zhě, wéi yù jiě. Mài rú gù，fǎn fú xián zhě jìng.

Fulminant distention and enlargement of the abdomen means that [the disease] is about to resolve. If the pulse remains as before or turns hidden and stringlike, this means tetany.

SYNOPSIS, LINE 2.8

This line describes the prognosis of tetanic disease by pulse and signs.

COMMENTARY, LINE 2.8

This line gives two outcomes for tetanic disease. "Fulminant distention and enlargement of the abdomen means [that the disease] is about to resolve" is a very much disputed part of the line. The pathomechanism of fulminant distention and enlargement of the abdomen is not clear, but these symptoms could possibly indicate that the evil is about to exit from the inside. It is thus a positive sign that the patient is about to recover. The phrase "The pulse remains as before" alludes to the pulse that is normally observed in tetany, i.e., as stated in the following line 2.9, "when pressed, tight like a string." If the pulse is tight like a string, this means that the tension in the sinews has not begun to abate. If instead the pulse is sunken, hidden, and stringlike, this means that the evil qì has penetrated deeply into the body and that the disease is continuing to advance, so that tetany can be expected to occur.

Line 2.9

夫痓脉，按之紧如弦，直上下行。[1]

Fū jìng mài, àn zhī jǐn rú xiān, zhí shàng xià xíng.

The pulse of tetany, when pressed, is tight like a string [2] from top to bottom.[3]

TEXT NOTES, LINE 2.9

[1] Another version of this text has "pounding and stringlike" (筑筑而弦 *zhù zhù ér xián*). The *Mài Jīng* ("The Pulse Canon") states: "People suffering from tetany have a pulse that is hidden and hard from top to bottom" (痓家其脉伏坚，直上下 *jìng jiā qí mài fú jiān, zhí shàng xià*).

[2] Tight like a string 紧如弦 *jǐn rú xián*: The *Jīn Guì Yù Hán Jīng* ("The Canon of the Golden Cabinet and Jade Sheath") and the *Mài Jīng* both have 紧而弦 *jǐn ér xián*, tight and stringlike. The characters 如 *rú* and 而 *ér* were commonly interchanged in ancient Chinese.

[3] From top to bottom 上下行 *shàng xià xíng*: From the inch position (寸部 *cùn bù*) to the cubit position (尺部 *chǐ bù*).

SYNOPSIS, LINE 2.9

This line describes the most commonly seen pulse of tetany.

COMMENTARY, LINE 2.9

Tetanic disease is caused by tension in the sinews. A stiff, straight pulse from the inch to the cubit corresponds to this and is therefore the most common pulse found in patients with tetany.

Line 2.10

痉病有灸疮，难治。

Jìng bìng yǒu jiǔ chuāng, nán zhì.

Tetanic disease with moxibustion sores[1] is difficult to treat.

TEXT NOTE, LINE 2.10

[1] Moxibustion sores 灸疮 *jiǔ chuāng*: Sores caused by burns the skin resulting from moxibustion.

SYNOPSIS, LINE 2.10

This line describes the prognosis of tetanic disease.

COMMENTARY, LINE 2.10

Moxibustion sores are burns on the skin from the application of moxibustion that turn into open, purulent sores. Purulent moxibustion sores cause damage to liquid and blood, which is a principal cause of tetanic disease. Hence if both conditions are affecting the patient simultaneously, the condition will be more serious than normal.

There has been disagreement among scholars as to whether the line implies that tetanic disease or moxibustion sores appear first. Some scholars, such as Yóu Zài-Jīng 尤在泾 and Zhāng Xū-Gǔ 章虚谷 believe that the sores come first. Others, notably Zhào Yǐ-Dé 赵以德, believe that the tetany comes first and is then complicated by moxibustion sores. The latter interpretation would imply that moxibustion is contraindicated in tetany. However, clinical practice suggests that unless there is extreme yīn depletion, it is not necessary to avoid the use of moxibustion. In view of this, the general opinion nowadays is that the line describes a preexisting condition of moxibustion sores that is complicated by subsequent tetany.

Line 2.11

太阳病，其证备，身体强，几几然脉反沉迟，此为痓。栝蒌桂枝汤主之。

栝蒌根二两，桂枝三两，芍药三两，甘草二两，生姜三两，大枣十二枚

右六味，以水九升，煮取三升，分温三服，取微汗。汗不出，食顷啜热粥发之。

Tài yáng bìng, qí zhèng bèi, shēn tǐ jiàng, shū shū rán mài fǎn chén chí, cǐ wéi jìng. Guā lóu guì zhī tāng zhǔ zhī.

Guā lóu gēn èr liǎng; guì zhī sān liǎng; sháo yào sān liǎng; gān cǎo èr liǎng; shēng jiāng sān liǎng; dà zǎo shí èr méi

Yòu liù wèi, yǐ shuǐ jiǔ shēng, zhǔ qǔ sān shēng, fēn wēn sān fú, qǔ wēi hàn. Hàn bù chū, shí qīng chuò rè zhōu fā zhī.

In greater yáng disease, if all signs are present and [in addition] the body is rigid and stretched[1] but the pulse is sunken and slow, this is tetany. Trichosanthes and Cinnamon Twig Decoction (栝楼桂枝汤 *guā lóu guì zhī tāng*) governs.[2]

Trichosanthes and Cinnamon Twig Decoction (栝楼桂枝汤 *guā lóu guì zhī tāng*)

- trichosanthes (栝楼 *guā lóu*, Trichosanthis Fructus) 2 *liǎng*
- cinnamon twig (桂枝 *guì zhī*, Cinnamomi Ramulus) 3 *liǎng*
- peony (芍药 *sháo yào*, Paeoniae Radix) 3 *liǎng*
- licorice (甘草 *gān cǎo*, Glycyrrhizae Radix) 2 *liǎng*
- fresh ginger (生姜 *shēng jiāng*, Zingiberis Rhizoma Recens) 3 *liǎng*
- jujube (大枣 *dà zǎo*, Jujubae Fructus) 12 pieces

Boil the above six ingredients in nine *shēng* of water to get three *shēng*. Divide into three doses and take warm to produce slight sweating. If the patient does not sweat, after a little while make them sip hot gruel to promote [sweating].

Text Notes, Line 2.11

[1] Stretched 几几然 *shū shū rán*: Stretched like the neck of a small bird trying in vain to fly.

[2] Govern 主之 *zhǔ zhī*: A decoction is said to "govern" a particular condition for which it is the main treatment.

Synopsis, Line 2.11

This line discusses the signs and treatment of soft tetany.

Commentary, Line 2.11

The text describes a condition where all the signs required to diagnose a patient as having greater yáng disease are present, and the body in addition is stiff and stretched. In other words, the patient has heat effusion, sweating, aversion to cold with headache and stiffness of the nape. In greater yáng disease with sweating and aversion to cold, the pulse is normally floating and moderate. In the present condition, however, it is sunken and slow, attesting to insufficiency of the fluids, which is preventing the sinews from being nourished adequately. A sunken pulse means that the disease evil is not only affecting the greater yáng exterior, but is also obstructing the sinews. A slow pulse indicates damage to liquid and inhibited movement of construction and defense. Since the condition is one of tetany with tension in the sinews, we can presume that the pulse would be not only sunken and slow, but also stringlike and tight—the typical pulse of tetanic disease. In sum, therefore, the condition is one of external evil obstructing the greater yáng sinews and insufficiency of the fluids depriving the sinews of moisture. The treatment is Trichosanthes and Cinnamon Twig Decoction (*guā lóu guì zhī tāng*), because it resolves the flesh, dispels the evil, engenders liquid, and enriches humor.

Line 2.12

太阳病，无汗，而小便反少，气上冲胸，口噤不得语，欲作刚痉，葛根汤主之。

葛根四两　麻黄（去节）三两　桂枝（去皮）二两　芍药二两　甘草（炙）二两 生姜三两　大枣十二枚

右七味, 㕮咀, 以水一斗, 先煮麻黄葛根减二升, 去沫, 内诸药, 煮取三升, 去滓, 温服一升, 覆取微似汗, 不须啜粥。余如桂枝汤法将息及禁忌。

Tài yáng bìng, wú hàn, ér xiǎo biàn fǎn shǎo, qì shàng chōng xiōng, kǒu jìn bù dé yǔ, yù zuò gāng jìng, gé gēn tāng zhǔ zhī.

Gé gēn sì liǎng; má huáng (qù jié) sān liǎng; guì zhī (qù pí) èr liǎng; sháo yào èr liǎng; gān cǎo (zhì) èr liǎng; shēng jiāng sān liǎng; dà zǎo shí èr méi

Yòu qī wèi, fǔ jǔ, yǐ shuǐ yī dǒu, xiān zhǔ má huáng gé gēn jiǎn èr shēng, qù mò, nà zhū yào, zhǔ qǔ sān shēng, qù zǐ, wēn fú yī shēng, fù qǔ wēi sì hàn, bù xū chuò zhōu. Yú rú guì zhī tāng fǎ jiāng xī jí jìn jì.

In greater yáng disease, if you see no sweating but scant urine, qì surging up into the chest, and a clenched jaw preventing speech, hard tetany is about to occur. Pueraria Decoction (*gé gēn tāng*) governs.

Pueraria Decoction
(葛根汤 *gé gēn tāng*)

- pueraria (葛根 *gé gēn*, Puerariae Radix) 4 *liǎng*
- ephedra (麻黄 *má huáng*, Ephedrae Herba) 3 *liang* (remove nodes)
- cinnamon twig (桂枝 *guì zhī*, Cinnamomi Ramulus) 2 *liǎng* (remove skin)
- peony (芍药 *sháo yào*, Paeoniae Radix) 2 *liǎng*
- licorice (甘草 *gān cǎo*, Glycyrrhizae Radix) 2 *liǎng* (mix-fry)
- fresh ginger (生姜 *shēng jiāng*, Zingiberis Rhizoma Recens) 3 *liǎng*
- jujube (大枣 *dà zǎo*, Jujubae Fructus) 12 pieces

Chew[1] the above seven ingredients. Then first boil the ephedra (*má huáng*) and pueraria (*gé gēn*) in one *dǒu* of water to get two *shēng*. Remove the foam. Add all [the other] agents and boil to get three *shēng*. Remove the dregs and take one *shēng* [per dose] warm. Cover [the patient with bedclothes] to obtain slight sweating. It is not necessary to sip gruel. Follow the rules for *guì zhī tāng* (Cinnamon Twig Decoction) regarding rest and contraindications.

TEXT NOTE, LINE 2.12

1. Chew 㕮咀 *fǔ jǔ*: In ancient times, the person preparing medicines would chew certain medicinals in preparation for boiling. In later times, this term was redefined. In the *Qiān Jīn Fāng* ("Thousand Gold Pieces Prescriptions"), it is defined in the first volume, section 7 on "Compounding Medicinals" as follows: "When the old formularies say "chew," it means that after weighing, you pound them [into a size] like soybeans. Then you blow to remove the fine powder." In more modern times, medicinal materials are cut and crushed rather than chewed.

SYNOPSIS, LINE 2.12

This line discusses the signs and treatment of impending hard tetany.

COMMENTARY, LINE 2.12

Greater yáng disease without sweating constitutes exterior repletion. It arises when cold fetters the fleshy exterior and blocks defense qì. Generally speaking, sweating causes a decrease in urine, while an absence of sweating causes an increase in urine. In the present condition, and contrary to expectation, absence of sweating is accompanied by scant urine. This reflects damage to fluids in the interior. Because of absence of sweating, the evil cannot reach the outer body; owing to scant urine it cannot descend. Instead, the evil surges upward into the chest. The clenched jaw preventing speech is a sign that the evil is starting to affect yáng brightness. If the disease advances, there will be arched-back rigidity and rigidity of the limbs; hence the text says "hard tetany is about to occur."

The present condition is caused by external evil obstructing greater yáng and yáng brightness and inhibiting the qì dynamic of construction-defense and the triple burner. Accordingly, the treatment is to promote sweating and dispel the evil, to harmonize construction and defense, and to upbear liquid and soothe the sinews. The formula that performs these actions is Pueraria Decoction (*gé gēn tāng*).

Pueraria (*gé gēn*) upbears liquid and soothes the sinews. Thus it is the chief medicinal of the formula. It is assisted by ephedra (*má huáng*), which opens the interstices. Cinnamon twig (*guì zhī*), peony (*sháo yào*), fresh ginger (*shēng jiāng*), and jujube (*dà zǎo*) harmonize construction and defense, while mix-fried licorice (*zhì gān cǎo*) helps peony (*sháo yào*) to relieve the tension of the sinews. The formula as a whole upbears liquid and effuses the exterior, while at the same time soothing the sinews and relieving tension.

Line 2.13

痉为病，胸满，口噤，卧不着席，脚挛急，必齘齿，可与大承气汤。

大黄（酒洗）四两　厚朴（炙，去皮）半斤　枳实（炙）五枚　芒硝三合

右四味，以水一斗，先煮二物取五升，去滓；内大黄煮取二升，去滓；内芒硝，更上火微一二沸，分温再服，得下止服。

Jìng wéi bìng, xiōng mǎn kǒu jìn, wò bù zhuó xí, jiǎo luán jí, bì xiè chǐ, kě yǔ dà chéng qì tāng.

Dà huáng (jiǔ xǐ) sì liǎng; hòu pò (jiǔ, qù pí) bàn jīn; zhǐ shí (zhì) wǔ méi; máng xiāo sān gě.

Yòu sì wèi, yǐ shuǐ yī dǒu, xiān zhǔ èr wù qǔ wǔ shēng, qù zǐ; nà dà huáng zhǔ qǔ èr shēng, qù zǐ; nà máng xiāo, gèng shàng huǒ wēi yī èr fèi, fēn wēn zài fú, dé xià zhǐ fú.

When tetany[1] is the disease and there is fullness in the chest, clenched jaw, lying without [the back] touching the mat,[2] and hypertonicity of the legs, there will be grinding of the teeth.[3] [In such cases,] you may give Major Qì-Coordinating Decoction (大承气汤 *dà chéng qì tāng*).

Major Qì-Coordinating Decoction (大承气汤 *dà chéng qì tāng*)
rhubarb (大黄 *dà huáng*, Rhei Radix et Rhizoma) 4 *liǎng* (rinse in wine)
officinal magnolia bark (厚朴 *hòu pò*, Magnoliae Officinalis Cortex) ½ *jīn* (mix-fry, remove skin)
unripe bitter orange (枳实 *zhǐ shí*, Aurantii Fructus Immaturus) 5 fruits (mix-fry)
mirabilite (芒硝 *máng xiāo*, Natrii Sulfas) 3 *gě*

Of the four above ingredients, boil the first two (officinal magnolia bark and unripe bitter orange in one *dǒu* of water to get five *shēng*. Remove the dregs, add the rhubarb and boil to get 2 *shēng*. Now add the mirabilite, return to the flame, and bring to a slight boil once or twice more. Remove the dregs. Divide into two doses and take warm. Stop taking [the formula] on defecation.

Text Notes, Line 2.13

[1] One variation of the text has "hard" before "tetany."

[2] Lying without [the back] touching the mat 卧不着席 *wò bù zháo xí*: The back does not touch the bed because it is in a state of arched rigidity.

[3] Grinding of the teeth 齘齿 *jiè chǐ*: Noisy grinding of the teeth due to severe clenched jaw.

Synopsis, Line 2.13

This line discusses the signs and treatment of interior heat giving rise to tetany.

Commentary, Line 2.13

This lines describes tetany that is caused by disease evil entering yáng brightness. An exterior pattern resolves when opening and discharge occurs, i.e., when the patient can sweat out the evil. If this fails to happen, the disease evil passes into yáng brightness in the interior. When exuberant yáng brightness heat scorches the sinews, tetany can arise. This is the situation described in the present line of the text.

The fullness in the chest is the result of exuberant heat causing congestion. The clenched jaw, arched-back rigidity (lying without the back touching the mat), hypertonicity of the legs, and grinding of the teeth are all signs of severe tetany.

The treatment involves freeing the bowels and discharging heat, combined with emergency precipitation to preserve yīn. These actions are performed by Major Qì-Coordinating Decoction (*dà chéng qì tāng*).

Line 2.14

太阳病，关节疼痛而烦，脉沉而细者，此名湿痹。湿痹之候，小便不利，大便反快，但当利其小便。

Tài yáng bìng, guān jié téng tòng ér fán, mài chén ér xì zhě, cǐ míng shī bì. Shī bì zhī hòu, xiǎo biàn bù lì, dà biàn fǎn kuài, dàn dāng lì qí xiǎo biàn.

In greater yáng disease, if there is vexing pain in the joints and a sunken and fine[1] pulse, this is called damp impediment. The sign of damp impediment is inhibited urination but free stool. [In such cases], disinhibit urine only.

Text Note, Line 2.14

1. Fine 細 *xì*: A textual variant has 緩 *huǎn*, "moderate" instead.

Synopsis, Line 2.14

This line discusses the signs and treatment principles of damp impediment.

Commentary, Line 2.14

Dampness is one of the six excesses. Thus like wind and cold it strikes greater yáng first. However, while wind and cold mostly damage the interstices, dampness easily flows into the joints. When dampness gets into the joints and obstructs the movement of yáng qì, there is pain and vexation. This condition is called damp impediment. Because the exterior is affected, the pulse is floating. Because the evil is dampness, the pulse is also moderate. Dampness affects the movement of construction and defense, so the pulse is also fine. In the present condition, the pulse is sunken, indicating that the interior is also affected by dampness. Interior dampness is usually attributable to dampness arising internally, which is mutually conducive with externally contracted dampness. The presence of internal dampness in the present condition is supported by the fact that the urine is inhibited but the stool is free. When dampness obstructs the center, it can cause impairment of qì transformation, which manifests in inhibited urination. It can also cause impairment of movement and transformation that manifests in "soggy diarrhea" (濡泻 *rú xiè*); hence the free stool.

The condition described in this line is treated by disinhibiting urine. Once the urine is disinhibited, the interior dampness will disappear and yáng qì will be freed. Consequently, the damp impediment will also be eliminated. The line mentions no formula, but most commentators recommend Poria Five Powder (*wǔ líng sǎn*) with double the amount of cinnamon twig (*guì zhī*).

Line 2.15

湿家之为病，一身尽疼，发热身色如熏黄也。

Shī jiā zhī wéi bìng, yī shēn jìn téng, fā rè shēn sè rú xūn huáng yě.

Dampness patients suffer from generalized pain throughout the whole body,[1] heat effusion, and a smoky yellow[2] complexion of the body.

Text Notes, Line 2.15

[1] A textual variant has "vexing pain."

[2] Smoky yellow 熏黄 *xūn huáng*: A dark yellow, like the yellowish black color of soot produced when burning wood or incense.

Synopsis, Line 2.15

This line discusses yellowing due to damp stagnation.

Commentary, Line 2.15

When dampness evil is contracted, the qì of the fleshy exterior fails to diffuse. This gives rise to qì stagnation and hence generalized pain. Dampness is a yīn evil and does not normally give rise to heat effusion. But heat effusion may occur when dampness is depressed in the qì aspect for a long time and consequently transforms into heat. A smoky yellow complexion reflects the presence of both dampness and heat, with dampness being more severe than the heat.

Line 2.16

湿家, 其人但头汗出, 背强欲得被覆向火, 若下之早则哕, 或胸满小便不利, 舌上如胎者, 以丹田有热, 胸中有寒, 渴欲得饮而不能饮, 则口燥烦也。

Shī jiā, qí rén dàn tóu hàn chū, bèi jiàng yù dé bèi fù xiàng huǒ, ruò xià zhī zǎo zé yuē, huò xiōng mǎn xiǎo biàn bù lì, shé shàng rú tāi zhě, yǐ dān tián yǒu rè, xiōng zhōng yǒu hán, kě yù dé yǐn ér bù néng yǐn, zé kǒu zào fán yě.

Dampness patients sweat only from the head, suffer from rigidity of the back, and desire to be covered with bedclothes and face the fire.[1] If precipitation is performed early, the result is hiccup or fullness in the chest with inhibited urination, and a tongue that resembles [one that has] fur. This is because there is heat in the cinnabar field[2] and cold on the chest. If there is thirst with a desire for water, but inability to drink, the result is vexing dryness of the mouth.[3]

Text Notes, Line 2.16

[1] Desire to be covered with bedcovers and face the fire 欲得被覆向火 *yù dé bèi fù xiàng huǒ*: Signs of aversion to cold.

[2] Cinnabar field 丹田 *dān tián*: A key location for vital physiological processes in the body in the lower abdomen. The term is also the name of an acupuncture point located below the umbilicus. Here, the term refers to the lower burner in its polarity with the chest.

[3] Vexing dryness of the mouth 口燥烦 *kǒu zào fán*: "Vexing" emphasizes the severity of "dryness." Vexing dryness of the mouth is understood to mean severe dryness and thirst with no desire to drink attributable to heat in the lower burner and dampness causing internal obstruction.

Synopsis, Line 2.16

This line discusses a transmuted pattern arising from inappropriate precipitation of damp disease.

Commentary, Line 2.16

When externally contracted cold-damp causes blockage of the interstices, yáng qì fails to reach the outer body and instead ascends counterflow, giving rise to sweating only from the head. When dampness encumbers the channels, there is stiffness in the back. When dampness obstructs yáng qì, the patient experiences aversion to cold and therefore desires to cover up well with bedclothes and get close to a source of heat. This condition is treated by warming the channels, dispersing dampness, and diffusing yáng qì.

If you inappropriately treat with offensive precipitation, you will not only have difficulty removing the disease evil, but you will furthermore damage yáng qì, giving rise to transmuted patterns. Offensive precipitation with cold and bitterness will damage center yáng and cause vacuity counterflow of stomach qì, which manifests in hiccup. When cold-damp stagnates in the upper burner, lung diffusion and depuration are impaired and the waterways are no longer properly regulated, so that the patient experiences fullness and oppression in the chest and inhibited urination. When depressed heat in the lower burner steams the cold-damp in the upper burner, the tongue surface will be damp, moist, white, and glossy, resembling a tongue coating, but not being a genuine tongue coating. This is attributable to cold in the upper burner and abnormal distribution of water and liquid, not to insufficiency of the fluids. Hence the patient experiences thirst but inability to swallow fluids.

Line 2.17

湿家，下之，额上汗出，微喘，小便利者死；若下利不止者，亦死。

Shī jiā, xià zhī, é shàng hàn chū, wēi chuǎn, xiǎo biàn lì zhě sǐ; ruò xià lì bù zhǐ zhě, yì sǐ.

When dampness patients manifest with sweating on the forehead, slight panting, and uninhibited urination[1] following precipitation treatment, they will die. If there is incessant diarrhea, they will also die.

TEXT NOTE, LINE 2.17

[1] Uninhibited urination 小便利 *xiǎo biàn lì*: Frequent long clear voidings of urine.

SYNOPSIS, LINE 2.17

This line describes critical signs occurring after inappropriate precipitation of damp disease.

COMMENTARY, LINE 2.17

This line describes an aggravated pattern resulting from inappropriate precipitation in dampness disease. Dampness is a yīn evil and can therefore easily damage yáng qì. If you treat this inappropriately with precipitation, you will damage interior yáng. Thus you create the situation of yīn exuberance and yáng vacuity. When vacuous yáng strays upward, there is sweating from the forehead and slight panting. When yīn cold is exuberant in the inner body, urination is uninhibited. This condition forms a critical pattern of yáng qì straying upward and yīn qì deserting downward, hence the text concludes that the patient will die. If after inappropriate precipitation the patient suffers from incessant diarrhea, this will deplete the fluids and prevent true yáng from keeping its composure. Thus uninhibited urination and incessant diarrhea entail similar pathomechanisms that lead to dual depletion of yīn and yáng, a critical condition that results in death.

Line 2.18

风湿相搏，一身尽疼痛，法当汗出而解，值天阴雨不止，医云：此可发汗。汗之病不愈者，何也？盖发其汗，汗大出者，但风气去，湿气在，是故不愈也。若治风湿者，发其汗，但微微似欲出汗者，风湿俱去也。

Fēng shī xiāng bó, yī shēn jìn téng tòng, fǎ dāng hàn chū ér jiě, zhí tiān yīn yǔ bù zhǐ, yī yún: Cǐ kě fā hàn. Hàn zhī bìng bù yú zhě, hé yě? Gài fā qí hàn, hàn dà chū zhě, dàn fēng qì qù, shī qì zài, shì gù bù yù yě. Ruò zhì fēng shī zhě, fā qí hàn, dàn wēi wēi sì yù chū hàn zhě, fēng shī jù qù yě.

Wind and dampness contending with each other [manifests in] generalized pain. The [treatment] method is to promote sweating and thus bring about resolution. If by chance there is incessant rainy, yīn weather, physicians say that this can be treated by promoting sweating. But if after promotion of sweating the patient does not recover, why [is this so]? In such cases, if promotion of sweating results in great sweating, only wind qì leaves while damp qì is still present. This is why [the patient] does not recover. If you treat wind-damp in such a way that you promote sweating only very slightly, to the point where the patient appears about to sweat, wind and dampness will both leave.

SYNOPSIS, LINE 2.18

This line explains the main points for using promotion of sweating in the treatment of wind-damp in the exterior.

COMMENTARY, LINE 2.18

When wind and dampness evils engage with each other, enter the fleshy exterior, and lodge in the sinews, bones, joints, skin, and flesh of the whole body, obstructing yáng qì, there will be generalized pain. This means wind-damp in the exterior. It should be treated by promoting sweating, so that the evil is resolved by perspiration. If a spell of of damp, rainy yīn-type weather occurs at the same time as the illness, it will exacerbate the external dampness and make the pain more severe. In such a case there is all the more need to promote sweating to cause the damp qì to evaporate. Yet if treatment is given to promote sweating and recovery does not ensue, this means that the treatment was not quite right.

Wind is a yáng evil and by nature light and buoyant, so it is easily dispersed. By contrast, dampness is a yīn evil and by nature clammy and stagnant, so it is difficult to remove. In the condition described in this line, sweating treatment caused great sweating. This successfully removed the wind, but not the dampness. Consequently not only did the patient not recover, but defensive yáng was damaged. In such a situation, we have to consider the specific nature of wind in combination with dampness. The treatment should aim to cause slight sweating, so that construction and defense are freed and the wind and dampness will be removed together. This is the key to the successful use of sweating in the treatment of externally contracted wind-damp.

Line 2.19

湿家病，身疼发热，面黄而喘，头痛鼻塞而烦，其脉大，自能饮食，腹中和无病，病在头中寒湿，故鼻塞，内药鼻中则愈。

Shī jiā bìng, shēn téng fā rè, miàn huáng ér chuǎn, tóu tòng bí sè ér fán, qí mài dà, zì néng yǐn shí, fù zhōng hé wú bìng, bìng zài tóu zhōng hán shī, gù bí sè, nà yào bí zhōng zé yù.

When dampness patients [present with] generalized pain, heat effusion, yellow face, panting, headache, nasal congestion and vexation, a large pulse, ability to eat and drink naturally, and harmony in the abdomen without disease, [this indicates that] the disease is cold-damp in the head; hence the nasal congestion. Insert medicine into the nose, and the patient will recover.

Synopsis, Line 2.19

This line describes the signs and treatment of cold damp damaging the head.

Commentary, Line 2.19

The condition described in this line is cold-damp affecting mainly the fleshy exterior and the upper body. When a patient contracts external cold-damp and the dampness evil stagnates in the flesh, sinew, and bone, there will be generalized pain. When cold fetters the exterior and causes yáng qì to become depressed, there is heat effusion. When dampness becomes depressed, this causes a yellow face. When cold-damp blocks the interstices and impairs lung qì diffusion, there is panting. When there is cold-damp in the upper body, clear yáng cannot bear upward. This results in nasal congestion and headache. In the condition described in this line, the stomach and intestines are well regulated and the interior is in harmony and unaffected by disease. Hence the pulse is large, and eating and drinking are normal. The emphasis in the line is on dampness in the upper body, since we are specifically told that "the disease is cold-damp in the head; hence the nasal congestion." The treatment suggested for this is to introduce medicinals into the nose. Acrid and fragrant medicines inserted in the nose have the effect of diffusing cold-damp, disinhibiting lung qì, and enabling clear yáng to reach upward, so that all the symptoms will be eliminated.

Line 2.20

湿家身烦疼，可与麻黄加朮汤发其汗为宜，慎不可以火攻之。

麻黄（去节）三两　桂枝（去皮）二两　甘草（炙）一两　杏仁（去皮尖）七十个　白朮四两

右五味，以水九升先煮麻黄，减二升，去上沫，内诸药煮取二升半，去滓，温服八合，覆取微似汗。

Shī jiā shēn fán téng, kě yǔ má huáng jiā zhú tāng fā qí hàn wéi yí, shèn bù kě yǐ huǒ gōng zhī.

Má huáng (qù jié) sān liǎng; guì zhī (qù pí) èr liǎng; gān cǎo (zhì) yī liǎng; xìng rén (qù pí jiān) qī shí ge; bái zhú sì liǎng

Yòu wǔ wèi, yǐ shuǐ jiǔ shēng xiān zhǔ má huáng, jiǎn èr shēng, qù shàng mò, nà zhū yào zhǔ qǔ èr shēng bàn, qù zǐ, wēn fú bā gě, fù qǔ wēi sì hàn.

When dampness patients [present with] generalized vexing pain,[1] you may give Ephedra Decoction Plus White Atractylodes (麻黄加朮汤 *má huáng jiā zhú tāng*) to promote sweating. Be careful not to attack with fire.[2]

Ephedra Decoction Plus White Atractylodes (麻黄加朮汤 *má huáng jiā zhú tāng*)

ephedra (麻黄 *má huáng*, Ephedrae Herba) 3 *liǎng* (remove nodes)

cinnamon twig (桂枝 *guì zhī*, Cinnamomi Ramulus) 2 *liǎng* (remove bark)

licorice (甘草 *gān cǎo*, Glycyrrhizae Radix) 1 *liǎng* (mix-fry)

apricot kernel (杏仁 *xìng rén*, Armeniacae Semen) 70 kernels (remove skin and tips)

white atractylodes (白朮 *bái zhú*, Atractylodis Macrocephalae Rhizoma) 4 ½ *liǎng*

Of the above five ingredients, first boil the ephedra (*má huáng*) in nine *shēng* of water and reduce to two *shēng*. Remove the foam from on top. Add all [other] medicines and boil down to two-and-a-half *shēng*. Remove the dregs and take eight *gě* [per dose] warm. Cover [the patient with bedclothes] to induce slight sweating.

Text Notes, Line 2.20

[1] Generalized vexing pain 身烦疼 *shēn fán téng*: Severe pain that makes the patient feel restless and frustrated.

[2] Attack with fire 火攻 *huǒ gōng*: Treat by fire methods, i.e., fumigation, hot pack, moxibustion, or warm needling.

Synopsis, Line 2.20

This line describes the signs, treatment, and contraindications of cold-damp in the exterior, which is an exterior repletion pattern.

Commentary, Line 2.20

When cold depresses the interstices and dampness stagnates in the sinews and bones, exterior yáng is obstructed and the movement of construction and defense is inhibited. This results in generalized pain. The use of Ephedra Decoction Plus White Atractylodes (*má huáng jiā zhú tāng*) here implies that dampness is complicated by wind-cold, which manifests in heat effusion, aversion to cold, and absence of sweating. While we generally treat wind-cold by promoting sweating, the presence of dampness evil counsels again excessive sweating. White atractylodes (*bái zhú*) combined with Ephedra Decoction (*má huáng tāng*) prevents the ephedra combination from causing excessive sweating and eliminates dampness in the exterior as well as in the interior. If you apply fire treatment (hot needling, fumigation, etc.), you will induce great sweating. You will thereby eliminate wind, but the dampness will remain.

Line 2.21

病者一身尽疼，发热，日晡所剧者, 名风湿。此病伤于汗出当风, 或久伤取冷所致也。可与麻黄杏仁薏苡甘草汤。

麻黄（去节，汤泡）半两　甘草（炙）一两　薏苡仁半两　杏仁（去皮尖，炒）十个

右剉麻豆大, 每服四钱匕, 水一盏半, 煮八分, 去滓, 温服, 有微汗, 避风。

Bìng zhě yī shēn jìn téng, fā rè, rì bū suǒ jù zhě, míng fēng shī. Cǐ bìng shāng yú hàn chū dāng fēng, huò jiǔ shāng qǔ lěng suǒ zhì yě. Kě yǔ má huáng xìng rén yì yǐ gān cǎo tāng.

Má huáng (qù jié, tāng pào) bàn liǎng; gān cǎo (zhì) yī liǎng; yì yǐ rén bàn liǎng; xìng rén (qù pí jiān, chǎo) shí gè

Yòu cuò má dòu dà, měi fú sì qián bǐ, shuǐ yī zhǎn bàn, zhǔ bā fēn, qù zǐ, wēn fú, yǒu wēi hàn, bì fēng.

When a patient [manifests with] pain throughout the whole body and heat effusion that becomes more severe in the late afternoon,[1] this is called wind-damp. This disease is [caused by] damage from exposure to wind during sweating, or by enduring damage from consumption of cold substances. You may give Ephedra, Apricot Kernel, Coix, and Licorice Decoction (麻黄杏仁薏苡甘草汤 *má huáng xìng rén yì yǐ gān cǎo tāng*).

Ephedra, Apricot Kernel, Coix, and Licorice Decoction (麻黄杏仁薏苡甘草汤 *má huáng xìng rén yì yǐ gān cǎo tāng*)

- ephedra (麻黄 *má huáng*, Ephedrae Herba) ½ *liǎng* (remove nodes and soak in hot water)
- licorice (甘草 *gān cǎo*, Glycyrrhizae Radix) 1 *liǎng* (mix-fry)
- coix (薏苡仁 *yì yǐ rén*, Coicis Semen) ½ *liǎng*
- apricot kernel (杏仁 *xìng rén*, Armeniacae Semen) 10 pieces (remove skin and tips and stir-fry)

Grate the above four ingredients to the size of hemp seeds (*má dòu*). For each dose, add four qián-spoonfuls[2] [of the mixed grated medicinals] to one-and-a-half cups of water and boil this [down to] eight tenths. Remove the dregs. Take warm and induce slight sweating. Avoid wind.

Text Notes, Line 2.21

[1] Late afternoon 日晡所 *rì bū suǒ*: 3–5 PM.

[2] *Qián*-spoonful 钱匕 *qián bǐ*: See Weights and Measures in the Introduction.

Synopsis, Line 2.21

This line describes the causes, signs, and treatment of wind-damp in the exterior.

Commentary, Line 2.21

When cold depresses the interstices, dampness stagnates in the sinews and bones, exterior yáng is obstructed, and the movement of construction and defense is inhibited. This results in generalized pain.

The reason for heat effusion becoming more severe in late afternoon has been explained by scholars in different ways. The most widely held view nowadays is that although dampness is a yīn evil, when it combines with the yáng evil wind, it tends to transform into heat and dryness. Since yáng brightness represents "dryness-earth" and late afternoon is the time when yáng brightness is most effulgent, the tendency toward heat and dryness is most pronounced at that time. An alternative explanation is that because the evil is in the skin and body hair, which are associated with the lung, and because lung-metal is associated with late afternoon, the activity of the evil is greatest at that time. Yet another is that because the disease is due to wind-damp and late afternoon is associated with greater yīn dampness-earth, the dampness is exacerbated at this time. All of the explanations given relate to the waxing and waning of evil and right throughout the day.

A characteristic of wind-damp is that is it often caused by sweating on exposure to wind or by habitual excessive consumption of cold foods and drinks. When there is wind-damp in the exterior, the aim of the treatment is to obtain resolution through slight sweating. In this line, we give Ephedra, Apricot Kernel, Coix, and Licorice Decoction (*má huáng xìng rén yì yǐ gān cǎo tāng*) to resolve the exterior and dispel dampness.

In the formula, ephedra (*má huáng*) promotes sweating and thereby resolves the exterior and disperses the wind-damp in the fleshy exterior. Apricot kernel (*xìng rén*) diffuses lung qì and therefore assists ephedra (*má huáng*) in its functions. Coix (*yì yǐ rén*) is sweet and bland in flavor and disinhibits dampness. Being slightly cold in nature, it counteracts the warm nature of ephedra (*má huáng*) and hence prevents the evil from transforming into heat and dryness. Licorice (*gān cǎo*) harmonizes the center. All of the ingredients together have a clear, light diffusing and transforming (轻清宣化 *qīng qīng xuān huà*) action that causes the wind-damp to resolve through slight sweating.

Line 2.22

风湿，脉浮，身重，汗出恶风者，防己黄芪汤主之。

防己一两　甘草(炒)半两　白朮七钱半　黄芪(去芦)一两一分

右剉麻豆大，每抄五钱匕，生姜四片，大枣一枚，水盏半，煎八分，去滓温服，良久再服。喘者加麻黄半两。胃中不和者加芍药三分，气上冲者加桂枝三分，下有陈寒者加细辛三分，服后当如虫行皮中，从腰下如冰，后坐被上，又以一被绕腰以下，温令微汗，差。

Fēng shī, mài fú, shēn zhòng, hàn chū wù fēng zhě, fáng jǐ huáng qí tāng zhǔ zhī.

Fáng jǐ yī liǎng; gān cǎo (chǎo) bàn liǎng; bái zhú qī qián bàn; huáng qí (qù lú) yī liǎng yī fēn

Yòu cuò má dòu dà, měi chāo wǔ qián bǐ, shēng jiāng sì piàn, dà zǎo yī méi, shuǐ zhǎn bàn, jiān bā fēn, qù zǐ wēn fú, liáng jiǔ zài fú. Chuǎn zhě jiā má huáng bàn liǎng. Wèi zhōng bù hé zhě jiā sháo yào sān fēn, qì shàng chōng zhě jiā guì zhī sān fēn, xià yǒu chén hán zhě jiā xì xīn sān fēn, fú hòu dāng rú chóng xíng pí zhōng, cóng yāo xià rú bīng, hòu zuò bèi shàng, yòu yǐ yī bèi rào yāo yǐ xià, wēn lìng wēi hàn, chài.

Wind-damp with a floating pulse, heavy body, sweating, and aversion to wind is governed by Fangji and Astragalus Decoction (防己黄芪汤 *fáng jǐ huáng qí tāng*).

Fangji and Astragalus Decoction (防己黄芪汤 *fáng jǐ huáng qí tāng*)
fangji (防己 *fáng jǐ*, Stephaniae Tetrandrae Radix) 1 *liǎng* licorice (甘草 *gān cǎo*, Glycyrrhizae Radix) ½ *liǎng* (stir-fry) white atractylodes (白朮 *bái zhú*, Atractylodis Macrocephalae Rhizoma) 7.5 *qián* astragalus (黄芪 *huáng qí*, Astragali Radix) 1 *liǎng* and 1 *fēn* (remove tops)

Cut the above [ingredients] to the size of hemp seeds (*má dòu*). Scoop up five qián-spoonfuls per dose [and add this with] four slices of fresh ginger (*shēng jiāng*) and one jujube (*dà zǎo*) to a cup-and-a-half of water. Boil this down to eight tenths and remove the dregs. Take warm and wait a good while before taking more. For panting, use an additional half *liǎng* of ephedra (*má huáng*). For disharmony in the stomach, add three *fēn* of peony (*sháo yào*). For qì surging upward, add three *fēn* of cinnamon twig (*guì zhī*). For old cold in the lower body, add three *fēn* of asarum (*xì xīn*). After taking [the formula, the patient should feel a sensation] like bugs crawling in the skin and icy coldness from the waist down. [To help the treatment, make the patient] sit on a bedcover and wrap another bedcover around them below the waist, to make them warm enough to cause a slight sweat. This will bring about recovery.

Synopsis, Line 2.22

This line describes the signs and treatment of wind-damp exterior vacuity.

Commentary, Line 2.22

A floating pulse and generalized heaviness are signs of wind-damp in the fleshy exterior. Sweating and aversion to wind are signs of exterior vacuity and insecurity of defense qì. Although the pattern is one of wind-damp, the exterior is already vacuous. Therefore, formulas like Ephedra Decoction (*má huáng tāng*) that are designed for exterior repletion are inappropriate. Instead, this line recommends Fangji and Astragalus Decoction (*fáng jǐ huáng qí tāng*), which boosts qì and eliminates dampness.

Within the formula, astragalus (*huáng qí*) boosts qì and secures the exterior. Fangji (*fáng jǐ*) and white atractylodes (*bái zhú*) eliminate wind-damp. Licorice (*gān cǎo*), fresh ginger (*shēng jiāng*), and jujube (*dà zǎo*) harmonize defense and construction, thereby addressing the exterior vacuity. Following the formula, the text states, "After taking [the formula, the patient should feel a sensation] like bugs crawling in the skin." This sensation is caused by the stirring of defensive yáng, a sign that the wind-damp is about to resolve.

Line 2.23

伤寒八九日，风湿相搏，身体疼烦，不能自转侧，不呕不渴，脉浮虚而濇者，桂枝附子汤主之；若大便坚，小便自利者，去桂加白朮汤主之。

桂枝（去皮）四两　生姜（切）三两　附子（炮去皮，破八片）三枚　甘草（炙）二两　大枣(擘)十二枚

右五味，以水六升，煮取二升，去滓，分温三服。

白朮二两　附子（炮去皮）一枚半　甘草（炙）一两　生姜（切）一两半　大枣（擘）六枚

右五味，以水三升，煮取一升，去滓，分温三服。一服觉身痹，半日许再服，三服都尽，其人如冒状，勿怪，即是朮附并走皮中，逐水气未得除故耳。

Shāng hán bā jiǔ rì, fēng shī xiāng bó, shēn tǐ téng fán, bù néng zì zhuǎn cè, bù ǒu bù kě, mài fú xū ér sè zhě, guì zhī fù zǐ tāng zhǔ zhī; ruò dà biàn jiān, xiǎo biàn zì lì zhě, qù guì jiā bái zhú tāng zhǔ zhī.

Guì zhī (qù pí) sì liǎng; shēng jiāng (qiē) sān liǎng; fù zǐ (pào qù pí, pò bā piàn) sān méi; gān cǎo (zhì) èr liǎng; dà zǎo (bò) shí èr méi

Yòu wǔ wèi, yǐ shuǐ liù shēng, zhǔ qǔ èr shēng, qù zǐ, fēn wēn sān fú.

Bái zhú èr liǎng; fù zǐ (pào qù pí) yī méi bàn; gān cǎo (zhì) yī liǎng; shēng jiāng (qiē) yī liǎng bàn; dà zǎo (bò) liù méi.

Yòu wǔ wèi, yǐ shuǐ sān shēng, zhǔ qǔ yī shēng, qù zǐ, fēn wēn sān fú. Yī fú jué shēn bì, bàn rì xǔ zài fú, sān fú dōu jìn, qí rén rú mào zhuàng, wù guài, jí shì zhú fù bìng zǒu pí zhōng, zhú shuǐ qì wèi dé chú gù ěr.

When cold damage [disease] persists for eight or nine days, wind and dampness are contending with each other. [If this manifests in] vexing generalized pain and inability to turn sides, but no retching and no thirst, with a pulse that is floating, vacuous and rough, Cinnamon Twig and Aconite Decoction (*guì zhī fù zǐ tāng*) governs. If the stool is hard but urination is uninhibited, [this] decoction minus cinnamon twig (*guì zhī*) plus white atractylodes (*bái zhú*) governs.

Cinnamon Twig and Aconite Decoction (桂枝附子 *guì zhī fù zǐ tāng*)

- cinnamon twig (桂枝 *guì zhī*, Cinnamomi Ramulus) 4 *liǎng* (remove bark)
- fresh ginger (生姜 *shēng jiāng*, Zingiberis Rhizoma Recens) 3 *liǎng* (cut)
- aconite (附子 *fù zǐ*, Aconiti Radix Lateralis Praeparata) 3 pieces (blast-fry, remove skin, and break into 8 slices)
- licorice (甘草 *gān cǎo*, Glycyrrhizae Radix) 2 *liǎng* (mix-fry)
- jujube (大枣 *dà zǎo*, Jujubae Fructus) 12 fruits (break)

Boil the above five ingredients in six *shēng* of water to get two *shēng*. Remove the dregs and divide into three [doses]. Take warm.

- white atractylodes (白朮 *bái zhú*, Atractylodis Macrocephalae Rhizoma) 2 *liǎng*
- aconite (附子 *fù zǐ*, Aconiti Radix Lateralis Praeparata) 1.5 pieces (blast-fry and remove skin)
- licorice (甘草 *gān cǎo*, Glycyrrhizae Radix) 1 *liǎng* (mix-fry)
- fresh ginger (生姜 *shēng jiāng*, Zingiberis Rhizoma Recens) 1.5 *liǎng* (cut)
- jujube (大枣 *dà zǎo*, Jujubae Fructus) 6 fruits

Boil the above five ingredients in three *shēng* of water to get one *shēng*. Remove the dregs and divide into three [doses].

Take warm. If after the first dose the person feels generalized impediment, take another dose in about half a day. If the patient finishes taking all three doses and experiences something like veiling, do not be surprised. This occurs because the white atractylodes (*bái zhú*) and aconite (*fù zǐ*) have penetrated into the skin to expel the water qì, which has not yet been eliminated.

Synopsis, Line 2.23

This line describes the signs and treatment of wind-damp exterior yáng vacuity.

Commentary, Line 2.23

When cold damage has lasted for eight or nine days without resolving, the reason is that wind, cold, and dampness are gathering together, impeding the fleshy exterior, and inhibiting the channels. This is reflected in the generalized pain and inability to turn sides. The absence of retching or vomiting suggests that the dampness evil has not passed into the interior to invade the stomach. Thus there is no depressed dampness transforming into heat. The pulse is floating, vacuous, and rough. "Floating" and "vacuous" mean floating without force. "Rough" reflects the dampness and cold stagnating in the fleshy exterior and the concurrent vacuity of yáng qì.

The formula used to treat this condition is Cinnamon Twig and Aconite Decoction (*guì zhī fù zǐ tāng*), because it warms the channels and assists yáng, as well as dispelling wind and transforming dampness. Within the formula, cinnamon twig (*guì zhī*) dispels wind. With the help of aconite (*fù zǐ*), it furthermore warms the channels and assists yáng. This combination is specifically designed for exterior vacuity with prevalent wind-cold-damp. Licorice (*gān cǎo*), fresh ginger (*shēng jiāng*), and jujube (*dà zǎo*) harmonize construction and defense, thus also addressing the exterior vacuity.

Line 2.12 states that inhibited urination with free stool is a sign of dampness in the interior. In this line we apparently have the opposite situation, i.e., hard stool and uninhibited urination. However, scholarly interpretation differs as to what this actually means.

One view, held by Xú Zhōng-Kě 徐忠可 is that "hard stool" does not imply constipation, but means normal stool (as opposed to the free stool described in line 2.12). Another view, held by Kē Yùn-Bó 柯韵伯 and others, is that "hard stool" means stool harder than normal, which is due to spleen vacuity and impaired movement and transformation as well as to impaired bladder qì transformation. The difference between normal stool and abnormally hard stool reflects a disagreement over whether the spleen is affected or not. Nevertheless, in either case the condition described in this line is understood to be chiefly one of dampness evil lodged in the exterior, which is what the proposed formula addresses.

Taking Cinnamon Twig and Aconite Decoction (*guì zhī fù zǐ tāng*) eliminates the wind, but can fail to eliminate all of the dampness. As a result, the body is still painful and turning sides is still difficult. In this case, we use White Atractylodes and Aconite Decoction (*bái zhú fù zǐ tāng*) to dispel dampness and warm the channels. Within the formula, white atractylodes (*bái zhú*) and aconite (*fù zǐ*) expel the dampness evil in the skin and warm the channels to restore yáng. Licorice (*gān cǎo*), fresh ginger (*shēng jiāng*), and jujube (*dà zǎo*) harmonize construction and defense, thus also addressing the exterior vacuity.

A commentary on the formula notes that "veiling" (clouded head) may occur after taking this formula and that this is due to yáng qì gaining the strength to expel water qì from the flesh and channels. This is a healthy reaction, not a cause for concern.

Line 2.24

风湿相搏，骨节疼烦掣痛，不得屈伸，近之则痛剧，汗出短气，小便不利，恶风不欲去衣，或身微肿者，甘草附子汤主之。

甘草（炙）二两　附子（炮去皮）二枚　白术二两　桂枝（去皮）四两

右四味，以水六升，煮取三升，去滓，温服一升，日三服，初服得微汗则解。能食汗出复烦者，服五合，恐一升多者，服六七合为妙。

Fēng shī xiāng bó, gǔ jié téng fán chè tòng, bù dé qū shēn, jìn zhī zé tòng jù, hàn chū duǎn qì, xiǎo biàn bù lì, wù fēng bù yù qù yī, huò shēn wēi zhǒng zhě, gān cǎo fù zǐ tāng zhǔ zhī.

Gān cǎo (zhì) èr liǎng; fù zǐ (pào qù pí) èr méi; bái zhú èr liǎng; guì zhī (qù pí) sì liǎng

Yòu sì wèi, yǐ shuǐ liù shēng, zhǔ qǔ sān shēng, qù zǐ, wēn fú yī shēng, rì sān fú, chū fú dé wēi hàn zé jiě. Néng shí hàn chū fù fán zhě, fú wǔ gě, kǒng yī shēng duō zhě, fú liù qī gě wéi miào.

Wind and dampness contending with each other manifests in vexing pain in the joints, pulling pain, inability to stretch, acute pain when touched, sweating and shortness of breath, inhibited urination, aversion to wind and reluctance to remove clothing, and in some cases, slight generalized swelling. Licorice and Aconite Decoction (*gān cǎo fù zǐ tāng*) governs.

Licorice and Aconite Decoction (*gān cǎo fù zǐ tāng*)

- licorice (甘草 *gān cǎo*, Glycyrrhizae Radix) 2 *liǎng* (mix-fry)
- aconite (附子 *fù zǐ*, Aconiti Radix Lateralis Praeparata) 2 pieces (blast-fry and remove skin)
- white atractylodes (白术 *bái zhú*, Atractylodis Macrocephalae Rhizoma) 2 *liǎng*
- cinnamon twig (桂枝 *guì zhī*, Cinnamomi Ramulus) 4 *liǎng* (remove bark)

Boil the above four ingredients in six *shēng* of water to get three *shēng*. Remove the dregs and take one *shēng* warm, three times a day. If you obtain slight sweating after taking [the medicine], the condition is resolved. If the patient can eat, but the sweating is followed by vexation, take [only] five *gě* [per dose]. If you fear that one *shēng* is too much, taking [only] six or seven *gě* [per dose] is fine.

Synopsis, Line 2.24

This line describes the signs and treatment of wind-damp dual vacuity of exterior and interior yáng qì.

COMMENTARY, LINE 2.24

"Vexing pain in the joints, pulling pain, and inability to stretch" reflects wind-damp that has already passed from the flesh into the joints and is giving rise to a condition more severe than in the preceding line. "Sweating and shortness of breath," "aversion to wind and reluctance to remove clothing" reflect the dual yáng vacuity of exterior and interior. "Inhibited urination" and "slight generalized swelling" reflects vacuous yáng failing to transform dampness. Thus the condition in this line is one of exuberant wind and dampness and dual vacuity of exterior and interior. The suggested formula uses cinnamon twig (*guì zhī*), white atractylodes (*bái zhú*), and aconite (*fù zǐ*). It addresses both the exterior and interior condition, assisting yáng qì to dispel wind and transform dampness.

Line 2.25

太阳中暍，发热恶寒，身重而疼痛，其脉弦细芤迟，小便已，洒洒然毛耸，手足逆冷，小有劳，身即热，口开前板齿燥，若发其汗，则恶寒甚；加温针则发热甚；数下之，则淋甚。

Tài yáng zhòng yè, fā rè wù hán, shēn zhòng ér téng tòng, qí mài xián xì kōu chí, xiǎo biàn yǐ, xiǎn xiǎn rán máo sǒng, shǒu zú nì lěng, xiǎo yǒu láo, shēn jí rè, kǒu kāi qián bǎn chǐ zào, ruò fā qí hàn, zé wù hán shèn; jiā wēn zhēn zé fā rè shèn; shù xià zhī, zé lìn shèn.

Greater yáng thermoplegia manifests in heat effusion and aversion to cold, generalized heaviness and pain, a stringlike, fine, scallion-stalk, and slow pulse, and shivering,[1] erect body hair, and counterflow cold of the extremities after urinating. [Even] slight taxation results in generalized heat, open mouth,[2] and dry front teeth.[3] Promotion of sweating aggravates the aversion to cold; application of warm needling aggravates the heat effusion; repeated precipitation treatment results in severe strangury.

TEXT NOTES, LINE 2.25

[1] Shivery 洒洒然 *xiǎn xiǎn rán*: Shaking with cold.

[2] Open mouth 口开 *kǒu kāi*: Open mouth and panting.

[3] Front teeth 板齿 *bǎn chǐ*: The two upper front teeth.

SYNOPSIS, LINE 2.25

This line introduces thermoplegia and describes the signs, treatment, and transmuted patterns resulting from inappropriate treatment.

COMMENTARY, LINE 2.25

Summerheat is one of the six excesses. In the initial stage, it affects greater yáng and is characterized by heat effusion and aversion to cold. However, summerheat often combines with dampness, which gives rise to generalized heaviness and pain. Because summerheat naturally causes sweating, it tends to cause dual vacuity of qì and yīn.

The commentator Yù Jiā-Yán 喻嘉言 notes: "In the summer months, the yáng of the human body discharges outward with sweat, and the yīn of the human body is consumed by heat. Thus yīn and yáng are both insufficient." This explains why summerheat causes dual vacuity of qì and yīn. The pulse is either stringlike and fine or scallion-stalk and slow. Both these pulses reflect dual vacuity of yīn and yáng.

Greater yáng is internally connected with the bladder and externally with the skin and body hair. Urination causes yáng qì to discharge downward, which in turn causes shivering and erect body hair and also makes the hands and feet turn cold. At the same time, the slightest exertion causes vacuous yáng to float astray, giving rise to generalized heat and panting with open mouth. When yīn liquid is consumed internally, this is reflected in dryness of the front teeth. This disease pattern is attributed to the body's inability to adapt to hot weather. It is marked by prominent vacuity signs, including a low-grade fever. This is different from the repletion patterns that are commonly observed in the initial period of external contractions.

Line 2.26

太阳中热者，暍是也，汗出恶寒，身热而渴，白虎加人参汤主之。

知母六两　石膏（碎）一斤　甘草二两　粳米六合　人参三两

右五味，以水一斗，煮米熟汤成，去滓，温服一升，日三服。

Tài yáng zhòng rè zhě, yè shì yě, hàn chū wù hán, shēn rè ér kě, bái hǔ jiā rén shēn tāng zhǔ zhī.

Zhī mǔ liù liǎng; shí gāo (suì) yī jīn gān cǎo èr liǎng; jīng mǐ liù gě; rén shēn sān liǎng.

Yòu wǔ wèi, yǐ shuǐ yī dǒu, zhǔ mǐ shóu tāng chéng, qù zǐ, wēn fú yī shēng, rì sān fú.

Thermoplegia means that greater yáng is struck by heat. [It is characterized by] sweating, aversion to cold, generalized heat [effusion], and thirst. White Tiger Decoction Plus Ginseng (*bái hǔ jiā rén shēn tāng*) governs.

White Tiger Decoction Plus Ginseng (*bái hǔ jiā rén shēn tāng*)
anemarrhena (知母 *zhī mǔ*, Anemarrhenae Rhizoma) 6 *liǎng*
gypsum (石膏 *shí gāo*, Gypsum Fibrosum) 1 *jīn* (crush)
licorice (甘草 *gān cǎo*, Glycyrrhizae Radix) 2 *liǎng*
non-glutinous rice (粳米 jīng mǐ, Oryzae Semen) 6 *gě*
ginseng (人参 *rén shēn*, Ginseng Radix) 3 *liǎng*

Boil the above five ingredients in one *dǒu* of water. When the rice is cooked, the decoction is ready. Remove the dregs and take one *shēng* warm, three times a day.

Synopsis, Line 2.26

This line describes the signs and treatment of summerheat-heat damaging liquid.

COMMENTARY, LINE 2.26

Thermoplegia is a disease caused by heat striking greater yáng, "heat" here meaning summerheat-heat. In the initial stages of summerheat disease, there is sweating. The sweating causes the interstices to open wide; hence there is also aversion to cold. It should be noted that in summerheat damage, sweating precedes and is the cause of aversion to cold. This is different from aversion to cold that is observed in, say, cold fettering the exterior, in which aversion to cold (or fear of cold) arises when defensive yáng is obstructed or interior yáng is insufficient. Summerheat-heat is an intense heat that damages yīn liquid, giving rise to generalized heat and to thirst.

The treatment for summerheat-heat is to clear heat and resolve summerheat and to boost qì and engender liquid. This line recommends White Tiger Decoction Plus Ginseng (*bái hǔ jiā rén shēn tāng*). Within the formula, gypsum (*shí gāo*) clears and drains summerheat-heat. Cool moistening anemarrhena (*zhī mǔ*) clears heat and engenders liquid. Ginseng (*rén shēn*) boosts qì and engenders liquid. Licorice (*gān cǎo*) and non-glutinous rice (*gēng mǐ*) boost the stomach and harmonize the center. Combined, the ingredients resolve summerheat-heat and restore qì and yīn.

Line 2.27

太阳中暍，身热疼重，而脉微弱，此以夏月伤冷水，水行皮中所致也。一物瓜蒂汤主之。

瓜蒂二十个

右剉, 以水一升, 煮取五合, 去滓顿服。

Tài yáng zhòng yè, shēn rè téng zhòng, ér mài wēi ruò, cǐ yǐ xià yuè shāng lěng shuǐ, shuǐ xíng pí zhōng suǒ zhì yě. Yī wù guā dì tāng zhǔ zhī.

Guā dì èr shí gè

Yòu cuò, yǐ shuǐ yī shēng, zhǔ qǔ wǔ gě, qù zǐ dùn fú.

When greater yáng thermoplegia manifests with generalized heat [effusion], pain, heaviness, and a faint and weak pulse, this is caused by damage from cold water in the summer months and by water moving in the skin. Single-Agent Melon Stalk Decoction (一物瓜蒂汤 *yī wù guā dì tāng*) governs.

Single-Agent Melon Stalk Decoction (一物瓜蒂汤 *yī wù guā dì tāng*)
melon stalk (瓜蒂 *guā dì*, Melonis Pedicellus) 20 stalks

Grate the above [ingredient] and boil in one *shēng* of water get five *gě*. Remove the dregs and quaff[1] [in a single dose].

TEXT NOTE

[1] Quaff 顿服 *dùn fú*: Swallow (the medicine) in one go.

SYNOPSIS, LINE 2.27

This line describes thermoplegia that is complicated by dampness.

COMMENTARY, LINE 2.27

Summerheat causes generalized heat. When it combines with dampness, it also causes pain and heaviness. Dampness is a yīn evil that damages yáng qì, hence summerheat-damp is characterized by a weak pulse. Summerheat-damp arises when people consume excessive amounts of cold drinks or enter cold water when sweating, to gain relief from the torrid heat of summer. As a result, they contract the evil of summerheat-damp. Furthermore, the dampness prevents exterior qì from diffusing and the summerheat from being discharged from the body.

The treatment is to dispel dampness and clear heat. This is achieved with Single-Agent Melon Stalk Decoction (*yī wù guā dì tāng*).

百合狐惑阴阳毒病脉证治第三

CHAPTER 3

Hundred-Union Disease, Fox-Creeper, and Yīn and Yáng Toxin

Pulses, Signs, Treatments

‡ Overview

This chapter describes three different disease categories: hundred-union disease, fox-creeper, and yīn and yáng toxin. From the time of the Zhāng Jī in the Eastern Hàn onward, these three diseases were discussed in numerous books including the *Zhǒu Hòu Bèi Jí Fāng* ("Emergency Standby Remedies"), *Mài Jīng* ("The Pulse Canon"), *Zhū Bìng Yuán Hòu Lùn* ("Te Origin and Indicators of Disease"), *Qiān Jīn Fāng* ("Thousand Gold Pieces Prescriptions"), and *Wài Tái Mì Yào* ("Secrets from the *Wài Tái* Library"). However, after the Táng, few references to them are found.

Despite their distinctive causes, key symptoms, and treatments, all three diseases are related to the pathomechanism of externally contracted febrile disease. In hundred-union disease, patients are "often taciturn; [they] desire to sleep [but] cannot sleep." This is similar to "taciturnity and desire to sleep… disquietude [when] lying [or] when up" of fox-creeper disease. At the same time the "erosion of the throat" of fox-creeper is similar to the sore throat of yīn-yáng toxin. Furthermore, although these diseases are related to externally contracted disease, none of them fit into the cold damage six-channel scheme. For these reasons, they are discussed together in the present chapter.

This chapter introduction describes not only the basic features of the three diseases, but also explains the significance of their unusual names.

HUNDRED-UNION DISEASE

Hundred-union disease can occur after febrile disease, if residual heat is still present. It can also result from emotional frustration giving rise to depression that transforms into fire. In either case, the pathomechanism involves damage to the humor of the heart, and lung and yīn vacuity with internal heat. Clinical manifestations also include mental abnormalities such as abstraction, as well as bitter taste in the mouth, reddish urine, and a pulse that is faint and rapid.

"Hundred-union disease" is a literal translation of the Chinese 百合病 *bǎi hé bìng*. Three reasons have been posited for this disease name. The first is that "hundred-union" means the "the hundred vessels," in reference to the locus of the disease. The disease is characterized by heart-lung vacuity heat. As we know, the heart governs the blood and vessels, while the lung assembles the hundred vessels. Thus, the disease involves the vessels in their relationship to the heart and lung. This interpretation is supported by the opening line of the chapter: "It is said that hundred-union disease [is so-called because] the hundred vessels [share] one [and the same] ancestor and all cause the disease." A second explanation of the name rests on the fact that "hundred union" 百合 *bǎi hé* is also the Chinese name for the lily bulb, the medicinal that is primarily used to treat this disease. The lily bulb is called "hundred-union" in allusion to its being composed of manifold converging layers.[1] A third explanation is that "hundred-union" refers to the complexity of the disease.

The three interpretations of the term are not mutually exclusive. The principle that a medicinal item is chosen to treat a certain disease because it has formal characteristics similar to those of the diseased body part has played an important role in the development of Chinese medicine. This is most clearly seen in the practice of consuming the penises of large and powerful animals such as seals and tigers to treat impotence. It surfaces indirectly in the use of red and bitter medicinals to treat heart disease, white and acrid medicinals to treat lung disease, etc. In this case, however, the characteristics are not observed in the organs themselves but in the phase to which they belong in the system of the five phases. In fact, the notion of meaningful connections between like phenomena lies at the basis of both the yīn-yáng and five-phase systems. Hence, it is very likely that ancient physicians such as Zhāng Jī would have seen a meaningful connection between the "hundred vessels" and the "hundred unions" of the lily bulb.

FOX-CREEPER

The term tentatively rendered here as "fox-creeper" appears in the received text as 狐惑 *hú huò*. The text of the *Jīn Guì Yào Lüè* itself explains the character 狐 *hú* as referring to the disease affecting the anus and/or genitals, and 惑 *huò* as referring to the disease in the throat. It is characterized by red eyes and by erosion of the throat and/or two yīn (anus and/or genitals), either occurring simultaneously or alternating.

---

[1] It is interesting to note that our word *onion* comes from the Old French *oignon*, in turn deriving from the Latin *unio*, reflects the very same logic for naming a bulb as the Chinese (百合) *bǎi hé*.

The *Jīn Guì* states that when the disease erodes the throat it is called "creeper" (惑 *huò*), while when it erodes the two yīn (anus and genitals) it is called "fox" (狐 *hú*). The use of the term 蚀 *shí*, literally "eat," "gnaw," and by extension, "erode," has given rise to a belief that "fox" and "creeper" may allude to worms believed to gnaw or erode the flesh. Since antiquity, many diseases have been explained by worms gnawing the flesh. However, in this case, the existence of "worms" would have been the product of speculation since the disease is associated with no animate life forms that can be seen with the naked eye. Many conditions traditionally attributable to worms were also associated with an underlying condition of damp-heat brewing internally. In the case of fox-creeper, the attributive cause of damp-heat is the now widely accepted explanation that avoids speculation.

Why the disease is so named has been the subject of dispute. The character 惑 *huò*, composed of a phonetic element on the top with a heart (心) signific below, means, among other things, "to deceive" or "beguile," suggesting that the disease name, when written in this way, literally means a disease bearing some elusive characteristics epitomized by a beguiling, sly fox.

Some scholars suggest that 惑 *huò* is a mistranscription of 蟚, now written as 蜮 and pronounced *huò* or *yù*, with the insect/reptile 虫 signific (also written as 蜮). This denotes a mystical turtle with three legs believed to kill or wound humans by shooting sand from its mouth. In the early seal (篆 *zhuàn*) script, the heart and insect/reptile signific look very similar and for this reason may have been confused. Supporting this interpretation is the fact that this turtle was also known as the 狐蟚 *hú huò/yù* ("fox-turtle)," or 短狐 *duǎn hú* ("short fox"), probably because it was believed to embody certain characteristics of the fox (e.g., slyness). If this is true, the disease is named after the mythical turtle.

Other scholars reject this explanation on the grounds that since the *Jīn Guì* text splits the term in two, explaining 狐 *hú* as erosion of the two yīn and 蟚 *huò/yù* as erosion of the throat, it is no longer clear whether the name was originally intended to refer to one animal or two. Furthermore, they point out that the connection between the fabulous turtle and possibly also the familiar fox and the disease is not clear either. In view of this, they prefer the explanation that the character 蟚 refers to worms nurtured by damp-heat which were originally regarded as the cause of the disease, rather than the attribution of a three-legged, sand-shooting turtle.

We render the term in English as "fox-creeper," because it can, just like the Chinese term, be interpreted to mean the turtle, the worms, the turtle as named after the fox, the turtle and the fox, or a disease as subtle and stealthy as a fox. In modern Chinese medicine, fox-creeper is sometimes used as a reference point for biomedical conditions such as Behçet's Disease.

Yīn-Yáng Toxin

Yīn-yáng toxin (阴阳毒 *yīn yáng dú*) is the generic designation for both yīn toxin and yáng toxin. It is generally believed to be caused by contraction of epidemic toxin that invades the blood. In clinic, its key symptoms are macular eruption and sore throat. It falls within the scope of acute febrile disease.

The term yīn-yáng toxin is at first encounter relatively self-explanatory, were it not for the vagueness of yīn and yáng. In this disease name, yīn and yáng refer not to cold and heat or interior and exterior respectively, but rather to the categories by which the presenting signs can be classified.

‡ Schematic Overview

Hundred Union Disease

1. Causes
   a) The signs may appear before any cold damage febrile disease (excessive emotional stimulus), or
   b) four or five days after the onset of disease, or
   c) gradually over twenty days or a month after the onset of disease. Each case is treated according to the signs.
2. Pathomechanism: The hundred vessels have a single ancestor, which can cause disease everywhere (heart-lung yīn vacuity with internal heat depriving the hundred vessels of nourishment).
3. Signs
   a) The disease manifests in desire but inability to eat; frequent taciturnity; desire but inability to sleep; desire but inability to walk; desire to eat and drink yet finding some foods delicious and others not even tolerable to smell; [signs] resembling a cold condition but without cold; [signs] resembling a heat condition but without heat; bitter taste in the mouth; and red urine. None of the various medicines can treat it. Taking medicine results in violent vomiting and diarrhea, as if [the patient] were possessed by a spirit. The physical form seems to be in harmony and the pulse is slightly rapid.
   b) Bitter taste in the mouth and red urine.
4. Prognosis
   a) If urination is always accompanied by headache, [the patient will] recover in sixty days.
   b) If urination is never accompanied by headache but there is [aversion to cold as if the patient were] wet, [the patient will] recover in forty days.
   c) If urination is fast and merely accompanied by dizziness, [the patient will] recover in twenty days.
5. Regular treatment: "If no vomiting, precipitation, or sweating [therapy] has been applied and the disease appears the same as in the beginning, Lily Bulb and Rehmannia Decoction (*bǎi hé dì huáng tāng*) governs."
6. Treatment after adverse treatment

a) After promotion of sweating: Lily Bulb and Anemarrhena Decoction (*bǎi hé zhī mǔ tāng*) to enrich the lung and stomach, to engender liquid, and to downbear counterflow.

b) After precipitation: Talcum and Hematite Decoction (*huá shí dài zhě tāng*) to nourish yīn and clear heat and to harmonize the stomach and downbear counterflow.

c) After ejection: Lily Bulb and Egg Yolk Decoction (*bǎi hé jī zǐ tāng*) to nourish the lung and stomach, to engender liquid, and downbear counterflow.

7. Treatment of transmuted patterns

a) Thirst: If the disease persists for a month without resolving and thirst appears, use Lily Bulb Wash (*bǎi hé xǐ fāng*) to nourish yīn and engender liquid, as well as Trichosanthes and Oyster Shell Powder (*guā lóu mǔ lì sǎn*).

b) Heat effusion: Lily Bulb and Talcum Powder (*bǎi hé huá shí sǎn*) to nourish yīn, clear heat, and inhibit urine.

FOX-CREEPER DISEASE

1. Cause: Damp-heat arising from worm toxin.

a) Arising after febrile disease, when residual heat has not been cleared.

b) Arising after measles, when residual heat is still present.

2. Pathomechanism: Damp-heat and worm toxin causing erosion.

3. Principles of treatment: Clearing heat and disinhibiting dampness; killing worms and resolving toxin.

4. Signs: Symptoms resembling cold damage, taciturnity and desire to sleep, inability to close the eyes, and disquietude whether lying down or being up. If it erodes the throat, it is called creeper; if it erodes the yīn [parts], it is called fox. [It further manifests with] no desire to eat or drink, aversion to the odor of food, and face and eyes that are now red, now black, now white.

5. Pattern identification.

a) Erosion in the upper body (throat): Husky voice. Licorice Heart-Draining Decoction (*gān cǎo xiè xīn tāng*) to clear heat and transform dampness and to quiet the center and resolve toxin.

b) Erosion in the lower body.

Anterior yīn: Ulceration of the genitals. Wash with Flavescent Sophora Decoction (*kǔ shēn tāng*) to clear heat and eliminate dampness and to kill worms and resolve toxin.

Posterior yīn: Erosion of the anus. Fumigate with realgar (*xióng huáng*) to dry dampness, kill worms, and resolve toxin.

6. Giving rise to welling-abscesses and suppuration.

a) Signs: Rapid pulse, absence of heat [effusion], slight vexation, taciturnity, desire only to sleep, and sweating. Initially, when [this condition] has lasted for only three or four days, the eyes become red like [those of a] turtledove. After seven or eight days, the four canthi of the eyes turn black. If [the patient] is able to eat, this indicates that pus has formed.

b) Treatment: Rice Bean and Chinese Angelica Powder (*chì xiăo dòu dāng guī săn*) to percolate dampness, clear heat, quicken the blood and expel pus.

YĪN-YÁNG TOXIN

1. Causes: Contraction of epidemic toxin.
2. Pathomechanism: Epidemic toxin entering the blood aspect:
   a) Exuberant heat in blood aspect and yáng toxin being forced upward.
   b) Internal putrefaction giving rise to pus: Yáng toxin.
   c) Static blood congealing and causing obstruction: Yīn toxin.
3. Pattern Identification.
   a) Yáng toxin: Face red with patches like brocade, sore throat, spitting of pus and blood.
   b) Yīn toxin: Green-blue face and eyes, generalized pain as though having been beaten by a stick, sore throat.
4. Prognosis.
   a) Within [the first] five days: treatable.
   b) [By the] seventh day: not treatable.
5. Treatment.
   a) Yáng toxin: Cimicifuga and Turtle Shell Decoction (*shēng má biē jiă tāng*) to clear heat, resolve toxin, and disperse stasis.
   b) Yīn toxin: Cimicifuga and Turtle Shell Decoction (*shēng má biē jiă tāng*) minus realgar (*xióng huáng*) and zanthoxylum (*shŭ jiāo*) to resolve toxin, quicken the blood, and disperse stasis.

Line 3.1

(1)论曰：百合病者，百脉一宗，悉致其病也。意欲食复不能食，常默默，欲卧不能卧，欲行不能行，欲饮食，或有美时，或有不用闻食臭时，如寒无寒，如热无热，口苦小便赤，诸药不能治，得药则剧吐利，如有神灵者，身形如和，其脉微数。

(2) 每溺时头痛者，六十日乃愈；若溺时头不痛，淅然者，四十日愈；若溺快然，但头眩者，二十日愈。

(3)其证或未病而预见，或病四五日而出，或病二十日或一月微见者，各随证治之。

(1) Lùn yuē: bǎi hé bìng zhě, bǎi mài yī zōng, xī zhì qí bìng yě. Yì yù shí fù bù néng shí, cháng mò mò, yù wò bù néng wò, yù xíng bù néng xíng, yù yǐn shí, huò yǒu měi shí, huò yǒu bù yòng wén shí chòu shí, rú hán wú hán, rú rè wú rè, kǒu kǔ xiǎo biàn chì, zhū yào bù néng zhì, dé yào zé jù tù lì, rú yǒu shén líng zhě, shēn xíng rú hé, qí mài wēi shuò.

(2) Měi niào shí tóu tòng zhě, liù shí rì nǎi yú; ruò niào shí tóu bù tòng, xī rán zhě, sì shí rì yú; ruò niào kuài rán, dàn tóu xuàn zhě, èr shí rì yú.

(3) Qí zhèng huò wèi bìng ér yù jiàn, huò bìng sì wǔ rì ér chū, huò bìng èr shí rì huò yī yuè wēi jiàn zhě, gè suí zhèng zhì zhī.

(1) It is said that hundred-union disease [is so-called because] the hundred vessels [share] one [and the same] ancestor, which can cause disease everywhere. It manifests in desire to eat but then not being able to, frequent taciturnity, desire to sleep but not being able to, desire to walk but not being able to, desire to eat and drink but finding some foods delicious and with others unable to bear even the smell, [signs] resembling a cold condition but without cold, [signs] resembling a heat condition but without heat, bitter taste in the mouth, and red urine. None of the various medicines can treat it. Taking medicine results in violent vomiting and diarrhea, as if [the patient] were possessed by a spirit. The physical form seems to be in harmony and the pulse is faint and rapid.

(2) If urination is always accompanied by headache, [the patient will] recover in sixty days. If urination is always accompanied by no headache but and [aversion to cold as if the body had been] wet, [the patient will] recover in forty days. If urination is fast and merely accompanied by dizziness, [the patient will] recover in twenty days.

(3) The signs [of hundred-union disease] may appear before the onset of any [cold damage heat] disease, or four or five days [after the onset of] disease, or gradually twenty days or a month [after the onset of] disease. Treat each case according to the signs.

Synopsis, Line 3.1

This line discusses hundred-union disease in terms of its location, pulse and symptoms, prognosis, and principles of treatment.

COMMENTARY, LINE 3.1

Hundred-union disease is characterized by heart-lung yīn vacuity with internal heat. The heart governs the blood and vessels, and the lung faces the hundred vessels. When the heart and lung are functioning normally, qì and blood are in harmony and the hundred vessels are all properly nourished. If, on the contrary, heart and lung yīn are vacuous as a result of unresolved heat after cold damage disease or depressed heat arising from affect-mind frustration (emotional problems), the hundred vessels are affected. Hence the text says, "The hundred vessels have a single ancestor, which can cause disease everywhere."

The first section of the line suggests that there are two main aspects to heart-lung yīn vacuity. First, insufficiency of yīn-blood affects the spirit and gives rise to abnormalities of the spirit-mind, speech, and movement, such as taciturnity and abstraction, desire to sleep but inability to sleep, desire to walk but inability to walk, desire to eat but inability to eat, and a good appetite sometimes yet poor appetite at other times. In addition, the patient suffers from conditions such as cold but not cold and heat but not heat. Second, yīn vacuity gives rise to internal heat; hence we see signs such as bitter taste in the mouth, reddish urine, and a faint and rapid pulse. This aspect of the disease is of central importance because the aim of effective treatment is to nourish yīn and clear heat.

The second section of the line discusses urination. It states that the patient may experience headache, aversion to wind, or dizziness upon urination. Since the condition primarily involves the lung and heart, we can explain the urinary symptoms in terms of the lung governing the regulation of the waterways and the passage of water down to the bladder. The bladder is connected to the head by its channel and is associated with the skin and body hair. It is through these connections that headache and dizziness on the one hand and aversion to wind on the other arise. The second section of the line also states that signs occurring upon urination are of significance in determining prognosis. Headache after urination suggests a long disease course, while aversion to cold and dizziness after urination imply shorter courses.

The third section of the line discusses the occurrence of hundred-union disease signs in relation to another disease. Although the text does not specifically mention cold damage febrile disease, most commentators take "disease" to mean cold damage. The implication is that heart-lung yīn vacuity is the result of damage to yīn fluids by febrile disease. In cases where hundred-union disease does not follow after heat disease, it is attributed to internal damage by the seven affects, causing qì to become depressed and bound, and consequently to transform into fire.

Line 3.2

百合病发汗后者，百合知母汤主之。
百合（擘）七枚　知母（切）三两。
右先以水洗百合，渍一宿，当白沫出去其水，更以泉水二升，煎取一升，去滓；别以泉水二升煎知母，取一升去滓；后合和煎取一升五合，分温再服。

Bǎi hé bìng fā hàn hòu zhě, bǎi hé zhī mǔ tāng zhǔ zhī.

Bǎi hé (bò) qī méi; zhī mǔ (qiē) sān liǎng.

Yòu xiān yǐ shuǐ xǐ bǎi hé, zì yī xiǔ, dāng bái mò chū qù qí shuǐ, gèng yǐ quán shuǐ èr shēng, jiān qǔ yī shēng, qù zǐ; bié yǐ quán shuǐ èr shēng jiān zhī mǔ, qǔ yī shēng qù zǐ; hòu hé huó jiān qǔ yī shēng wǔ gě, fēn wēn zài fú.

After sweating has been induced in hundred-union disease, Lily Bulb and Anemarrhena Decoction (百合知母汤 *bǎi hé zhī mǔ tāng*) governs.

Lily Bulb and Anemarrhena Decoction (百合知母汤 *bǎi hé zhī mǔ tāng*)
lily bulb (百合 *bǎi hé*, Lilii Bulbus) 7 bulbs (break) anemarrhena (知母 *zhī mǔ*, Anemarrhenae Rhizoma) 3 *liǎng* (cut)

Taking the above [ingredients], first wash the lily bulb (*bǎi hé*) and steep overnight. This should produce a white foam. Discard the water and boil [the lily bulb] in two *shēng* of spring water to get one *shēng*. Remove the dregs. Boil the anemarrhena (*zhī mǔ*) separately in another two *shēng* of spring water to get one *shēng*, and remove the dregs. Now blend [the two decoctions] and boil to get one *shēng* and five *gě*. Divide into two [doses] and take warm.

Synopsis, Line 3.2

This line discusses the treatment of hundred-union disease after inappropriate precipitation.

Commentary, Line 3.2

Hundred-union disease is attributed to heart-lung yīn vacuity with internal dryness and heat. You should never treat such patterns by sweating. If the practitioner mistakes "[signs] resembling a cold condition but without cold," and "[signs] resembling a heat condition but without heat" for exterior repletion and promotes sweating, yīn humor will undergo further damage, giving rise to heart vexation and thirst. After inappropriate sweating, the correct treatment is to supplement vacuity and clear heat and to nourish yīn and moisten dryness. Lily Bulb and Anemarrhena Decoction (*bǎi hé zhī mǔ tāng*) is the recommended formula.

Within the formula, lily bulb (*bǎi hé*) moistens the lung and clears the heart, boosts qì and quiets the spirit; anemarrhena (*zhī mǔ*) nourishes yīn and clears heat, and eliminates vexation and moistens dryness. The formula uses spring water because of its ability to help clear internal heat.

Line 3.3

百合病下之后者，滑石代赭汤主之。

百合（擘）七枚　滑石（碎绵裹）三两 代赭石（如弹丸大一枚，碎绵裹）

右先以水洗百合，渍一宿，当白沫出，去其水，更以泉水二升煎取一升，去滓；别以泉水二升煎滑石、代赭，取一升去滓；后合和重煎取一升五合，分温服。

Bǎi hé bìng xià zhī hòu zhě, huá shí dài zhě tāng zhǔ zhī.

Bǎi hé (bò) qī méi; huá shí (suì mián guǒ) sān liǎng; dài zhě shí (rú dàn wán dà yī méi, suì mián guǒ)

Yòu xiān yǐ shuǐ xǐ bǎi hé, zì yī xiǔ, dāng bái mò chū, qù qí shuǐ, gèng yǐ quán shuǐ èr shēng jiān qǔ yī shēng, qù zǐ; bié yǐ quán shuǐ èr shēng jiān huá shí, dài zhě, qǔ yī shēng qù zǐ; hòu hé huó chóng jiān qǔ yī shēng wǔ gě, fēn wēn fú.

In hundred-union disease, when precipitation has been promoted, Talcum and Hematite Decoction (滑石代赭汤 *huá shí dài zhě tāng*) governs.

Talcum and Hematite Decoction (滑石代赭汤 *huá shí dài zhě tāng*)

lily bulb (百合 *bǎi hé*, Lilii Bulbus) 7 bulbs (break)
talcum (滑石 *huá shí*, Talcum) 3 *liǎng* (crush and wrap in cotton gauze)
hematite (代赭石 *dài zhě shí*, Haematitum) 1 pellet-sized piece (crush and wrap in cotton)

Of the above [ingredients], first wash the lily bulb (*bǎi hé*) and steep overnight. This should produce a white foam. Discard the water and boil [the lily bulb] in two *shēng* of spring water to get one *shēng*. Remove the dregs. Boil the talcum (*huá shí*) and hematite (*dài zhě shí*) separately in another two *shēng* of spring water to get one *shēng*, and remove the dregs. Now blend [the two decoctions] and boil to get one *shēng* and five *gě*. Divide into two [doses] and take warm.

SYNOPSIS, LINE 3.3

This line describes the treatment of hundred-union disease after inappropriate precipitation.

COMMENTARY, LINE 3.3

Conditions of yīn vacuity with internal heat should be treated by clearing and moistening, not by precipitation. Since precipitation makes the stool more fluid and frequent, it entails loss of fluids. For this reason, it is classically used for repletion patterns in patients who have the yīn-humor resources to withstand the treatment. A practitioner might mistake the symptom described in the first line of this section as "desire to eat and drink but finding some foods delicious and with others unable to bear even the smell" for a repletion pattern of evil heat in the interior and apply precipitation. This will have two consequences. One is further damage to liquid and humor, which exacerbates the internal heat and hence results in short voidings of urine. The other is damage to stomach qì, which gives rise to counterflow ascent of stomach qì. This manifests in retching, vomiting, or hiccup.

After a patient has undergone inappropriate precipitation, treatment should aim to nourish yīn and clear heat and to disinhibit urine and downbear counterflow. The suggested formula is Talcum and Hematite Decoction (*huá shí dài zhě tāng*).

Within the formula, lily bulb (*bǎi hé*) nourishes and moistens the heart and lung, and hence addresses the root of the disease. Talcum (*huá shí*) clears heat and disinhibits urine, thereby conducting the vacuity heat out through the urine. It also enables hematite (*dài zhě shí*), which is heavy and settling by nature, to downbear counterflow and harmonize the stomach. Both these medicinals act together to treat the tip of the disease caused by the inappropriate precipitation. Spring water helps the talcum (*huá shí*) clear heat and disinhibit urine. Altogether these ingredients restore yīn humor, abate vacuity heat, and harmonize stomach qì. Thus addressing both the root and tip of the disease.

Line 3.4

百合病吐之后者，用后方主之。

百合（擘）七枚　鸡子黄一枚

右先以水洗百合，渍一宿，当白沫出，去其水，更以泉水二升煎取一升，去滓，内鸡子黄，搅匀煎五分，温服。

Bǎi hé bìng tù zhī hòu zhě, yòng hòu fāng zhǔ zhī.

Bǎi hé (bò) qī méi; jī zǐ huáng yī méi

Yòu xiān yǐ shuǐ xǐ bǎi hé, zì yī xiǔ, dāng bái mò chū, qù qí shuǐ, gèng yǐ quán shuǐ èr shēng jiān qǔ yī shēng, qù zǐ, nà jī zǐ huáng, jiǎo yún jiān wǔ fēn, wēn fú.

Once vomiting has been promoted in hundred-union disease, use the following formula to govern [this condition].

Lily Bulb and Egg Yolk Decoction (百合鸡子汤 *bǎi hé jī zǐ tāng*)

lily bulb (百合 *bǎi hé*, Lilii Bulbus) 7 bulbs (break)
egg yolk (鸡子黄 *jī zǐ huáng*, Galli Vitellus) 1 yolk

Of the above [ingredients], first wash the lily bulb (*bǎi hé*) and steep overnight. This should produce a white foam. Discard the water and boil [the lily bulb] in two *shēng* of spring water to get one *shēng*. Remove the dregs. Add the egg yolk, blend until smooth, and boil down to five tenths. Take warm.

Synopsis

This line describes the treatment of hundred-union disease after inappropriate ejection [has been promoted].

Commentary

Ejection should not be used to treat yīn vacuity with internal heat. If the practitioner mistakes "inability to bear even the smell of food" for abiding food in the upper stomach duct, and applies ejection, the result will be further damage to the fluids and heart yīn and disquietude of the heart spirit, manifesting as heart palpitation, vacuity vexation, and difficulty sleeping. Ejection will also damage the stomach by causing disharmony, manifesting as clamoring stomach and dry retching. When adverse ejection treatment has been applied, you have to correct it by enriching yīn humor, quieting the spirit, and harmonizing the stomach.

The formula suggested is Lily Bulb and Egg Yolk Decoction (百合鸡子汤 *bǎi hé jī zǐ tāng*).

Within the formula, lily bulb (*bǎi hé*) boosts yīn and clears heat, and moistens and nourishes the heart and lung. Egg yolk (*jī zǐ huáng*) enriches yīn, nourishes the blood, and quiets the spirit on the one hand, and supplements the center to harmonize the stomach on the other hand. Thus the formula as a whole has the action of nourishing yīn and clearing heat, as well as quieting the spirit and harmonizing the stomach.

Line 3.5

百合病不经吐下发汗，病形如初者，百合地黄汤主之。

百合（擘）七枚　生地黄汁一升

右以水洗百合渍一宿，当白沫出，去其水，更以泉水二升煎取一升，去滓，内地黄汁煎取一升五合，分温再服。中病，勿更服。大便当如漆。

Bǎi hé bìng bù jīng tù xià fā hàn, bìng xing rú chū zhě, bǎi hé dì huáng tāng zhǔ zhī.

Bǎi hé (bò) qī méi; shēng dì huáng zhī yī shēng

Yòu yǐ shuǐ xǐ bǎi hé zì yī xiǔ, dāng bái mò chū, qù qí shuǐ, gèng yǐ quán shuǐ èr shēng jiān qǔ yī shēng, qù zǐ, nà dì huáng zhī jiān qǔ yī shēng wǔ gě, fēn wēn zài fú. Zhòng bìng, wù gèng fú. Dà biàn dāng rú qī.

In hundred-union disease, if neither vomiting, precipitation, nor sweating have been effected and the disease appears the same as in the beginning, Lily Bulb and Rehmannia Decoction (百合地黄汤 ***bǎi hé dì huáng tāng***) governs.

Lily Bulb and Rehmannia Decoction (百合地黄汤 *bǎi hé dì huáng tāng*)
lily bulb (百合 *bǎi hé*, Lilii Bulbus) 7 bulbs (break) fresh rehmannia juice (生地黄汁 *shēng dì huáng zhī*, Rehmanniae Radix Recentis Succus) 1 *shēng*

Of the above [ingredients], first wash the lily bulb (*bǎi hé*) and steep overnight. This should produce a white foam. Discard the water and boil [the lily bulb] in two *shēng* of spring water to get one *shēng*. Remove the dregs. Add the rehmannia juice (*dì huáng zhī*) and boil to get one *shēng* and five *gě*. Divide into two [doses] and take warm. When the disease is struck, do not take any more. The stool should be like lacquer.[1]

Text Note, Line 3.5

[1] The stool should be like lacquer 大便当如漆 *dà biàn dāng rú qī*: The stool will be black as a result of the rehmannia.

Synopsis, Line 3.5

This line describes the direct treatment of hundred-union disease.

COMMENTARY, LINE 3.5

Hundred-union disease that has not been inappropriately treated by ejection, precipitation, or sweating, and that long continues to manifest in the original signs described in the first line of the chapter, reflects a straightforward case of heart-lung yīn vacuity with internal heat. The appropriate treatment is Lily Bulb and Rehmannia Decoction (*bǎi hé dì huáng tāng*).

Within the formula, lily bulb (*bǎi hé*) moistens and nourishes the heart and lung, and clears vacuity heat in the qì aspect. Dried/fresh rehmannia (*shēng dì huáng*) nourishes heart yīn and clears vacuity heat in the blood aspect. Spring water is used to help the yīn-nourishing and heat-clearing action and to conduct the heat out through the urine. The formula as a whole moistens and nourishes the heart and lung, treats both qì and blood, and restores yīn and clears heat as well.

The meaning of the second to last sentence (中病，勿更服 *zhòng bìng, wù gèng fú*) is still subject to debate. In the translation above, we have followed the practice of most commentators who interpret the character 更 *gèng* as "more." Thus, the sentence tells us to stop taking the formula after the formula has achieved results. This is most likely related to the fact that fresh rehmannia juice is sweet and moistening and can over time cause diarrhea. However, an alternative view reads 更 as "to change," in which case the sentence means: "After the disease is struck, do not change the formula," that is, continue taking the same formula. Proponents of this view emphasize the chronic slow nature of hundred-union disease, because of which the patient should continue taking the formula for a while. After taking this medicine, the stool will turn black. This is the color of the rehmannia and will disappear when the medicine is discontinued. It is no cause for worry.

Line 3.6

百合病一月不解，变成渴者，百合洗方主之。

百合一升

右以水一斗渍之一宿，以洗身，洗已，食煮饼，勿以盐豉也。

Bǎi hé bìng yī yuè bù jiě, biàn chéng kě zhě, bǎi hé xǐ fāng zhǔ zhī.

Bǎi hé yī shēng

Yòu yǐ shuǐ yī dǒu zì zhī yī xiǔ, yǐ xǐ shēn, xǐ yǐ, shí zhǔ bǐng, wù yǐ yán chǐ yě.

If hundred-union disease fails to resolve within one month and transmutes into thirst, Lily Bulb Wash (百合洗方 *bǎi hé xǐ fāng*) governs.

Lily Bulb Wash (百合洗方 *bǎi hé xǐ fāng*)
lily bulb (百合 *bǎi hé*, Lilii Bulbus) 1 *shēng*

Steep the above [ingredient] in 1 *dǒu* of water overnight. Use this to bathe the body. After bathing, eat boiled cake,[1] but avoid salty fermented beans.

TEXT NOTE, LINE 3.6

[1] Boiled cake 煮饼 *zhǔ bǐng*: This is believed to be a generic term for foods made from flour and water paste, prominently including noodles.

SYNOPSIS, LINE 3.6

This line describes the external treatment of enduring hundred-union disease that has transmuted into thirst.

Normally hundred-union disease does not include thirst among its presenting signs. However, if the disease is not eliminated after a month or so and thirst appears as an additional symptom, this means that the yīn vacuity and internal heat have become more pronounced. In this situation, Lily Bulb and Rehmannia Decoction (*bǎi hé dì huáng tāng*) is not powerful enough to restore the patient to health. Thus the present line suggests that in addition to oral medication, the patient should also be given a bathing formula. Because the lung is connected with the skin and body hair their qì communicate. Soaking the body in Lily Bulb Wash (*bǎi hé xǐ fāng*) can reinforce the yīn-nourishing and heat-clearing effect of the oral medication.

The directions furthermore recommend eating boiled cake (noodles), as the qì of wheat is able to nourish the humor of the heart; and warn against consuming salty fermented beans, an aged condiment that can damage yīn-blood.

Line 3.7

百合病渴不差者，栝蒌牡蛎散主之。

栝蒌根　牡蛎（熬）等分

右为细末，饮服方寸匕，日三服。

Bǎi hé bìng kě bù chài zhě, guā lóu mǔ lì sǎn zhǔ zhī.

Guā lóu gēn; mǔ lì (áo) děng fèn

Yòu wéi xì mò, yǐn fú fāng cùn bǐ, rì sān fú.

If hundred-union disease with thirst fails to improve, Trichosanthes and Oyster Shell Powder (栝蒌牡蛎散 *guā lóu mǔ lì sǎn*) governs.

Trichosanthes and Oyster Shell Powder (栝蒌牡蛎散 *guā lóu mǔ lì sǎn*)
trichosanthes (栝楼 *guā lóu*, Trichosanthis Fructus) oyster shell (牡蛎 *mǔ lì*, Ostreae Concha) (simmer)

Make a fine powder with equal amounts of the above [ingredients]. Take a square-inch-spoonful in liquid,[1] three times a day.

TEXT NOTE, LINE 3.7

[1] Take a square-inch-spoonful 服方寸匕 *fú fāng cùn bǐ*: See Weights and Measures in the Introduction.

SYNOPSIS, LINE 3.7

This line describes the treatment in cases where a patient fails to recover from hundred-union disease with thirst.

COMMENTARY, LINE 3.7

This line is a continuation of the two previous lines. It explains how to treat persistent hundred-union disease with thirst that fails to resolve even after the patient has taken the two preceding internal and external medications recommended. The fact that the patient fails to recover suggests that the heat is exuberant and damage to liquid is severe; stronger medication is needed. The formula suggested here is Trichosanthes and Oyster Shell Powder (*guā lóu mǔ lì sǎn*).

Within the formula, cold bitter trichosanthes (*guā lóu*) clears lung and stomach heat, while also engendering liquid and allaying thirst. Cold salty oyster shell (*mǔ lì*) conducts the heat downwards, so that it does not flame upward and scorch the fluids. After the formula has engendered fluids and cleared the vacuity heat, the thirst resolves of its own accord.

Line 3.8

百合病变发热者，百合滑石散主之。

百合（炙）一两　滑石三两

右为散，饮服方寸匕，日三服，当微利者，止服，热则除。

Bǎi hé bìng biàn fā rè zhě, bǎi hé huá shí sǎn zhǔ zhī.

Bǎi hé (zhì) yī liǎng; huá shí sān liǎng

Yòu wéi sǎn, yǐn fú fāng cùn bǐ, rì sān fú, dāng wēi lì zhěn, zhǐ fú, rè zé chú.

If hundred-union disease transmutes into heat effusion,[1] Lily Bulb and Talcum Powder (百合滑石散 *bǎi hé huá shí sǎn*) governs.

Lily Bulb and Talcum Powder (百合滑石散 *bǎi hé huá shí sǎn*)
lily bulb (百合 *bǎi hé*, Lilii Bulbus) 1 *liǎng* (mix-fry) talcum (滑石 *huá shí*, Talcum) 3 *liǎng*

Pulverize the above [ingredients]. Take a square-inch-spoonful in liquid, three times a day. When slight diarrhea appears, stop taking [this formula]. The heat has been eliminated.

TEXT NOTE, LINE 3.8

1. An alternative version of the text has: 发寒热 *fā hán rè* "[aversion] to cold and heat effusion," that is, alternating fever and chills.

SYNOPSIS, LINE 3.8

This line describes the treatment of hundred-union disease that has transmuted into heat effusion.

COMMENTARY, LINE 3.8

Hundred-union disease is characterized by "[signs] resembling a cold condition but without cold," and "[signs] resembling a heat condition but without heat." If heat effusion arises, it is because the disease has lasted for a long time and the internal heat has grown more exuberant, so that it reaches out to the skin. The resulting heat effusion takes the form of heat in the five hearts (soles, palms, and chest) and post-meridian generalized heat effusion. It is accompanied by short rough voidings of scant urine. This condition is treated with Lily Bulb and Talcum Powder (*bǎi hé huá shí sǎn*).

Within this formula, lily bulb (*bǎi hé*) is the chief medicinal, nourishing lung yīn and clearing the upper source of heat. It is supported by talcum (*huá shí*), which clears the internal heat and disinhibits urine, allowing the heat to be discharged through the urine. When the urine is freed, the internal heat is eliminated and the exterior heat resolves naturally.

Line 3.9

百合病见于阴者，以阳法救之；见于阳者，以阴法救之。见阳攻阴，复发其汗，此为逆；见阴攻阳乃复下之，此亦为逆。

Bǎi hé bìng jiàn yú yīn zhě, yǐ yáng fǎ jiù zhī; jiàn yú yáng zhě, yǐ yīn fǎ jiù zhī. Jiàn yáng gōng yīn, fù fā qí hàn, cǐ wéi nì; jiàn yīn gōng yáng nǎi fù xià zhī, cǐ yì wéi nì.

If hundred-union disease manifests in yīn, rescue it by the yáng method; if it manifests in yáng, rescue it by the yīn method. If it manifests in yáng and you attack yīn and further promote sweating, this is an adverse treatment. If it manifests in yīn and you attack yáng and further precipitate, this is also an adverse treatment.

SYNOPSIS, LINE 3.9

This line discusses principles for treating hundred-union disease.

COMMENTARY, LINE 3.9

The use of the terms yīn and yáng in this line is ambiguous and has given rise to disagreement among scholars. There are three interpretations:

According to Xú Zhōng-Kě 徐忠可, "yīn" and "yáng" means vacuity of yīn liquid and exuberant yáng heat respectively, while "yáng method" and "yīn method" are taken to mean draining heat and nourishing yīn respectively.

According to Táng Róng-Chuān 唐容川 and Táo Bǎo-Sūn 陶葆荪, "yīn" and "yáng" mean exterior and interior respectively, while "yáng method" means clearing the exterior and "yīn method" means clearing the interior.

According to Wèi Niàn-Tíng 魏念庭 and Wú Qiān 吴謙, "yīn" and "yáng" refer to yīn exuberance due to yáng vacuity and yáng hyperactivity due to yīn vacuity, while "yáng method" and "yīn method" mean warming yáng and nourishing yīn respectively.

In every one of the variations of hundred-union disease discussed in the eight preceding lines, the disease takes the form of yīn vacuity with internal heat, which is treated by nourishing yīn and clearing heat. Of the above three interpretations, the first therefore makes fullest sense: "Manifesting in yīn" means that the disease manifests primarily as vacuity of yīn liquid, while "manifesting in yáng" means that it manifests primarily as exuberant yáng heat. In this case, "yáng method" means discharging heat, while "yīn method" means nourishing yīn.

Line 3.10

狐惑之为病，状如伤寒，默默欲眠，目不得闭，卧起不安。蚀于喉为惑，蚀于阴为狐，不欲饮食，恶闻食臭，其面目乍赤、乍黑、乍白，蚀于上部则声喝，甘草泻心汤主之。

甘草四两　黄芩　人参　干姜各三两
黄连一两　大枣十二枚　半夏半升

右七味，水一斗，煮取六升，去滓，再煎温服一升，日三服。

Hú huò zhī wéi bìng, zhuàng rú shāng hán, mò mò yù mián, mù bù dé bì, wò qǐ bù ān. Shí yú hóu wéi huò, shí yú yīn wéi hú, bù yù yǐn shí, wù wén shí chòu, qí miàn mù zhà chì, zhà hēi, zhà bái, shí yú shàng bù zé shēng yè, gān cǎo xiè xīn tāng zhǔ zhī.

Gān cǎo sì liǎng; huáng qín sān liǎng; rén shēn sān liǎng; gān jiāng gè sān liǎng; huáng lián yī liǎng; dà zǎo shí èr méi; bàn xià bàn shēng.

Yòu qī wèi, shuǐ yī dǒu, zhǔ qǔ liù shēng, qù zǐ, zài jiān wēn fú yī shēng, rì sān fú.

The disease of fox-creeper manifests in signs resembling cold damage, with taciturnity and desire to sleep, inability to close the eyes, and disquietude whether lying down or being up. If it erodes the throat, it is called "creeper";[1] if it erodes the yīn [parts],[2] it is called "fox." [It further manifests with] no desire to eat or drink, aversion to the odor of food, and face and eyes that are now red, now black, now white. If [the disease] erodes the upper [body][3] and the voice is husky, Licorice Heart-Draining Decoction (甘草泻心汤 *gān cǎo xiè xīn tāng*) governs.

Licorice Heart-Draining Decoction (甘草泻心汤 *gān cǎo xiè xīn tāng*)
licorice (甘草 *gān cǎo*, Glycyrrhizae Radix) 4 *liǎng* scutellaria (黄芩 *huáng qín*, Scutellariae Radix) 3 *liǎng*

ginseng (人参 *rén shēn*, Ginseng Radix) 3 *liǎng*
dried ginger (干姜 *gān jiāng*, Zingiberis Rhizoma) 3 *liǎng*
coptis (黄连 *huáng lián*, Coptidis Rhizoma) 1 *liǎng*
jujube (大枣 *dà zǎo*, Jujubae Fructus) 12 fruits
pinellia (半夏 *bàn xià*, Pinelliae Rhizoma) ½ *shēng*

Boil the above [ingredients] with one *dǒu* of water to get six *shēng*. Remove the dregs and boil again. Take a dose of one *shēng* warm three times a day.

TEXT NOTES, LINE 3.10

[1] Fox-creeper 狐惑 *hú huò*: See the introduction to this chapter.

[2] Yīn [parts] 阴 *yīn*: The anus and genitals.

[3] The upper [body] 上 *shàng*: The throat.

SYNOPSIS, LINE 3.10

This line discusses the signs of fox-creeper and the method of treating erosion of the throat.

COMMENTARY, LINE 3.10

Fox-creeper is a disease characterized by ulceration of the flesh in the throat and two yīn. As the text says, erosion of the throat is called "creeper," while erosion of the two yīn (anus and genitals) is called "fox." As pointed out in the introduction, the term "fox" and "creeper" may allude to worms believed to gnaw or erode the flesh. The only evidence we have for Zhāng-Jī's belief in such worms is his use of 蚀 *shí*, literally "eat," "gnaw," and by extension, "erode." In any event, the existence of such "worms" would have been the product of speculation since the disease is associated with no living organisms that can be seen with the naked eye.

The lesions associated with fox-creeper are the result of damp-heat congesting the qì dynamic. Commentators interpret the resemblance to cold damage as referring to heat effusion and aversion to cold, which arises as right qì and evil qì vie for supremacy. Brewing damp-heat affects the heart spirit, giving rise to taciturnity and desire to sleep. However, the patient is fidgety and cannot close the eyes or sleep in peace.

Damp-heat obstructs the qì dynamic of the spleen and stomach, hence there is no thought of food and drink, and in serious cases the patient does not even want to smell food. When damp-heat has lain depressed for a long time, construction-blood is damaged, hence the face and eyes are sometimes red, sometimes black, and sometimes white. When the damp-heat lies depressed in the upper body, it causes ulceration of the throat, a condition that is called creeper; when damp-heat flows downward, it causes ulceration of the two yīn, in which case the condition is called "fox." When the throat is affected, the voice turns hoarse. This is treated by clearing heat and drying dampness, and by resolving toxin and supporting right. The suggested formula is Licorice Heart-Draining Decoction (*gān cǎo xiè xīn tāng*).

Within the formula, licorice (*gān cǎo*) clears heat and resolves toxin. It is combined with scutellaria (*huáng qín*) and coptis (*huáng lián*), which are both bitter and downbearing. They clear heat, dry dampness, and resolve toxin. Dried ginger (*gān jiāng*) and pinellia (*bàn xià*) are acrid opening medicinals; they not only dry dampness, but also regulate the qì dynamic. This combination as a whole achieves the goal of transforming dampness, clearing heat, and regulating the qì dynamic, thereby eliminating evil and restoring right.

Line 3.11

蚀于下部则咽干，苦参汤洗之。

苦参一升以水一斗，煎取七升，去滓熏洗，日三服。

Shí yú xià bù zé yān gān, kǔ shēn tāng xǐ zhī.

Kǔ shēn yī shēng yǐ shuǐ yī dǒu, jiān qǔ qī shēng, qù zǐ xūn xǐ, rì sān fú.

If [the disease] erodes the lower parts, the pharynx becomes dry. [Treat this by] bathing it with Flavescent Sophora Decoction (苦参汤 *kǔ shēn tāng*).

Boil one *shēng* of flavescent sophora (*kǔ shēn*) in one *dǒu* of water to get seven *shēng*. Remove the dregs. [Use this to] steam and bathe [the genitals] three times a day.

Synopsis, Line 3.11

This line offers a method of treating erosion of the anterior yīn (genitals) in fox-creeper.

Commentary, Line 3.11

The foot reverting yīn liver vessel skirts around the genitals and also passes alongside the throat. We can explain the presence of ulceration of the genitals in combination with dry throat as heat toxin surging up the liver channel into the throat. When Flavescent Sophora Decoction (*kǔ shēn tāng*) is used to steam and bathe the genitals, it kills worms, resolves toxin, and transforms dampness. Since this formula addressed the root of the disease, when the ulceration heals, the dryness of the throat naturally disappears.

Line 3.12

蚀于肛者，雄黄熏之。

雄黄

右一味为末，筒瓦二枚合之，烧向肛熏之。

Shí yú gāng zhě, xióng huáng xūn zhī.

Xióng huáng

Yòu yī wèi wéi mò, tǒng wǎ èr méi gě zhī, shāo xiàng gāng xūn zhī.

If [the disease] erodes the anus, fumigate with realgar (*xióng huáng*).

realgar (雄黄 *xióng huáng*)

Pulverize the realgar (*xióng huáng*). Place two concave tiles together to form a tube and burn [the realgar] in this to fumigate the anus.

SYNOPSIS, LINE 3.12

This line describes the treatment of fox-creeper eroding the anus.

COMMENTARY, LINE 3.12

When fox-creeper affects the anus to the point of causing ulceration, the text recommends fumigation with realgar (*xióng huáng*). Similar to the action of flavescent sophora (*kǔ shēn*) in the preceding line, realgar has a strong worm-killing, toxin-resolving, and dampness-drying action that is effective for this condition. Since erosion of the anus is caused by damp-heat toxin flowing into the lower body, external fumigation with realgar can therefore be successfully combined with internal consumption of heat-clearing, dampness-drying, and toxin-resolving medicinals.

Line 3.13

病者脉数，无热微烦，默默但欲卧，汗出。初得之三四日，目赤如鸠眼，七八日目四眦黑；若能食者，脓已成也。赤小豆当归散主之。

赤小豆（浸令芽出，曝干）三升当归

右二味，杵为散，浆水服方寸匕，日三服。

Bìng zhě mài shuò, wú rè wēi fán, mò mò dàn yù wò, hàn chū. Chū dé zhī sān sì rì, mù chì rú jiū yǎn, qī bā rì mù sì zì hēi; ruò néng shí zhě, nóng yǐ chéng yě. Chì xiǎo dòu dāng guī sǎn zhǔ zhī.

Chì xiǎo dòu (jìn lìng yá chū, pù gān) sān shēng; dāng guī

Yòu èr wèi, chǔ wéi sǎn, jiāng shuǐ fú fāng cùn bǐ, rì sān fú.

This disease can manifest in a rapid pulse, absence of heat [effusion],[1] slight vexation, taciturnity, desire only to sleep, and sweating. Initially, when [this condition] has lasted only for three or four days, the eyes become red like [those of a] turtle-dove.[2] After seven or eight days, the four canthi[3] of the eyes turn black.[4] If [the patient] is able to eat, this indicates that pus has formed. Rice Bean and Chinese Angelica Powder (赤小豆当归散 *chì xiǎo dòu dāng guī sǎn*) governs.

Rice Bean and Chinese Angelica Powder (赤小豆当归散 *chì xiǎo dòu dāng guī sǎn*)
rice bean (赤小豆 *chì xiǎo dòu*, Phaseoli Semen) 3 *shēng* (soak, allow to sprout, and sun-dry)

Chinese angelica (当归 *dāng guī*, Angelicae Sinensis Radix) [no quantity given in source text]

Pestle the above two [ingredients] into a powder. Take a square-inch-spoonful in sour rice milk,[5] three times a day.

TEXT NOTES, LINE 3.13

[1] Absence of heat [effusion] 无热 *wú rè*: Most commentators interpret this as absence of [aversion to] cold and heat [effusion] (无寒热 *wú hán rè*).

[2] Eyes become red like [those of] turtledoves 目赤如鸠 *mù chì rú bān jiū*: The turtledove has red eyes.

[3] Four canthi 四眦 *sì zì*: The inner and outer canthi (i.e., corners) of each eye.

[4] 目四眦黑 *mù sì zì hēi*: An alternative version of this text has "yellow" (黄 *huáng*) instead of black.

[5] Sour rice milk 浆水 *jiāng shuǐ*: The *Běn Cǎo Gāng Mù* ("Herbal Foundation Compendium") gives *jiāng shuǐ* as a synonym for 酸浆 *suān jiāng* and explains that this substance is prepared by steaming rice and letting it soak in cold water for 5 or 6 days until it is fermented to the point of resembling starch water. Some modern texts wrongly equate this product with vinegar. Although the synonym 醋浆水 *cù jiāng shuǐ* contain the word 醋 *cù* meaning vinegar (as in line 20.10), the process described does not result in what would be called vinegar.

SYNOPSIS, LINE 3.13

This line discusses the signs and treatment of fox-creeper that brews and binds to produce pus.

COMMENTARY, LINE 3.13

In line 3.10 above, fox-creeper disease was described as resembling cold damage. However, it is not caused by cold damage, but by damp-heat binding into toxin and invading the blood aspect. Hence in this line, "absence of heat [effusion]" indicates that there is no heat effusion (or aversion to cold) in the fleshy exterior. The heat toxin has entered the interior, harassing the spirit and giving rise to a rapid pulse, absence of heat [effusion], slight vexation, taciturnity, and desire only to sleep.

The liver stores the blood and opens at the eyes. When heat toxin harasses the blood aspect, it flames upward along the liver channel, giving rise to red eyes that look like the eyes of a turtledove. When heat toxin brews and binds in the blood aspect, it causes heat stasis and putrefaction of the blood. After seven or eight days of this, the canthi therefore turn black as a result. If the patient is able to eat at this stage, it means that the qì dynamic in the spleen and stomach is barely affected, because the heat toxin is binding primarily in the blood aspect.

In this condition, the appropriate formula is Rice Bean and Chinese Angelica Powder (*chì xiǎo dòu dāng guī sǎn*). Within this formula, rice bean (*chì xiǎo dòu*) percolates dampness and clears heat; it also resolves toxin and expels pus. Chinese angelica (*dāng guī*) quickens the blood, eliminates stasis, and engenders the new. Sour rice milk (*jiāng shuǐ*) has a clearing, cooling, toxin-resolving action.

Line 3.14

阳毒之为病，面赤斑斑如锦纹，咽喉痛，唾脓血。五日可治，七日不可治，升麻鳖甲汤主之。

升麻二两　当归一两　蜀椒（炒去汗）一两　甘草二两　鳖甲（炙）手指大一片　雄黄（研）半两

右六味，以水四升煮取一升，顿服之，老小再服。取汗。

Yáng dú zhī wéi bìng, miàn chì bān bān rú jǐn wén, yān hóu tòng, tuò nóng xuè. Wǔ rì kě zhì, qī rì bù kě zhì, shēng má biē jiǎ tāng zhǔ zhī.

Shēng má èr liǎng; dāng guī yī liǎng; shǔ jiāo (chǎo qù hàn) yī liǎng gān cǎo èr liǎng; biē jiǎ (zhì) shǒu zhǐ dà yī piàn; xióng huáng (yán) bàn liǎng.

Yòu liù wèi, yǐ shuǐ sì shēng zhǔ qǔ yī shēng, dùn fú zhī, lǎo xiǎo zài fú. Qǔ hàn.

The disease of yáng toxin manifests in a face that is red with patches like brocade, sore throat, and spitting of pus and blood. It is treatable within [the first] five days [but by the] seventh day it cannot be treated. Cimicifuga and Turtle Shell Decoction (升麻鳖甲汤 *shēng má biē jiǎ tāng*) governs.

Cimicifuga and Turtle Shell Decoction (升麻鳖甲汤 *shēng má biē jiǎ tāng*)

- cimicifuga (升麻 *shēng má*, Cimicifugae Rhizoma) 2 *liǎng*
- Chinese angelica (当归 *dāng guī*, Angelicae Sinensis Radix) 1 *liǎng*
- zanthoxylum (蜀椒 *shǔ jiāo*, Zanthoxyli Pericarpium) 1 *liǎng* (stir-fry to remove sweat[1])
- licorice (甘草 *gān cǎo*, Glycyrrhizae Radix) 2 *liǎng*
- turtle shell (鳖甲 *biē jiǎ*, Trionycis Carapax) 1 finger-sized piece (mix-fry)
- realgar (雄黄 *xióng huáng*, Realgar) ½ *liǎng* (grind finely)

Boil the six above ingredients in four *shēng* of water to get one *shēng*. Quaff in one go. Old and young patients should take it in two doses. Promote sweating.[2]

TEXT NOTES, LINE 3.14

[1] Remove sweat 去汗 *qù hàn*: Remove the water and oil.

[2] The *Qiān Jīn Fāng* ("Thousand Gold Pieces Prescriptions") and (*Zhǒu Hòu Bèi Jí Fāng* ("Emergency Standby Remedies") here add: "For yáng toxin, use Cimicifuga Decoction (*shēng má tāng*) minus turtle shell (*biē jiǎ*) and plus cinnamon twig (*guì zhī*); for yīn toxin, use Licorice Decoction (*gān cǎo tāng*) minus realgar (*xióng huáng*)."

SYNOPSIS, LINE 3.14

This line discusses the signs and treatment of yáng toxin.

COMMENTARY, LINE 3.14

Yīn-yáng toxin is caused by contracting epidemic heat toxin. The disease can take two forms: yīn toxin and yáng toxin. As mentioned in the chapter introduction, the significance of yīn and yáng in this context is not completely clear, but the two forms are differentiated by their specific symptoms, particularly the depth to which the toxin has penetrated and the color of the facial complexion.

The present line deals with yáng toxin. The main signs of yáng toxin are red face with patches like brocade, sore throat, and spitting of pus and blood. These signs are due to epidemic toxin affecting the construction aspect. When heat forces construction-blood outward, the face becomes red and blotchy. The sore throat is due to epidemic toxin gathering and binding in the throat and causing local qì stagnation and blood stasis. When epidemic heat toxin exuberates, it cause putrefaction of the blood and flesh; hence we see spitting of pus and blood.

Disease caused by epidemic toxin develops rapidly, so it requires early treatment. As it progresses, it becomes harder to treat. This is why the text says that it can be treated within the first five days, but not after the seventh. The number of days is only a rough guide.

The principles of treating disease caused by epidemic toxin are to clear heat and resolve toxin. When the epidemic toxin reaches construction-blood, it can cause blood stasis. This requires treatment by enriching yīn and moving the blood. The recommended formula is Cimicifuga and Turtle Shell Decoction (*shēng má biē jiǎ tāng*), which can be varied according to need. Within the formula, cimicifuga (*shēng má*) and licorice (*gān cǎo*) clear heat and resolve toxin. Turtle shell (*biē jiǎ*) and Chinese angelica (*dāng guī*) enrich yīn and disperse stasis. Because the disease is in the case of yáng toxin located in the exterior, realgar (*xióng huáng*) and zanthoxylum (*shǔ jiāo*) are used for their acrid nature to outthrust the toxin. In the case of yīn toxin, the disease is located in the interior and cannot be outthrust. Therefore the acrid medicinals realgar and zanthoxylum are removed from the formula for yīn toxin, because these can consume blood and damage yīn.

Line 3.15

阴毒之为病，面目青，身痛如被杖，咽喉痛。五日可治，七日不可治，升麻鳖甲汤去雄黄、蜀椒主之。

Yīn dú zhī wéi bìng, miàn mù qīng, shēn tòng rú bèi zhàng, yān hóu tòng. Wǔ rì kě zhì, qī rì bù kě zhì, shēng má biē jiǎ tāng qù xióng huáng, shǔ jiāo zhǔ zhī.

The disease of yīn toxin manifests in a green-blue face and eyes, generalized pain as though having been beaten by a stick, and sore throat. Within [the first] five days it can be treated, [but by the] seventh day, it cannot be treated. Cimicifuga and Turtle Shell Decoction (*shēng má biē jiǎ tāng*) minus realgar (*xióng huáng*) and zanthoxylum (*shǔ jiāo*) governs.

Synopsis, Line 3.15

This line discusses the signs and treatment of yīn toxin.

Commentary, Line 3.15

The present line deals with yīn toxin. The main signs of yīn toxin are blue-green facial complexion, generalized pain, and sore throat. When the disease toxin invades the blood and vessels, blood stasis arises and causes blockage, hence the green-blue facial complexion. In accordance with the principle "when there is stoppage, there is pain," this blockage due to blood stasis also accounts for the generalized pain. When the epidemic toxin binds in the throat, there is local pain.

The text in this line recommends the same toxin-resolving stasis-dispersing formula, Cimicifuga and Turtle Shell Decoction (*shēng má biē jiǎ tāng*) as for yáng toxin in the preceding line. However, we should remove realgar (*xióng huáng*) and zanthoxylum (*huā jiāo*) from the formula to prevent damage to yīn qì. Again, as in the preceding line, the disease becomes more difficult to treat as it advances.

疟病脉证治第四

CHAPTER 4

Malaria

Pulses, Signs, Treatments

‡ Overview

The present chapter concerns the diagnosis and treatment of malaria, a disease that is here characterized by episodes of vigorous heat effusion followed by aversion to cold and shivering resolved by sweating. This traditional notion is wider than the modern medical concept denoted by the English term malaria and the Chinese term 瘧疾 *nüè jí*. For this reason, while retaining the familiar term malaria, we suggest the literal translation "torment disease" as a possibly superior term.

The oldest Chinese character dictionary, the *Shuō Wén Jiě Zì* ("Explanation of Simple Graphs and Complex Characters"), explains the Chinese term 疟 *nüè*, translated here as malaria, as "cold and heat occurring at intervals" (寒热休作 *hán rè xiū zuò*, literally "pausing and arising"). The *Shì Míng* ("Explanation of Terms") explains the literal meaning of the character as "cruel torment" (酷虐 *kù nüè*). The character is composed of 虐, meaning to abuse or torment, combined with the illness signific (疒). The literal meaning of the character thus reflects the continuing torture that the disease often inflicts on its victims. Note that the English term malaria is derived from the Italian for "bad air," reflecting the environmental conditions it is associated with in the European tradition. Malaria was recognized in China (as in the pre-modern West) by presenting signs. In modern times, the term malaria has been redefined to mean a disease caused by the various protozoans of the genus *Plasmodium*—a somewhat narrower interpretation than that of traditional Chinese medicine.

On the basis of different pulse presentations, the present chapter offers specific treatments including sweating, ejection, precipitation, warming, needling, moxibustion, and dietary adjustment. The *Jīn Guì Yào Lüè* therefore represents an impressive advance in knowledge over the *Nèi Jīng* ("The Inner Canon"), which merely noted its characteristic sign of alternating heat and cold. The *Jīn Guì Yào Lüè* classifies malaria into three types as pure-heat malaria (瘅疟 *dàn nüè*), warm malaria (温疟 *wēn nüè*), and female malaria (牝疟 *pìn nüè*) according to the relative dominance of heat effusion and aversion to cold. It also points out that malaria, when persisting for a long time, can cause mother of malaria (疟母 *nüè mǔ*), an abdominal mass that is now referred to as splenomegaly in modern medicine.

The present chapter consists of comparatively few lines. However, it builds on the *Nèi Jīng* understanding to present a comprehensive explanation of the pathomechanisms, signs, pulses, and various forms of the disease. Thus the *Jīn Guì Yào Lüè* provided the basis for the development of discourse on malaria for subsequent generations of physicians.

Schematic Overview

Malaria

1. Pulse and treatment method

   a) Main pulse: naturally stringlike—evil in the liver and gallbladder

   b) Concurrent pulse

      Stringlike and slightly tight: Disease in the interior; treat with precipitation.

      Stringlike and tight: Disease in the exterior; promote sweating (with acupuncture or medicinals).

      Stringlike and slow: disease due to cold; treat by warming.

      Stringlike and rapid: Disease due to heat; wind is erupting. Treat by clearing; judicious eating.

      Floating and large: Disease in the upper body; treat with ejection.

2. Prognosis and outcomes: Malaria that breaks out on the first of each month should subside by the fifteenth day. If not, it should resolve by the end of the month. If the patient does not recover… this [means that the disease] is binding into a concretion or conglomeration. It is called mother of malaria.

3. Pattern identification

   a) Pure-heat malaria

      Pathomechanism: Heat in both exterior and interior with severe heat damaging liquid.

      Main signs: Heat only without cold.

      Method of treatment: Clear heat and engender liquid.

      Formula: White Tiger Decoction Plus Ginseng (*bái hǔ jiā rén shēn tāng*), etc.

b) Warm malaria

Pathomechanism: Intense internal heat with unresolved exterior evil.

Main signs: Generalized heat with slight aversion to cold, vexing pain in the joints, with a pulse that sometimes tends to be stringlike.

Method of treatment: Clear heat and engender liquid; resolve the exterior and dispel evil.

Formula: White Tiger Decoction Plus Cinnamon Twig (*bái hǔ jiā guì zhī tāng*), etc.

c) Female malaria

Pathomechanism: Phlegm-rheum collecting internally with yáng qì becoming depressed.

Main signs: Pronounced cold with mild heat.

Method of treatment: Dispel phlegm and check malaria.

Formula: Dichroa Leaf Powder (*shǔ qī sǎn*). For slight heat, use Bupleurum, Cinnamon Twig, and Dried Ginger Decoction (*chái hú guì jiāng tāng*); if there are exterior signs, use Oyster Shell Decoction (*mǔ lì tāng*).

d) Mother of malaria

Pathomechanism: Enduring illness with vacuity of right qì and phlegm-stasis gathering and binding.

Main signs: Glomus lump under the rib-sides.

Method of treatment: Break stasis and transform phlegm; support right and clear the concretion.

Formula: Turtle Shell Decocted Pill (*biē jiǎ jiān wán*).

e) Taxation malaria

Pathomechanism: Evil in lesser yáng, severe heat damaging liquid.

Main signs: Alternating heat and cold occurring at set times, with thirst and desire to drink.

Method of treatment: Harmonize lesser yáng; clear heat and engender liquid.

Formula: Bupleurum Decoction Minus Pinellia Plus Trichosanthes Root (*chái hú qù bàn xià jiā guā lóu tāng*).

Line 4.1

师曰：疟脉自弦，弦数者多热，弦迟者多寒。弦小紧者下之差，弦迟者可温之，弦紧者可发汗、针灸也，浮大者可吐之，弦数者风发也，以饮食消息止之。

Shī yuē: Nüè mài zì xiān, xián shuò zhě duō rè, xián chí zhě duō hán. Xián xiǎo jǐn zhě xià zhī chài, xián chí zhě kě wēn zhī, xián jǐn zhě kě fā hàn, zhēn jiǔ yě, fú dà zhě kě tù zhī, xián shuò zhě fēng fā yě, yǐ yǐn shí xiāo xī zhǐ zhī.

The Master says: "The pulse of malaria is naturally stringlike. When it is stringlike and rapid, [this indicates] mostly heat [effusion]; when it is stringlike and slow, [this indicates] mostly [aversion to] cold. When it is stringlike, small, and tight, [treat] it with precipitation, and [the patient] will recover. When it is stringlike and slow, you can [treat it by] warming. When it is stringlike and tight, you can [treat it by] promoting sweating, and with acupuncture and moxibustion. When it is floating and large, you can [treat it with] ejection. When it is stringlike and rapid, [this indicates that] wind is erupting.[1] You can stop this with a judicious diet."

TEXT NOTE, CHAPTER 4.1

[1] Wind is erupting 风发 *fēng fā*: "Wind" denotes a specific evil qì (as in "wind-damp," "wind-cold"), but can also refer to yáng evils as a whole, or evil qì in general. Here it refers to the exuberant heat of malaria.

SYNOPSIS, CHAPTER 4.1

This line identifies the patterns of malaria and explains its etiology through the pulse.

COMMENTARY, CHAPTER 4.1

The basic pathomechanism of malaria is evil in lesser yáng, which is usually characterized by a stringlike pulse. Thus the text says, "The pulse of malaria is naturally stringlike." However, due to different constitutions and causes of the disease, the stringlike pulse invariably appears in combination with other pulse conditions. For example, when heat effusion is more pronounced than aversion to cold, the pulse is stringlike and rapid; if aversion to cold is more pronounced, the pulse will be stringlike and slow.

Malaria can affect the patient in different ways and undergo a number of transmutations and transformations. It may tend to affect the exterior or the interior, the upper body or the lower body; it may tend toward heat or cold. A pulse that is stringlike, small, and tight indicates that the disease is primarily in the interior. There is usually concurrent food stagnation, which can be treated by judicious use of precipitation (although not necessarily precipitation of the powerful variety as exemplified by qì-coordinating formulas).

A pulse that is floating and large indicates that the disease tends to be in the exterior and can be treated by the judicious use of ejection. Stringlike and tight, and stringlike and slow pulses both indicate cold. However, a stringlike and tight pulse suggests that the disease tends to be in the exterior and is associated with contraction of wind-cold. This can be treated by promoting sweating, if necessary in combination with acupuncture and moxibustion. A stringlike and slow pulse indicates interior cold, which is treated by warming. A pulse that is stringlike and rapid indicates intense interior heat and that the evil is yáng in nature and may engender wind. Hence the text says "wind is erupting." This can be treated by a diet of sweet and cold foods.

Line 4.2

病疟，以月一日发，当以十五日愈；设不差，当月尽解；如其不差，当云何？师曰：此结为癥瘕，名曰疟母，急治之，宜鳖甲煎丸。

鳖甲（炙）十二分　乌扇（烧）三分　黄芩三分　柴胡六分　鼠妇（熬）三分　干姜三分　大黄三分　芍药五分　桂枝三分　葶苈（熬）一分　石苇（去毛）三分　厚朴三分 牡丹（去心）五分瞿麦二分　紫葳三分　半夏一分　人参一分　蟅虫（熬）五分　阿胶（炙）三分　蜂窝（炙）四分　赤硝十二分　蜣螂（熬）六分　桃仁二分

右二十三味，为末，取煅灶下灰一斗，清酒一斛五斗，浸灰，候酒尽一半，着鳖甲于中，煮令泛烂如胶漆，绞取汁，内诸药，煎为丸如梧子大，空心服七丸，日三服。

Bìng nüè, yǐ yuè yī rì fā, dāng yǐ shí wǔ rì yù shè bù chài, dāng yuè jìn jiě; rú qí bù chài, dāng yún hé? Shī yuē: Cǐ jié wéi zhēng jiǎ, míng yuē nüè mǔ, jí zhì zhī, yí biē jiǎ jiān wán.

Biē jiǎ (zhì) shí èr fēn; wū shàn (shāo) sān fēn; huáng qín sān fēn; chái hú liù fēn; shǔ fù (áo) sān fēn; gān jiāng sān fēn; dà huáng sān fēn; sháo yào wǔ fēn guì zhī sān fēn; tíng lì (áo) yī fēn; shí wěi (qù máo) sān fēn; hòu pò sān fēn mǔ dān (qù xīn) wǔ fēn; qú mài èr fēn zǐ wēi sān fēn; bàn xià yī fēn; rén shēn yī fēn; zhè chóng (áo) wǔ fēn; ē jiāo (zhì) sān fēn; fēng cháo (zhì) sì fēn; chì xiāo shí èr fēn; qiāng láng (áo) liù fēn; táo rén èr fēn.

Yòu èr shí sān wèi, wéi mò, qǔ duàn zào xià huī yī dǒu, qīng jiǔ yī hú wǔ dǒu, jìn huī, hòu jiǔ jìn yī bàn, zhù biē jiǎ yú zhōng, zhǔ lìng fàn làn rú jiāo qī, jiǎo qǔ zhī, nà zhū yào, jiān wéi wán rú wú zǐ dà, kōng xīn fú qī wán, rì sān fú.

"Malaria that erupts on the first of each month[1] should subside by the fifteenth day. If not, it should resolve by the end of the month. If the patient does not recover, what should we call this [disease]?" The Master says: "This [means that the disease] is binding into concretions or conglomerations.[2] It is called mother of malaria. Treat this urgently. Turtle Shell Decocted Pill (鳖甲煎丸 *biē jiǎ jiān wán*) is appropriate."

Turtle Shell Decocted Pill
(鳖甲煎丸 *biē jiǎ jiān wán*)

turtle shell (鳖甲 *biē jiǎ*, Trionycis Carapax) 12 parts (mix-fry)
belamcanda (乌扇 *wū shàn*, Belamcandae Rhizoma)[3] 3 parts (burn)
scutellaria (黄芩 *huáng qín*, Scutellariae Radix) 3 parts
bupleurum (柴胡 *chái hú*, Bupleuri Radix) 6 parts
wood louse (鼠妇 *shǔ fù*, Armadillidium) 3 parts (simmer)
dried ginger (干姜 *gān jiāng*, Zingiberis Rhizoma) 3 parts
rhubarb (大黄 *dà huáng*, Rhei Radix et Rhizoma) 3 parts
peony (芍药 *sháo yào*, Paeoniae Radix) 5 parts
cinnamon twig (桂枝 *guì zhī*, Cinnamomi Ramulus) 3 parts
lepidium/descurainiae (葶苈 *tíng lì*, Lepidii/Descurainiae Semen) 1 part (simmer)
pyrrosia (石韦 *shí wéi*, Pyrrosiae Folium) 3 parts (remove hair)
officinal magnolia bark (厚朴 *hòu pò*, Magnoliae Officinalis Cortex) 3 parts
moutan (牡丹 *mǔ dān*, Moutan Cortex) 5 parts (remove heart)
dianthus (瞿麦 *qú mài*, Dianthi Herba) 2 parts
campsis flower (紫葳 *zǐ wēi*, Campsis Flos)[4] 3 parts
pinellia (半夏 *bàn xià*, Pinelliae Rhizoma) 1 parts
ginseng (人参 *rén shēn*, Ginseng Radix) 1 parts
ground beetle (蟅虫 *zhè chóng*, Eupolyphaga seu Steleophaga) 5 parts (simmer)
ass hide glue (阿胶 *ē jiāo*, Asini Corii Colla) 3 parts (mix-fry)
hornet's nest (蜂窝 *fēng wō*, Vespae Nidus)[5] 4 parts (simmer)
red niter (赤消 *chì xiāo*, Nitrum Rubrum) 12 parts
dung beetle (蜣螂 *qiāng láng*, Catharsius) 6 parts (simmer)
peach kernel (桃仁 *táo rén*, Persicae Semen) 2 parts

Pulverize the above 23 ingredients. Soak one *dǒu* of furnace ash (*zào xià huī*) in one *hú* and five *dǒu* of clear wine (*qīng jiǔ*). Wait until half of the wine has disappeared, then add the turtle shell (*biē jiǎ*) and boil until it is mushy like gluey lacquer. Wring out to obtain the juice. Add all the [other] medicinals to this, boil, and make pills the size of firmiana seeds. Take seven pills on an empty stomach, three times a day.[6]

TEXT NOTES, LINE 4.2

[1] Month 月 *yuè*: A month in the lunar calendar.

[2] Concretions and conglomerations 癥瘕 *zhēng jiǎ*: Concretions are hard glomus lumps that do not move, while conglomerations are glomus lumps that come and go. By this definition, the lump that forms in malaria is actually a concretion.

[3] Belamcanda 屋扇 *wū shàn* (Belamcandae Rhizoma): Nowadays, this medicinal is usually referred to in Chinese as 射干 *shè gān*.

[4] Campsis flower 紫葳 *zǐ wēi* (Campsis Flos): Nowadays, this medicinal is usually referred to in Chinese as 凌霄花 *líng xiāo huā*.

[5] Hornet's nest 蜂窝 *fēng wō* (Vespae Nidus): Nowadays, this medicinal is usually referred to in Chinese as 露蜂房 *lù fēng fáng*.

[6] A comment included in the received text reads:《千金方》用鳖甲十二片，又有海藻三分，大戟一分，蟅虫五分，无鼠妇、赤消二味，以鳖甲煎和

诸药为丸。*«Qiān Jīn Fāng» yòng biē jiǎ shí èr piàn, yòu yǒu hǎi zǎo sān fèn, dà jǐ yī fèn, zhè chóng wǔ fèn, wú shǔ fù, chì xiāo èr wèi, yǐ biē jiǎ jiān huó zhū yào wéi wán.* "The *Qiān Jīn Fāng* ("Thousand Gold Pieces Prescriptions") uses 12 pieces of turtle shell (*biē jiǎ*), 3 parts of sargassum (*hǎi zǎo*), 1 part of euphorbia/knoxia (大戟 *dà jǐ*), 5 parts of ground beetle (*zhè chóng*), but not the two ingredients wood louse (*shǔ fù*) and red niter (*chì xiāo*). All ingredients are boiled with the turtle shell (*biē jiǎ*) and made into pills."

SYNOPSIS, LINE 4.2

This line discusses the prognosis of malaria and the formation and treatment of mother of malaria.

COMMENTARY, LINE 4.2

The present line states that a patient in whom malaria starts on the first day of a lunar month should recover by the 15th day of the month. Failing that, he or she will recover by the end of the month (i.e., after 30 days). In the ancient Chinese calendar, five days formed a *hòu* (候), and three *hòu* formed a solar term (节气 *jié qì*). The early classics emphasized that the human body was closely related to the seasons and that construction, defense, qì, and blood were renewed in each solar term. Hence, we can understand the notion that malaria that is not resolved on the 15th will be resolved on the 30th of the month in terms of the natural waxing and waning of the body's right qì.

If the patient does not recover after a month, this is because a concretion or conglomeration is forming. "Concretion and conglomeration" (癥瘕 *zhēng jiǎ*) is an expression used to denote abdominal masses. The abdominal mass that forms in malaria, which is equivalent to splenomegaly in Western medicine, is given the specific name "mother of malaria" (瘧母 *nüè mǔ*). Mother of malaria forms when the disease persists or when it is inappropriately treated, and right qì weakens gradually, allowing phlegm and static blood to form under the rib-side.

Mother of malaria is a condition of right vacuity and evil repletion. It is a condition that needs to be treated swiftly if it is not to worsen. Hence the text warns the practitioner to treat it urgently. The suggested formula is Turtle Shell Decocted Pill (*biē jiǎ jiān wán*), which both supports right and dispels evil. Since the evil is a combination of phlegm and static blood, the evil-dispelling action of the formula accords with the *Nèi Jīng*'s ("The Inner Canon") principle that "hardness is to be whittled away" (坚者削之 *jiān zhě xiāo zhī*). The formula softens hardness and transforms phlegm on the one hand, and quickens blood and transforms stasis on the other.

Within the formula, turtle shell (*biē jiǎ*) softens hardness and disperses binds; furnace ash (*zào xià huī*) disperses concretions and transforms accumulations. These two medicinals in combination address the problem of the mother of malaria. Peach kernel (*táo rén*), moutan (*mǔ dān pí*), peony (*sháo yào*), campsis flower (*líng xiāo huā*), red niter (*chì xiāo*), rhubarb (*dà huáng*), ground beetle (*zhè chóng*), dung beetle (*qiāng láng*), and hornet's nest (*lù fēng fáng*) break blood and expel stasis, i.e., they have a powerful stasis-dispelling action. Belamcanda (*shè gān*), lepidium/descurainiae (*tíng lì zǐ*), pinellia (*bàn xià*), officinal magnolia bark (*hòu pò*), and bupleurum (*chái hú*) disperse phlegm and rectify qì. Dianthus (*qú mài*) and pyrrosia (*shí wéi*) disinhibit water and thereby guide the evil to be discharged with urine. Dried ginger (*gān jiāng*), cinnamon twig (*guì zhī*), and scutellaria (*huáng qín*) resolve the alternating aversion to cold and heat effusion. Ginseng (*rén shēn*) and ass hide glue (*ē jiāo*) supplement qì and blood. Clear wine (*qīng jiǔ*) frees the blood vessels. Thus the formula as a whole has the effect of dispersing the phlegm and static blood and gradually restoring right qì so that the malaria has no place where it can linger.

Line 4.3

师曰：阴气孤绝，阳气独发，则热而少气烦冤，手足热而欲呕，名曰瘅疟。若但热不寒者，邪气内藏于心，外舍分肉之间，令人消铄肌肉。

Shī yuē: Yīn qì gū jué, yáng qì dú fā, zé rè ér shǎo qì fán yuān, shǒu zú rè ér yù ǒu, míng yuē dàn nüè. Ruò dàn rè bù hán zhě, xié qì nèi cáng yú xīn, wài shè fēn ròu zhī jiān, lìng rén xiāo shuò jī ròu.

The Master says: "When yīn qì[1] alone expires and yáng qì[2] alone effuses, the result is heat [effusion] and shortage of qì with vexation and oppression, heat in the extremities, and desire to retch. [This] is called pure-heat malaria.[3] If there is only heat and no cold, evil qì internally hides in the heart and externally abides in the seams of the flesh.[4] This causes wasting of the person's flesh."

Text Notes, Line 4.3

[1] Yīn qì 阴气 *yīn qì*: The body's yīn humor.

[2] Yáng qì 阳气 *yáng qì*: Heat evil.

[3] Pure-heat malaria 瘅疟 *dān nüè*: Malaria characterized by heat without cold.

[4] Seams of the flesh 分肉 *fēn ròu*: The Chinese concept of flesh includes both white layers of flesh (fat) and red layers (muscle) in clearly distinct seams. The term "seams of the flesh" here refers to both seams, i.e., the flesh as a whole.

Synopsis, Line 4.3

This line describes the pathomechanism and signs of pure-heat malaria.

Commentary, Line 4.3

When the body's fluids are depleted and yáng heat is overly exuberant, the patient suffers only heat effusion and no aversion to cold. Exuberant heat damages qì, hence there is shortage of qì and vexation and oppression. Since the extremities are the root of yáng, exuberant heat gives rise to heat in the extremities. When heat damages yīn humor, stomach qì ascends counterflow, giving rise to vomiting and retching. "Evil qì internally hides in the heart and externally abides in the seams of the flesh" means that heat is exuberant in both the viscera and the fleshy exterior. Dual heat in the exterior and interior causes wasting of the flesh, i.e., emaciation.

Line 4.4

温疟者，其脉如平，身无寒但热，骨节疼烦，时呕，白虎加桂枝汤主之。

知母六两　甘草（炙）二两　石膏一斤　粳米二合　桂枝（去皮）三两

右剉，每五钱，水一盏半，煎至八分，去滓，温服，汗出愈。

Wēn nüè zhě, qí mài rú píng, shēn wú hán dàn rè, gǔ jié téng fán, shí ǒu, bái hǔ jiā guì zhī tāng zhǔ zhī.

Zhī mǔ liù liǎng; gān cǎo (zhì) èr liǎng; shí gāo yī jīn; jīng mǐ èr gě; guì zhī (qù pí) sān liǎng

Yòu cuò, měi wǔ qián, shuǐ yī zhǎn bàn, jiān zhì bā fēn, qù zǐ, wēn fú, hàn chū yù.

Warm malaria manifests in a pulse that is as normal, no cold but only heat in the body, vexing pain in the joints, and periodic retching. White Tiger Decoction Plus Cinnamon Twig (白虎加桂枝汤 *bái hǔ jiā guì zhī tāng*) governs.

White Tiger Decoction Plus Cinnamon Twig (白虎加桂枝汤 *bái hǔ jiā guì zhī tāng*)

- anemarrhena (知母 *zhī mǔ*, Anemarrhenae Rhizoma) 6 *liǎng*
- licorice (甘草 *gān cǎo*, Glycyrrhizae Radix) 2 liǎng (mix-fry)
- gypsum (石膏 *shí gāo*, Gypsum Fibrosum) 1 *jīn*
- non-glutinous rice (粳米 *jīng mǐ*, Oryzae Semen) 2 *gě*
- cinnamon twig (桂枝 *guì zhī*, Cinnamomi Ramulus) 3 *liǎng* (remove bark)

Grate the above ingredients. For each dose, [measure] five *qián* and boil in one-and-a-half cups of water until reduced to eight tenths. Remove the dregs. Take warm. When [the patient] sweats, recovery will ensue.

Synopsis, Line 4.4

This line discusses the signs and treatment of warm malaria.

Commentary, Line 4.4

The first phrase in this line states that warm malaria is characterized by a normal pulse. The meaning of "normal" has been the subject of controversy. There are three distinct interpretations: (a) The pulse resembles that of a normal healthy person; (b) the pulse is not stringlike as is usually the case in malaria, but it still differs from that of a healthy person; and (c) the pulse is stringlike as is normally the case in malaria. According to clinical practice, warm malaria manifests with a stringlike rapid pulse during episodes, but with a moderate (i.e., not stringlike) pulse as in healthy people before and after episodes. Hence there is no definitive answer as to which interpretation is correct.

Heat effusion without aversion to cold needs to be understood in a relative sense. As stated already in the *Nèi Jīng* ("The Inner Canon"), malaria is always characterized by alternating heat and cold. In cases of warm malaria, exuberant internal heat makes the aversion to cold very slight while making the heat effusion much more pronounced. Vexing pain in the joints indicates that the exterior has not resolved. When heat damages the stomach, there is frequent retching.

The treatment proposed for warm malaria is White Tiger Decoction Plus Cinnamon Twig (*bái hǔ jiā guì zhī tāng*). White Tiger Decoction (*bái hǔ tāng*) clears heat, engenders liquid, and checks retching. Cinnamon twig (*guì zhī*) is added to resolve the exterior evil.

Line 4.5

疟多寒者，名曰牡疟，蜀漆散主之。

蜀漆（洗去腥）云母（烧二日夜）
龙骨等分

右三味，杵为散，未发前以浆水服半钱。温疟加蜀漆半分，临发时服一钱匕。

Nüè duō hán zhě, míng yuē mǔ nüè, shǔ qī sǎn zhǔ zhī.

Shǔ qī (xǐ qù xīng); yún mǔ (shāo èr rì yè); lóng gǔ děng fēn

Yòu sān wèi, chǔ wéi sǎn, wèi fā qián yǐ jiāng shuǐ fú bàn qián. Wēn nüè jiā shǔ qī bàn fēn, lín fā shí fú yī qián bǐ.

Malaria with predominant [aversion to] cold is called female malaria.[1] Dichroa Leaf Powder (蜀漆散 *shǔ qī sǎn*) governs.

Dichroa Leaf Powder (蜀漆散 *shǔ qī sǎn*)

- dichroa leaf (蜀漆 *shǔ qī*, Dichroae Folium) (wash to remove fishy smell)
- muscovite (云母 *yún mǔ*, Muscovitum) (roast for 2 days and nights)
- dragon bone (龙骨 *lóng gǔ*, Mastodi Ossis Fossilia)

Pestle equal amounts of the above three ingredients into a powder. Before a malaria attack, take half a *qián*[2] in sour rice milk. For warm malaria, add half a part of dichroa leaf (*shǔ qī*) and take one qián-spoonful right before an attack.[3]

Text Notes, Line 4.5

[1] Female malaria 牝疟 *pìn nüè*: This refers to malaria in patients with yáng vacuity, where the malarial evil lies in the lesser yīn channel. This type of malaria is characterized by pronounced shivering with little or no heat effusion, pale white complexion, and regular episodes. The term "female" means "yīn," i.e., characterized by cold rather than heat. There is also a corresponding term, male malaria (牡疟 *mǔ nüè*), which is not mentioned in the text, but appears in the appended formulas from the *Wài Tái Mì Yào* ("Secrets from the *Wài Tái* Library") at the end of this chapter.

[2] Qián 钱: This is probably an abbreviation for 钱匕 *qián bǐ*, qián-spoonful.

[3] A textual variation has Mysore thorn seed (云实 *yún shí*) instead of muscovite (云母 *yún mǔ*).

Synopsis, Line 4.5

This line describes the signs and treatment of female malaria.

Commentary, Line 4.5

Female malaria is a type of malaria that is characterized by pronounced aversion to cold with only mild heat effusion. It arises as a result of constitutional yáng vacuity and preexisting phlegm-rheum that obstructs yáng qì.

Treatment of female malaria involves dispelling phlegm and freeing yáng using Dichroa Leaf Powder (*shǔ qī sǎn*). Within the formula, dichroa leaf (*shǔ qī*) dispels phlegm and interrupts malaria. Muscovite (*yún mǔ*) and dragon bone (*lóng gǔ*) assist yáng and support right, as well as settle fright and calm the spirit. The formula is taken in sour rice milk (*jiāng shuǐ*) just before an episode for best results. This timing of treatment is also mentioned in "Treatise on Needling Malaria" (刺疟篇 *cì nüè piān*) in the *Sù Wèn*.

附《外台秘要》方 *Fù «Wài Tài Mì Yào» fāng*

Formulas from the Wài Tái Mì Yào ("Secrets from the Wài Tái Library")

治牝虐。

牡蛎（熬）四两 麻黄(去节)四两 甘草二两 蜀漆三两

右四味，以水八升先煮蜀漆、麻黄，去上沫，得六升，内诸药煮取二升，温服一升。若吐，则勿更服。

Zhì pìn nüè.

Mǔ lì tāng

Mǔ lì (áo) sì liǎng; má huáng (qù jié) sì liǎng; gān cǎo èr liǎng; shǔ qī sān liǎng

Yòu sì wèi, yǐ shuǐ bā shēng xiān zhǔ shǔ qī, má huáng, qù shàng mò, dé liù shēng, nà zhū yào zhǔ qǔ èr shēng, wēn fú yī shēng. Ruò tù, zé wù gèng fú.

A treatment for male malaria.

Oyster Shell Decoction (牡蛎汤 *mǔ lì tāng*)

- oyster shell (牡蛎 *mǔ lì*, Ostreae Concha) 4 *liǎng* (simmer)
- ephedra (麻黄 *má huáng*, Ephedrae Herba) 4 liǎng (remove nodes)
- licorice (甘草 *gān cǎo*, Glycyrrhizae Radix) 2 *liǎng*
- dichroa leaf (蜀漆 shǔ qī, Dichroae Folium) 3 *liǎng*

Of the above four ingredients, first boil the dichroa leaf (*shǔ qī*) and ephedra (*má huáng*) in eight *shēng* of water. Remove the scum off the top. Reduce to six *shēng*. Add all the [other] ingredients and boil to get two *shēng*. Take one *shēng* [per dose] warm. If vomiting results, do not take more.

治疟病以发渴者，亦治劳疟。

柴胡八两 人参 黄芩 甘草各三两 栝蒌根四两 生姜二两 大枣十二枚

右七味, 以水一斗二升, 煮取六升, 去滓, 再煎取三升, 温服一升, 日二服。

Zhì nüè bìng yǐ fā kě zhě, yì zhì láo nüè.

Chái hú bā liǎng; rén shēn huáng qín gān cǎo gè sān liǎng; guā lóu gēn sì liǎng; shēng jiāng èr liǎng; dà zǎo shí èr méi

Yòu qī wèi, yǐ shuǐ yī dǒu èr shēng, zhǔ qǔ liù shēng, qù zǐ, zài jiān qǔ sān shēng, wēn fú yī shēng, rì èr fú.

A treatment for malarial disease with thirst, as well as for taxation malaria.

Bupleurum Decoction Minus Pinellia Plus Trichosanthes Root (柴胡去半夏加栝楼汤 *chái hú qù bàn xià jiā guā lóu tāng*)

bupleurum (柴胡 *chái hú*, Bupleuri Radix) 8 *liǎng*
ginseng (人参 *rén shēn*, Ginseng Radix) 3 *liǎng*
scutellaria (黄芩 *huáng* qín, Scutellariae Radix) 3 *liǎng*
licorice (甘草 *gān cǎo*, Glycyrrhizae Radix) 3 *liǎng*
trichosanthes root (栝蒌 *guā lóu gēn*, Trichosanthis Radix) 4 *liǎng*
fresh ginger (生姜 *shēng jiāng*, Zingiberis Rhizoma Recens) 2 *liǎng*
jujube (大枣 *dà zǎo*, Jujubae Fructus) 12 fruits

Boil the above seven ingredients in one *dǒu* and two *shēng* of water to get six *shēng*. Remove the dregs and boil again to get three *shēng*. Take one *shēng* [per dose] warm, two times a day.

治疟寒多微有热，或但寒不热。

柴胡半斤 桂枝三两（去皮） 干姜二两 栝蒌根四两 黄芩三两 牡蛎三两（熬） 甘草二两（炙）

右七味，以水一斗二升，煮取六升，去滓，再煎取三升，温服一升，日三服。初服微烦，复服汗出便愈。

Zhì nüè hán duō wēi yǒu rè, huò dàn hán bù rè.

Chái hú bàn jīn; jīn guì zhī (qù pí) sān liǎng; gān jiāng èr liǎng; guā lóu gēn sì liǎng; huáng qín sān liǎng; mǔ lì (áo) sān liǎng; gān cǎo (zhì) èr liǎng

Yòu qī wèi, yǐ shuǐ yī dǒu èr shēng, zhǔ qǔ liù shēng, qù zhā, zài jiān qǔ sān shēng, wēn fú yī shēng, rì sān fú. Chū fú wēi fán, fù fú hàn chū biàn yù.

A treatment for malaria with predominant cold and slight heat, or with only cold and no heat.[1]

Bupleurum, Cinnamon Twig, and Dried Ginger Decoction (柴胡桂姜汤 *chái hú guì jiāng tāng*)

bupleurum (柴胡 *chái hú*, Bupleuri Radix) ½ *jīn*
cinnamon twig (桂枝 *guì zhī*, Cinnamomi Ramulus) 3 *liǎng* (remove bark)
dried ginger (干姜 *gān jiāng*, Zingiberis Rhizoma) 2 *liǎng*
trichosanthes root (栝蒌 *guā lóu gēn*, Trichosanthis Radix) 4 *liǎng*
scutellaria (黄芩 *huáng qín*, Scutellariae Radix) 3 *liǎng*
oyster shell (牡蛎 *mǔ lì*, Ostreae Concha) 3 *liǎng* (simmer)
licorice (甘草 *gān cǎo*, Glycyrrhizae Radix) 2 *liǎng* (mix-fry)

Boil the above seven ingredients in one *dǒu* and two *shēng* of water to get six *shēng*. Remove the dregs and boil again to get three *shēng*. Take one *shēng* warm, three times a day. [If] the first dose causes slight vexation and the second dose sweating, recovery will ensue.

FORMULA NOTE

[1] The commentary here states: Taking one preparation works like magic (服一剂如神 *fú yī jì rú shén*).

中风历节脉证治第五

CHAPTER 5

Wind-Stroke and Joint-Running

Pulses, Signs, Treatments

‡ Overview

As the title specifies, this chapter concerns wind-stroke and joint-running. The diseases of wind-stroke and joint-running are both caused by contraction of wind evil in patients suffering from depletion of right qì. The diseases also have similar manifestations in that they involve physical handicap. These similarities explain why they are discussed together in the same chapter.

Wind-Stroke

Wind-stroke is a disease characterized by sudden clouding collapse and loss of consciousness, which leaves the patient with deviated eyes and mouth and hemiplegia. It corresponds to what modern medicine calls stroke, apoplexy, or now more commonly cerebrovascular accident. In the Jīn Guì Yào Lüè ("Essential Prescriptions of the Golden Cabinet") and in medical literature up until the Táng period, wind-stroke was attributed to "evil striking [patients with] internal vacuity" (内虚邪中 *nèi xū xié zhòng*), in other words, contraction of external evil by patients suffering from depletion of right qì. Later physicians offered new explanations for the disease, so that the discussions on the subject in modern literature only partially resemble those of the *Jīn Guì Yào Lüè* ("Essential Prescriptions of the Golden Cabinet").

The Chinese term 中风 *zhòng fēng* is duplicated in the literal English translation wind-stroke. Like our English term "stroke," it suggests a disease that afflicts the body suddenly and forcefully. Unlike the term "stroke," it suggests a causative agent originally recognized in Chinese medicine—wind. It should further be noted that the term wind-stroke has two different meanings in Chinese medicine, even as early as in the writings of Zhāng Jī. In the context of cold damage disease, it refers to greater yáng wind-strike, which is an external contraction of wind evil giving rise to a condition characterized by heat effusion and sweating, aversion to wind, and a moderate floating pulse. In the context of miscellaneous diseases, it refers to stroke or apoplexy.

JOINT-RUNNING

Joint-running is a disease characterized by pain and stiffness in multiple joints of the body. It is attributed to contraction of wind, cold, and dampness evil in patients suffering from internal damage to the liver and kidney. The evils invade the channels and lodge in the joints, causing obstruction of the channels and painful swelling of the joints. Wind is considered the most important of the offending evils because wind is swift and changeable and in this disease swiftly spreads through the joints of the whole body. For this reason, Cháo Yuán-Fāng (巢原方), the author of the *Zhū Bìng Yuán Hòu Lùn* ("The Origin and Indicators of Disease"), called it "joint-running wind" (历节风 *lì jié fēng*), the name more commonly used today.

Nowadays, joint-running (wind) falls within the scope of impediment patterns (痹证 *bì zhèng*), although in certain medical texts of the past, notably the *Zhū Bìng Yuán Hòu Lùn* ("The Origin and Indicators of Disease"), *Qiān Jīn Yào Fāng* ("A Thousand Gold Pieces Prescriptions"), and *Sān Yīn Fāng* ("Three Causes Prescriptions"), it was considered separate. The word 痹 *bì*, translated as impediment, originally means obstruction. In the *Jīn Guì Yào Lüè* ("Essential Prescriptions of the Golden Cabinet"), it appears in wind-stroke in this chapter (where it denotes a condition differentiated from wind-stroke). It also occurs in 血痹 *xuè bì*, blood impediment (Chapter 6) and 胸痹 *xiōng bì*, chest impediment (Chapter 9). These latter two conditions involve obstruction, but not by wind-cold-damp.

SCHEMATIC OVERVIEW

WIND-STROKE

1. Main signs: hemiplegia, deviated face, faint and rapid pulse.
2. Differentiation from similar conditions:

   Hemiplegia with pain sensation—wind-stroke.

   Local paralysis of arms without loss of pain sensation—impediment pattern.
3. Wind invited by vacuity

   a) Wind-stroke

   Slow pulse—cold.

   Moderate pulse—vacuity.

b) Dormant papules: Insufficiency of channel qì, insufficiency of heart qì allowing evil qì to enter the center giving rise to itching and dormant papules, fullness in the chest and shortness of breath.

4. Signs

a) Mild pattern

Main sign: deviated eyes and mouth.

Pulse: floating and tight.

Pathomechanism: cold and vacuity contending with each other, evil in the skin, emptiness of the network vessels. Bandit evil failing to be discharged, either on the left or right. Evil qì causes slackness, while right qì causes tension, pulling the evil qì toward it.

b) Severe wind-stroke

Evil in the network vessels. Insensitivity of the skin.

Evil in the channels: body heavy and unwieldy.

Evil in the bowels: failure to recognize people.

Evil in the viscera: difficulty in speaking; drooling.

5. Principles of treatment

a) Wind-cold

Signs: vexing heaviness of the limbs, aversion to cold and insufficiency in the heart.

Formula: Hóu's Black Powder (*hóu shì hēi sǎn*).

b) Wind-heat

Signs: Wind pulling in adults and fright epilepsy with tugging and slackening in children, with episodes occurring several dozens of times a day.

Formula: Wind-Drawing Decoction (*fēng yǐn tāng*).

c) Blood vacuity and wind-heat:

Signs: manic appearance, reckless behavior, incessant soliloquy, absence of cold and heat, and a floating pulse.

Formula: Fangji and Rehmannia Decoction (*fáng jǐ dì huáng tāng*).

d) Topical treatment for head wind: Head Wind Rubbing Powder (*tóu fēng mó sǎn*).

Joint Running

1. Pattern identification:

a) Entering water while sweating, in liver-kidney vacuity.

Pulse: at the inch opening, sunken (bones, kidney) and weak (sinew, liver)

Signs: Joint-running pain and yellow sweat.

b) Sweating during exposure to wind, in insufficiency of qì and blood.

Pulse: at the inch opening, floating (spontaneous sweating) and slippery (replete grain qì).

Pulse at lesser yīn, floating (exuberant wind qì) and weak (insufficiency of blood). Wind and blood contending with each other: pulling pain.

Exuberant physique: Pulse rough and small; shortness of breath; spontaneous sweating, joint-running pain with difficulty in bending and stretching.

c) Intemperate consumption of rich food damaging the liver and kidney

Food and drink: Excessive sourness damaging the sinews causing them to slacken (called discharge); excessive saltiness damaging the bones, causing wilting and limpness (called desiccation).

Pathomechanism: [When] construction qì does not flow freely, defense qì cannot move alone. Construction and defense are both debilitated, the triple burner is not controlled, and the four ascriptions are cut off.

Signs: Marked emaciation with enlarged swollen feet and yellow sweat.

Differentiation: cold lower legs—yellow sweat; hot lower legs—joint running.

2. Treatment

a) Wind-damp pattern

Signs: limb joint pain, marked emaciation, feet swollen as if about to drop off, dizzy vision, shortness of breath, seething desire to vomit.

Formula: Cinnamon Twig, Peony, and Anemarrhena Decoction (*guì zhī sháo yào zhī mǔ tāng*).

b) Cold-damp pattern

Signs: joint-running pain with inability to bend and stretch.

Formula: Aconite Main Root Decoction (*wū tóu tāng*)

Line 5.1

夫风之为病，当半身不遂，或但臂不遂者，此为痹。脉微而数，中风使然。

Fū fēng zhī wéi bìng, dāng bàn shēn bù suì, huò dàn bèi bù suì zhě, cǐ wéi bì. Mài wēi ér shuò, zhòng fēng shǐ rán.

All diseases caused by wind must [manifest with] hemiplegia.[1] In some cases, if we see paralysis of the arm only,[2] this is impediment. A faint and rapid pulse is caused by wind-stroke.

TEXT NOTES, LINE 5.1

[1] Hemiplegia 半身不遂 *bàn shēn bù suì*: Half-body paralysis, that is, loss of voluntary movement of the limbs on one side of the body.

[2] Paralysis of the arm only 但臂不遂 *dà bì bù suì*: Loss of voluntary movement of the upper limb only. Again, the implication is that only one side of the body is affected.

SYNOPSIS, LINE 5.1

This line describes the pulse and signs of wind-stroke and the way to distinguish it from impediment.

COMMENTARY, LINE 5.1

Wind-stroke is characterized by loss of voluntary movement of both limbs on either side of the body. If only an upper limb is affected, this is not wind-stroke but impediment. The hemiplegia of wind-stroke is attributed to depletion of blood and qì and to static blood obstructing the network vessels. Loss of the use of limbs in impediment is attributed to wind, cold, and dampness impeding the channel vessels. Hence, the slight and rapid pulse that the text associates with wind-stroke hints at the contributing factors of wind-stroke hemiplegia. The slight pulse reflects insufficiency of qì and blood. The rapidity of the pulse reflects the evil repletion.

Yù Jiā-Yán 喻嘉言 and Zhāng Lù 张璐 have argued that "impediment" here does not refer to the specific disease that is caused by a combination of wind, cold, and dampness that is characterized by pain and numbness, but to a mild form of wind-stroke. This argument is not without reason. However, quite apart from how the text should be interpreted, wind-stroke in clinical practice is distinguished from impediment disease not only by which limbs are affected, but also by the presence or absence of pain. While both diseases may be characterized by numbness and loss of movement, only impediment is associated with pain.

Line 5.2

(1)寸口脉浮而紧，紧则为寒，浮则为虚，寒虚相搏，邪在皮肤。浮者血虚，络脉空虚，贼邪不泻，或左或右，邪气反缓，正气即急，正气引邪，㖞僻不遂。

(2)邪在于络，肌肤不仁；邪在于经，即重不胜；邪入于腑，即不识人；邪入于脏，舌即难言，口吐涎。

治大风，四肢烦重，心中恶寒不足者。

菊花四十分 白朮十分 细辛三分 茯苓三分 牡蛎三分 桔梗八分 防风十分 人参三分 矾石三分 黄芩五分 当归三分 干姜三分 芎藭三分 桂枝三分

右十四味，杵为散，酒服方寸匕，日一服。初服二十日，温酒调服，禁一切鱼肉大蒜，常宜冷食，六十日止，即药积在腹中不下也，热食即下矣，冷食自能助药力。

(1) Cùn kǒu mài fú ér jǐn, jǐn zé wéi hán, fú zé wéi xū, hán xū xiāng bó, xié zài pí fū. Fú zhě xuè xū, luò mài kōng xū, zéi xié bù xiè, huò zuǒ huò yòu, xié qì fǎn huǎn, zhèng qì jí jí, zhèng qì yǐn xié, wāi pì bù suì.

(2) Xié zài yú luò, jī fū bù rén; xié zài yú jīng, jí zhòng bù shèng; xié rù yú fǔ, jí bù shì rén; xié rù yú zàng, shé jí nán yán, kǒu tù xián.

Zhì dà fēng, sì zhī fán zhòng, xīn zhōng wù hán bù zú zhě.

Jú huā sì shí fèn; bái zhú shí fèn; xì xīn sān fèn; fú líng sān fèn; mǔ lì sān fèn; jié gěng bā fèn; fáng fēng shí fèn; rén shēn sān fèn; fán shí sān fèn; huáng qín wǔ fèn; dāng guī sān fèn; gān jiāng sān fèn; xiōng qióng sān fèn; guì zhī sān fèn

yòu shí sì wèi, chǔ wéi sǎn, jiǔ fú fāng cùn bǐ, rì yī fú. Chū fú èr shí rì, wēn jiǔ tiáo fú, jìn yī qiè yú ròu dà suàn, cháng yí lěng shí, liù shí rì zhǐ, jí yào jī zài fù zhōng bù xià yě, rè shí jí xià yǐ, lěng shí zì néng zhù yào lì.

(1) When the inch opening pulse is floating and tight, the tightness means cold, while the floating means vacuity. Cold and vacuity contend with each other,[1] and the evil is in the skin. [In a patient with] a floating pulse, blood is vacuous, the network vessels are empty, and the bandit evil fails to drain,[2] whether on the left or the right [side of the body]. When the evil qì slackens, right qì becomes tense and draws the evil to it, [giving rise to] deviation [of the eyes and mouth].

(2) When the evil is the network vessels, the skin is numb. When the evil is the channels, [the body is] heavy and unwieldy. When the evil enters the bowels, [the patient] fails to recognize people. When the evil enters the viscera, the tongue has difficulty in speaking and the mouth drools.

[Hóu's Black Powder] Treats great wind[1] with vexing heaviness[2] of the limbs, and aversion to cold and insufficiency in the heart.[3]

Hóu's Black Powder
侯氏黑散 *hóu shì hēi sǎn*

- chrysanthemum (菊花 *jú huā*, Chrysanthemi Flos) 40 parts
- white atractylodes (白朮 *bái zhú*, Atractylodis Macrocephalae Rhizoma) 10 parts
- poria (茯苓 *fú líng*, Poria) 3 parts
- oyster shell (牡蛎 *mǔ lì*, Ostreae Concha) 3 parts
- platycodon (桔梗 *jié gěng*, Platycodonis Radix) 8 parts
- saposhnikovia (防风 *fáng fēng*, Saposhnikoviae Radix) 10 parts

ginseng (人参 *rén shēn*, Ginseng Radix) 3 parts
alum (矾石 fán shí, Alumen) 3 parts
scutellaria (黄芩 *huáng qín*, Scutellariae Radix) 5 parts
Chinese angelica (当归 *dāng guī*, Angelicae Sinensis Radix) 3 parts
dried ginger (干姜 *gān jiāng*, Zingiberis Rhizoma) 3 parts
xiongqiong (芎藭 *xiōng qióng*, Chuanxiong Rhizoma) 3 parts
cinnamon twig (桂枝 *guì zhī*, Cinnamomi Ramulus) 3 parts

Pestle the above fourteen ingredients into a powder and take a square-inch-spoonful in wine, once a day. Initially, take it for 20 days, balancing it with the consumption of warm wine. Exclude [from the diet] all fish, meat, and garlic, and eat cold food often. Stop after sixty days, when the medicine has accumulated in the abdomen and will not descend. Warm food will cause it to descend; cold food will naturally help the strength of the medicine.

TEXT NOTES, LINE 5.2

1. Cold and vacuity contend with each other 寒虚相博 *hán xū xiāng bó*: This means that there is vacuity of right qì and contraction of external evil.

2. The bandit evil fails to drain 贼邪不泻 *zéi xiè bù xiè*: The evil fails to leave the body.

SYNOPSIS, LINE 5.2

This line discusses the pathomechanism of wind-stroke on the basis of the pulse and identifies deep and shallow wind-stroke patterns.

COMMENTARY, LINE 5.2

The first section of the line discusses the pathomechanism by which the mouth and eyes become deviated. When the inch opening pulse is floating and tight, the tightness reflects the presence of cold evil, while the floating quality reflects vacuity of right qì. When external evil invades the body of a patient suffering from vacuity of right qì, it will first stagnate in the skin and flesh. Because qì and blood are depleted, right qì lacks the strength to dispel the evil, so that the external evil cannot be eliminated from the body. The evil affects one side of the body or the other. The affected side, owing to damage to the channel vessels, becomes flaccid, while the unaffected side is relatively tense. Because the unaffected side is tense, it pulls the slack unaffected side over toward it, giving rise to deviated mouth and eyes.

The second section explains the depth of the disease. The first level of penetration is that of the network vessels. The network vessels are the fine vessels that are distributed throughout the skin and flesh. Hence, they represent the shallowest penetration of the disease. Invasion of the network vessels by the disease evil gives rise to numbness of the skin. The second level of penetration is that of the channels. The channels are the larger vessels of the body. They connect with the sinew and bones. When the evil penetrates the channels, it moves deeper into the body, causing the limbs to become heavy and limp.

The deepest level of penetration is invasion of the viscera and bowels, which is characterized by clouded spirit, sluggish speech, and drooling from the mouth. Zhāng Jī actually states that when the evil invades the bowels there is failure to recognize people, and when it enters the viscera there is sluggish speech and drooling from the mouth. However, this latter distinction has never been satisfactorily explained.

Some commentators explain invasion of the bowels giving rise to failure to recognize people by the fact that the stomach vessel connects with the heart. When the evil obstructs the stomach, it affects the stomach's function of free downward flow, so that turbid qì rises and clouds the heart spirit. Invasion of the viscera giving rise to sluggish speech can be more directly explained in terms of the tongue being the sprout of the heart. However, it is unclear why disease affecting the bowels should be characterized by a visceral sign rather than a true bowel sign and why different heart signs should be variously attributed to disease affecting the bowels and disease affecting the viscera. The relevant arguments may have been devised solely to justify Zhāng Jī's statements.

Of note is that later physicians did not find the distinction between bowel strike and visceral strike to be clinically valuable. Modern textbooks tend to present only a broad distinction between channel and network vessel strike on the one hand and bowel and visceral strike on the other.

Formula Notes, Line 5.2

[1] Great wind 大风 *dà fēng*: A disease category used in early texts. Commentators disagree on the exact connotation of this term, explaining it either as wind striking the bowels and viscera directly or as invading the extremities and from there affecting the heart.

[2] Vexing heaviness 烦重 *fán zhòng*: Severe heaviness.

[3] Aversion to cold and insufficiency in the heart 心中恶寒不足 *xīn zhōng wù hán bù zú*: This refers to insufficiency of center yáng and aversion to cold in the chest.

Formula Commentary, Line 5.2

Commentators have noted that the attached formula for Hóu's Black Powder (*hóu shì hēi sǎn*) differs in style from the other formulas in this text. They have therefore suggested that it might have been added to the text several centuries later during the Suí or Táng periods. Nevertheless, in clinical practice it is of definite value in the treatment of wind-stroke and is therefore included here. The *Wài Tái Mì Yào* ("Secrets from the *Wài Tái* Library") recommends this formula as a treatment for wind epilepsy.

When right qì is vacuous and blood and qì are insufficient, the wind-cold external evil can easily overcome the vacuity and invade the body. The evil obstructs the movement of qì and blood in the channels and network vessels, and the sinews, bones, and flesh are deprived of warmth and nourishment. Therefore, the extremities feel particularly heavy. Yáng vacuity in the spleen and stomach causes aversion of cold in the chest and stomach duct.

In the formula, saposhnikovia (*fáng fēng*), chrysanthemum (*jú huā*), cinnamon twig (*guì zhī*), platycodon (*jié gěng*), and asarum (*xì xīn*) course wind and resolve the exterior, thereby expelling the external evil. Ginseng (*rén shēn*), white atractylodes (*bái zhú*), poria (*fú líng*), and dried ginger (*gān jiāng*) warm the center and boost qì, thereby supplementing the vacuity of center yáng. Chuanxiong (*chuān xiōng*) and Chinese angelica (*dāng guī*) nourish blood and quicken the network vessels. Although we do not see clear heat signs, wind is a yáng evil and has a tendency to transform into heat. Thus, the formula uses astragalus (*huáng qín*) to discharge heat. Oyster shell (*mǔ* lì) and alum (*fán shí*) are used to disperse phlegm. All these ingredients work together to resolve the exterior and expel wind, supplement and nourish qì and blood, and disperse phlegm and quicken the network vessels.

Line 5.3

寸口脉迟而缓，迟则为寒，缓则为虚。营缓则为亡血，卫缓则为中风。邪气中经，则身痒而瘾疹；心气不足，邪气入中，则胸满而短气。

Cùn kǒu mài chí ér huǎn, chí zé wéi hán, huǎn zé wéi xū. Róng huǎn zé wéi wáng xuè, wèi huǎn zé wéi zhōng fēng. Xié qì zhòng jīng, zé shēn yǎng ér yǐn zhěn; xīn qì bù zú, xié qì rù zhōng, zé xiōng mǎn ér duǎn qì.

When the inch opening pulse is slow and moderate, the slowness means cold and the moderateness means vacuity. If it is moderate in the construction [aspect],[1] this is blood collapse;[2] if it is moderate in the defense [aspect],[3] this is wind-stroke. When evil qì strikes the channels, the result is generalized itching and dormant papules.[4] When heart qì is insufficient[5] and evil qì enters the center, the result is fullness in the chest and shortness of breath.

Text Notes, Line 5.3

[1] Moderate in the construction [aspect] 营缓 *yíng huǎn*: This refers to a pulse that is sunken and moderate, indicating insufficiency of construction qì.

[2] Blood collapse 亡血 *wǎng xuè*: Blood vacuity.

[3] Moderate in the defense [aspect] 卫缓 *wèi huǎn*: This refers to a pulse that is floating and moderate, indicating insufficiency of defense qì.

[4] Dormant papules 瘾疹 *yǐn zhěn:* Itchy wheals that come and go.

[5] Heart qì is insufficient 心气不足 *xīn qì bù zú*: "Heart qì" loosely denotes heart and lung qì in the chest.

Synopsis, Line 5.3

This line discusses insufficiency of construction-defense qì and blood as the internal cause of wind-stroke.

Commentary, Line 5.3

The present line discusses the internal causes of wind-stroke on the basis of a slow and moderate pulse. We are told that the inch opening pulse is slow and moderate. A pulse that is slow usually indicates cold. When we consider the present line against the background of the preceding statement that a tight pulse indicates an external contraction of wind-cold, we understand that "slowness means cold" actually refers to an external assault by wind-cold. A moderate pulse reflects insufficiency of right qì, wherein a moderate pulse that is also floating signifies vacuity of defense qì and a moderate pulse that is sunken signifies vacuity of construction-blood. Because of this insufficiency of construction and defense qì and blood, the fleshy exterior is insecure and can therefore easily attract the external evils wind and cold. Since right qì is unable to fight evil, this can turn into the disease of wind-stroke.

If right qì is still strong when wind-cold invades the channels and network vessels, the disease evil stagnates there and impedes construction and defense. This results in itching of the skin, and because it is the nature of wind to stir, in dormant papules. If right qì is insufficient and heart-lung qì is vacuous, the disease evil exploits the vacuity and enters the body, congesting yáng qì in the chest. This manifests in fullness of the chest and shortness of breath.

Formulas, Line 5.3

风引汤

除热瘫痫。

大黄 干姜 龙骨 各四两 桂枝三两 甘草 牡蛎各二两 寒水石 滑石 赤石脂 白石脂 紫石英 石膏各六两

右十二味, 杵, 粗筛, 以韦囊盛之。取三指撮, 井花水三升, 煮三沸, 温服一升。

Fēng yǐn tāng

Chú rè tān xián.

Dà huáng sì liǎng; gān jiāng sì liǎng; lóng gǔ gè sì liǎng; guì zhī sān liǎng; gān cǎo èr liǎng; mǔ lì gè èr liǎng; hán shuǐ shí liù liǎng; huá shí liù liǎng; chì shí zhī[liù liǎng; bái shí zhī liù liǎng; zǐ shí yīng liù liǎng; shí gāo gè liù liǎng.

Yòu shí èr wèi, chǔ, cū shāi, yǐ wéi náng chéng zhī. Qǔ sān zhǐ cuò, jǐng huā shuǐ sān shēng, zhǔ sān fèi, wēn fú yī shēng.

Wind-Pulling[1] Decoction

Eliminates heat paralysis[2] and epilepsy.

Wind-Pulling Decoction (风引汤 *fēng yǐn tāng*)
rhubarb (大黄 *dà huáng*, Rhei Radix et Rhizoma) 4 *liǎng*
dried ginger (干姜 *gān jiāng*, Zingiberis Rhizoma) 4 *liǎng*
dragon bone (龙骨 *lóng gǔ*, Mastodi Ossis Fossilia) 4 *liǎng*
cinnamon twig (桂枝 *guì zhī*, Cinnamomi Ramulus) 3 *liǎng*
licorice (甘草 *gān cǎo*, Glycyrrhizae Radix) 2 *liǎng*
oyster shell (牡蛎 *mǔ lì*, Ostreae Concha) 2 *liǎng*
glauberite (寒水石 *hán shuǐ shí*, Gypsum seu Calcitum) 6 *liǎng*
talcum (滑石 *huá shí*, Talcum) 6 *liǎng*
halloysite (赤石脂 *chì shí zhī*, Halloysitum Rubrum) 6 *liǎng*
kaolin (白石脂 *bái shí zhī*, Kaolin) 6 *liǎng*
fluorite (紫石英 *zǐ shí yīng*, Fluoritum) 6 *liǎng*
gypsum (石膏 *shí gāo*, Gypsum Fibrosum) 6 *liǎng*

Pestle and coarsely sift the above 12 ingredients. Place in a medicinal bag.[3] Take out a three-finger pinch, [add to] three *shēng* of well-flower water[4] and bring to a boil three times. [For each dose], take one *shēng* warm.[5]

Formula Notes, Line 5.3

[1] Wind pulling 风引 *fēng yǐn*: The convulsions (抽搐 *chōu chù*) of wind-epilepsy.

[2] Paralysis 瘫 *tān*: Here refers to 风瘫 *fēng tān* ("wind paralysis"), a common expression for hemiplegia.

[3] Medicinal bag 韦囊 *wéi náng*: A leather bag used in ancient China for keeping medicinals.

[4] Well-flower water 井花水 *jǐng huā shuǐ*: Clear water that is drawn from a well early in the morning.

[5] The commentary adds: "A wind-eliminating formula for conditions doctors cannot cure, treating wind pulling in adults and fright epilepsy with tugging and slackening in children, with episodes ocurring several dozens of times a day. Dr. Cháo states that Wind-Drawing Decoction (*fēng yǐn tāng*) is appropriate for leg qì."

Formula Commentary, Line 5.3

As the name and indications of this formula show, Wind-Pulling Decoction (*fēng yǐn tāng*) is recommended for paralysis and epilepsy that is related to the presence of heat. The specific pathomechanism is yáng heat exuberance with internal stirring of wind evil, which is treated by clearing heat and extinguishing wind.

In the formula, oyster shell (*mǔ* lì) and dragon bone (*lóng gǔ*) subdue yáng and extinguish wind; halloysite (*chì shí zhī*), kaolin (*bái shí zhī*), and fluorite (*zǐ shí yīng*) settle fright and quiet the spirit; gypsum (*shí gāo*), talcum (*huá shí*), and glauberite (*hán shuǐ shí*) clear heat and disperse fire; and rhubarb (*dà huáng*) conducts heat downward.

Because these ingredients are cold and sagging and therefore dangerous for the spleen and stomach, dried ginger (*gān jiāng*) and cinnamon twig (*guì zhī*) are added to warm and move the spleen, and licorice (*gān cǎo*) is added to harmonize all the other medicinals, thereby avoiding damage to the spleen and stomach. This formula is recommended for any condition with exuberant heat and stirring wind, regardless of whether it is hemilateral paralysis in adults with wind-stroke or tugging and slackening of the limbs in children with fright epilepsy.

防己地黄汤

治病如狂状妄行，独语不休，无寒热，其脉浮。

防己一分　桂枝三分　防风三分　甘草二分

右四味，以酒一杯，浸之一宿，绞取汁；生地黄二斤，㕮咀，蒸之如斗米饭久；以铜器盛其汁，更绞地黄汁，和分再服。

Fáng jǐ dì huáng tāng

Zhì bìng rú kuáng zhuàng wàng xíng, dú yǔ bù xiū, wú hán rè, qí mài fú.

Fáng jǐ yī fēn; guì zhī sān fēn; fáng fēng sān fēn; gān cǎo èr fēn

Yòu sì wèi, yǐ jiǔ yī bēi, jìn zhī yī xiǔ, jiǎo qǔ zhī; shēng dì huáng èr jīn, fǔ jǔ, zhēng zhī rú dǒu mǐ fàn jiǔ; yǐ tóng qì chéng qí zhī, gèng jiǎo dì huáng zhī, huó fēn zài fú.

Fangji and Rehmannia Decoction

Treats disease [that manifests] like mania with reckless behavior, incessant soliloquy,[1] absence of cold and heat, and a floating pulse.

Fangji and Rehmannia Decoction (防己地黄汤 *Fáng jǐ dì huáng tāng*)

fangji (防己 *fáng jǐ*, Stephaniae Tetrandrae Radix) 1 parts
cinnamon twig (桂枝 *guì zhī*, Cinnamomi Ramulus) 3 parts
saposhnikovia (防风 *fáng fēng*, Saposhnikoviae Radix) 3 parts
licorice (甘草 *gān cǎo*, Glycyrrhizae Radix) 2 parts

Steep the four above ingredients for one night in a cup of wine and then wring out the juice. Chew two *jīn* of rehmannia (*dì huáng*) and steam for the length of time [that it takes to cook] a dipper-full (*dǒu*) of rice. Pour the juice into a copper vessel, wring the rehmannia (*dì huáng*) out to get more juice, and combine [the two lots of juice]. Divide into two doses.

FORMULA NOTE, LINE 5.3

[1] Incessant soliloquy 独语不休 *dú yǔ bù xiū*: Continual talking to oneself.

COMMENTARY, LINE 5.3

This formula is used to treat conditions characterized by mania, agitation, and disquietude, abnormal behavior, and soliloquy, with neither heat nor cold and a floating pulse. These symptoms are caused by an insufficiency of heart blood that is exploited by external evil, resulting in blockage in the network vessels. The agitation, abnormal behavior, and soliloquy (talking to self) are due to the fact that the heart is without a ruler. The floating pulse and absence of heat and cold indicate that the disease is not in the exterior, but related to blood vacuity and emptiness of the vessels. Therefore, the formula mainly aims at nourishing blood and supporting right, with dispelling wind, overcoming dampness, and warming and moving blood as secondary goals.

Among the formula ingredients, fangji (*fáng jǐ*) and saposhnikovia (*fáng fēng*) are able to dispel wind and overcome dampness; cinnamon twig (*guì zhī*) in conjunction with licorice (*gān cǎo*), after soaking in wine, warm and free the blood vessels. These ingredients are used in rather small amounts, whereas a large amount of rehmannia (*dì huáng*) is added after being steamed. Thereby increased in strength, it enriches yīn and nourishes blood. All together, the medicinals nourish yīn blood, dispel wind-damp, and free blood.

头风摩散

大附子（炮）一枚　盐等分

右二味为散，沐了，以方寸匕，已摩疾上，令药力行。

Tóu fēng mó sǎn

Dà fù zǐ (pào) yī méi; yán děng fèn

Yòu èr wèi wéi sǎn, mù liǎo, yǐ fāng cùn bǐ, yǐ mó jí shàng, lìng yào lì xíng.

Head Wind[1] Rubbing Powder (头风摩散 *tóu fēng mó sǎn*)

aconite (附子 *fù zǐ*, Aconiti Radix Lateralis Praeparata) 1 piece (blast-fry)
salt (盐 *yán*, Sal)

Make a powder with equal amounts of the above two ingredients. Wash the head and afterwards rub a square-inch-spoonful on the diseased [area]. Make the strength of the medicine move [through the scalp].

FORMULA NOTE, LINE 5.3

[1] Head wind 头风 *tóu fēng*: Enduring recurrent headache and dizziness.

FORMULA COMMENTARY, LINE 5.3

Head wind is primarily caused by an external assault of wind-cold, which results in obstruction in the channels and network vessels. Its special characteristics are recurring headache, dizziness, and symptoms aggravated on exposure to wind-damp. The present formula dispels wind, disperses cold, and relieves pain.

Line 5.4

寸口脉沉而弱，沉即主骨，弱即主筋，沉即为肾，弱即为肝。汗出入水中，如水伤心，历节黄汗出，故曰历节。

Cùn kǒu mài chén ér ruò, chén jí zhǔ gǔ, ruò jí zhǔ jīn, chén jí wéi shèn, ruò jí wéi gān, hàn chū rù shuǐ zhōng. Rú shuǐ shāng xīn, lì jié huáng hàn chū, gù yuē lì jié.

[When] the inch pulse is sunken and weak, the sunkenness is a symptom of the bones, and the weakness is a symptom of the sinews, because sunkenness means the kidney, and weakness means the liver. [When people] enter water when sweating, if water damages the heart,[1] the disease will run through the joints of the body [giving rise to] yellow sweating; hence [this is] called joint-running.[2]

TEXT NOTES, LINE 5.4

[1] If water damages the heart 如水伤心 *rú shuǐ shāng xīn*: The heart governs the blood and vessels. Water damaging the heart therefore refers to water-damp damaging the blood and vessels.

[2] Joint-running 历节 *lì jié*: Pain in numerous joints preventing normal bending and stretching.

SYNOPSIS, LINE 5.4

This line discusses the pathomechanism of joint-running.

COMMENTARY, LINE 5.4

This line describes how joint-running arises due to cold-damp invading the inner body in patients with liver-kidney vacuity. The pulse in such cases is sunken and weak. The sunken quality reflects the fact that disease is in the interior and specifically indicates kidney qì vacuity. Because the kidney governs the bones, a sunken pulse can also mean disease of the bone. A weak pulse means insufficiency of liver blood. Since the liver governs the sinews, it also means disease of the sinews. Both kidney qì vacuity and liver blood vacuity are internal factors in the development of joint-running.

When a person sweats, the interstices open. If a person with kidney qì vacuity and liver blood vacuity bathes, works in water, encounters rainy weather, or otherwise is exposed to water while sweating, water-damp can exploit the vacuity and enter the body. When a person is affected by cold, the skin contracts, the interstices are blocked, the person is unable to sweat, and the evil cannot be discharged outward. Instead, it flows into the flesh, sinews, and bone and damages the blood and vessels, causing multiple joints to become painful and swollen. If cold-damp lies depressed for a long time, it can transform into heat. Damp-heat steaming in the bones and joints results in the discharge of yellow sweat in the swollen painful joints. This differs from the disease of yellow sweat, caused by damp-heat lying depressed in the skin, in which yellow sweat is discharged all over the body, in combination with swelling of the extremities, head, and face.

Line 5.5

趺阳脉浮而滑，滑则谷气实，浮则汗自出。

Fū yáng mài fú ér huá, huá zé gǔ qì shí, fú zé hàn zì chū.

[When] the instep yáng[1] pulse is floating and slippery, the slippery quality means that grain qì is replete, and the floating quality means spontaneous sweating.

Text Note, Line 5.5

[1] Instep yáng 跗阳 *fū yáng*: The pulsating vessel felt on the dorsum of the foot at Surging Yáng (*chōng yáng*, ST-42), one of the six positions and nine indicators (六補九候 *liù bù jiǔ hòu*).

Synopsis, Line 5.5

This line discusses heat brewing in the stomach on the basis of a slippery and floating pulse.

Commentary, Line 5.5

The instep yáng pulse reflects stomach qì. When this pulse is slippery, it means "replete grain qì," which here indicates exuberant stomach heat. A floating pulse is a sign of wind, but it can also be a sign of interior heat steaming outward. A floating pulse at the inch opening (wrist) primarily means wind and secondarily means interior. A floating pulse at the instep yáng means either vacuity or exuberant qì. When floating and slippery qualities are detected at the instep yáng, this strongly suggests interior heat steaming. The reason why the line associates sweating with this floating pulse is because the interior heat is also causing the fluids to discharge outward. When a patient is exposed to wind or enters water under these circumstances, the contention between interior heat and external evil can give rise to joint-running.

Line 5.6

少阴脉浮而弱，弱则血不足，浮则为风，风血相搏，即疼痛如掣。

Shào yīn mài fú ér ruò, ruò zé xuè bù zú, fú zé wéi fēng, fēng xuè xiāng bó, jí téng tòng rú chè.

[When] the lesser yīn pulse[1] is floating and weak, the weak quality means that blood is insufficient, [while] the floating quality means wind. When wind and blood contend with each other, there is pain as if from pulling.[2]

TEXT NOTES, LINE 5.6

[1] Lesser yīn pulse 少阴脉 *shào yīn mài*: The pulse felt at Spirit Gate (*shén mén*, HT-7) and Great Ravine (*tài xī*, KI-3).

[2] Pain as if from pulling 疼痛如掣 *téng tòng rú chè*: Pain associated with a pulling sensation.

SYNOPSIS, LINE 5.6

This line discusses yīn-blood vacuity with contraction of wind evil, which gives rise to joint-running.

COMMENTARY, LINE 5.6

The significance of "lesser yīn pulse" is not entirely clear. Given the particular context here and the reference to the inch opening and instep yáng pulses above, it most likely refers to diagnosing the foot lesser yīn kidney channel at Great Ravine (*tài xī*, KI-3) and the hand lesser yīn heart channel at Spirit Gate (*shén mén*, HT-7). Thus it reflects the condition of the heart and kidney, and a weak lesser yīn pulse specifically expresses an insufficiency of heart-kidney yīn blood. Given that the floating characteristic further indicates wind, this line discusses conditions of yīn-blood vacuity complicated by wind evil entering the blood vessels. The struggle between right and evil causes impediment in the channels and stagnation of qì and blood, which results in tugging pain in the joints and inability to bend and stretch.

Line 5.7

盛人脉濇小，短气自汗出，历节痛，不可屈伸，此皆饮酒汗出当风所致。

Shèng rén mài sè xiǎo, duǎn qì zì hàn chū, lì jié tòng, bù kě qū shēn, cǐ jiē yǐn jiǔ hàn chū dāng fēng suǒ zhì.

[When] people of exuberant [physique][1] [present with] a pulse that is rough and small, shortness of breath, spontaneous sweating, joint-running pain, and inability to bend and stretch, this is always [due to] drinking wine, sweating, and exposure to wind.

TEXT NOTE, LINE 5.7

1. People of exuberant physique 盛人 *shèng rén*: Obese people.

SYNOPSIS, LINE 5.7

This line discusses the signs and pathomechanisms of joint-running in the obese.

COMMENTARY, LINE 5.7

Fat people with strong, firm bodies and plentiful qì and blood should present with a slippery and large pulse. In the present line however, the pulse is rough and small, indicating an exuberant physique in conjunction with qì vacuity. Despite the outward superabundance, there is internal insufficiency. The qì vacuity is reflected in shortness of breath and insecurity of defense qì that manifests in spontaneous sweating. When defense qì is vacuous and the interstices are loose and empty, a person is prone to contraction of external wind. Furthermore, obese people tend toward dampness, which is exacerbated by drinking alcohol. If such a person sweats after drinking and then is exposed to wind, the wind and dampness will combine internally and externally and stagnate in the sinews and bones, obstructing the movement of qì and blood. This gives rise to pain in the joints and inhibited bending and stretching.

Line 5.8

诸肢节疼痛，身体魁羸，脚肿如脱，头眩短气，温温欲吐，桂枝芍药知母汤主之。

桂枝四两　芍药三两　甘草二两　麻黄二两　生姜五两　白朮五两　知母四两　防风四两 附子（炮）二枚

右九味，以水七升，煮取二升，温服七合，日三服。

Zhū zhī jié téng tòng, shēn tǐ kuí léi, jiǎo zhǒng rú tuō, tóu xuàn duǎn qì, yùn yùn yù tù, guì zhī sháo yào zhī mǔ tāng zhǔ zhī.

Guì zhī sì liǎng; sháo yào sān liǎng; gān cǎo èr liǎng; má huáng èr liǎng; shēng jiāng wǔ liǎng; bái zhú wǔ liǎng; zhī mǔ sì liǎng; fáng fēng sì liǎng; fù zǐ (pào) èr méi

Yòu jiǔ wèi, yǐ shuǐ qī shēng, zhǔ qǔ èr shēng, wēn fú qī gě, rì sān fú.

All types of joint pain with marked emaciation[1] of the body, feet swollen as [if about to] drop off,[2] dizzy head, shortness of breath, and seething desire to vomit[3] are governed by Cinnamon Twig, Peony, and Anemarrhena Decoction (桂枝芍药知母汤 *guì zhī sháo yào zhī mǔ tāng*).

Cinnamon Twig, Peony, and Anemarrhena Decoction (桂枝芍药知母汤 *guì zhī sháo yào zhī mǔ tāng*)
cinnamon twig (桂枝 *guì zhī*, Cinnamomi Ramulus) 4 *liǎng* peony (芍药 *sháo yào*, Paeoniae Radix) 3 *liǎng* licorice (甘草 *gān cǎo*, Glycyrrhizae Radix) 2 *liǎng*

ephedra (麻黄 *má huáng*, Ephedrae Herba) 2 *liǎng*
fresh ginger (生姜 *shēng jiāng*, Zingiberis Rhizoma Recens) 5 *liǎng*
white atractylodes (白朮 *bái zhú*, Atractylodis Macrocephalae Rhizoma) 5 *liǎng*
anemarrhena (知母 *zhī mǔ*, Anemarrhenae Rhizoma) 4 *liǎng*
saposhnikovia (防风 *fáng fēng*, Saposhnikoviae Radix) 4 *liǎng*
aconite (附子 *fù zǐ*, Aconiti Radix Lateralis Praeparata) 2 pieces (blast-fry)

Boil the above nine ingredients in 7 *shēng* of water to get 2 *shēng*. Take seven *gě* warm, three times a day.

TEXT NOTES, LINE 5.8

[1] Marked emaciation 魁羸 *kuí léi*: It is agreed that this term means marked emaciation, it is not clear why the word 魁 *kuí*, "large" or "prominent" appears here. Some have suggested that it may be a mistranscription of 尪 *wāng*, which also denotes emaciation.

[2] Feet swollen as [if about to] drop off 脚肿欲脱 *jiǎo zhǒng yù tuō*: Swelling of the feet and lower legs with a sense of distention and numbness, as though they were about to detach themselves from the body.

[3] Seething desire to vomit 温温欲吐 *yùn yùn yù tù*: Desire to vomit with depression and ill-being in the heart.

SYNOPSIS, LINE 5.8

This line discusses the signs and treatment of wind-damp joint-running.

COMMENTARY, LINE 5.8

When wind-damp flows into the sinews and joints, it inhibits the flow of qì and blood; hence the joints become painful and swollen. When wind-damp lies depressed for a long time, it transforms into heat, consuming qì and damaging yīn. As a result, the body becomes progressively emaciated. When damp turbidity pours downward and has no way out, the feet become swollen. When dampness brews internally, it obstructs the upbearing and downbearing of qì, giving rise to shortness of breath. When clear yáng fails to bear upward, there is dizziness. When dampness harasses the stomach, it impairs the harmonious downbearing of the stomach; hence there is a desire to vomit. Because wind-damp is transforming into heat, which damages yīn, the condition is complicated by yīn vacuity internal heat, which manifests in heat effusion. Thus as a whole the pathomechanism is one of lodged dampness evil lying depressed for a long time and transforming into heat, which damages yīn. The evils impede the sinews vessels, giving rise to joint-running disease.

The treatment for this condition is to address both the evil and right. You must dispel wind and eliminate dampness on the one hand, and free yáng and diffuse impediment on the other. At the same time, you must clear heat and nourish yīn.

The proposed formula is Cinnamon Twig, Peony, and Anemarrhena Decoction (*guì zhī sháo yào zhī mǔ tāng*). The cinnamon twig (*guì zhī*) and aconite (*fù zǐ*) free yáng and diffuse impediment, while also warming the channels and dispersing cold. Cinnamon twig (*guì zhī*) combined with ephedra (*má huáng*) and saposhnikovia (*fáng fēng*) dispels wind and disperses exterior dampness. White atractylodes (*bái zhú*) fortifies the spleen and dries internal dampness. Anemarrhena (*zhī mǔ*) and peony (*sháo yào*) boost yīn and clear the blood. Fresh ginger (*shēng jiāng*) downbears counterflow and checks retching. Licorice (*gān cǎo*) harmonizes the stomach and regulates the center.

The ingeniousness of the formula is that it treats both the evil and right, and applies both cold and heat. It includes warm/hot ephedra (*má huáng*), cinnamon twig (*guì zhī*), and aconite (*fù zǐ*) to dispel wind and cold, and white atractylodes (*bái zhú*) to eliminate exterior and interior dampness. It also includes cold/cool anemarrhena (*zhī mǔ*) and peony (*sháo yào*) to support right and nourish yīn.

In this combination, the cold/cool medicines prevent the warm acrid medicines from transforming into dryness and damaging yīn, while warm/hot medicinals prevent the cold/cool agents from assisting the cold and damaging yáng.

Line 5.9

味酸则伤筋，筋伤则缓，名曰泄，咸则伤骨，骨伤则痿，名曰枯。枯泄相搏，名曰断泄。营气不通，卫不独行，营卫俱微，三焦无所御，四属断绝，身体羸瘦，独足肿大，黄汗出，胫冷。 假令发热，便为历节也。

Wèi suān zé shāng jīn, jīn shāng zé huǎn, míng yuē xiè, xián zé shāng gǔ, gǔ shāng zé wěi, míng yuē kū. Kū xiè xiāng bó, míng yuē duàn xiè. Yíng qì bù tōng, wèi bù dú xíng, yíng wèi jù wēi, sān jiāo wú suǒ yù, sì shǔ duàn jué, shēn tǐ léi sòu, dú zú zhǒng dà, huáng hàn chū, jìng lěng. Jiǎ lìng fā rè, biàn wéi lì jié yě.

Sour flavor damages the sinews, and when the sinews are damaged, they slacken. This is called "discharge." Saltiness damages the bones, and when the bones are damaged, they wilt. This is called "desiccation." When desiccation and discharge contend with each other, this is called "severing [and] discharge."[1] [When] construction qì does not flow freely, defense qì cannot move alone. Construction and defense are both debilitated, the triple burner is not controlled, and the four ascriptions[2] are cut off.[3] The body is markedly emaciated, the feet only are swollen, yellow sweat issues, and the lower legs are cold. If [the lower legs] effuse heat, this is joint-running.

TEXT NOTES, LINE 5.9

[1] Severing [and] discharge 断泄 *duàn xiè*: See Commentary below.

[2] The four ascriptions 四属 *sì shǔ*: The skin, flesh, fat, and marrow.

[3] Cut off 断绝 *duàn jué*: They are deprived of the nourishment of essential qì.

SYNOPSIS, LINE 5.9

This line discusses liking for sour and salty food as the cause of joint-running, differentiating this from yellow sweat disease.

COMMENTARY, LINE 5.9

The human body needs foods of the five flavors to maintain health. Excessive consumption of one particular flavor can be damaging. Sourness generally supplements the liver, but when eaten in excess can damage it instead. The liver stores the blood and governs the sinews. When the liver is damaged, the blood is no longer stored by the liver but discharges, while the sinews slacken and fail to perform their function. Damage to the liver function is referred to in the text as "discharge."

Similarly, saltiness usually supplements the kidney, but when eaten in excess it can damage the kidney. The kidney governs the bones and engenders marrow. When the kidney is damaged, the bones and marrow are also affected. They become weak, which is referred to in the text as "desiccation." A combination of these two conditions is called "severing and discharge." When liver-kidney vacuity persists, essence and blood become debilitated, which affects construction, defense, qì, and blood. Vacuity of construction and defense deprives the skin, flesh, fat, and marrow (the four ascriptions) of nourishment and warmth. As a result, the body becomes increasingly emaciated. When the triple burner fails to perform its function and the sluices fail to operate, damp turbidity flows downward rather than being discharged, hence the feet are swollen.

The last part of the line hints at a distinction between yellow sweat disease and joint-running. Yellow sweat may occur in yellow sweat disease as well as in joint-running. In yellow sweat disease, the lower legs are cold, while in joint-running with yellow sweat, the lower legs effuse heat. Not mentioned in the line is the fact that with joint-running the joints are painful and swollen, and the yellow sweat is confined to the joints. In yellow sweat disease, there is no pain and swelling of the joints, and the yellow sweat is generalized.

Line 5.10

病历节不可屈伸, 疼痛, 乌头汤主之。

治脚气疼痛, 不可屈伸。

麻黄 芍药 黄芪各三两 甘草（炙）川乌（㕮咀, 以蜜二升, 煎取一升, 即出乌头）五枚

右五味，㕮咀四味，以水三升，煮取一升，去滓，内蜜煎中，更煎之，服七合，不知，尽服之。

治脚气冲心。

矾石二两

右一味，一浆水一斗五升，煎三五沸，浸脚良。

Bìng lì jié bù kě qū shēn, téng tòng, wū tóu tāng zhǔ zhī.

Zhì jiǎo qì téng tòng, bù kě qū shēn.

Má huáng sháo yào huáng qí gè sān liǎng; gān cǎo (zhì); chuān wū (fǔ jǔ, yǐ mì èr shēng, jiān qǔ yī shēng, jí chū wū tóu) wǔ méi

Yòu wǔ wèi, fǔ qǔ sì wèi, yǐ shuǐ sān shēng, zhǔ qǔ yī shēng, qù zǐ, nà mì jiān zhōng, gèng jiān zhī, fú qī gě, bù zhī, jìn fú zhī.

Zhì jiǎo qì chōng xīn.

Fán shí èr liǎng

Yòu yī wèi, yī jiāng shuǐ yī dǒu wǔ shēng, jiān sān wǔ fèi, jìn jiǎo liáng.

[For] joint-running with inability to bend and stretch and with pain, Aconite Main Root Decoction (乌头汤 *wū tóu tāng*) governs.

Treats leg qì with pain and inability to bend and stretch.

Aconite Main Root Decoction (乌头汤 *wū tóu tāng*)
ephedra (麻黄 *má huáng*, Ephedrae Herba) peony (芍药 *sháo yào*, Paeoniae Radix) astragalus (黄芪 *huáng qí*, Astragali Radix) 3 *liǎng* each licorice (甘草 *gān cǎo*, Glycyrrhizae Radix) (mix-fry) aconite main root (川乌 *chuān wū*, Aconiti Radix) 5 pieces (chew and boil in two *shēng* of honey to get one *sheng*, then remove the aconite)

Of the above five ingredients, chew [the first] four and boil in three *shēng* of water to get one *shēng*. Remove the dregs. Add the honey to the brew and boil again. Take seven *gě* [per dose]. If no effect is noticed, use it all.

To treat leg qì surging into the heart.[1]

Alum Decoction (矾石汤 *fán shí tāng*)
alum (矾石 *fán shí*, Alumen) 2 *liǎng*

Boil the single ingredient above in one *dǒu* and five *shēng* of sour rice milk, bringing to a boil three to five times. Soaking the legs is good.

TEXT NOTE, LINE 5.10

[1] Leg qì surging into the heart 脚气冲心 *jiǎo qì chōng xīn*: Leg qì disease with heart palpitation, panting, and vomiting. This is explained in terms of the qì of the disease surging into the region of the heart and disturbing not only the function of the heart but also that of the stomach.

SYNOPSIS, LINE 5.10

This line discusses the signs and treatment of cold-damp joint-running.

COMMENTARY, LINE 5.10

When cold-damp becomes lodged in the joints, impeding the channel vessels and inhibiting the movement of qì and blood, the joints become acutely painful and cannot bend and stretch. Aconite Main Root Decoction (*wū tóu tāng*) is used here to warm the channels and dispel cold and to eliminate dampness and resolve pain. Within the formula, ephedra (*má huáng*) effuses sweat and diffuses impediment. Aconite main root (*wū tóu*) dispels cold and resolves pain. Peony (*sháo yào*) and licorice (*gān cǎo*) moderate tension and soothe the sinews. Astragalus (*huáng qí*) boosts qì and secures the exteriror, helping ephedra (*má huáng*) and main tuber (*wū tóu*) to warm the channels relieve pain and reducing the dispersing effect of ephedra (*má huáng*). Honey (*mì*) is sweet and moderating, and resolves the toxin of aconite main root (*wū tóu*). The formula as a whole causes cold-damp to resolve through light sweating, so that right qì will naturally be restored by eliminating the disease.

Leg qì surging into the heart refers to severe cases of leg qì. Leg qì alone is a disease that manifests in painful swollen legs, possibly with weakness and numbness. If these symptoms are complicated by disturbances in the chest like heart palpitation, panting, oppression in the chest, and vomiting, this is due to devitalized heart yáng and dual vacuity of the spleen and kidney. When the spleen is vacuous, it fails to move water-damp; when the kidney is vacuous, qì transformation breaks down. As a result, damp turbidity exuberates internally and, when compounded by a vacuity of heart yáng, surges up into the heart. Alum Decoction (*fán shí tāng*) applied externally as a soak dries dampness, downbears turbidity, clears heat, and resolves toxin.

附方 Appended Formulas, Line 5.10

《古今录验》续命汤 Life Prolonging Decoction (续命汤 *xù mìng tāng*) from the *Gŭ Jīn Lù Yàn* ("Ancient and Modern Records Tested")

治中风痱，身体不能自收持，口不能言，冒昧不知痛处，或拘急不得转侧。

麻黄 桂枝 当归 人参 石膏 干姜 甘草各三两 芎藭一两 杏仁四十枚

右九味，以水一斗，煮取四升，温服一升，当小汗，薄覆脊，凭几坐，汗出则愈，不汗更服，无所禁，勿当风。并治但伏不得卧，咳逆上气，面目浮肿。

Xù mìng tāng

Zhì zhōng fēng féi, shēn tǐ bù néng zì shōu chí, kǒu bù néng yán, mào mèi bù zhī tòng chù, huò jū jí bù dé zhuǎn cè.

Má huáng guì zhī dāng guī rén shēn shí gāo gān jiāng gān cǎo gè sān liǎng xiōng qióng yī liǎng xìng rén sì shí méi

Yòu jiǔ wèi, yǐ shuǐ yī dǒu, zhǔ qǔ sì shēng, wēn fú yī shēng, dāng xiǎo hàn, bó fù jǐ, píng jī zuò, hàn chū zé yù, bù hàn gèng fú, wú suǒ jìn, wù dāng fēng. Bìng zhì dàn fú bù dé wò, ké nì shàng qì, miàn mù fú zhǒng.

For treating wind-stroke disability[1] [manifesting in] inability of the body to hold itself together, inability to speak, veiling confusion[2] not knowing the location of the pain, and possibly hypertonicity with inability to turn sides.[3]

Life-Prolonging Decoction (*xù mìng tāng* 续命汤)
ephedra (麻黄 *má huáng*, Ephedrae Herba) 3 *liǎng*
cinnamon twig (桂枝 *guì zhī*, Cinnamomi Ramulus) 3 *liǎng*
Chinese angelica (当归 *dāng guī*, Angelicae Sinensis Radix) 3 *liǎng*
ginseng (人参 *rén shēn*, Ginseng Radix) 3 *liǎng*
gypsum (石膏 *shí gāo*, Gypsum Fibrosum) 3 *liǎng*
dried ginger (干姜 *gān jiāng*, Zingiberis Rhizoma) 3 *liǎng*
licorice (甘草 *gān cǎo*, Glycyrrhizae Radix) 3 *liǎng*
xiongqiong (芎藭 *xiōng qióng*, Chuanxiong Rhizoma)1 *liǎng*
apricot kernel (杏仁 *xìng rén*, Armeniacae Semen) 40 kernels

Boil the above nine ingredients with one *dǒu* of water to get four *shēng*. Take one shēng [per dose] warm, which should induce slight sweating. Thinly cover the back and sit leaning over a small table. If [the patient] sweats, recovery will ensue.

If there is no sweating, take another dose. There are no contraindications other than to avoid exposure to wind. [This formula] also treats only being able to bend over, but not to lie down, counterflow ascent cough, and puffy swelling of the face and eyes.

FORMULA NOTES, LINE 5.10

1 Wind-stroke disability 中风痱 *zhòng fēng féi*: Inhibited movement of the body with inability to feel pain or itching. It is also called 风痱 *fēng féi*, wind disability.

2 Veiling confusion 冒昧 *mào mèi*: Clouded head and confused mind.

3 The commentary adds: "Yáo states: This is the same as Major Life-Prolonging Decoction (*dà xù mìng tāng*). It also treats postpartum bleeding in women, and the elderly and young."

THREE YELLOWS DECOCTION (三黄汤 *sān huáng tāng*) from the *Qiān Jīn Fāng* ("Thousand Gold Pieces Prescriptions")

治中风手足拘急，百节疼痛，烦热心乱，恶寒，经日不欲饮食。

麻黄五分　独活四分　细辛二分　黄芪二分　黄芩三分

右五味，以水六升，煮取二升，分温三服。一服小汗，二服大汗。心热加大黄二分，腹满加枳实一枚，气逆加人参三分，悸加牡蛎三分，渴加栝蒌根三分，先有寒加附子一枚。

Zhì zhōng fēng shǒu zú jū jí, bǎi jié téng tòng, fán rè xīn luàn, wù hán, jīng rì bù yù yǐn shí.

Má huáng wǔ fèn; dú huó sì fèn; xì xīn èr fèn; huáng qí èr fèn; huáng qín sān fèn

Yòu wǔ wèi, yǐ shuǐ liù shēng, zhǔ qǔ èr shēng, fēn wēn sān fú. Yī fú xiǎo hàn, èr fú dà hàn. Xīn rè jiā dà huáng èr fēn, fù mǎn jiā zhǐ shí yī méi, qì nì jiā rén shēn sān fēn, jì jiā mǔ lì sān fēn, kě jiā guā lóu gēn sān fēn, xiān yǒu hán jiā fù zǐ yī méi.

For treating wind-stroke with hypertonicity of the extremities, pain in the hundred joints, heat vexation and aversion to cold, and no desire for food and drink for several days.

Three Yellows Decoction (三黄汤 *sān huáng tāng*)
ephedra (麻黄 *má huáng*, Ephedrae Herba) 5 parts
pubescent angelica (独活 *dú huó*, Angelicae Pubescentis Radix) 4 parts
asarum (细辛 *xì xīn*, Asari Radix et Rhizoma) 2 parts
astragalus (黄芪 *huáng qí*, Astragali Radix) 2 parts
scutellaria (黄芩 *huáng qín*, Scutellariae Radix) 3 parts

Boil the above five ingredients in six *shēng* of water to get two *shēng*. Separate into three doses and take warm. The first dose induces slight sweating; the second dose induces great sweating. For heat in the heart, add two parts of rhubarb (*dà huáng*); for abdominal fullness, add one piece of unripe bitter orange (*zhǐ shí*); for qì counterflow, add three parts of ginseng (*rén shēn*); for palpitation, add three parts of oyster shell (*mǔ lì*); for thirst, add three parts of trichosanthes root (*guā lóu gěn*); for preexisting cold, add one piece of aconite (*fù zǐ*).

WHITE ATRACTYLODES AND ACONITE DECOCTION (朮附汤 *zhú fù tāng*) from the *Jìn Xiào Fāng* ("Handy and Effective Formulas")

治风虚头重眩，苦极，不知食味，暖肌补中，益精气。

白朮二两 附子(炮去皮)一枚半 甘草（炙）一两

右三味，剉，每五钱匕，姜五片，枣一枚，水盏半，煎七分，去滓温服。

Zhì fēng xū tóu zhòng xuàn, kǔ jí, bù zhī shí wèi, nuǎn jī bǔ zhōng, yì jīng qì.

Bái zhú èr liǎng fù zǐ (pào qù pí) yī méi bàn gān cǎo (zhì) yī liǎng

Yòu sān wèi, cuò, měi wǔ qián bǐ, jiāng wǔ piàn, zǎo yī méi, shuǐ zhǎn bàn, jiān qī fēn, qù zǐ wēn fú.

For treating wind vacuity, heaviness of the head and dizziness, extreme suffering, and inability to taste the flavor of food. It warms the flesh, supplements the center, and boosts essential qì.

White Atractylodes and Aconite Decoction (朮附汤 *zhú fù tāng*)
white atractylodes (白朮 *bái zhú*, Atractylodis Macrocephalae Rhizoma) 2 *liǎng*
aconite (附子 *fù zǐ*, Aconiti Radix Lateralis Praeparata) 1.5 pieces (blast-fry and remove skin)
licorice (甘草 *gān cǎo*, Glycyrrhizae Radix) 1 *liǎng* (mix-fry)

Grate the above three ingredients. For each [dose], boil five qián-spoonfuls in half a cup of water with five slices of ginger and one jujube until reduced to seven tenths. Remove dregs and take warm.

CUĪ'S EIGHT-INGREDIENT PILL (崔氏八味丸 *cuī shì bā wèi wán*)

治脚气上入，少腹不仁。

干地黄八两 山茱萸 薯蓣各四两 泽泻 茯苓 牡丹皮各三两 桂枝 附子（炮）各一两

右八味，末之，炼蜜和丸梧子大，酒下十五丸，日再服。

Zhì jiǎo qì shàng rù, shào fù bù rén.

Gān dì huáng bā liǎng shān zhū yú shǔ yù gè sì liǎng zé xiè fú líng mǔ dān pí gè sān liǎng guì zhī fù zǐ (pào) gè yī liǎng

Yòu bā wèi, mò zhī, liàn mì huò wán wú zǐ dà, jiǔ xià shí wǔ wán, rì zài fú.

For treating leg qì entering the upper body and insensitivity of the lesser abdomen.

Cuī's Eight-Ingredient Pill (崔氏八味丸 *cuī shì bā wèi wán*)
dried rehmannia (干地黄 *gān dì huáng*, Rehmanniae Radix) 8 *liǎng*
cornus (山茱萸 *shān zhū yú*, Corni Fructus) 4 *liǎng*
dioscorea (薯蓣 *shǔ yù*, Dioscoreae Rhizoma) 4 *liǎng*
alisma (泽泻 *zé xiè*, Alismatis Rhizoma) 3 *liǎng*
poria (茯苓 *fú líng*, Poria) 3 *liǎng*
moutan (牡丹皮 *mǔ dān* pí, Moutan Cortex) 3 *liǎng*
cinnamon twig (桂枝 *guì zhī*, Cinnamomi Ramulus)1 *liǎng*
aconite (附子 *fù zǐ*, Aconiti Radix Lateralis Praeparata)1 *liǎng* (blast-fry)

Grind the above eight ingredients and blend with processed honey (*liàn mì*). Form into pills the size of firmiana seeds. Swallow 15 pills in wine twice a day.

SPLEEN-EFFUSING DECOCTION PLUS WHITE ATRACTYLODES (越婢加朮汤 *yuè bì jiā zhú tāng*) from the *Qiān Jīn Fāng* ("Thousand Gold Pieces Prescriptions")

治肉极，热则身体津脱，腠理开，汗大泄，厉风气，下焦脚弱。

麻黄六两 石膏半斤 生姜二两 甘草二两 白朮四两 大枣十五枚

右六味，以水六升，先煮麻黄，去上沫，内诸药，煮取三升，分温三服，恶风加附子一枚，炮。

Zhì ròu jí, rè zé shēn tǐ jīn tuō, còu lǐ kāi, hàn dà xiè, lì fēng qì, xià jiāo jiǎo ruò.

Má huáng liù liǎng shí gāo bàn jīn shēng jiāng èr liǎng gān cǎo èr liǎng bái zhú sì liǎng dà zǎo shí wǔ méi

Yòu liù wèi, yǐ shuǐ liù shēng, xiān zhǔ má huáng, qù shàng mò, nà zhū yào, zhǔ qǔ sān shēng, fēn wēn sān fú, wù fēng jiā fù zǐ yī méi, pào.

For treating extreme of the flesh,[1] heat causing generalized desertion of liquid, opening of the interstices, great discharge of sweat, pestilential wind qì, and weakness of the lower burner and legs.

Spleen-Effusing Decoction Plus White Atractylodes (越婢加朮汤 *yuè bì jiā zhú tāng*)

- ephedra (麻黄 *má huáng*, Ephedrae Herba) 6 *liǎng*
- gypsum (石膏 *shí gāo*, Gypsum Fibrosum) ½ *jīn*
- fresh ginger (生姜 *shēng jiāng*, Zingiberis Rhizoma Recens) 2 *liǎng*
- licorice (甘草 *gān cǎo*, Glycyrrhizae Radix) 2 *liǎng*
- white atractylodes (白朮 *bái zhú*, Atractylodis Macrocephalae Rhizoma) 4 *liǎng*
- jujube (大枣 *dà zǎo*, Jujubae Fructus) 15 pieces

Of the above six ingredients, first boil the ephedra in six *shēng* of water. Remove the scum, add all [the other] medicinals, and boil to get three *shēng*. Separate into three doses and take warm. For aversion to cold, add one piece of blast-fried aconite (*pào fù zǐ*).

FORMULA NOTE, LINE 5.10

[1] Extreme of the flesh 肉极 *ròu jí*: This is the name of a disease that manifests in emaciation of the flesh in the extremities and in fatigue and lack of strength.

血痹虚劳病脉证治第六

CHAPTER 6

Blood Impediment and Vacuity Taxation

Pulses, Signs, Treatments

‡ OVERVIEW

This chapter discusses blood impediment and vacuity taxation, with emphasis on vacuity taxation. The two disease categories are placed together in one chapter because both are vacuity patterns.

BLOOD IMPEDIMENT

Blood impediment is mainly characterized by numbness in parts of the body. It arises when patients suffering from qì and blood vacuity contract external wind evil, which causes stagnation in the flow of blood. It is called "blood impediment," but differs from classical impediment patterns, which are caused by a combination of wind, cold, and dampness and are characterized chiefly by pain in the sinews, bones, flesh, and joints. Blood impediment is also caused by external evil, but not necessarily by a combination of wind, cold, and dampness. Furthermore its chief sign is numbness rather than pain.

VACUITY TAXATION

Vacuity taxation is broad in scope and refers to conditions of chronic debilitation that arise from a variety of causes and manifest in numerous symptoms. It includes any severe and chronic form of vacuity that results from taxation fatigue, i.e., excessive taxing of the body by overexertion, sexual intemperance, or dietary irregularities, and over time turns into detriment. It involves depletion of yīn and yáng, qì and blood, and bowels and viscera. It can be divided into qì vacuity, blood vacuity, dual vacuity of qì and blood, yīn vacuity, and yáng vacuity. Because detriment to yīn affects yáng and detriment to yáng affects yīn, any severe, chronic form of yīn or yáng vacuity results in dual vacuity of yīn and yáng, which is a fundamental feature of vacuity taxation patterns. Vacuity detriment is treated by supplementing qì, nourishing the blood, enriching yīn, and warming yáng. Supplementing the spleen and kidney figure prominently.

Vacuity detriment refers to conditions that have been variously named as "the five taxations" and "five detriments" in the *Nèi Jīng* ("The Inner Canon") and as "six [dire] extremes" and "seven damages" in later literature. Vacuity detriment is sometimes confused with pulmonary consumption (肺痨 *fèi láo*, 痨瘵 *láo zhài*), a contagious disease characterized by cough, expectoration of blood, tidal heat effusion, night sweating, and emaciation. However, contagiousness and expectoration of blood are not features of vacuity detriment patterns, and the two diseases need to be differentiated clearly.

Schematic Overview

Blood Impediment

1. Cause: [This disease affects] respected and honored people with weak bones and exuberant flesh. Because they are heavy and encumbered, they are easily fatigued and sweat and they frequently toss and turn in their sleep. If they are exposed to [even] slight wind, they contract this disease as a result.
2. Pulses:
   a) Main pulse
      Yīn and yáng are both faint.
      Faint on the inch opening.
   b) Concurrent pulse
      Slightly tight at the bar.
      Slightly tight at the cubit.
3. External signs
   a) Generalized insensitivity, as in wind impediment.
4. Treatment
   a) Acupuncture: Use needles to conduct yáng qì. [This will] make the pulse harmonious and remove the tightness, [so that the patient will] then recover.
   b) Formula: Astragalus and Cinnamon Twig Five Agents Decoction (*huáng qí guì zhī wǔ wù tāng*).

Vacuity Taxation

1. Pattern identification

   a) Main pulse and signs: In men who [appear] healthy, a large pulse means taxation; an extremely vacuous one also means taxation.

   b) Blood vacuity

   Pulse: floating.

   Complexion: Thin white.

   Disease pattern: blood collapse, interior vacuity, thirst, sudden panting and palpitation.

   c) Qì vacuity and blood desertion

   Pulse: in males, vacuous, sunken, and stringlike.

   Complexion: White.

   Signs: shortness of breath, abdominal urgency, inhibited urination, white facial complexion, periodic dimness of vision, concurrent spontaneous external bleeding, lesser abdominal fullness.

   d) Vacuous yīn and floating yang

   Pulse: Floating and large.

   Signs: vexation in the extremities, genital cold, spontaneous loss of semen, aching pain and wasting with inability to walk.

   Mechanism: Aggravated in the spring and summer; remission in the autumn and winter.

   e) Dual vacuity of fire and water in the kidney

   Pulse: In males, floating, weak, and rough.

   Signs: Essential qì clear and cold—childlessness.

   f) Yáng qì floating outward

   Pulse: In a person of fifty or sixty years of age, a pathologically large pulse.

   Signs: Impediment along the furrows of the back, rumbling intestines, saber and pearl-string lumps.

   g) Dual vacuity of yīn and yáng

   Pulse: In men [who appear] normal healthy, a pulse that is vacuous, weak, fine, or faint.

   Signs: Night sweating.

   h) Spleen qì vacuity cold

   Pulse: sunken, small, slow.

   Pathomechanism: deserting qì.

   Signs: Noisy panting when walking fast, counterflow cold of the extremities, abdominal fullness, in severe cases sloppy diarrhea, and food failing to disperse and transform.

   i) Depletion of essential qì

Pulse: stringlike = reduced = cold; large = scallion-stalk = vacuity; cold + vacuity = drumskin.

Disease: In women, it manifests in mid-term delivery (late miscarriage) and spotting; in men, in blood collapse and seminal loss.

2) Treatment

a) Spleen-kidney vacuity cold

Pulse: Extremely vacuous, scallion-stalk, and slow.

Signs: Seminal loss with stringlike tension in the lesser abdomen, yīn-head cold, hair loss = clear grain, blood collapse, and seminal loss.

Formula: Tiānxiōng Aconite Powder (*tiān xióng sǎn*).

b) Liver-kidney vacuity cold

Pulse: scallion-stalk, stirring, and slightly tight.

Signs: Seminal loss with stringlike tension in the lesser abdomen, yīn-head cold, hair loss = in men seminal loss and in women dreaming of intercourse.

Formula: Cinnamon Twig Decoction Plus Dragon Bone and Oyster Shell (*guì zhī jiā lóng gǔ mǔ lì tāng*).

c) Kidney yáng depletion

Signs: Vacuity taxation lumbar pain, hypertonicity in the lesser abdomen, inhibited urination.

Formula: Eight-Ingredient Kidney Qì Pill (*bā wèi shèn qì wán*).

d) Yīn vacuity and yáng exuberance

Signs: Vacuity taxation with vexation and sleeplessness.

Formula: Spiny Jujube Decoction (*suān zǎo rén tāng*).

e) Concurrent contraction of wind qì

Signs: Vacuity taxation with insufficiency of everything and the hundred diseases of wind qì.

Formula: Dioscorea Pill (*shǔ yù wán*).

f) Dry blood in the inner body

Signs: Marked emaciation, encrusted skin, dark eyes, abdominal fullness with inability to eat.

Formula: Rhubarb and Ground Beetle Pill (*dà huáng zhè chóng wán*).

Line 6.1

问曰：血痹病从何得之？师曰：夫尊荣人骨弱肌肤盛，重困疲劳汗出，卧不时动摇，加被微风遂得之。但以脉自微濇，在寸口，关上小紧，宜针引阳气，令脉和紧去则愈。

Wèn yuē: xuè bì bìng cóng hé dé zhī? Shī yuē: Fū zūn róng rén gǔ ruò jī fū shèng, zhòng kùn pí láo hàn chū, wò bù shí dòng yáo, jiā bèi wēi fēng suì dé zhī. Dàn yǐ mài zì wēi sè zài cùn kǒu, guān shàng xiǎo jǐn, yí zhēn yǐn yáng qì, lìng mài hé, jǐn qù zé yú.

Question: "How is blood impediment disease acquired?"

The Master says: "[This disease affects] respected and honored people[1] with weak bones and exuberant flesh.[2] Because they are heavy and encumbered, they are easily fatigued and sweat and they frequently toss and turn in their sleep. If they are exposed to [even] slight wind, they contract this disease as a result. [In such patients, if] the pulse is normally slightly rough, but is slightly tight[3] on the inch opening and bar,[4] it is appropriate to use needles to conduct yáng qì.[5] [This will] make the pulse harmonious and remove the tightness. Recovery will ensue.

TEXT NOTES, LINE 6.1

[1] Respected and honored people 尊荣人 *zūn róng rén*: People of high social status. As the text hints, these are people who tend to be overfed and lacking in exercise.

[2] Weak bones and exuberant flesh 骨弱肌肤盛 *gǔ ruò jī fū shèng*: Fundamentally unhealthy and overfed.

[3] Slightly tight 小紧 *xiǎo jǐn*: The Chinese literally states "small tight." This could be taken to mean "small [i.e., fine] and tight," but *xiǎo* can also be used adverbially (slightly).

[4] On the inch opening and bar 寸口关上 *cùn kǒu guān shàng*: The inch opening usually refers to the area of the wrist pulse as a whole. From the context here, however, it refers to the inch position (寸部 *cùn bù*), which is closest to the hand (see Chapter 1, line 1.7, note 1, and compare to the next line (6.2).

[5] Conduct *yáng qì* 引阳气 *yǐn yáng qì*: Incite yáng qì to move.

SYNOPSIS, LINE 6.1

This line discusses the cause, pathomechanism, pulse, and treatment of blood impediment.

COMMENTARY, LINE 6.1

The present line discusses how blood impediment arises. The disease primarily affects people who are well fed but do not engage in manual labor. Although they have exuberant flesh, they have weak sinews and bones—a condition often described as "external superabundance and internal insufficiency" (有余于外，不足于内 *yǒu yú yú wài, bù zú yú nèi*). Such people suffer from insecure interstices, which makes their resistance to disease poor. Because they lack healthful exercise and, having little to do, tend to think a lot, they have difficulty getting to sleep or do not sleep soundly, hence they tend to toss and turn. People who are externally superabundant and internally insufficient tend to sweat at the slightest exertion. In people constitutionally prone to fatigue, sweating can exacerbate yáng vacuity and increase susceptibility to contraction of external evils. It is precisely people of this kind who are susceptible to blood impediment since this disease arises when a person with blood and qì vacuity contracts external wind evil, which then causes inhibited movement of blood.

Line 6.2

血痹阴阳俱微，寸口关上微，尺中小紧，外证身体不仁，如风痹状，黄芪桂枝五物汤主之。

黄芪三两　芍药三两　桂枝三两　生姜六两　大枣十二枚

右五味，以水六升，煮取二升，温服七合，日三服。

Xuè bì yīn yáng jù wēi, cùn kǒu guān shàng wēi, chǐ zhōng xiǎo jǐn, wài zhèng shēn tǐ bù rén, rú fēng bì zhuàng, huáng qí guì zhī wǔ wù tāng zhǔ zhī.

Huáng qí sān liǎng; sháo yào sān liǎng; guì zhī sān liǎng; shēng jiāng liù liǎng; dà zǎo shí èr méi

Yòu wǔ wèi, yǐ shuǐ liù shēng, zhǔ qǔ èr shēng, wēn fú qī gě, rì sān fú.

In blood impediment, when yīn and yáng are both faint,[1] when [the pulse is] faint on the inch opening and bar and small and tight in the cubit, and when the external signs are generalized numbness and an appearance as in wind impediment,[2] [then] Astragalus and Cinnamon Twig Five Agents Decoction (*huáng qí guì zhī wǔ wù tāng*) governs.

Astragalus and Cinnamon Twig Five Agents Decoction (黄芪桂枝五物汤 *huáng qí guì zhī wǔ wù tāng*)

- astragalus (黄芪 *huáng qí*, Astragali Radix) 3 *liǎng*
- peony (芍药 *sháo yào*, Paeoniae Radix) 3 *liǎng*
- cinnamon twig (桂枝 *guì zhī*, Cinnamomi Ramulus) 3 *liǎng*
- fresh ginger (生姜 *shēng jiāng*, Zingiberis Rhizoma Recens) 6 *liǎng*
- jujube (大枣 dà zǎo, Jujubae Fructus) 12 pieces

Boil the above five ingredients with six *shēng* of water to get two *shēng*. Take seven *gě* three times a day.[3]

TEXT NOTES, LINE 6.2

[1] Yīn and yáng are both faint 阴阳俱微 *yīn yáng jù wēi*: The yīn and yáng aspects of the body are both weak.

[2] Wind impediment 风痹 *fēng bì*: An impediment pattern attributed to wind-cold-damp invading the limbs and channels. It is characterized by wandering pain, which indicates that wind is the dominant evil.

[3] A commentary included in the received text adds: An alternative version of this formula includes ginseng (*rén shēn*).

SYNOPSIS, LINE 6.2

Continuing from the preceding line, this line describes a severe form of blood impediment and its treatment.

COMMENTARY, LINE 6.2

Debilitation of yīn and yáng means that construction, defense, qì and blood are insufficient. When the pulse is faint at the inch opening and bar and tight at the cubit, this means that yáng qì is insufficient and that blood is stagnant. As a result, the skin is deprived of nourishment and warmth, and tingling and numbness arise. Blood impediment is characterized mainly by tingling and numbness of the flesh. In cases of severe contraction of external evil, there may also be pain. Hence the text refers to an "appearance as in wind impediment." However, blood impediment and wind impediment are different, the former being principally characterized by numbness and the latter by pain.

Line 6.3

夫男子平人，脉大为劳，极虚亦为劳。

Fū nán zǐ píng rén, mài dà wéi láo, jí xū yì wéi láo.

In men [who appear] healthy, a large pulsē means taxation;[2] an extremely vacuous one also means taxation.

TEXT NOTES, LINE 6.3

[1] Large pulse 脉大 *mài dà*: A broad pulse, i.e., the opposite of a fine pulse.

[2] Taxation 劳 *láo*: Vacuity taxation, any pattern of severe vacuity (of qì, blood, bowels, or viscera).

SYNOPSIS, LINE 6.3

This line describes the main pulses of vacuity taxation.

COMMENTARY, LINE 6.3

In this line, we learn how to diagnose vacuity taxation in "men [who appear] healthy" by the pulse. It should be noted that vacuity taxation is by no means limited to males. However, vacuity of yīn essence and of yáng qì is the most common pathology of vacuity taxation and is caused primarily by excessive sexual taxation. Thus, this line refers to patients who have damaged essence and consumed yīn through excessive sexual intercourse.

A large pulse means a pulse that is large, floating, and forceless, characteristics that reflect external superabundance and internal insufficiency. This pulse is often observed in patterns of yīn vacuity with floating yáng. "Extremely vacuous" means that when lightly pressed, the pulse is soft, and when heavily pressed, it is extremely forceless. This is a sign that essence and qì are severely damaged. A large pulse is different from an extremely vacuous one, but they are both signs of vacuity taxation.

Line 6.4

男子面色薄者，主渴及亡血，卒喘悸，脉浮者，里虚也。

Nán zǐ miàn sè bó zhě, zhǔ kě jí wáng xuè, zú chuǎn jì, mài fú zhě, lǐ xū yě.

In men, a thin complexion[1] in combination with the symptoms of thirst and blood collapse,[2] sudden panting and palpitation,[3] and a floating pulse mean interior vacuity.

TEXT NOTES, LINE 6.4

[1] Thin complexion 面色薄 *miàn sè bó*: A pale white and lusterless complexion.

[2] Blood collapse 亡血 *wáng xuè*: In modern texts, this compound is used as a technical term to refer to critical blood vacuity. However, in the *Jīn Guì Yào Lüè* as in the *Shāng Hán Lùn*, "blood collapse" simply refers to loss of blood.

[3] Sudden panting and palpitation 卒喘悸 *cù chuǎn jì*: Panting and palpitation at the slightest exertion.

SYNOPSIS, LINE 6.4

This line describes the signs of vacuity taxation with dual vacuity of qì and blood.

COMMENTARY, LINE 6.4

The heart governs the blood, and its bloom is in the face. When yīn-blood is vacuous and fails to rise to luxuriate the face, the facial complexion is pale white and lusterless. When yīn-blood is insufficient, the fluids are also scant, so there is also thirst. When qì is vacuous and cannot contain the blood, the result is loss of blood. When kidney qì is vacuous, it cannot ensure qì absorption. When heart blood is scant, it cannot nourish the heart. Thus there is panting and palpitation. Because the blood is vacuous and qì is floating, the pulse is floating and forceless. In combination, all these signs indicate a pattern of interior vacuity.

Line 6.5

男子脉虚沉弦，无寒热，短气，里急，小便不利，面色白，时目瞑，兼衄，少腹满，此为劳使之然。

Nán zǐ mài xū chén xián, wú hán rè, duǎn qì, lǐ jí, xiǎo biàn bù lì, miàn sè bái, shí mù míng, jiān nǜ, shào fù mǎn, cǐ wéi láo shǐ zhī rán.

For men [with] a vacuous, sunken, and stringlike pulse, absence of cold and heat,[1] shortness of breath, abdominal urgency, inhibited urination, a white facial complexion, periodic dimness of vision[2] with concurrent spontaneous external bleeding,[3] and lesser abdominal fullness, these signs are caused by taxation.

TEXT NOTES, LINE 6.5

[1] Absence of cold and heat 无寒热 *wú hán rè*: Aversion to cold and heat effusion appearing together are signs of externally contracted disease. By stressing the absence of these signs, the author emphasizes that the condition he is describing is due entirely to internal causes.

[2] Periodic dimness of vision 时目瞑 *shí mù míng*: Periodic loss of visual acuity. The term 瞑 *míng* has two meanings. One is "heavy eyes" and the other is "dimness of vision." The latter applies here.

[3] Spontaneous external bleeding 衄 *nǜ*: Bleeding that is not attributable to external injury, especially nosebleed.

SYNOPSIS, LINE 6.5

This line further describes the signs of vacuity taxation with dual vacuity of qì and blood.

COMMENTARY, LINE 6.5

In vacuity taxation, a pulse that is slightly stringlike and forceless at the deep level means dual vacuity of qì and blood, when it is not accompanied by signs of external contraction. A white face, periodic dimness of vision, and spontaneous external bleeding are signs of liver-spleen blood vacuity. Shortness of breath, abdominal urgency, inhibited urination, and lesser abdominal fullness are signs that kidney yáng is insufficient and unable to warm and transform the fluids. Whenever the pulse and signs described in this line appear, they indicate vacuity taxation. Hence the text says, "These signs are caused by taxation."

Line 6.6

劳之为病, 其脉浮大, 手足烦, 春夏剧, 秋冬瘥, 阴寒精自出, 酸削不能行。

Láo zhī wéi bìng, qí mài fú dà, shǒu zú fán, chūn xià jù, qiū dōng chài, yīn hán jīng zì chū, suān xuē bù néng xíng.

Taxation disease manifests in a floating and large pulse, vexation in the extremities,[1] aggravation in summer and remission in winter, genital cold,[2] spontaneous loss of semen, and aching and wasting with inability to walk.

TEXT NOTES, LINE 6.6

[1] Vexation in the extremities 手足烦 *shǒu zú fán*: Vexing heat in the extremities.

[2] Genital cold 阴寒 *yīn hán*: The Chinese says 'yīn cold', but yīn here refers not to the nature of cold but to the yīn region, i.e., the genitals.

[3] Aching pain and wasting with inability to walk 酸削不能行 *suān xuè bù néng xíng*: Lǐ Kè-Guāng 李克光 argues that 酸削 *suān xuē* means simply aching pain of the legs, with no implication of wasting.

SYNOPSIS, LINE 6.6

This line describes vacuity taxation with yīn vacuity affecting yáng, mentioning its relationship with the seasons.

COMMENTARY, LINE 6.6

When yáng is vacuous, it floats to the outside and therefore makes the pulse floating and large. Yīn vacuity engenders internal heat. Because the limbs are the root of all yáng, yáng hyperactivity due to yīn vacuity manifests in vexing heat of the extremities. In the spring and summer, wood and fire are exuberant and yáng qì floats outward. This causes even greater yīn vacuity. Hence in these seasons, the disease is more severe. In the autumn and winter, metal and water are exuberant and the yīn of the body receives the aid of the seasons, so that the disease is alleviated. As yīn vacuity affects yáng, kidney yáng also becomes vacuous and fails to warm the body. When kidney yáng is vacuous, the essence gate is insecure and there is seminal efflux. The loss of essence through seminal efflux makes kidney essences even more vacuous, so that bone and marrow are deprived of nourishment. This causes pain in the lower limbs and difficulty in walking.

Line 6.7

男子脉浮弱而濇，为无子，精气清冷。

Nán zǐ mài fú ruò ér sè, wéi wú zǐ, jīng qì qīngíng.

In men, a floating, weak, and rough pulse means sterility and that essential qì is [clear and] cold.[1]

TEXT NOTE, LINE 6.7

[1] Essential qì is [clear and] cold 精气清冷 *jīng qì qīng lěng*: The term 精气 *jīng qì* normally refers to a physiological entity present in both men and women (essential qì); here, however, it refers to seminal fluid. We do not know whether 清 *qīng* is to be taken in the sense of clear and colorless or in the sense of cool.

A textual variation that lacks this character suggests that the emphasis is on coldness. Seminal cold is characterized by cold, thin, scant semen and is considered a cause of male sterility.

SYNOPSIS, LINE 6.7

This line discusses sterility due to vacuity taxation on the basis of the pulse.

COMMENTARY, LINE 6.7

When true yáng is insufficient, the pulse is floating and weak. A rough pulse, that is, one that flows intermittently instead of freely, is a sign of debilitation of essence-blood. In men, this pulse indicates scantness of essential qì and insufficiency of both true yīn and true yáng. When the pulse is floating and forceless and at the same time inhibited, this is caused by depleted essence and qì exacerbating each other. Hence the semen is thin and cold and cannot produce a fetus.

Line 6.8

夫失精家，少腹弦急，阴头寒，目眩，发落，脉极虚芤迟，为清谷亡血失精；脉得诸芤动微紧，男子失精，女子梦交，桂枝龙骨牡蛎汤主之。

桂枝　芍药　生姜各三两　甘草二两　大枣十二枚　龙骨　牡蛎各三两

右七味，以水七升，煮取三升，分温三服。

天雄（炮）三两　白朮八两　桂枝六两　龙骨三两

右四味，杵为散，酒服半钱匕，日三服，不知，稍增之。

Fū shī jīng jiā, shào fù xián jí, yīn tóu hán, mù xuàn, fà luò, mài jí xū kōu chí, wéi qīng gǔ wáng xuè shī jīng; mài dé zhū kōu dòng wēi jǐn, nán zǐ shī jīng, nǚ zǐ mèng jiāo, guì zhī lóng gǔ mǔ lì tāng zhǔ zhī.

Guì zhī, sháo yào, shēng jiāng gè sān liǎng; gān cǎo èr liǎng; dà zǎo shí èr méi; lóng gǔ, mǔ lì gè sān liǎng

Yòu qī wèi, yǐ shuǐ qī shēng, zhǔ qǔ sān shēng, fēn wēn sān fú.

Tiān xióng (pào) sān liǎng; bái zhú bā liǎng; guì zhī liù liǎng; lóng gǔ sān liǎng

Yòu sì wèi, chǔ wéi sǎn, jiǔ fú bàn qián bǐ, rì sān fú, bù zhī, shāo zēng zhī.

If patients suffering from seminal loss present with stringlike tension in the lesser abdomen,[1] yīn-head cold,[2] dizzy vision,[3] hair loss, and a pulse that is extremely vacuous, scallion-stalk, and slow, this means clear grain,[4] blood collapse, and seminal loss. Whenever you see a pulse that is scallion-stalk and stirring or faint and tight, this means seminal loss in men and dreaming of intercourse in women.[5] Cinnamon Twig Decoction Plus Dragon Bone and Oyster Shell (*guì zhī jiā lóng gǔ mǔ lì tāng*) governs.[6]

Cinnamon Twig Decoction Plus Dragon Bone and Oyster Shell (桂枝加龙骨牡蛎汤 *guì zhī jiā lóng gǔ mǔ lì tāng*)
cinnamon twig (桂枝 *guì zhī*, Cinnamomi Ramulus) 3 *liǎng*

peony (芍药 *sháo yào*, Paeoniae Radix) 3 *liǎng*
fresh ginger (生姜 *shēng jiāng*, Zingiberis Rhizoma Recens) 3 *liǎng*
licorice (甘草 *gān cǎo*, Glycyrrhizae Radix) 2 *liǎng*
jujube (大枣 *dà zǎo*, Jujubae Fructus) 12 pieces
dragon bone (龙骨 *lóng gǔ*, Mastodi Ossis Fossilia) 3 *liǎng*
oyster shell (牡蛎 *mǔ lì*, Ostreae Concha) 3 *liǎng*

Boil the above seven ingredients in seven *shēng* of water to get three *shēng*. Divide into three doses and take warm.

Tiānxiōng Aconite Powder (天雄散 *tiān xióng sǎn*)

tiānxióng aconite (天雄 *tiān xióng*, Aconiti Radix Lateralis Tianxiong) 3 *liǎng* (blast-fry)
white atractylodes (白朮 *bái zhú*, Atractylodis Macrocephalae Rhizoma) 8 *liǎng*
cinnamon twig (桂枝 *guì zhī*, Cinnamomi Ramulus) 6 *liǎng*
dragon bone (龙骨 *lóng* gǔ, Mastodi Ossis Fossilia) 3 *liǎng*

Pestle the above four ingredients into a powder. Take half a qián-spoonful in wine, three times a day. If no change is noticed, increase the dose slightly.

TEXT NOTES, LINE 6.8

[1] Stringlike tension in the lesser abdomen 少腹弦急 *shào fù xián jí*: An uncomfortable feeling of tension in the lesser abdomen (the part of the abdomen below the umbilicus).

[2] Yīn-head cold 阴头寒 *yīn tóu lěng*: Cold in the yīn head (i.e., the glans penis); genital cold.

[3] A textual variation instead has "pain in the eye sockets" (目眶痛 *mù kuàng tòng*).

[4] Clear grain 清谷 *qīng gǔ*: Clear-grain diarrhea. This refers to diarrhea that is characterized by watery, light brown stool containing partially digested food and having no malodor. Clear-food diarrhea is accompanied by aversion to cold and cold limbs, and is a sign of kidney and spleen yáng vacuity.

[5] Dreaming of intercourse 梦交 *mèng jiāo*: Nighttime dreaming of sexual intercourse.

[6] The *Xiǎo Pǐn Fāng* ("Small Formulary") here comments: "In patients with vacuity, floating heat, and sweating, leave out the cinnamon twig (*guì zhī*) and add 3 liǎng each of black swallowwort (*bái wēi*) and aconite (*fù zǐ*). Consequently, [this formula] is called 'Two Additions Dragon Bone Decoction' (*èr jiā lóng gǔ tāng*)."

SYNOPSIS, LINE 6.8

This line discusses the signs and treatment of seminal loss due to dual vacuity of yīn and yáng, arising when yīn vacuity affects yáng.

COMMENTARY, LINE 6.8

Frequent dream emission can cause damage to yīn that affects yáng, giving rise to stringlike tension in the lesser abdomen and cold in the exterior genitals. Essence-blood depletion causes dizziness and hair loss. The statement that a vacuous, scallion-stalk, and slow pulse indicates clear grain, blood collapse, and seminal loss is an intercalation meaning that this kind of pulse may be seen not only in patients suffering from seminal loss, but also in people suffering from clear-grain diarrhea and loss of blood.

A scallion-stalk, stirring pulse is a large floating pulse that is empty in the center and forceless. It is mainly associated with the bar position and indicates yīn-blood depletion and unconstrained heart spirit. A pulse that is slightly tight is one that is vacuous and stringlike. It indicates yáng vacuity and interior cold. Thus these two pulses together indicate dual vacuity of yīn and yáng, which lies at the root of seminal emission in males and dreaming of intercourse in females. When yīn is left unsecured by yáng, the result is seminal emission. When yáng is not nourished by yīn, it floats unconstrained, giving rise to dreaming of intercourse.

In both males and females, yīn and yáng can be brought into harmony using Cinnamon Twig Decoction Plus Dragon Bone and Oyster Shell (*guì zhī jiā lóng gǔ mǔ lì tāng*). Within the formula, cinnamon twig (*guì zhī*) harmonizes yīn and yáng. Dragon bone (*lóng gǔ*) and oyster shell (*mǔ lì*) subdue yáng to yīn, and have a securing, containing action that checks seminal emission. When yīn and yáng are in harmony, yáng is able to secure and contain, and yīn can be constrained internally. Thus, seminal emission and dreaming of intercourse are cured.

Line 6.9

男子平人，脉虚弱细微者，善盗汗也。

Nán zǐ píng rén, mài xū ruò xì wēi zhě, shàn dào hàn yě.

In men [who appear] healthy, a pulse that is vacuous, weak, fine, or faint indicates a tendency to night sweating.[1]

Text Note, Line 6.9

[1] Tendency to night sweating 喜盗汗 *xǐ dào hàn*: Sweat regularly during sleep.

Synopsis, Line 6.9

This line discusses the pulse that is associated with vacuity taxation night sweating.

Commentary, Line 6.9

"Men [who appear] healthy" has the same meaning as the same phrase occurring in line 6.3 above, namely a patient who appears healthy on the outside but presents with an abnormal pulse. Vacuity taxation is by no means confined to men, but males given to excessive bedroom activity are especially prone to it.

This line speaks of a pulse that is vacuous, weak, fine, or faint. "Vacuous" and "weak" both refer to a pulse that lacks force, but a vacuous pulse is floating and large, indicating yáng vacuity, while a weak pulse is sunken and small, indicating dual vacuity of qì and blood. These two characteristics cannot manifest simultaneously. A fine pulse indicates yīn-blood vacuity. A faint pulse is one that is extremely fine and forceless, indicating yáng qì vacuity. These two characteristics can manifest simultaneously. The pulse characteristics described in this line express a pathomechanism of dual vacuity of yīn and yáng. When yáng qì is vacuous and fails to secure and yīn is vacuous and unconstrained, frequent night sweating results.

Line 6.10

人年五六十，其病脉大者，痹侠背行，若肠鸣，马刀侠瘿者，皆为劳得之。

Rén nián wǔ liù shí, qí bìng mài dà zhě, bì xiá bèi háng, ruò cháng míng, mǎ dāo jiā yǐng zhě, jiē wéi láo dé zhī.

If a person of fifty or sixty years of age with a pathologically large pulse and impediment along the furrows of the back[1] suffers from rumbling intestines or saber and pearl-string lumps,[2] all [these conditions] are acquired as a result of taxation.

Text Notes, Line 6.10

[1] Impediment along the furrows of the back 痹侠背行 *bì jiā bèi háng*: The term 痹 *bì* (impediment) has several meanings and usages: First, it denotes impeded physical movement, and specifically a disease characterized by impeded physical movement and caused by wind-cold-dampness (including conditions classed in Western medicine as arthritis). Second, it describes blockage of qì in the body. And third, it refer to numbness, which is the meaning it carries in the present line.

[2] Saber and pearl-string lumps 马刀侠瘿 *mǎ dāo jiā yǐng*: Scrofula. Saber lumps (马刀 *mǎ dāo*) are scrofula occurring in a configuration that looks like the shape of a saber (a curved cavalry sword); pearl-string lumps (侠瘿 *jiā yǐng*) occur on the neck giving the appearance of a pearl necklace.

Synopsis, Line 6.10

This line discusses the manifestation of vacuity heat and vacuity cold in patients with a large pulse.

Commentary, Line 6.10

When a person reaches the age of fifty or sixty, essential qì gradually weakens. Qì becomes vacuous and cannot warm the body, and blood becomes scant and fails to provide nourishment. As a result, the channel vessels become impeded; hence there numbness on either side of the spine. If a floating, large, and forceless pulse is accompanied by rumbling intestines, this is usually due to vacuous and cold spleen qì failing to move and transform. Thus the pathomechanism is one of vacuity cold. On the other hand, if this type of pulse manifests with saber and pearl-string lumps, this is usually due to phlegm-fire that arises in patients with yīn vacuity with floating yáng when internal heat scorches the fluids so that they turn into phlegm. Hence the pathomechanism is one of vacuity heat. These two disease patterns differ in nature, but they both develop out of vacuity and are both characterized by a pulse that is floating, large, and forceless.

Line 6.11

脉沉小迟，名脱气，其人疾行则喘喝，手足逆寒，腹满，甚则溏泄，食不消化也。

Mài chén xiǎo chí, míng tuō qì, qí rén jí xíng zé chuǎn hē, shǒu zú nì hán, fù mǎn, shèn zé táng xiè, shí bù xiāo huà yě.

[When the] pulse is sunken, small, and slow, [this is] called "deserting qì."[1] Such a person manifests with noisy panting when walking fast, counterflow cold of the extremities,[2] abdominal fullness, and in severe cases sloppy diarrhea and food failing to disperse and transform.[3]

Text Notes, Line 6.11

[1] Deserting qì 脱气 *tuō qì*: Debilitation of yáng qì.

[2] Counterflow cold of the extremities 手足逆寒 *shǒu zú nì hán*: Pronounced cold in the extremities up to the knees and elbows or beyond, as occurs in yáng collapse or internal heat evil block.

[3] Food failing to disperse and transform 食不消化 *shí bù xiāo huà*: Food failing to be digested properly.

Synopsis, Line 6.11

This line describes the pulse and signs of spleen-kidney debilitation in vacuity taxation.

Commentary, Line 6.11

A sunken, small, and slow pulse reflects spleen-kidney yáng vacuity. Panting when walking fast indicates kidney qì vacuity. Counterflow cold of the extremities reflects yáng vacuity since yáng vacuity results in external cold (陽虛則外寒 *yáng xū zé wài hán*). Abdominal fullness, sloppy stool, and non-transformation of food are all signs that the stomach is failing to ripen and decompose food properly and that the spleen is failing to move and transform.

Line 6.12

脉弦而大，弦则为减，大则为芤，减则为寒，芤则为虚，虚寒相搏，此名为革。妇人则半产漏下，男子则亡血失精。

Mài xián ér dà, xián zé wéi jiǎn, dà zé wéi kōu, jiǎn zé wéi hán, kōu zé wéi xū, xū hán xiāng bó, cǐ míng wéi gé. Fù rén zé bàn chǎn lòu xià, nán zǐ zé wáng xuè shī jīng.

When a pulse is both stringlike and large, stringlike means reduced,[1] and large means scallion-stalk; reduced means cold, and scallion-stalk means vacuity. Vacuity and cold contend with each other, and this is called a drumskin [pulse]. In women, [this type of pulse] means mid-term delivery[2] and spotting;[3] in men, it means blood collapse and seminal loss.

TEXT NOTES, LINE 6.12

[1] Reduced 減 *jiǎn*: Lacking in force when pressure is applied.

[2] Mid-term delivery 半产 *bàn chǎn*: Late miscarriage. The Chinese term means "half delivery," i.e., delivery in mid-pregnancy, before the normal term.

[3] Spotting 漏下 *lòu xià*: The Chinese term literally means "leaking down." It denotes a slight, often continual loss of the blood via the vagina.

SYNOPSIS, LINE 6.12

This line describes the pathomechanism and particular manifestations of a drumskin pulse in vacuity taxation.

COMMENTARY, LINE 6.12

A drumskin pulse includes two characteristics, namely stringlike and large. A pulse that is stringlike only does not change when pressure is applied, while the stringlike quality of the drumskin pulse is markedly reduced when pressure is applied. A large pulse normally refers to a large, surging, and forceful pulse, but the large quality of the drumskin pulse is characterized by hollowness in the center, similar to a scallion-stalk pulse.

Pulse types that are reduced when pressed heavily indicate cold; pulses that are large and empty in the center indicate vacuity. Therefore, we see how both cold and vacuity are reflected in a drumskin pulse. The drumskin pulse is large, urgent on the outside, and empty in the center. It arises when yīn-blood is depleted and fails to constrain yáng, so that vacuous yáng floats outward. Hence, when it appears in women, it is usually the result of a late miscarriage or spotting, while in men it is usually due to loss of blood or semen.

Line 6.13

虚劳里急，悸，衄，腹中痛，梦失精，四肢痠疼，手足烦热，咽干口燥，小建中汤主之。

桂枝（去皮）三两　甘草三两（炙）
大枣十二枚　芍药六两　生姜二两
胶饴一升

右六味，以水七升，煮取三升，去滓，内胶饴，更上微火消解，温服一升，日三服。

Xū láo lǐ jí, jì, nǜ, fù zhōng tòng, mèng shī jīng, sì zhī suān téng, shǒu zú fán rè, yān gān kǒu zào, xiǎo jiàn zhōng tāng zhǔ zhī.

Guì zhī (qù pí) sān liǎng; gān cǎo sān liǎng (zhì); dà zǎo shí èr méi; sháo yào liù liǎng; shēng jiāng èr liǎng; jiāo yí yī shēng

Yòu liù wèi, yǐ shuǐ qī shēng, zhǔ qǔ sān shēng, qù zǐ, nèi jiāo yí, gèng shàng wēi huǒ xiāo jiě, wēn fú yī shēng, rì sān fú.

In vacuity taxation with abdominal urgency, palpitation, spontaneous external bleeding, pain in the abdomen, seminal loss while dreaming, aching pain in the limbs, vexing heat in the hands and feet, and dry throat and mouth, Minor Center-Fortifying Decoction (小建中汤 *xiǎo jiàn zhōng tāng*) governs.

Minor Center-Fortifying Decoction (小建中汤 *xiǎo jiàn zhōng tāng*)

cinnamon twig (桂枝 *guì zhī*, Cinnamomi Ramulus) 3 *liǎng* (remove bark)
licorice (甘草 *gān cǎo*, Glycyrrhizae Radix) 3 *liǎng* (mix-fry)
jujube (大枣 *dà zǎo*, Jujubae Fructus) 12 pieces
peony (芍药 *sháo yào*, Paeoniae Radix) 6 *liǎng*
fresh ginger (生姜 *shēng jiāng*, Zingiberis Rhizoma Recens) 2 *liǎng*
malt sugar (胶饴 *jiāo yí*, Maltosum) 1 *shēng*

Boil the above six ingredients with seven *shēng* of water to get three *shēng*. Remove the dregs. Add the malt sugar (*jiāo yí*) and return to the fire to melt it over a small flame. Take one *shēng* warm, three times a day.[1]

TEXT NOTE, LINE 6.13

[1] The commentary here adds an extensive note: "Patients suffering from retching should not take Center-Fortifying Decoction (*jiàn zhōng tāng*) because it is sweet. The *Qiān Jīn Fāng* ("Thousand Gold Pieces Prescriptions") uses this formula to treat the following symptoms in men and women, caused by accumulated cold and qì stagnation or by failure to recover from a major illness: heaviness of the limbs, aching pain in the flesh and bones, breathing with shortage of qì, panting upon physical activity, fullness in the chest and rapid breathing, rigidity and pain in the lumbus and back, vacuity palpitation in the heart, dry throat and lips, lack of color in the face and body, possibly no taste for food and drink, distention in the rib-side and abdomen, heaviness of the head and inability to lift it, and lying down more than being up. In severe cases, this lasts for many years; in light cases for a hundred days. If it gradually causes emaciation, weakness, and exhaustion of qì in the five viscera, recovery is difficult. The result is insufficiency in all six vessels, vacuity cold and lack of qì, hypertonicity in the lesser abdomen, marked emaciation and weakness, and the hundred diseases. [The formula for this condition] is called Astragalus Center-Fortifying Decoction (*huáng qí jiàn zhōng tāng*) and it includes two *liǎng* of ginseng (*rén shēn*)."

Synopsis, Line 6.13

This line describes the signs and treatment of vacuity taxation with dual vacuity of yīn and yáng.

Commentary, Line 6.13

Vacuity taxation usually develops by a pathomechanism of yīn vacuity affecting yáng or yáng vacuity affecting yīn, giving rise to dual vacuity of yīn and yáng and therefore marked by both heat and cold signs. However, yīn vacuity or yáng vacuity is always more marked than the other, and so are the heat and cold signs. Yīn vacuity engenders heat, giving rise to spontaneous external bleeding (nosebleed), vexing heat in the extremities, and dry pharynx and mouth. Yáng vacuity engenders cold, giving rise to abdominal urgency and abdominal pain. There are other signs of yīn-yáng disharmony. When heart-construction is insufficient, the result is heart palpitation. When kidney yīn is insufficient and cannot be contained, there is seminal loss. When qì and blood are vacuous and cannot nourish the four limbs, there is aching pain in the limbs.

We cannot simply treat dual vacuity of yīn and yáng by the principle of treating cold with heat or heat with cold. Instead, we have to enhance center qì. Hence, this line recommends Minor Center-Fortifying Decoction (*xiǎo jiàn zhōng tāng*). Within this formula, the sweetness of licorice (*gān cǎo*), jujube (*dà zǎo*), and malt sugar (*yí táng*) fortifies the center and relaxes tension. The acridity of fresh ginger (*shēng jiāng*) and cinnamon twig (*guì zhī*) frees yáng and regulates defense qì. The sourness of peony (*sháo yào*) astringes and harmonizes construction qì. When center qì is fortified, it can move to all parts of the body. By fortifying the center, we restore the source of qì and blood production and supplement and harmonize yīn and yáng. When this happens, the cold-heat complex gradually disappears.

Line 6.14

虚劳里急，诸不足，黄芪建中汤主之。

Xū láo lǐ jí, zhū bù zú, huáng qí jiàn zhōng tāng zhǔ zhī.

In vacuity taxation with abdominal urgency and insufficiency of everything,[1] Astragalus Center-Fortifying Decoction (*huáng qí jiàn zhōng tāng*) governs.[2]

Text Notes, Line 6.14

[1] Insufficiency of everything 诸不足 *zhū bù zú*: This means that qì, blood, yīn, and yáng are all insufficient.

[2] The commentary here adds: "Add one-and-a-half liǎng of astragalus (*huáng qí*) to Minor Center-Fortifying Decoction (*xiǎo jiàn zhōng tāng*), and follow the directions above. For shortness of breath and fullness in the chest, add fresh ginger (*shēng jiāng*); for abdominal fullness, leave out the jujube (*dà zǎo*) and add two and half liǎng of poria (*fú líng*); for vacuity detriment of the lung, add three liǎng of pinellia (*bàn xià*)."

SYNOPSIS, LINE 6.14

This line discusses the treatment of dual vacuity of yīn and yáng with relatively pronounced qì vacuity.

COMMENTARY, LINE 6.14

This line continues the line of thought from the last line. It seems to describe the same condition, but this time prescribes Astragalus Center-Fortifying Decoction (*huáng qí jiàn zhōng tāng*) instead of Minor Center-Fortifying Decoction (*xiǎo jiàn zhōng tāng*). We can infer that Zhāng Jī added astragalus (*huáng qí*) here for its effect of supplementing the center and boosting qì, to treat particularly pronounced signs of qì vacuity such as spontaneous sweating, fatigue, aversion to wind, a vacuous pulse, and shortage of qì, or numbness and insensitivity.

Line 6.15

虚劳腰痛，少腹拘急，小便不利者，八味肾气丸主之。

干地黄八两　山药　山茱萸各四两
泽泻三两　茯苓三两　牡丹皮三两
桂枝　附子（炮）各一两

右八味，末之，炼蜜和丸梧子大，酒下十五丸，加至二十五丸，日再服。

Xū láo yāo tòng, shào fù jū jí, xiǎo biàn bù lì zhě, bā wèi shèn qì wán zhǔ zhī.

Gān dì huáng bā liǎng; shǔ yù sì liǎng; shān zhū yú sì liǎng; zé xiè sān liǎng; fú líng sān liǎng; mǔ dān pí sān liǎng; guì zhī fù zǐ (pào) gè yī liǎng

Yòu bā wèi, mò zhī, liàn mì huò wán wú zǐ dà, jiǔ xià shí wǔ wán, jiā zhì èr shí wǔ wán, rì zài fú.

In vacuity taxation with lumbar pain, hypertonicity in the lesser abdomen, and inhibited urination, Eight-Ingredient Kidney Qì Pill (*bā wèi shèn qì wán*) governs.[1]

Eight-Ingredient Kidney Qì Pill
(*bā wèi shèn qì wán*)

- dried rehmannia (干地黄 *gān dì huáng*, Rehmanniae Radix) 8 *liǎng*
- dioscorea (山药 *shān yào*, Dioscoreae Rhizoma) 4 *liǎng*
- cornus (山茱萸 *shān zhū yú*, Corni Fructus) 4 *liǎng*
- alisma (泽泻 *zé xiè*, Alismatis Rhizoma) 3 *liǎng*
- poria (茯苓 *fú líng*, Poria) 3 *liǎng*
- moutan (牡丹皮 *mǔ dān pí*, Moutan Cortex) 3 *liǎng*
- cinnamon twig (桂枝 *guì zhī*, Cinnamomi Ramulus) 1 *liǎng*
- aconite (附子 *fù zǐ*, Aconiti Radix Lateralis Praeparata) 1 *liǎng* (blast-fry)

Pulverize the above eight ingredients. Blend with processed honey (*liàn mì*), and form into pills the size of firmiana seeds. Swallow fifteen pills in wine twice a day. Increase [the dosage] up to twenty-five pills.

TEXT NOTE, LINE 6.15

1. The commentary here adds a note that the formula is found under the section on "Foot Qì." However, since the formula that is attached to this line in this edition

is called Kidney Qì Pill (*shèn qì wán*) and contains eight ingredients, the commentary must have come from an edition where this formula was placed in a different section.

SYNOPSIS, LINE 6.15

This line discusses the signs and treatment of vacuity taxation with kidney yáng vacuity.

COMMENTARY, LINE 6.15

The lumbus is the house of the kidney, and kidney yáng vacuity therefore results in lumbar pain. When kidney qì is insufficient, qì transformation in the bladder is inhibited, so that there is hypertonicity of the lesser abdomen with inhibited urination.

This condition is treated with Eight-Ingredient Kidney Qì Pill (*bā wèi shèn qì wán*), which assists yáng to transform water, while enriching yīn to help engender qì. Thereby, the formula arouses kidney qì and cures this condition.

Line 6.16

虚劳诸不足，风气百疾，薯蓣丸主之。
薯蓣三十分　当归 桂枝　曲　干地黄　豆黄卷各十分　甘草二十八分　人参七分　芎藭　芍药　白朮 麦门冬　杏仁各六分　柴胡　桔梗　茯苓各五分　阿胶七分　干姜三分　白蔹二分　防风六分　大枣（为膏）百枚
右二十一味，末之，炼蜜和丸如弹子大，空腹酒服一丸，一百丸为剂。

Xū láo zhū bù zú, fēng qì bǎi jí, shǔ yù wán zhǔ zhī.

Shǔ yù sān shí fēn; dāng guī guì zhī qū gān dì huáng dòu huáng juàn gè shí fēn gān cǎo èr shí bā fēn; rén shēn qī fēn; xiōng qióng sháo yào bái zhú mài mén dōng xìng rén gè liù fēn;chái hú jié gěng fú líng gè wǔ fēn; ē jiāo qī fēn; gān jiāng sān fēn; bái liǎn èr fēn; fáng fēng liù fēn; dà zǎo (wéi gāo) bǎi méi

Yòu èr shí yī wèi, mò zhī, liàn mì huò wán rú dàn zǐ dà, kōng fù jiǔ fú yī wán, yī bǎi wán wéi jì.

For vacuity taxation with insufficiency of everything and the hundred diseases of wind qì,[1] Dioscorea Pill (薯蓣丸 *shǔ yù wán*) governs.

Dioscorea Pill (薯蓣丸 *shǔ yù wán*)
dioscorea (薯蓣 *shǔ yù*, Dioscoreae Rhizoma) 30 parts
Chinese angelica (当归 *dāng guī*, Angelicae Sinensis Radix) 10 parts
medicated leaven (曲 *qū*, Massa Medicata Fermentata) 10 parts
dried rehmannia (干地黄 *gān dì huáng*, Rehmanniae Radix) 10 parts
dried soybean sprout (豆黄卷 *dòu huáng juǎn*, Sojae Semen Germinatum) 10 parts
licorice (甘草 *gān cǎo*, Glycyrrhizae Radix) 28 parts
ginseng (人参 *rén shēn*, Ginseng Radix) 7 parts
chuanxiong (芎藭 *xiōng qióng*, Chuanxiong Rhizoma) 6 parts

peony (芍药 *sháo yào*, Paeoniae Radix) 6 parts
white atractylodes (白术 *bái zhú*, Atractylodis Macrocephalae Rhizoma) 6 parts
ophiopogon (麦门冬 *mài mén dōng*, Ophiopogonis Radix) 6 parts
apricot kernel (杏仁 *xìng rén*, Armeniacae Semen) 6 parts
bupleurum (柴胡 *chái hú*, Bupleuri Radix) 5 parts
platycodon (桔梗 *jié gěng*, Platycodonis Radix) 5 parts
poria (茯苓 *fú líng*, Poria) 5 parts
ass hide glue (阿胶 *ē jiāo*, Asini Corii Colla) 7 parts
dried ginger (干姜 *gān jiāng*, Zingiberis Rhizoma) 3 parts
ampelopsis (白蔹 *bái liǎn*, Ampelopsis Radix) 2 parts
saposhnikovia (防风 *fáng fēng*, Saposhnikoviae Radix) 6 parts
jujube (大枣 *dà zǎo*, Jujubae Fructus) 100 pieces (make into a paste)

Pulverize the above 21 ingredients. Blend with processed honey (*liàn mì*) and form into pills the size of slingshot pellets. On an empty stomach, take one pill [per dose] in wine. A hundred pills make one preparation [of this formula].

TEXT NOTE, LINE 6.16

[1] Wind qì 风气 *fēng qì*: Here, this refers to any externally contracted evil.

SYNOPSIS, LINE 6.16

This line describes the treatment of vacuity taxation with concurrent wind qì.

COMMENTARY, LINE 6.16

In vacuity taxation, when qì, blood, yīn, and yáng are all insufficient, the patient's right qì is weak and therefore unable to resist the invasion of external evils. To treat the many diseases caused by external evils in patients suffering from vacuity taxation, you must not limit treatment either to supplementing the vacuity or to dispelling the evil, but rather fortify the spleen with Dioscorea Pill (*shǔ yù wán*). The spleen and stomach are later heaven, the source of engendering transformation of qì, blood, construction, and defense. When qì, blood, yīn, and yáng are all insufficient, unless splenic movement and transformation is healthy and the patient eats more, there is no way he can recover.

Within the formula, dioscorea (*shān yào*) rectifies the stomach and spleen. Ginseng (*rén shēn*), white atractylodes (*bái zhú*), poria (*fú líng*), dried ginger (*gān jiāng*), dried soybean sprout (*dà dòu huáng juǎn*), jujube (*dà zǎo*), and medicated leaven (*shén qū*) boost qì and regulate the center. Chinese angelica (*dāng guī*), chuanxiong (*chuān xiōng*), peony (*sháo yào*), rehmannia (*dì huáng*), ophiopogon (*mài mén dōng*), ass hide glue (*ē jiāo*) nourish the blood and enrich yīn. Bupleurum (*chái hú*), cinnamon twig (*guì zhī*), and saposhnikovia (*fáng fēng*) dispel wind and disperse evils. Apricot kernel (*xìng rén*), platycodon (*jié gěng*), and ampelopsis (*bái liǎn*) rectify qì and open depression. This combination as a whole supports right qì and dispels the evil.

Line 6.17

虚劳虚烦不得眠，酸枣仁汤主之。

酸枣仁二升　甘草一两　知母二两
茯苓二两　芎藭二两

右五味，以水八升，煮酸枣仁得六升，内诸药煮取三升，分温三服。

Xū láo xū fán bù dé mián, suān zǎo rén tāng zhǔ zhī.

Suān zǎo rén èr shēng; gān cǎo yī liǎng zhī mǔ èr liǎng; fú líng èr liǎng; xiōng qióng èr liǎng

Yòu wǔ wèi, yǐ shuǐ bā shēng, zhǔ suān zǎo rén dé liù shēng, nà zhū yào zhǔ qǔ sān shēng, fēn wēn sān fú.

For vacuity taxation with vacuity vexation[1] and inability to sleep, Spiny Jujube Decoction (酸枣仁汤 *suān zǎo rén tāng*) governs.

Spiny Jujube Decoction (酸枣仁汤 *suān zǎo rén tāng*)

spiny jujube (酸枣仁 *suān zǎo rén*, Ziziphi Spinosi Semen) 2 *shēng*
licorice (甘草 *gān cǎo*, Glycyrrhizae Radix) 1 *liǎng*
anemarrhena (知母 *zhī mǔ*, Anemarrhenae Rhizoma) 2 *liǎng*
poria (茯苓 *fú líng*, Poria) 2 *liǎng*
chuanxiong (芎藭 *xiōng qióng*, Chuanxiong Rhizoma) 2 *liǎng*

Of the above five ingredients, boil the spiny jujube (*suān zǎo rén*) in eight *shēng* of water to get six *shēng*. Then add all the [other] ingredients and boil to get three *shēng*. Divide into three [doses] and take warm.

TEXT NOTES, LINE 6.17

[1] Vacuity vexation 虚烦 *xū fán*: Heat vexation due to vacuity fire harassing the inner body. Vacuity vexation is a feeling of unease and listlessness in the heart, accompanied by unquiet sleep.

[2] Here the commentary adds, "Master Shēn also includes 2 *liǎng* of fresh ginger (生姜 *shēng jiāng*, Zingiberis Rhizoma Recens)."

SYNOPSIS, LINE 6.17

This line discusses the signs and treatment of insomnia in vacuity taxation due to yīn vacuity.

COMMENTARY, LINE 6.17

The special characteristic of "vacuity vexation and inability to sleep" is depression in the heart, disquietude, and inability to fall asleep when lying down. These symptoms are caused by insufficiency of liver yīn and internally harassing vacuity heat. When liver yīn is sufficient, the liver is able to store the ethereal soul; hence the person is able to sleep. When liver yīn is insufficient, the liver cannot store the ethereal soul; hence there is insomnia. Yīn vacuity engenders heat, and this vacuity heat harasses the heart spirit; hence there is depression in the heart, vexation, and disquietude. The root cause of this condition is therefore found in the liver, but also affects the heart, and is related to yīn vacuity. In treatment, we therefore nourish yīn and supplement the vacuity, while also clearing heat and eliminating the vexation.

In the formula, spiny jujube (*suān zǎo rén*) nourishes liver yīn and settles the heart spirit; anemarrhena (*zhī mǔ*) nourishes yīn, clears heat, and eliminates vexation; poria (*fú ling*) settles the spirit and quiets the heart; chuanxiong (*chuān xiōng*) courses and regulates qì and blood in the liver; and licorice (*gān cǎo*) harmonizes all the other ingredients. Thus the formula has the effect of nourishing the liver, quieting the heart, clearing heat, and eliminating vexation.

Line 6.18

五劳虚极，羸瘦腹满，不能饮食，食伤、忧伤、饮伤、房室伤、饥伤、劳伤、经络营卫气伤，内有干血，肌肤甲错，两目黯黑，缓中补虚，大黄蟅虫丸主之。

大黄（蒸）十分 黄芩二两 甘草三两 桃仁一升 杏仁一升 芍药四两 干漆一两 虻虫一升 水蛭百枚 蟅虫半斤 蛴螬一升 干地黄十两

右十二味，末之，炼蜜和丸小豆大，酒饮服五丸，日三服。

Wǔ láo xū jí, léi sòu fù mǎn, bù néng yǐn shí, shí shāng, yōu shāng, yǐn shāng, fáng shì shāng, jī shāng, láo shāng, jīng luò yíng wèi qì shāng, nèi yǒu gān xuè, jī fū jiǎ cuò, liǎng mù àn hēi, huǎn zhōng bǔ xū, dà huáng zhè chóng wán zhǔ zhī.

Dà huáng (zhēng) shí fèn; huáng qín èr liǎng; gān cǎo sān liǎng; táo rén yī shēng; xìng rén yī shēng; sháo yào sì liǎng; gān qī yī liǎng; méng chóng yī shēng; shuǐ zhì bǎi méi; zhè chóng bàn; jīn qí cáo yī shēng; gān dì huáng shí liǎng

Yòu shí èr wèi, mò zhī, liàn mì huò wán xiǎo dòu dà, jiǔ yǐn fú wǔ wán, rì sān fú.

For the five taxations[1] with extreme vacuity, marked emaciation, abdominal fullness, inability to eat and drink, food damage, anxiety damage, drink damage,[2] bedroom damage,[3] hunger damage, taxation damage,[4] channel, network [vessel], construction and defense qì damage, dry blood in the inner body, encrusted skin,[5] and dark eyes,[6] moderate the center and supplement vacuity.[7] Rhubarb and Ground Beetle Pill (大黄蟅虫丸 *dà huáng zhè chóng wán*) governs.

Rhubarb and Ground Beetle Pill (大黄蟅虫丸 *dà huáng zhè chóng wán*)

rhubarb (大黄 *dà huáng*, Rhei Radix et Rhizoma) 10 parts (steam)
scutellaria (黄芩 *huáng qín*, Scutellariae Radix) 2 *liǎng*
licorice (甘草 *gān cǎo*, Glycyrrhizae Radix) 3 *liǎng*
peach kernel (桃仁 *táo rén*, Persicae Semen) 1 *shēng*
apricot kernel (杏仁 *xìng rén*, Armeniacae Semen) 1 *shēng*
peony (芍药 *sháo yào*, Paeoniae Radix) 4 *liǎng*
lacquer (干漆 *gān qī*, Toxicodendri Resina) 1 *liǎng*
tabanus (虻虫 *méng chóng*, Tabanus) 1 *shēng*

leech (水蛭 *shuǐ zhì*, Hirudo) 100 pieces
ground beetle (蟅虫 *zhè chóng*, Eupolyphaga seu Steleophaga) ½ *jīn*
June beetle grub (蛴螬 *qí cáo*, Holotrichiae Vermiculus) 1 *shēng*
dried rehmannia (干地黄 *gān dì huáng*, Rehmanniae Radix) 10 *liǎng*

Pulverize the above twelve ingredients. Blend with processed honey (*liàn mì*) and form into pills the size of small beans. Take five pills with wine, three times a day.

TEXT NOTES, LINE 6.18

[1] Five taxations 五劳 *wǔ láo*: As the Treatise Explaining the Five Qì (*xuān míng wǔ qì lùn*) of the *Sù Wèn* ("Plain Questions") states: "Long seeing damages the blood; long lying damages qì; long sitting damages the flesh; long standing damages the bones; long walking damages the sinews."

[2] Drink damage 饮伤 *yǐn shāng*: Damage to the body from excessive consumption of alcohol.

[3] Bedroom damage 房室伤 *fáng shì shāng*: Damage to the body from excessive sexual activity.

[4] Taxation damage 劳伤 *láo shāng*: This term is often used in the wider sense of overexertion, intemperate living (including dietary irregularities and sexual intemperance), or the seven affects (emotional imbalance) as a cause of disease. In the present context, it seems to refer specifically to overexertion.

[5] Encrusted skin 肌肤甲错 *jī fū jiǎ cuò*: Dry rough skin with a scaly appearance.

[6] Dark eyes 两目黯黑 *liǎng mù àn hēi*: This phrase could have two meanings: (1) Dark coloration of the whites of the eyes. (2) A subjective sensation that things are dark and unclear, which is a sign of static blood collecting internally.

[7] Moderate the center and supplement vacuity 緩中補虛 *huǎn zhōng bǔ xū*: Moderate (gentle) attack in which static blood is gently eliminated and new blood is gradually engendered.

[8] Small beans 小豆 *xiǎo dòu*: Beans such as adzuki beans or mung beans.

SYNOPSIS, LINE 6.18

This line discusses the signs and treatment of blood stasis occurring in vacuity taxation.

COMMENTARY, LINE 6.18

The symptoms described in this line are related to extreme vacuity as a result of the five taxations and the seven damages. The seven types of damage are listed here as: food damage; anxiety damage; drink damage; bedroom damage; hunger damage; taxation damage; and channel, network vessel, construction, and defense qì damage. Note that the first six are causes, while the last is an effect. These causes of taxation over time result in detriment to the viscera and bowels.

Marked emaciation is a sign of extreme vacuity taxation. Abdominal fullness and inability to eat or drink is the manifestation of abnormal spleen-stomach movement and transformation. When vacuity taxation persists, it affects the qì and blood of channels and network vessels, resulting in static blood. In the text, static blood is referred to as "dry blood." Static blood manifests in encrusted skin and dark eyes because the skin and eyes are deprived of nourishment from yīn-blood.

The formula suggested is Rhubarb and Ground Beetle Pill (*dà huáng zhè chóng wán*). In this formula, rhubarb (*dà huáng*), ground beetle (*zhè chóng*), peach kernel (*táo rén*), tabanus (*méng chóng*), leech (*shuǐ zhì*), June beetle grub (*qí cáo*), and lacquer (*gān qī*) quicken the blood and transform stasis; peony (*sháo yào*) and rehmannia (*dì huáng*) nourish the blood and supplement vacuity; apricot kernel (*xìng rén*) rectifies qì; scutellaria (*huáng qín*) clears heat; licorice (*gān cǎo*) and processed honey (*liàn mì*) boost qì and harmonize the center. Even though this formula consists a number of powerful ingredients to attack static blood, these are combined with qì boosting, yīn-blood-enriching ingredients and mixed with honey into pills to moderate the attack.

This combination thus constitutes a "moderate formula" (缓方 *huǎn fāng*) to treat static blood as a result of enduring illness. Applying the principle of simultaneous supplementation and attack, it is a powerful formula in the form of a slow-acting pill. It supports right without leaving any stasis and dispels stasis without damaging right. For this reason the text says that it "moderates the center and supplements vacuity."

附方 APPENDED FORMULAS, LINE 6.18

HONEY-FRIED LICORICE DECOCTION (炙甘草汤 *zhì gān cǎo tāng*) from the *Qiān Jīn Yì* ("Wings of the Thousand Gold Pieces Prescriptions")[1]

治虚劳不足，汗出而闷，脉结悸，行动如常，不出百日，危急者十一日死。

甘草四两（炙） 桂枝 生姜各三两 麦门冬半升 麻仁半升 人参 阿胶各二两 大枣三十枚 生地黄 一斤

右九味，以酒七升、水八升，先煮八味，取三升，去滓，内胶消尽，温服一升，日三服。

Zhì xū láo bù zú, hàn chū ér mèn, mài jié jì, xíng dòng rú cháng, bù chū bǎi rì, wēi jí zhě shí yī rì sǐ.

Gān cǎo sì liǎng (zhì); guì zhī, shēng jiāng gè sān liǎng; mài mén dōng bàn shēng; má rén bàn shēng; rén shēn, ē jiāo gè èr liǎng; dà zǎo sān shí méi; shēng dì huáng yī jīn

Yòu jiǔ wèi, yǐ jiǔ qī shēng, shuǐ bā shēng, xiān zhǔ bā wèi, qǔ sān shēng, qù zǐ, nà jiāo xiāo jìn, wēn fú yī shēng, rì sān fú.

For treating vacuity taxation and insufficiency, with sweating and oppression, a bound pulse, and palpitation. [Even though] the patient engages in activity as if healthy, death will ensue in no more than a hundred days, and in critical cases in eleven days.

Honey-Fried Licorice Decoction (炙甘草汤 *zhì gān cǎo tāng*)
licorice (甘草 *gān cǎo*, Glycyrrhizae Radix) 4 *liǎng* (mix-fry) cinnamon twig (桂枝 *guì zhī*, Cinnamomi Ramulus) 3 *liǎng* fresh ginger (生姜 *shēng jiāng*, Zingiberis Rhizoma Recens) 3 *liǎng* ophiopogon (麦门冬 *mài mén dōng*, Ophiopogonis Radix) ½ *shēng* cannabis seed (麻仁 *má rén*, Cannabis Semen) ½ *shēng* ginseng (人参 *rén shēn*, Ginseng Radix) 2 *liǎng* ass hide glue (阿胶 *ē jiāo*, Asini Corii Colla) 2 *liǎng* jujube (大枣 *dà zǎo*, Jujubae Fructus) 30 pieces dried/fresh rehmannia (生地黄 *shēng dì huáng*, Rehmanniae Radix) 1 *jīn*

Of the above nine ingredients boil the first eight, excepting the ass hide glue (*ē jiāo*), in seven *shēng* of wine and eight *shēng* of water to get three *shēng*. Remove the dregs, and add the ass hide glue (*ē jiāo*) to melt completely. Take one *shēng* warm, three times a day.

FORMULA NOTE, LINE 6.18

[1] The commentary states here, "The formula is also called Pulse-Restorative Decoction (*fù mài tāng*)."

FORMULA COMMENTARY, LINE 6.18

Vacuity taxation and general insufficiency refers to patterns where qì, blood, yīn, and yáng are all vacuous. Sweating is a symptom of yáng being vacuous and therefore unable to secure defense so that yīn liquid is not guarded internally. Oppression in the chest indicates that heart qì is vacuous and devitalized. When qì is vacuous and blood scant, the heart is deprived of nourishment; hence there is heart palpitation and ill-being. A bound pulse, lastly, suggests that both qì and blood fail to move freely because they are vacuous.

Altogether these symptoms point to vacuity detriment of qì, blood, yīn, and yáng. Right qì is already debilitated even if the patient still acts like a healthy person. This is in fact a life-threatening condition that needs to be treated urgently by boosting heart qì and nourishing heart blood.

OTTER'S LIVER POWDER (獭肝散 *tǎ gān sǎn*)
from the *Zhǒu Hòu Bèi Jí Fāng* ("Emergency Standby Remedies")

治冷劳，又主鬼疰一门相染。

獭肝一具，炙干末之，水服方寸匕，日三服。

Zhì lěng láo, yòu zhǔ guǐ zhù yī mén xiāng rǎn.

Tǎ gān yī jù, zhì gān mò zhī, shuǐ fú fāng cùn bǐ, rì sān fú.

For treating cold taxation, and also for governing demonic influx that has been contracted from another household.

Otter's Liver Powder (獭肝散 *tǎ gān sǎn*)
otter's liver (獭肝 *tǎ gān*, Lutrae Iecur) 1 whole liver

Fry until dry and pulverize. Take a square-inch-spoonful in water, three times a day.

FORMULA COMMENTARY, LINE 6.18

Otter's liver is sweet, salty, and neutral, and is used to treat conditions of coughing. Having a supplementing and cough-calming effect, it is therefore appropriate for treating cold taxation. Demonic influx is a chronic disease contracted through contagion from corpses. The reason why it is listed here as an indication for this formula is unclear.

肺痿肺痈咳嗽上气病脉证治第七

CHAPTER 7

Lung Wilting, Pulmonary Welling-Abscess, and Cough with Qì Ascent

Pulses, Signs, Treatments

‡ OVERVIEW

This chapter covers lung wilting, pulmonary welling-abscess, and cough with qì ascent. Although these three diseases are attributable to different causes, they all affect the lung, manifest in cough, and have related and interconnected pathomechanisms. For this reason, they are discussed together in this chapter.

LUNG WILTING

Lung wilting is a chronic condition that involves weakness and devitalization of lung qì and wilting of the lobes of the lung. It is characterized chiefly by ejection of foamy drool and secondarily by cough, panting, and emaciation. The present chapter distinguishes vacuity heat and vacuity cold lung wilting. Vacuity heat lung wilting results from severe collapse of fluids with vacuity heat scorching the lung, causing dual damage to qì and yīn. Vacuity cold lung wilting arises from vacuity cold in the lung, qì failing to distribute liquid, and the upper body failing to restrain the lower body. The two forms have different pathomechanisms, but both are characterized by the same chief sign (ejection of foamy drool), are chronic diseases, and are usually the result of another disease or inappropriate treatment.

Pulmonary Abscess

Pulmonary welling-abscess refers to suppurating lesions of the lung. It is caused by contraction of wind evil and heat toxin, which gather in the lung, cause the blood and flesh to putrefy, and give rise to pus. The disease generally falls into three stages: the exterior-pattern stage, the suppurative stage, and the rupture stage. The exterior-pattern stage is characterized by heat effusion, aversion to cold, cough, and a floating pulse, i.e., signs similar to those of externally contracted wind-heat. The suppurative stage is characterized by shivering, rapid pulse, cough, chest pain, and ejection of fishy-smelling purulent phlegm. The rupture stage is characterized by ejection of phlegm and blood. While lung wilting manifests as vacuity, pulmonary welling-abscess classically manifests as repletion. However, in its later stages, pulmonary welling-abscess can convert into vacuity.

Cough with Qì Ascent

Cough with qì ascent means cough with counterflow ascent of lung qì. It manifests in panting, inability to lie flat, and phlegm rale in the throat. The term "qì ascent" denotes a pathomechanism of counterflow ascent of lung qì developing when the lung's depurative downbearing function is severely compromised. Since this phenomenon can be subjectively experienced by the patient as an upward force in the respiratory tract that makes it uncomfortable to lie flat, qì ascent can also be considered as a sign. Cough with qì counterflow ascent can be divided into vacuity and repletion patterns. The vacuity form is usually due to the kidney failing to absorb qì. The repletion form, which is the focus of the present chapter, usually takes the form of pulmonary distention resulting from a pathomechanism of evil repletion and qì block that arises when internally collecting water-rheum is complicated by externally contracted wind-cold. It is characterized by cough, panting, inability to lie flat, and frog rale in the throat.

‡ Schematic Overview

Lung Wilting

1) Vacuity heat type
   a) Causes: Wearing of fluids, yīn vacuity with internal heat.
   b) Main signs: cough, ejection of turbid phlegm, foamy drool, marked emaciation.
   c) Pulse: Vacuous, rapid.
   d) Treatment principle: clear and nourish the lung and stomach—Ophiopogon Decoction (*mài mén dōng tāng*)
   d) Appended formulas

      Honey-Fried Licorice Decoction (*zhì gān cǎo tāng*) to boost qì, engender liquid, and moisten dryness.

      Licorice Decoction (*gān cǎo tāng*) to enrich dryness and moisten the lung.
2) Vacuity cold type

a) Causes: upper burner yáng vacuity with cold in the lung.

b) Main signs: No cough, no thirst, ejection of foamy drool, frequent urination, dizzy head, enuresis.

c) Treatment principle: Warm the lung and disperse cold—Licorice and Dried Ginger Decoction (*gān cǎo gān jiāng tāng*).

d) Appended formula: Fresh Ginger and Licorice Decoction (*shēng jiāng gān cǎo tāng*) from the *Qiān Jīn Fāng* ("Thousand Gold Pieces Prescriptions") to bank up earth and moisten dryness.

Pulmonary Welling-Abscess

1) Causes

a) Wind striking defense; exhaling prevents [the evil from] entering further—wind damaging the skin and body hair.

b) Heat encroaching on construction; inhaling prevents [the evil from] exiting—heat damaging the blood and vessels.

2) Pathomechanisms

a) Wind dwelling in the lung.

b) Heat encroaching, causing blood to congeal, and amassing and binding to form a suppurating welling-abscess.

3) Pulses

a) Inch opening

Floating = wind—sweating.

Rapid = heat—aversion to cold.

Slippery and rapid—rapid and replete.

4) Main Signs

a) Exterior pattern stage: Heat effusion, aversion to cold, cough, fullness in the chest.

b) Suppurative stage: Intensifying chest pain, vigorous fever, quivering with cold, rapid pulse, frequent spitting of turbid foam.

c) Rupture stage: turbid spittle with fishy odor, ejection of pus and blood that resembles rice gruel.

5) Treatment

a) Exterior pattern stage: resolve the exterior with coolness and acridity while clearing internal heat.

b) Pus formation stage: Lepidium/Descurainiae and Jujube Lung-Draining Decoction (*tíng lì dà zǎo xiè fèi tāng*) and Phragmites Stem Decoction (*wěi jīng tāng*) from the *Qiān Jīn Fāng* ("Thousand Gold Pieces Prescriptions") to clear heat and drain the lung.

c) Rupture stage: Platycodon Decoction (*jié gěng tāng*) to expel pus and resolve toxin.

6) Prognosis

a) In the bud, [the patient] can be saved.

b) When pus has formed, [the patient] dies.

Cough and Qì Ascent

1) Causes: Water-rheum collecting internally and wind-cold fettering the outer body.

2) Pattern identification

a) Pulmonary distention

Main signs: Panting and agitation.

Mechanism: Imminent wind swelling. When sweat effuses, recovery ensues.

b) Critical signs: Qì ascent, puffy swollen face, raised-shoulder breathing, and a large floating pulse (cannot be treated). Diarrhea means that it is even more severe.

3) Pattern Identification and Treatment

a) Cold rheum depressing the lung

Main signs: Cough and qì ascent; frog rale in the throat.

Formula: Belamcanda and Ephedra Decoction (*shè gān má huáng tāng*) to disperse cold and flush rheum.

b) Rheum evil being forced upward

Main signs: Cough and counterflow qì ascent, fullness in the chest, inhibited throat, frog rale, floating pulse.

Formula: Officinal Magnolia Bark and Ephedra Decoction (*hòu pò má huáng tāng*) to clear heat and discharge fullness.

c) Water-rheum binding internally

Main signs: Cough and qì ascent, sunken pulse.

Formula: Sun Spurge Decoction (*zé qī tāng*) to expel water and flush rheum.

d) Thick phlegm causing obstruction

Main signs: Cough and counterflow qì ascent, frequently spitting turbid spittle, only sitting, and inability to sleep.

Formula: Gleditsia Fruit Pill (*zào jiá wán*) to flush turbid phlegm.

e) Depressed evil in the outer body with water-rheum in the inner body

Main signs: Cough and qì ascent, vexation and agitation, panting, floating pulse

Formula: Minor Black Dragon Decoction Plus Gypsum (*xiǎo qīng lóng jiā shí gāo tāng*) to disperse rheum and eliminate vexation.

f) Phlegm-heat depressing the lung

Main signs: Cough and qì ascent with eyes as if fit to burst from their sockets, floating and large pulse.

Formula: Spleen-Effusing Decoction Plus Pinellia (*yuè bì jiā bàn xià tāng*) to clear heat and flush rheum.

Line 7.1

(1) 问曰：热在上焦者，因咳为肺痿，肺痿之病，从何得之？师曰：或从汗出，或从呕吐，或从消渴，小便利数，或从便难，又被快药下利，重亡津液，故得之。

(2) 曰：寸口脉数，其人咳，口中反有浊唾涎沫者何？师曰：为肺痿之病。若口中辟辟燥，咳即胸中隐隐痛，脉反滑数，此为肺痈咳唾脓血。

(3) 脉数虚者为肺痿，数实者为肺痈。

(1) Wèn yuē: Rè zài shàng jiāo zhě, yīn ké wéi fèi wěi, fèi wěi zhī bìng, cóng hé dé zhī? Shī yuē: Huò cóng hàn chū, huò cóng ǒu tù, huò cóng xiāo kě, xiǎo biàn lì shuò, huò cóng biàn nán, yòu bèi kuài yào xià lì, zhòng wáng jīn yè, fù dé zhī.

(2) Yuē: Cùn kǒu mài shuò, qí rén ké, kǒu zhōng fǎn yǒu zhuó tuò xián mò zhě hé? Shī yuē: Wéi fèi wěi zhī bìng. Ruò kǒu zhōng pì pì zào, ké jí xiōng zhōng yǐn yǐn tòng, mài fǎn huá shuò, cǐ wéi fèi yōng ké tuò nóng xuè.

(3) Mài shuò xū zhě wéi fèi wěi, shuò shí zhě wéi fèi yōng.

(1) Question: "In patients with heat in the upper burner, cough causes lung wilting. Where does the disease of lung wilting come from?" The Master says: "It comes from sweating, from vomiting and retching, from dispersion-thirst[1] and frequent uninhibited urination, or from difficult defecation that was precipitated by means of quickening medicines,[2] which caused severe collapse of the fluids."

(2) Question: "When a person has a rapid pulse at the inch opening, and coughs, but has turbid spittle and foamy drool in the mouth, what does this mean?" The Master says: "This is the disease of lung wilting. If the mouth is sapless and dry,[3] and coughing causes dull pain in the chest, but the pulse is slippery and rapid, [this] is pulmonary welling-abscess with coughing of pus and blood.

(3) [If the] pulse is rapid and vacuous, it is lung wilting; if it is rapid and replete, it is pulmonary welling-abscess."

Text Notes, Line 7.1

[1] Dispersion-thirst 消渴 *xiāo kě*: This disease name first occurred in the *Sù Wèn* ("Plain Questions"). It describes severe thirst that is the result of internal heat consuming the fluids.

[2] Quickening medicines 快药 *kuài yào*: Drastic precipitating medicines like rhubarb (*dà huáng*).

[1] Sapless and dry 辟辟燥 *pī pī zào*: Commentators explain the Chinese *pī pī* as an onomatopoeic description of the sound made when sucking to draw saliva with dry lips.

Synopsis, Line 7.1

This line describes the causes, pulses, and signs of lung wilting, differentiating it from pulmonary welling-abscess.

Commentary, Line 7.1

This line is divided into three sections. The first section describes the causes of lung wilting. The second describes the pulses of lung wilting and pulmonary welling-abscess. The third further describes how lung wilting and pulmonary welling-abscess are distinguished in diagnosis.

In the first line, we learn how lung wilting arises. Although the disease can take the form of either vacuity heat or vacuity cold, vacuity heat is more commonly observed. Its pathomechanism is discussed here.

Heat in the upper burner that scorches the lung can cause qì counterflow with cough. When the cough persists for a long time, the lung becomes weak and devitalized, so that lung wilting develops. The reasons for the heat are numerous. It may be due to excessive sweating, to frequent vomiting, to dispersion-thirst with frequent, uninhibited urination, or to excessive use of precipitating medicines to treat constipation. Any of these cause damage to liquid and yīn vacuity, which in turn can give rise to internal heat that scorches the lung.

The lung is the delicate viscus. It likes moisture and is averse to dryness. When vacuity heat scorches the lung, the lung's function of diffusion and depurative downbearing is impaired and lung qì ascends counterflow, giving rise to cough. When the cough persists for a long time, it damages both qì and yīn in the lung. When lung qì is damaged, the lung becomes weak and is unable to distribute fluids. Instead, the fluids are boiled by the heat and form phlegm. When lung yīn is deprived of nourishment, the lobes of the lung become desiccated and wilted.

The second section describes the main signs of lung wilting and pulmonary welling-abscess. The main sign of lung wilting is coughing up of turbid spittle and foamy drool, with a pulse that is rapid at the inch position. The inch position reflects the upper burner; a rapid pulse there indicates heat. Hence a pulse that is rapid at the inch position reflects heat in the upper burner. However, heat is not the only problem, because the patient presents not only with a rapid pulse, but also with "turbid spittle and foamy drool in the mouth." We cannot explain this latter sign by heat alone, but must take into account the effect of heat on the fluids. The character 反 *fǎn* ("but") is significant here. It emphasizes the special characteristic of lung wilting wherein there is phlegm present in a condition of heat in the upper burner and "severe collapse of the fluids." This phlegm is a result of fluids collecting and steaming in the lung when lung qì is too vacuous to distribute them. Ascending counterflow with lung qì, they are expelled during coughing. While lung wilting is characterized by a rapid pulse at the inch position and by turbid spittle and foamy drool in the mouth, pulmonary welling-abscess is characterized by dryness in the mouth, cough that causes a dull pain in the chest, coughing up of pus and blood, as a well a rapid pulse.

The last section describes the difference between lung wilting and pulmonary welling-abscess in the pulse. In lung wilting, the pulse is vacuous, rapid, and forceless, reflecting a vacuity condition characterized by yīn vacuity with heat, collapse of the fluids, and damage to both qì and yīn. By contrast, pulmonary welling-abscess is characterized by a pulse that is slippery, rapid, and forceful, reflecting a repletion condition arising when evil heat gathers in the lung, qì and blood become congested, and right qì is not yet markedly weakened.

Line 7.2

问曰：病咳逆，脉之，何以知此为肺痈？当有脓血，吐之则死，其脉何类？师曰：寸口脉微而数，微则为风，数则为热；微则汗出，数则恶寒。风中于卫，呼气不入；热过于营，吸而不出；风伤皮毛，热伤血脉；风舍于肺，其人则咳，口干喘满，咽燥不渴，多唾浊沫，时时振寒。热之所过，血为之凝滞，蓄结痈脓，吐如米粥。始萌可救，脓成则死。

Wèn yuē: Bìng ké nì, mài zhī, hé yǐ zhī cǐ wéi fèi yōng? dāng yǒu nóng xuè, tù zhī zé sǐ? qí mài hé lèi? Shī yuē: Cùn kǒu mài wēi ér shuò, wēi zé wéi fēng, shuò zé wéi rè; wēi zé hàn chū, shuò zé wù hán. Fēng zhōng yú wèi, hū qì bù rù; rè guò yú yíng, xī ér bù chū; fēng shāng pí máo, rè shāng xuè mài; fēng shè yú fèi, qí rén zé ké, kǒu gān chuǎn mǎn, yān zào bù kě, duō tuò zhuó mò, shí shí zhèn hán. Rè zhī suǒ guò, xuè wéi zhī níng zhì, xù jié yōng nóng, tù rú mǐ zhōu. Shǐ méng kě jiù, nóng chéng zé sǐ.

Question: "When a patient presents with cough counterflow, how do you know from the pulse whether this is a pulmonary welling-abscess? There must be pus and blood, and if the patient vomits it up, death will ensue. What type of pulse does such a patient have?" The Master says: "The inch opening pulse will be faint[1] and rapid. A faint pulse means wind; a rapid pulse means heat. When the pulse is faint, there will be sweating; when it is rapid, there will be aversion to cold. When wind strikes the defense, exhaling of qì prevents [the evil] from entering; when heat encroaches[2] into construction, inhaling qì prevents [the evil] from exiting. Wind damages the skin and [body] hair; heat damages the blood and vessels. When wind abides in the lung, the person suffers from cough, dry mouth, panting and fullness, dry pharynx but no thirst, increased spitting of turbid foam,[3] and frequent quivering with cold. When heat encroaches, blood congeals and stagnates, amassing to bind into a welling-abscess with pus that when ejected looks like rice gruel. In the bud,[4] [the patient] can be saved; when pus has formed, [the patient] dies."

Text Notes, Line 7.2

[1] Faint 微 *wēi*: A faint pulse is here understood to mean a floating pulse.

[2] Encroach 过 *guò*: Invasion.

[3] Turbid foam 濁沫 *zhuó mò*: This is the turbid spittle and foamy drool mentioned in the previous line.

[4] In the bud 始萌 *shǐ méng*: In the initial stage.

Synopsis, Line 7.2

This line discusses the causes, pathomechanism, pulse and signs, and prognosis of pulmonary welling-abscess.

COMMENTARY, LINE 7.2

Pulmonary welling-abscess is caused by contraction of wind-heat evil, which is reflected in a pulse that is rapid and faint (floating). This line also tells us that a faint (floating) pulse means sweating, and a rapid one means aversion to cold. When wind-heat invades the body, defense qì is damaged and the interstices become loose. There is heat effusion, aversion to cold, and sweating. When the interstices are loose, they open and discharge, i.e., they allow sweat to flow forth. Because there is sweating, there is aversion to cold, despite the heat effusion. There is no direct relationship between sweating and a floating pulse or between aversion to cold and a rapid pulse. Sweating and aversion to cold are associated with wind-heat, which also gives rise to a pulse that is floating and rapid.

We are told that "wind damages the skin and body hair." "The skin and body hair" denotes the exterior, and when wind-heat assails the exterior, the result is aversion to cold, heat effusion, sweating, dry itchy throat, cough, and a floating and rapid pulse. These signs are like those of any other exterior pattern when defense qì is affected. However, in pulmonary welling-abscess, heat is entering construction-blood. Hence the text says that wind damages the skin and body hair, heat damages the blood and vessels. Damage to the blood and vessels is an important element of pulmonary welling-abscess over the whole course of its development.

The line suggests that pulmonary welling-abscess can be divided into three stages: an exterior-pattern stage, a suppurative stage, and a rupture stage.

The exterior-pattern stage is the initial stage, which arises when wind-heat assails the exterior. The signs, as already described, are aversion to cold, heat effusion, sweating, dry itchy throat, cough, and a floating and rapid pulse. Both wind and heat are present. However, we are told, "When wind strikes defense, exhaling of qì prevents [the evil] from entering; when heat penetrates construction, inhaling qì prevents [the evil] from getting out." This means that wind affecting the exterior is relatively easy to expel from the body, while heat affecting the blood and vessels represents a deeper penetration that is less easily eliminated. From the point of view of treatment, this means that in pulmonary welling-abscess the simple use of exterior-resolving formulas will be to no avail. To address the issue of heat affecting the blood and vessels, a heat-clearing toxin-resolving action is required. Clearing heat and resolving toxin is an important element in the treatment of pulmonary welling-abscess throughout its whole course.

The suppurative stage is described in the sentence that begins "when wind abides in the lung..." In this stage, the heat evil congests and stagnates, inhibiting lung qì and giving rise to panting and fullness. As a result of the inhibition of lung qì, the liquid of the lung is not distributed. Hence phlegm and drool bind internally, causing frequent spitting of turbid foam. When heat enters construction-blood, construction-yīn is damaged, so that the throat becomes dry. Shivering is a major sign of suppuration. It is often difficult to distinguish from the aversion to cold associated with the exterior-pattern stage. Evil affecting the exterior of the body prevents defense qì from adequately performing its warming function. When there is exuberant interior heat, right and evil are engaging in a fierce struggle in the interior. In addition, the inhibited diffusion of lung qì caused by heat also affects the function of exterior defense. This gives rise to pronounced shivering.

The rupture stage occurs when the putrefaction of the flesh and suppuration reach a point when pus is released into the airways. It is characterized by ejection of gruel-like fishy-smelling pus and blood, by pain in the chest, and again by shivering and a rapid pulse. By this stage, both evil qì and right qì have weakened, so that the pace of development becomes less urgent.

The final sentence reads, "In the bud, [the patient] can be saved; when pus has formed, [the patient] dies." This is a warning that pulmonary welling-abscess is ideally treated in its earlier stages. As the disease progresses, treatment becomes more difficult.

Line 7.3

上气，面浮肿，肩息，其脉浮大，不治，又加利，尤甚。

Shàng qì, miàn fú zhǒng, jiān xī, qí mài fú dà, bù zhì, yòu jiā lì, yóu shèn.

Qì ascent[1] with a puffy swollen face, raised-shoulder breathing,[2] and a large floating pulse cannot be treated. If it is further complicated by diarrhea, it is even more severe.

TEXT NOTES, LINE 7.3

[1] Qì ascent 上气 *shàng qì*: Upward counterflow of qì. This terms means both the upward movement of qì and the rapid breathing to which it gives rise.

[2] Raised-shoulder breathing 肩息 *jiàn xī*: Lifting the shoulders in order to breathe; a sign of extremely labored breathing.

SYNOPSIS, LINE 7.3

This line discusses qì ascent in vacuity patterns.

COMMENTARY, LINE 7.3

Qì ascent patterns can take the form of vacuity or repletion. The present line describes a vacuity pattern of puffy swelling of the face, raised shoulder breathing, and a pulse that is floating and large. Both puffy swelling of the face and raised shoulder breathing may occur in either vacuity or repletion patterns, but in the present line, the mention of a pulse that is floating and large is a clear indication of vacuity. A pulse that is floating, large, and without root indicates depleted kidney qì failing to ensure qì absorption and yáng qì floating upward. In enduring illness with rapid panting, yáng qì is dispersed, so that lung qì and kidney yáng both become depleted. When lung qì is vacuous and therefore fails to distribute fluid, and when the kidney is vacuous and therefore fails to transform water-damp, water qì spills upward into the face, causing puffy swelling. When lung vacuity causes inhibited breathing and kidney vacuity impairs proper qì absorption, breathing becomes difficult, so there is raised shoulder breathing, i.e., gaping mouth and raised shoulders. When vacuous yáng strays outward, the pulse is floating, large, and without root. Such a serious condition that affects both lung and kidney is very likely to also cause spleen vacuity, which may manifest in diarrhea. Severe vacuity of the lung, kidney, and spleen is difficult to treat.

Line 7.4

上气，喘而躁者，属肺胀，欲作风水，发汗则愈。

Shàng qì, chuǎn ér zào zhě, shǔ fèi zhàng, yù zuò fēng shuǐ, fā hàn zé yù.

Qì ascent with panting and agitation is ascribed to pulmonary distention.[1] Wind water is imminent.[2] If you promote sweating, recovery will ensue.

Text Notes, Line 7.4

[1] Pulmonary distention 肺胀 *fèi zhàng*: A disease name referring to the key symptom of distention and fullness of lung qì. It is caused by the patient's inability to diffuse and depurate qì.

[2] Wind water 风水 *fēng shuǐ*: A disease name that identifies a type of water qì that is caused by water qì spilling into the fleshy exterior as a result of lung qì congestion obstructing wind and water. See the chapter on "Water Qì" for more detail.

Synopsis, Line 7.4

This line discusses qì ascent in repletion patterns.

Commentary, Line 7.4

This line describes qì ascent in a repletion pattern with pulmonary distention and panting. This usually arises when wind-cold fetters the outer body in a patient who suffers from water-rheum collecting internally. It occurs in people with existing cough and panting due to water-rheum impairing normal diffusion and depuration of the lung. When such people contract wind-cold, it fetters the exterior and also stirs the phlegm-rheum internally. As a result, phlegm and drool congest, and the qì dynamic becomes depressed. The result is oppression in the chest with vexation and agitation. When lung qì is blocked, it can no longer keep the waterways clear, so that water qì spills into the exterior instead of descending to the bladder. Wind water develops as a result. This condition is treated by promoting sweating, to resolve the water-rheum and external evil by passing it outward through the sweat, thereby freeing lung qì and the waterways and reversing the counterflow.

Line 7.5

肺痿吐涎沫而不咳者，其人不渴，必遗尿、小便数。所以然者，以上虚不能制下故也。此为肺中冷，必眩、多涎唾，甘草干姜汤以温之。若服汤已渴者，属消渴。

甘草（炙）四两　干姜（炮）二两

右㕮咀，以水三升，煮取一升五合，去滓，分温再服。

Fèi wěi tù xián mò ér bù ké zhě, qí rén bù kě, bì yí niào, xiǎo biàn shuò. Suǒ yǐ rán zhě, yǐ shàng xū bù néng zhì xià gù yě. Cǐ wéi fèi zhōng lěng, bì xuàn, duō xián tuò, gān cǎo gān jiāng tāng yǐ wēn zhī. Ruò fú tāng yǐ kě zhě, shǔ xiāo kě.

Gān cǎo (zhì) sì liǎng; gān jiāng (pào) èr liǎng

Yòu fǔ jǔ, yǐ shuǐ sān shēng, zhǔ qǔ yī shēng wǔ gě, qù zǐ, fēn wēn zài fú.

In lung wilting with ejection of foamy drool and without cough, the patient will not experience thirst, but inevitably enuresis and frequent urination. The reason for this is that the upper body is vacuous and therefore unable to restrain the lower body. This means that there is cold in the lung. It invariably manifests in dizziness and increased drool and spittle. Use Licorice and Dried Ginger Decoction (甘草干姜汤 *gān cǎo gān jiāng tāng*) to warm [the lung]. If there is thirst after taking the decoction, this is ascribed to dispersion-thirst.

Licorice and Dried Ginger Decoction (甘草干姜汤 *gān cǎo gān jiāng tāng*)
licorice (甘草 *gān cǎo*, Glycyrrhizae Radix) 4 *liǎng* (mix-fry) dried ginger (干姜 *gān jiāng*, Zingiberis Rhizoma) 2 *liǎng* (blast-fry)

Chew the above ingredients and boil with three *shēng* of water to get one *shēng* and five *gě*. Remove the dregs. Divide into two [doses] and take warm.

Synopsis, Line 7.5

This line discusses the signs and treatment of lung wilting due to vacuity cold.

Commentary, Line 7.5

In contrast to the development of vacuity heat lung wilting, which was described above in line 7.1, the current line describes vacuity cold lung wilting, a condition that develops from upper burner yáng vacuity and vacuity cold in the lung. Lung wilting due to vacuity cold may develop from pre-existing yáng vacuity, but it can also develop when vacuity heat lung wilting persists for a long time, and yīn damages yáng. Because yáng is vacuous and cannot form qì, and because qì is vacuous and cannot contain or distribute liquid, fluids collecting in the lung transform into drool. The result is ejection of foamy drool without thirst. In lung qì vacuity cold, lung qì lacks the strength to ascend counterflow, hence there is no cough. Because of the upper burner vacuity cold, fluid tends to flow straight down to the lower burner. This results in enuresis or frequent urination, hence the text says that "the upper body is vacuous and therefore unable to restrain the lower body." This is the opposite of cases where blocked lung qì fails to ensure the free regulation of the waterways, giving rise to urinary stoppage. It is also quite different from the frequent urination in dispersion-thirst, which is accompanied by thirst and large intake of water. As already mentioned, in vacuity cold lung wilting, there is no thirst.

Vacuity cold lung wilting is here treated with Licorice and Dried Ginger Decoction (*gān cǎo gān jiāng tāng*). In this formula, licorice (*gān cǎo*) is sweet and warm and supplements vacuity, while dried ginger (*gān jiāng*) is acrid and warm and disperses cold. Acridity and sweetness in combination can restore yáng qì, warm lung qì, and normalize qì transformation. By warming the center and supplementing spleen-earth, which is the mother of lung-metal, this formula also engenders metal and supplements the vacuity of the lung.

Line 7.6

咳而上气，喉中水鸡声，射干麻黄汤主之。

射干十三枚　麻黄四两　生姜四两　细辛　紫苑　款冬花各三两　五味子半升　大枣七枚　半夏（大者洗）八枚

右九味，以水一斗二升，先煮麻黄两沸，去上沫，内诸药煮取三升，分温三服。

Ké ér shàng qì, hóu zhōng shuǐ jī shēng, shè gān má huáng tāng zhǔ zhī.

Shè gān shí sān méi; má huáng sì liǎng; shēng jiāng sì liǎng; xì xīn, zǐ wǎn, kuǎn dōng huā, gè sān liǎng; wǔ wèi zǐ bàn shēng; dà zǎo qī méi; bàn xià (dà zhě xǐ) bā méi

Yòu jiǔ wèi, yǐ shuǐ yī dǒu èr shēng, xiān zhǔ má huáng liǎng fèi, qù shàng mò, nà zhū yào zhǔ qǔ sān shēng, fēn wēn sān fú.

For cough with qì ascent and a frog ralē in the throat, Belamcanda and Ephedra Decoction (射干麻黄汤 *shè gān má huáng tāng*) governs.

Belamcanda and Ephedra Decoction (射干麻黄汤 *shè gān má huáng tāng*)

- belamcanda (射干 *shè gān*, Belamcandae Rhizoma) 13 pieces[2]
- ephedra (麻黄 *má huáng*, Ephedrae Herba) 4 *liǎng*
- fresh ginger (生姜 *shēng jiāng*, Zingiberis Rhizoma Recens) 4 *liǎng*
- asarum (细辛 *xì xīn*, Asari Radix et Rhizoma) 3 *liǎng*
- aster (紫菀 *zǐ wǎn*, Asteris Radix) 3 *liǎng*
- coltsfoot (款冬花 *kuǎn dōng huā*, Farfarae Flos) 3 *liǎng*
- schisandra (五味子 *wǔ wèi zǐ*, Schisandrae Fructus) ½ *shēng*
- jujube (大枣 *dà zǎo*, Jujubae Fructus) 7 pieces
- pinellia (半夏 *bàn xià*, Pinelliae Rhizoma) 8 pieces (3 large ones, washed)

Of the nine above ingredients, first boil the ephedra (*má huáng*) in one *dǒu* and two *shēng* of water, bringing it to a boil twice. Remove the scum, add all the [other] medicinals, and boil down to three *shēng*. Divide into three [doses] and take warm.

TEXT NOTES, LINE 7.6

[1] Frog rale 水鸡声 *shuǐ jī shēng*: Lit. "the sound of frogs," this describes the continuous rale of phlegm in the throat.

[2] A textual variation here recommends three *liǎng* instead.

[3] A textual variation here recommends ½ *shēng* instead.

SYNOPSIS, LINE 7.6

This line discusses the signs and treatment of cold rheum depressing the lung.

COMMENTARY, LINE 7.6

Cough with qì ascent and phlegm rale in the throat, which falls within the scope of what biomedicine calls asthma, is commonly seen in clinical practice. When cold rheum depresses the lung and prevents lung qì from diffusing, there is counterflow ascent with panting and cough. When phlegm obstructs the airways and is disturbed by the breath, we hear a phlegm rale in the throat, which is often described as "frog rale" because it sounds like a chorus of frogs.

Wheezing and panting due to cold rheum depressing the lung is treated by dispersing cold and diffusing the lung and by downbearing counterflow and transforming phlegm. The formula presented in this line is Belamcanda and Ephedra Decoction (*shè gān má huáng tāng*). Within this formula, belamcanda (*shè gān*) disperses phlegm and opens binds; ephedra (*má huáng*) diffuses the lung and calms panting; fresh ginger (*shēng jiāng*) and asarum (*xì xīn*) disperse cold and move water; coltsfoot (*kuǎn dōng huā*), aster (*zǐ wǎn*), and pinellia (*bàn xià*) downbear qì and transform phlegm; schisandra (*wǔ wèi zǐ*) constrains lung qì and combined with the ephedra (*má huáng*), asarum (*xì xīn*), fresh ginger (*shēng jiāng*), and pinellia (*bàn xià*) ensures contraction within dispersion; jujube (*dà zǎo*) calms the center and harmonizes all the medicinals. This formula is commonly used to treat cold-rheum cough and panting. It has the advantage of eliminating evil without damaging right.

Line 7.7

咳逆上气，时时吐浊，但坐不得眠，皂荚丸主之。

皂荚（刮去皮，用酥炙）八两

右一味，末之，蜜丸梧子大，以枣膏和汤服三丸，日三夜一服。

Ké nì shàng qì, shí shí tǔ zhuó, dàn zuò bù dé mián, zào jiá wán zhǔ zhī.

Zào jiá (guā qù pí, yòng sū zhì) bā liǎng.

Yòu yī wèi, mò zhī, mì wán wú zǐ dà, yǐ zǎo gāo huó tāng fú sān wán, rì sān yè yī fú.

For cough and counterflow qì ascent, [in which the patient] frequently spits turbid [spittle], can only sit, and is unable to sleep,[1] Gleditsia Fruit Pill (皂荚丸 *zào jiá wán*) governs.

Gleditsia Fruit Pill (皂荚丸 *zào jiá wán*)
gleditsia (皂荚 *zào jiá*, Gleditsiae Fructus) 8 *liǎng* (scrape off the skin and mix-fry in butter)

Pulverize the single ingredient above and make honey pills the size of firmiana seeds. Take three pills [per dose], three times a day and once at night, mixed with jujube paste and hot water.

TEXT NOTES, LINE 7.7

[1] "Can only sit, and is unable to sleep" 但坐不得眠 *dàn zuò bù dé mián*: This describes a pathological state where the patient's lung is so congested by phlegm they are unable to breathe lying flat and even in a sitting position are still unable to fall asleep.

[2] Butter 酥 *sū*: The *Běn Cǎo Gāng Mù* ("Herbal Foundation Compendium") describes how this product is obtained by scalding milk repeatedly, taking the skin floating on the top, boiling this again until the fat comes out, and finally separating it into solids and pure oil. It stresses that the highest grade is made from cow's milk and is cool in nature, while sheep and water buffalo milk are of inferior quality and are hot in nature (*Běn Cǎo Gāng Mù* 50:1785-6).

SYNOPSIS, LINE 7.7

This line describes the signs and treatment of panting and cough due to phlegm turbidity congestion the lungs.

COMMENTARY, LINE 7.7

When the lung fails to depurate and turbid phlegm congests the airways, there is cough and panting. Thick phlegm in the lung is forced upward by qì, causing frequent cough and expectoration of phlegm. However, coughing never manages to clear the lung of phlegm, so that cough counterflow, panting, and fullness persist. These signs are exacerbated when the patient lies down, so that sleep is also affected.

This condition requires a powerful phlegm-eliminating action, which is provided by Gleditsia Fruit Pill (*zào jiá wán*).

When the phlegm is eliminated, the panting and cough spontaneously stop. Within the formula, acrid and salty gleditsia (*zào jiá*) flushes phlegm and disinhibits the orifices, diffusing congestion and abducting stagnation. Because gleditsia is drastic and harsh in its action, it is mix-fried with butter, made into honey pills, and taken with jujube paste. This helps to ensure that the phlegm is eliminated without damaging the stomach and spleen or right qì.

Line 7.8

咳而脉浮者，厚朴麻黄汤主之。

厚朴五两　麻黄四两　石膏如鸡子大

杏仁半升　半夏半升　干姜二两

细辛二两　小麦一升　五味子半升

右九味，以水一斗二升，先煮小麦熟，去滓，内诸药煮取三升，温服一升，日三服。

Ké ér mài fú zhě, hòu pò má huáng tāng zhǔ zhī.

Hòu pò wǔ liǎng; má huáng sì liǎng; shí gāo rú jī zǐ dà; xìng rén bàn shēng; bàn xià bàn shēng; gān jiāng èr liǎng; xì xīn èr liǎng; xiǎo mài yī shēng; wǔ wèi zǐ bàn shēng

Yòu jiǔ wèi, yǐ shuǐ yī dǒu èr shēng, xiān zhǔ xiǎo mài shóu, qù zǐ, nà zhū yào zhǔ qǔ sān shēng, wēn fú yī shēng, rì sān fú.

For cough with a floating pulse, Officinal Magnolia Bark and Ephedra Decoction (厚朴麻黄汤 *hòu pò má huáng tāng*) governs.

Officinal Magnolia Bark & Ephedra Decoction (厚朴麻黄汤 *hòu pò má huáng tāng*)

- officinal magnolia bark (厚朴 *hòu pò*, Magnoliae Officinalis Cortex) 5 *liǎng*
- ephedra (麻黄 *má huáng*, Ephedrae Herba) 4 *liǎng*
- gypsum (石膏 *shí gāo*, Gypsum Fibrosum) a lump the size of a chicken egg
- apricot kernel (杏仁 *xìng rén*, Armeniacae Semen) ½ *shēng*
- pinellia (半夏 *bàn xià*, Pinelliae Rhizoma) ½ *shēng*
- dried ginger (干姜 *gān jiāng*, Zingiberis Rhizoma) 2 *liǎng*
- asarum (细辛 *xì xīn*, Asari Radix et Rhizoma) 2 *liǎng*
- wheat (小麦 *xiǎo mài*, Tritici Semen) 1 *shēng*
- schisandra (五味子 *wǔ wèi zǐ*, Schisandrae Fructus) ½ *shēng*

Of the nine above ingredients, first boil the wheat in one *dǒu* and two *shēng* of water until cooked. Remove the dregs, add [the other] medicinals, and boil down to three *shēng*. Take one *shēng* [per dose] warm, three times a day.

Synopsis, Line 7.8

This line describes the location and treatment of cough and panting on the basis of the pulse.

Commentary, Line 7.8

When cough is accompanied by a floating pulse, this tells us the condition and the pathomechanism: A floating pulse indicates disease of the exterior. When the disease evil is in the upper body, the pulse is also floating. From this we can tell that the disease is near the exterior and that there is an exuberant evil in the upper body. This condition also manifests in signs such as cough and panting counterflow, fullness in the chest, vexation and agitation, inhibition in the throat, gurgling sound of phlegm, sweating from the head only, propped breathing (倚息 *yǐ xī*, ability to breathe comfortably only in a propped up position, not lying down), a floating pulse, and a slippery tongue fur.

The treatment proposed for this condition is Officinal Magnolia Bark and Ephedra Decoction (*hòu pò má huáng tāng*), which disperses rheum and downbears counterflow, thereby relieving cough and calming panting. Within the formula, officinal magnolia bark (*hòu pò*), ephedra (*má huáng*), and apricot kernel (*xìng rén*) diffuse the lung and disinhibit qì; asarum (*xì xīn*), dried ginger (*gān jiāng*), and pinellia (*bàn xià*) transform phlegm and relieve cough; gypsum (*shí gāo*) clears heat and eliminates vexation; wheat (*xiǎo mài*) nourishes right and quiets the center; and schisandra (*wǔ wèi zǐ*) constrains lung qì.

Line 7.9

脉沉者，泽漆汤主之。

半夏半升　紫参五两　泽漆（以东流水五斗煮取一斗五升）三斤　生姜五两　白前五两　甘草 黄芩　人参 桂枝各三两

右九味，㕮咀，内泽漆汁中煮取五升，温服五合，至夜尽。

Mài chén zhě, zé qī tāng zhǔ zhī.

Bàn xià bàn shēng; zǐ shēn wǔ liǎng; zé qī (yǐ dōng liú shuǐ wǔ dǒu zhǔ qǔ yī dǒu wǔ shēng) sān jīn; shēng jiāng wǔ liǎng; bái qián wǔ liǎng; gān cǎo huáng; qín rén shēn guì zhī gè sān liǎng

Yòu jiǔ wèi, fǔ jǔ, nà zé qī zhī zhōng zhǔ qǔ wǔ shēng, wēn fú wǔ gě, zhì yè jìn.

When the pulse is sunken, Sun Spurge Decoction (泽漆汤 *zé qī tāng*) governs.

Sun Spurge Decoction
(泽漆汤 *zé qī tāng*)

pinellia (半夏 *bàn xià*, Pinelliae Rhizoma) ½ *shēng*
zǐ shēn (紫参)[1] 5 *liǎng* [see below]
sun spurge (泽漆 *zé qī*, Euphorbiae Helioscopiae Herba) 3 *jīn* (boil in 5 *dǒu* of east-flowing water to get 1 *dǒu* and five *shēng*)
fresh ginger (*shēng jiāng*) 5 *liǎng*
willowleaf swallowwort (白前 *bái qián*, Cynanchi Stauntonii Rhizoma) 5 *liǎng*
licorice (甘草 *gān cǎo*, Glycyrrhizae Radix) 3 *liǎng*
scutellaria (黄芩 *huáng qín*, Scutellariae Radix) 3 *liǎng*
ginseng (人参 *rén shēn*, Ginseng Radix) 3 *liǎng*
cinnamon twig (桂枝 *guì zhī*, Cinnamomi Ramulus) 3 *liǎng*

Chew the nine above ingredients. Boil them in the sun spurge (*zé qī*) liquid to get five *shēng*. Take five *gě* [per dose] warm, finishing [the entire preparation] by nighttime.

TEXT NOTES, LINE 7.9

[1] 紫参 *zǐ shēn*: Modern scholars are unsure what *zǐ shēn* denotes and whether in fact it was what Zhāng Jī wrote. The term 紫参 *zǐ shēn* appears in the *Shén Nóng Běn Cǎo Jīng* ("The Divine Husbandman's Herbal Foundation Canon"), where it is described in the following way: "Also called 杜蒙 *dù méng*. Bitter in flavor, cold, non-toxic. Treats concretions and gatherings in the heart and abdomen, cold and heat evil qì. Frees the nine orifices and disinhibits the stool and urine. Treats ox disease. Grows in valleys."

The *Běn Cǎo Gāng Mù* ("Herbal Foundation Compendium") says that it treats all blood diseases. Whether the *zǐ shēn* in these two references is the same is unsure; no modern *Jīn Guì* texts specify the botanical name of the plant from which it is derived.

The *Zhōng Yào Dà Cí Diǎn* ("Great Encyclopedia of Chinese Medicinals") gives 紫参 *zǐ shēn* as an alternate names for 红骨参 *hóng gǔ shēn*, Salviae Plectranthoidis Radix, and 拳参 *quán shēn*, Bistortae Rhizoma. *Hóng gǔ shēn* is warm, bitter, and sweet; it quickens the network vessels and strengthens the sinews and warms the channels and the network vessels; it treats wind-cold impediment, numbness of the limbs, sinew and bone pain, and hemiplegia. *Quán shēn* is bitter and cool, clears heat and settles fright, rectifies dampness and disperses swelling, and treats fright convulvsions, lockjaw, red dysentery, swollen welling-abscesses, and scrofula.

A commentary in the received text states, "In one version, aster (紫菀 *zǐ wǎn*, Asteris Radix)," which warms the lung, precipitates qì, disperses phlegm, and relieves cough, treats wind-cold cough and panting, coughing of blood and pus in vacuity taxation, throat impediment (*hóu bì*), and inhibited urination. Aster is now commonly used in place of 紫参 *zǐ shēn* in modern clinical practice.

[2] East-flowing water 东流水 *dōng liú shuǐ*: Water from an eastward flowing river.

SYNOPSIS, LINE 7.9

This line continues the discussion of the location and treatment of cough and panting on the basis of the pulse.

COMMENTARY, LINE 7.9

The preceding line discussed the treatment of cough with a floating pulse. This line discusses cough with a sunken pulse. A sunken pulse means that the disease is in the interior, while also indicating water. Hence, in a patient suffering from cough, this pulse indicates water-rheum collecting internally. Water-rheum collecting internally manifests in panting and cough. When the water-rheum spills outward, there is generalized heaviness. The reason why water-rheum is collecting is because of spleen vacuity. Hence the physician needs to treat not only the tip (i.e. water-rheum collecting), but also the root, namely spleen vacuity.

Within the formula, sun spurge (*zé qī*) disperses phlegm and expels water; *zǐ shēn* quickens blood, and in combination with sun spurge (*zé qī*) expels water and disperses swelling; fresh ginger (*shēng jiāng*), pinellia (*bàn xià*), and cinnamon twig (*guì zhī*) disperse water and downbear counterflow; willowleaf swallowwort (*bái qián*) calms panting and relieves cough; ginseng (*rén shēn*) and licorice (*gān cǎo*) support right and bank up the spleen, so that the formula as a whole treats the root as well as the tip. Scutellaria (*huáng qín*) is added to discharge heat that develops when water-rheum remains for a long time. As a whole, the formula expels water and frees yáng, while relieving cough and calming panting.

Line 7.10

大逆上气，咽喉不利，止逆下气者，麦门冬汤主之。

麦门冬七升半夏一升　人参二两　甘草二两粳米三合　大枣十二枚

右六味，以水一斗二升，煮取六升，温服一升，日三、夜一服。

Dà nì shàng qì, yān hóu bù lì, zhǐ nì xià qì zhě, mài mén dōng tāng zhǔ zhī.

Mài mén dōng qī shēng; bàn xià yī shēng; rén shēn èr liǎng; gān cǎo èr liǎng; jīng mǐ sān gě; dà zǎo shí èr méi

Yòu liù wèi, yǐ shuǐ yī dǒu èr shēng, zhǔ qǔ liù shēng, wēn fú yī shēng, rì sān, yè yī fú.

For great counterflow qì ascent with inhibited throat, to stop counterflow and precipitate qì, Ophiopogon Decoction (麦门冬汤 *mài mén dōng tāng*) governs.

Ophiopogon Decoction (麦门冬汤 *mài mén dōng tāng*)
ophiopogon (麦门冬 *mài mén dōng*, Ophiopogonis Radix) 7 *shēng*
pinellia (半夏 *bàn xià*, Pinelliae Rhizoma) 1 *shēng*
ginseng (人参 *rén shēn*, Ginseng Radix) 2 *liǎng*
licorice (甘草 *gān cǎo*, Glycyrrhizae Radix) 2 *liǎng*
non-glutinous rice (粳米 *jīng mǐ*, Oryzae Semen) 3 *gě*
jujube (大枣 *dà zǎo*, Jujubae Fructus) 12 pieces

Boil the above six ingredients in one *dǒu* and two *shēng* of water to get six *shēng*. Take one *shēng* [per dose] warm, three times a day and once at night.

SYNOPSIS, LINE 7.10

This line discusses the signs and treatment of cough and panting due to vacuity fire.

COMMENTARY, LINE 7.10

When lung and stomach fluid are consumed, yīn vacuity develops. As a result of this, fire effulges and flames upward. This vacuity fire scorches the lung and affects its depurative downbearing function. This manifests in panting and cough. When vacuity fire scorches liquid, the throat lacks moisture and therefore becomes dry and inhibited, with ungratifying expectoration of thick sticky phlegm.

From the description of the pathomechanism and the formula used to treat the condition, we can infer that accompanying symptoms also include dry mouth with a desire for cooling and moistening drinks, a red tongue with scant fur, and a pulse that is vacuous and rapid. Although the disease affects the lung, it is rooted in insufficiency of stomach yīn; hence the treatment needs to address both the lung and stomach.

The recommended formula is Ophiopogon Decoction (*mài mén dōng tāng*), which clears and nourishes the lung and stomach, as well as checks counterflow and downbears qì. The actions of the individual ingredients of the formula are as follows: Ophiopogon (*mài mén dōng*) moistens the lung and nourishes the stomach, while also clearing vacuity fire. Pinellia (*bàn xià*) precipitates qì and transforms phlegm. The formula uses only a small quantity relative to the much larger amounts of clearing and moistening medicinals, so there is no fear of excessive dryness. Ginseng (*rén shēn*), licorice (*gān cǎo*), jujube (*dà zǎo*), and non-glutinous rice (*jīng mǐ*) nourish the stomach and boost qì, enabling the spleen and stomach to engender liquid. If fire counterflow is pronounced, lophatherum (*dàn zhú yè*) and gypsum (*shí gāo*) can be added to enhance the heat-clearing action.

Line 7.11

肺痈喘不得卧，葶苈大枣泻肺汤主之。

葶苈（熬令黄色，捣丸如弹子大）

大枣十二枚

右先以水三升，煮枣取二升，去枣内葶苈，煮取一升，顿服。

Fèi yōng chuǎn bù dé wò, tíng lì dà zǎo xiè fèi tāng zhǔ zhī.

Tíng lì (áo lìng huáng sè, dǎo wán rú dǎn zi dà); dà zǎo shí èr mei

Yòu xiān yǐ shuǐ sān shēng, zhǔ zǎo qǔ èr shēng, qù zǎo nà tíng lì, zhǔ qǔ yī shēng, dùn fú.

For pulmonary welling-abscess with inability to lie down, Lepidium/Descurainiae and Jujube Lung-Draining Decoction (葶苈大枣泻肺汤 *tíng lì dà zǎo xiè fèi tāng*) governs.

Lepidium/Descurainiae and Jujube Lung-Draining Decoction (葶苈大枣泻肺汤 *tíng lì dà zǎo xiè fèi tāng*)
lepidium/descurainiae (葶苈 *tíng lì*, Lepidii/Descurainiae Semen) (simmer until yellow, crush [and form into] pills the size of slingshot pellets) jujube (大枣 *dà zǎo*, Jujubae Fructus) 12 pieces

Of the above ingredients, first boil the jujube (*dà zǎo*) in three *shēng* of water to get two *shēng*. Remove the jujube (*dà zǎo*), add the lepidium/descurainiae (*tíng lì zǐ*), and boil to get one *shēng*. Quaff.

Synopsis, Line 7.11

This line discusses the treatment of repletion-pattern panting due to pulmonary welling-abscess.

Commentary, Line 7.11

In the initial stage of pulmonary welling-abscess, disease evil enters the lung and scorches liquid, turning it into phlegm. This causes congestion, which manifests in panting. In severe cases, the congestion is exacerbated when the patient lies down; hence a powerful formula is called for. The formula suggested is Lepidium/Descurainiae and Jujube Lung-Draining Decoction (*tíng lì dà zǎo xiè fèi tāng*), which is used as an emergency treatment to drain the repletion evil in the lung.

The actions of the individual ingredients of the formula are as follows: Lepidium/Descurainiae (*tíng lì zǐ*) is bitter and cold. It is a draining precipitant as well as phlegm-expelling medicinal. It is also an extremely powerful agent and is therefore combined with sweet, warm jujube (*dà zǎo*). This not only moderates the nature of the lepidium/descurainiae (*tíng lì zǐ*), but also quiets the center, that is, limits the formula's side-effects on the digestive tract. Jujube is thus included in this formula for the same reason that it is included in Ten Jujubes Decoction (*shí zǎo tāng*, see 12.22) and as a paste, in Gleditsia Fruit Pill (*zào jiá wán*, see line 7.7 above).

Line 7.12

咳而胸满，振寒，脉数，咽干不渴，时出浊唾腥臭，久久吐脓如米粥者，为肺痈，桔梗汤主之。

桔梗一两　甘草二两

右二味，以水三升，煮取一升，分温再服，则吐脓血也。

Ké ér xiōng mǎn, zhèn hán, mài shuò, yān gān bù kě, shí chū zhuó tuò xīng chòu, jiǔ jiǔ tù nóng rú mǐ zhōu zhě, wéi fèi yōng, jié gēng tāng zhǔ zhī.

Jié gēng yī liǎng; gān cǎo èr liǎng

Yòu èr wèi, yǐ shuǐ sān shēng, zhǔ qǔ yī shēng, fēn wēn zài fú, zé tù nóng xuè yě.

Cough with fullness in the chest, quivering with cold, a rapid pulse, a dry pharynx but no thirst, periodic ejection of turbid fishy-smelling spittle, and, after a longer time, ejection of pus like rice gruel constitutes pulmonary welling-abscess. Platycodon Decoction (桔梗汤 *jié gěng tāng*)[1] governs.

Platycodon Decoction (桔梗汤 *jié gěng tāng*)
platycodon (桔梗 *jié gěng*, Platycodonis Radix) 1 *liǎng*
licorice (甘草 *gān cǎo*, Glycyrrhizae Radix) 2 *liǎng*

Boil the above two ingredients in three *shēng* of water to get one *shēng*. Divide into two [doses] and take warm. As a result, [the patient] will eject pus and blood.

TEXT NOTE, LINE 7.12

[1] The commentary here adds: "It also treats blood impediment."

SYNOPSIS, LINE 7.12

This line discusses the signs and treatment of pulmonary welling-abscess in the suppurative and rupture stage.

COMMENTARY, LINE 7.12

This line follows the theme from line 7.2, which described the pathomechanism and development of pulmonary welling-abscess. The present line adds information about the suppurative and rupture stage and its treatment.

When wind-heat lodges in the lung and inhibits lung qì, there is cough and fullness in the chest. Shivering, a rapid pulse, a dry pharynx, and absence of thirst are signs indicating that the disease has developed to the stage where heat is damaging the blood and vessels and where heat toxin is brewing. Over time, depressed evil heat becomes toxic, qì and blood vanquish, and welling-abscess with pus forms. This manifests in frequent ejection of fishy-smelling pus, which over time takes on the appearance of rice gruel.

The formula proposed is Platycodon Decoction (*jié gěng tāng*), which is composed of two ingredients only. Platycodon (*jié gěng*) opens and lifts lung qì and expels pus, while licorice (*gān cǎo*) resolves toxin. The combination therefore has the action of clearing heat and resolving toxin and of dispelling phlegm and expelling pus. It is a sweet, moderate, light formula.

Note that when this formula says that the patient will "eject" (吐 *tù*) pus and blood, this does not meant that one should treat the patient with ejection therapy, but that ejection of pus and blood is a symptom to be expected as a sign of the formula's efficacy.

Line 7.13

咳而上气，此为肺胀，其人喘，目如脱状，脉浮大者，越婢加半夏汤主之。

麻黄六两　石膏半斤　生姜三两　大枣十五枚　甘草二两　半夏半升

右六味，以水六升先煮麻黄，去上沫，内诸药，煮取三升，分温三服。

Ké ér shàng qì, cǐ wéi fèi zhàng, qí rén chuǎn, mù rú tuō zhuàng, mài fú dà zhě, yuè bì jiā bàn xià tāng zhǔ zhī.

Má huáng liù liang; shí gāo bàn jīn; shēng jiāng sān liǎng; dà zǎo shí wǔ méi; gān cǎo èr liǎng; bàn xià bàn shēng

Yòu liù wèi, yǐ shuǐ liù shēng xiān zhǔ má huáng, qù shàng mò, nà zhū yào, zhǔ qǔ sān shēng, fēn wēn sān fú.

Cough with qì ascent constitutes pulmonary distention. If the eyes of a patient [with this condition] look like they are about to burst from their sockets, and if the pulse is floating and large, Spleen-Effusing Decoction Plus Pinellia (越婢加半夏汤 *yuè bì jiā bàn xià tāng*) governs.

Spleen-Effusing Decoction Plus Pinellia (越婢加半夏汤 *yuè bì jiā bàn xià tāng*)

- ephedra (麻黄 *má huáng*, Ephedrae Herba) 6 *liǎng*
- gypsum (石膏 *shí gāo*, Gypsum Fibrosum) ½ *jīn*
- fresh ginger (生姜 *shēng jiāng*, Zingiberis Rhizoma Recens) 3 *liǎng*
- jujube (大枣 *dà zǎo*, Jujubae Fructus) 15 pieces
- licorice (甘草 *gān cǎo*, Glycyrrhizae Radix) 2 *liǎng*
- pinellia (半夏 *bàn xià*, Pinelliae Rhizoma) ½ *shēng*

Of the above six ingredients, first boil the ephedra (*má huáng*) in six *shēng* of water. Remove the scum, add all [the other] medicinals, and boil to get three *shēng*. Divide into three [doses] and take warm.

Synopsis, Line 7.13

This line describes the signs and treatment of cough and panting due to rheum-heat (饮热 *yǐn rè*) depressing the lung.

Commentary, Line 7.13

When externally contracted wind-heat combines with water-rheum that has collected internally, the water-rheum and the heat ascend counterflow giving rise to cough and panting and in severe cases protrusion of the eyes. The combination of these evils can be deduced from the pulse: A floating pulse indicates disease in the exterior or upper body. A large pulse indicates heat. A floating and large pulse therefore indicates wind-heat ascending counterflow with rheum evil. This is treated by swiftly giving the patient Spleen-Effusing Decoction Plus

Pinellia (*yuè bì jiā bàn xià tāng*) to diffuse the lung and discharge heat, and to downbear counterflow and calm panting.

Within the formula, acrid ephedra (*má huáng*) and cool gypsum (*shí gāo*) combine to bring up water qì and to clear the interior heat. Fresh ginger (*shēng jiāng*) and pinellia (*bàn xià*) disperse water and downbear counterflow. Licorice (*gān cǎo*) and jujube (*dà zǎo*) harmonize all the medicinals in the formula.

Line 7.14

肺胀咳而上气，烦躁而喘，脉浮者，心下有水，小青龙加石膏汤主之。

麻黄　芍药　桂枝　细辛　甘草　干姜各三两　五味子　半夏各半升　石膏二两

右九味，以水一斗，先煮麻黄，去上沫，内诸药，煮取三升，强人服一升，羸者减之，日三服，小儿服四合。

Fèi zhàng ké ér shàng qì, fán zào ér chuǎn, mài fú zhě, xīn xià yǒu shuǐ, xiǎo qīng lóng jiā shí gāo tāng zhǔ zhī.

Má huáng sháo yào; guì zhī, xì xīn, gān cǎo, gān jiāng gè sān liǎng; wǔ wèi zǐ, bàn xià gè bàn shēng; shí gāo èr liǎng

Yòu jiǔ wèi, yǐ shuǐ yī dǒu, xiān zhǔ má huáng, qù shàng mò, nà zhū yào, zhǔ qǔ sān shēng, qiáng rén fú yī shēng, léi zhě jiǎn zhī, rì sān fú, xiǎo ér fú sì gě.

Pulmonary distention with cough and qì ascent, vexation and agitation with panting, and a floating pulse indicate the presence of water below the heart. Minor Black Dragon Decoction Plus Gypsum (小青龙加石膏汤 *xiǎo qīng lóng jiā shí gāo tāng*)[1] governs.

Minor Black Dragon Decoction Plus Gypsum (小青龙加石膏汤 *xiǎo qīng lóng jiā shí gāo tāng*)

- ephedra (麻黄 *má huáng*, Ephedrae Herba) 3 *liǎng*
- peony (芍药 *sháo yào*, Paeoniae Radix) 3 *liǎng*
- cinnamon twig (桂枝 *guì zhī*, Cinnamomi Ramulus) 3 *liǎng*
- asarum (细辛 xì xīn, Asari Radix et Rhizoma) 3 *liǎng*
- licorice (甘草 *gān cǎo*, Glycyrrhizae Radix) 3 liǎng
- dried ginger (干姜 *gān jiāng*, Zingiberis Rhizoma) 3 *liǎng*
- schisandra (五味子 *wǔ wèi zǐ*, Schisandrae Fructus) ½ *shēng*
- pinellia (半夏 *bàn xià*, Pinelliae Rhizoma) ½ *shēng*
- gypsum (石膏 *shí gāo*, Gypsum Fibrosum) 2 *liǎng*

Of the above nine ingredients, first boil the ephedra (*má huáng*) in one *dǒu* of water. Remove the scum, add all [the other] ingredients, and boil to get three *shēng*. For strong patients, give one *shēng* per dose; for markedly emaciated patients, reduce the amount. Take three doses a day. For children, the dose is four *gě*.

Text Note, Line 7.14

[1] A comment included in the received text reads, "The *Qiān Jīn Fāng* offers the same [description of] pattern and treatment, but additionally includes [the symptom of] pain under the rib-side stretching into the empty basin." "Empty basin" 缺盆 *quē pén* refers to the supraclavicular fossa.

SYNOPSIS, LINE 7.14

This line discusses the signs and treatment of cough and panting due to cold rheum.

COMMENTARY, LINE 7.14

The present line describes a situation in which pre-existing water-rheum below the heart is stirred by externally contracted wind-cold. When wind-cold fetters the exterior, the pulse is floating. Water-rheum below the heart can seep into the lung and thereby affect the diffusion and downbearing functions of the lung. This manifests in cough and panting. When the rheum evil lies depressed for a long time, it transforms into heat, which manifests in vexation and agitation. The key element in the condition is water below the heart, because this is the direct cause of not only the cough and panting but also the vexation and agitation.

The recommended formula is Minor Black Dragon Decoction Plus Gypsum (*xiǎo qīng lóng jiā shí gāo tāng*), to resolvs the exterior and transform phlegm, downbear counterflow and calm panting, and clear heat and eliminate vexation. The actions of the individual ingredients are as follows: Ephedra (*má huáng*) and cinnamon twig (*guì zhī*) resolve the exterior and disperse cold, as well as diffusing the lung and calming panting. Peony (*sháo yào*) and cinnamon twig (*guì zhī*) harmonize construction and defense. Asarum (*xì xīn*) and dried ginger (*gān jiāng*) warm the lung and transform rheum. Pinellia (*bàn xià*) downbears counterflow and transforms phlegm. Schisandra (*wǔ wèi zǐ*) has an astringent action that prevents lung qì from dispersing excessively. Gypsum (*shí gāo*) clears and disperses depressed heat to eliminate the vexation. It also helps ephedra (*má huáng*) in bringing up water qì. Finally, licorice (*gān cǎo*) harmonizes all the medicinals in the formula.

附方 APPENDED FORMULAS, LINE 7.14

HONEY-FRIED LICORICE DECOCTION (炙甘草汤 *zhì gān cǎo tāng*)
from the *Qiān Jīn Yì* ("Wings of the Thousand Gold Pieces Prescriptions")

治肺痿涎唾多，心中温温液液者。

Zhì fèi wěi xián tuò duō, xīn zhōng yùn yùn yè yè zhě.

For treating lung wilting with copious drool and spittle, and pervasive nausea in the heart.[1]

FORMULA NOTE, LINE 7.14

[1] Pervasive nausea 温温液液 *yùn yùn yè yè*: The commentary explains this as a feeling of constant retching in the heart [region]. After this sentence, the commentary adds: "For the formula, see the chapter on Vacuity Taxation." (Chapter 6).

Licorice Decoction (甘草汤 *gān cǎo tāng*) from the *Qiān Jīn Yào Fāng* ("A Thousand Gold Pieces Prescriptions")

甘草
右一味，以水三升煮减半，分温三服。

Gān cǎo

Yòu yī wèi, yǐ shuǐ sān shēng zhǔ jiǎn bàn, fēn wēn sān fú.

Licorice Decoction (甘草汤 *gān cǎo tāng*)
licorice (甘草 *gān cǎo*, Glycyrrhizae Radix)

Boil the single above ingredient in three *shēng* of water until reduced by half. Divide into three [doses] and take warm.

Fresh Ginger and Licorice Decoction (生姜甘草汤 *shēng jiāng gān cǎo tāng*) from the *Qiān Jīn Yào Fāng* ("A Thousand Gold Pieces Prescriptions")

治肺痿咳唾涎沫不止，咽燥而渴。
生姜五两 人参三两 甘草四两 大枣十五枚
右四味，以水七升，煮取三升，分温三服。

Zhì fèi wěi ké tuò, xián mò bù zhǐ, yān zào ér kě.

Shēng jiāng wǔ liǎng; rén shēn sān liǎng; gān cǎo sì liǎng; dà zǎo shí wǔ méi.

Yòu sì wèi, yǐ shuǐ qī shēng, zhǔ qǔ sān shēng, fēn wēn sān fú.

For treating lung wilting with cough and incessant spitting of foamy drool, dry pharynx, and thirst.

Fresh Ginger and Licorice Decoction (生姜甘草汤 *shēng jiāng gān cǎo tāng*)
fresh ginger (生姜 *shēng jiāng*, Zingiberis Rhizoma Recens) 5 *liǎng* ginseng (人参 *rén shēn*, Ginseng Radix) 3 *liǎng* licorice (甘草 *gān cǎo*, Glycyrrhizae Radix) 4 *liǎng* jujube (大枣 *dà zǎo*, Jujubae Fructus) 15 pieces

Boil the above four ingredients in seven *shēng* of water to get three *shēng*. Divide into three [doses] and take warm.

Cinnamon Twig Decoction Minus Peony Plus Gleditsia (桂枝去芍药加皂荚汤 *guì zhī qù sháo yào jiā zào jiá tāng*) from the *Qiān Jīn Yào Fāng*

治肺痿吐涎沫。
桂枝 生姜各三两 甘草二两 大枣十枚
皂荚（去皮子，炙焦）一枚
右五味，以水七升，微微火煮取三升，分温三服。

Zhì fèi wěi tù xián mò.

Guì zhī, shēng jiāng gè sān liǎng ; gān cǎo èr liǎng ; dà zǎo shí méi; zào jiá (qù pí zǐ, zhì jiāo) yī méi.

Yòu wǔ wèi, yǐ shuǐ qī shēng, wēi wēi huǒ zhǔ qǔ sān shēng, fēn wēn sān fú.

For treating lung wilting with ejection of foamy drool.

Cinnamon Twig Decoction Minus Peony Plus Gleditsia (桂枝去芍药加皂荚汤 *guì zhī qù sháo yào jiā zào jiá tāng*)
cinnamon twig (桂枝 *guì zhī*, Cinnamomi Ramulus) 3 *liǎng* fresh ginger (生姜 *shēng jiāng*, Zingiberis Rhizoma Recens) 3 *liǎng* licorice (甘草 *gān cǎo*, Glycyrrhizae Radix) 2 *liǎng* jujube (大枣 *dà zǎo*, Jujubae Fructus) 10 pieces gleditsia (皂荚 *zào jiá*, Gleditsiae Fructus) 1 piece (remove skin and seeds, mix-fry until scorched) 1 piece

Boil the above five ingredients in seven *shēng* of water over a very small flame to get three *shēng*. Divide into three [doses] and take warm.

PLATYCODON WHITE POWDER (桔梗白散 *jié gěng bái sǎn*)
from the *Wài Tái Mì Yào* ("Secrets from the *Wài Tái* Library")

治咳而胸满，振寒，脉数，咽干不渴，时出浊唾腥臭，久久吐脓如米粥者，为肺痈。

桔梗　贝母各三分　巴豆（去皮，熬研如脂）一分

右三味, 为散, 强人饮服半钱匕, 羸者减之。病在膈上者, 吐脓血, 膈下者泻出; 若下多不止, 饮冷水一杯则定。

Zhì ké ér xiōng mǎn, zhèn hán, mài shuò, yān gān bù kě, shí chū zhuó tuò xīng chòu, jiǔ jiǔ tù nóng rú mǐ zhōu zhě, wéi fèi yōng.

Jié gēng, bèi mǔ gè sān fèn; bā dòu (qù pí, áo yán rú zhī) yī fen

Yòu sān wèi, wéi sǎn, qiáng rén yǐn fú bàn qián bǐ, léi zhě jiǎn zhī. Bìng zài gé shàng zhě, tù nóng xuè, gé xià zhě xiè chū; ruò xià duō bù zhǐ, yǐn lěng shuǐ yī bēi zé dìng.

For treating cough with fullness in the chest, quivering with cold, a rapid pulse, dry pharynx but no thirst, periodic ejection of turbid fishy-smelling spittle, and, over time, ejection of pus like rice gruel, which constitutes pulmonary welling-abscess.

Platycodon White Powder (桔梗白散 *jié gěng bái sǎn*)
platycodon (桔梗 *jié gěng*, Platycodonis Radix) 3 parts
fritillaria (贝母 *bèi mǔ*, Fritillariae Bulbus) 3 parts
croton (巴豆 *bā dòu*, Crotonis Fructus) 1 part (remove skin, simmer, and grind to a fatty paste)

Make a powder of the above three ingredients. Strong patients should take half a qián-spoonful in liquid; markedly emaciated patients should reduce the amount. If the disease is above the diaphragm, it manifests with ejection of pus and blood. If the disease is below the diaphragm, it manifests with diarrhea. If there is profuse incessant precipitation, drink a cup of cold water to settle it.

PHRAGMITES STEM DECOCTION (苇茎汤 *wěi jīng tāng*)
from the *Qiān Jīn Yào Fāng* ("A Thousand Gold Pieces Prescriptions)

治咳有微热，烦满，胸中甲错，是为肺痈。

苇茎二升 薏苡仁半升 桃仁五十枚 瓜瓣半升

右四味，以水一斗，先煮苇茎得五升，去滓，内诸药，煮取二升，服一升，再服，当吐如脓。

Zhì ké yǒu wēi rè, fán mǎn, xiōng zhōng jiǎ cuò, shì wéi fèi yōng.

Wěi jīng èr shēng; yì yǐ rén bàn shēng; táo rén wǔ shí méi; guā bàn bàn shēng

Yòu sì wèi, yǐ shuǐ yī dǒu, xiān zhǔ wěi jīng dé wǔ shēng, qù zǐ, nà zhū yào, zhǔ qǔ èr shēng, fú yī shēng, zài fú, dāng tù rú nóng.

For treating cough with slight heat, vexation and fullness, and encrusted skin on the chest, this being pulmonary welling-abscess.

Phragmites Stem Decoction (苇茎汤 *wěi jīng tāng*)
phragmites stem (苇茎 *wěi jīng*, Phragmitis Rhizoma) 2 *shēng*

coix (薏苡仁 *yì yǐ rén*, Coicis Semen) ½ *shēng*
peach kernel (桃仁 *táo rén*, Persicae Semen) 50 pieces
wax gourd seed (瓜瓣 *guā bàn*) ½ *shēng*

Of the above four ingredients, first boil the phragmites stem (*wěi jīng*) in one *dǒu* of water to get five *shēng*. Remove the dregs, add all [the other] medicinals, and boil to get two *shēng*. Take two doses of one *shēng* each. This should cause ejection of pus-like [matter].

Line 7.15

肺痈胸满胀，一身面目浮肿，鼻塞清涕出，不闻香臭酸辛，咳逆上气，喘鸣迫塞，葶苈大枣泻肺汤主之。

Fèi yōng xiōng mǎn zhàng, yī shēn miàn mù fú zhǒng, bí sè qīng tì chū, bù wén xiāng chòu suān xīn, ké nì shàng qì, chuǎn míng pò sè, tíng lì dà zǎo xiè fèi tāng zhǔ zhī.

For pulmonary welling-abscess with fullness and distention in the chest; puffy swelling of the whole body, face, and eyes; nasal congestion with clear snivel and inability to smell fragrance, fetor, sourness, or acridity; cough and counterflow qì ascent; and panting with rale, distress, and congestion. Lepidium/Descurainiae and Jujube Lung-Draining Decoction (*tíng lì dà zǎo xiè fèi tāng*) governs.[1]

Formula Note, Line 7.15

[1] Following this, the commentary adds: "For the formula, see above. Take one pack in three days to a total of three or four packs. First take one pack of Minor Black Dragon Decoction (*xiǎo qīng lóng tāng*) and then take [this formula]. For the formula for Minor Black Dragon Decoction (*xiǎo qīng lóng tāng*), see the chapter on cough."

Synopsis, Line 7.15

This line further describes the clinical manifestations and application of Lepidium/Descurainiae and Jujube Lung-Draining Decoction (*tíng lì dà zǎo xiè fèi tāng*).

Commentary, Line 7.15

Although this line mentions pulmonary welling-abscess, the symptoms described here are actually quite different from this disease. Physicians throughout the ages have therefore questioned its meaning. On the basis of the constellation of symptoms and the recommended treatment, it is possible that the term 痈 *yōng* ("welling-abscess") here should actually be read as 壅 *yōng* ("congestion").

The treatment recommended here consists of first administering Minor Black Dragon Decoction (*xiǎo qīng lóng tāng*) to resolve the exterior, and then give Lepidium/Descurainiae and Jujube Lung-Draining Decoction (*tíng lì dà zǎo xiè fèi tāng*) to precipitate water-rheum.

奔豚气病脉证治第八

CHAPTER 8

Running Piglet Qì

Pulses, Signs, Treatments

‡ Overview

This chapter describes the causes, pathomechanisms, signs, and treatment for running piglet qì. Because the disease has special characteristics that make it easy to identify, it is given its own chapter. This chapter also mentions three other diseases—ejection of pus, fright, and fire evil. However, these are dealt with more fully in other chapters, and hence are not discussed in this introduction.

The term "running piglet qì" denotes a surging from the lesser abdomen to the throat that occurs in repeated episodes of sudden onset. "Running piglet qì" is a literal translation of the Chinese 奔豚气 *bēn tún qì*: 奔 is an alternate character for 賁, which is here used in the sense of "to run"; 豚 *tún* refers to a small pig; and 气 *qì* is the character for qì. The image of the running piglet figuratively describes the surging sensation. The word qì figures in the name because this is considered to be a disease of qì. Thus, the special feature of the pathomechanism is the derangement and upward surging of qì.

As described in this chapter, "running piglet disease" refers to a surging from the lesser abdomen to the throat. During attacks, [the patient seems as if] about to die; then [the qì] returns and the disease stops." It is different from the condition of "qì surging up from the lesser abdomen" that characterizes "surging mounting" (冲疝 *chōng shàn*) as described in the *Sù Wèn* ("Plain Questions"). It also differs from the condition of "kidney accumulation running piglet" (肾积贲豚 *shèn jī bēn tún*) that is described in the *Nàn Jīng* ("The Classic of Difficult Issues"). In contrast to running piglet disease, surging mounting manifests with urinary and fecal stoppage in addition to the chief sign of qì surging upward. Kidney accumulation running piglet is essential an accumulation-gathering condition with lumps in the lesser abdomen, which is quite different from the pathomechanism of running piglet qì.

The pathomechanism of running piglet qì disease is complex. Although it is usually associated with abnormalities of the affect-mind, it is also involves the liver and the kidney, and we need to distinguish between cold and heat. In clinical practice, the condition therefore has to be diagnosed and identified with care.

Schematic Overview

Running Piglet Qì Disease

1. Causes and Pathomechanisms

   Emotional stimuli such as fright and fear ⇨ liver depression transforming into fire ⇨ qì and fire surging upward.

   Yáng vacuity after sweating: Further contraction of cold evil or pre-existing water-rheum in patients suffering from kidney yáng vacuity ⇨ water-cold surging upward.

2. Patterns and Treatment

   Liver qì running piglet: Characterized by qì surging up into the chest, abdominal pain, and alternating cold and heat. Treated by discharging liver depression and by downbearing counterflow and relieving pain using Running Piglet Pill (*bēn tūn wán*).

   Kidney qì running piglet

   Running piglet that has already occurred: Characterized by qì surging up from the lower abdomen into the heart, with abdominal pain. Treated by assisting yáng, dispersing cold, and downbearing counterflow, using Cinnamon Twig Decoction Plus Extra Cinnamon (*guì zhī jiā guì tāng*).

   Running piglet about to occur: Characterized by palpitation below the umbilicus. Treated by warming yáng, supplementing earth, and disinhibiting water, using Poria, Cinnamon Twig, Licorice, and Jujube Decoction (*fú líng guì zhī gān cǎo dà zào tāng*).

Line 8.1

师曰：病有奔豚，有吐脓，有惊怖，有火邪，此四部病，皆从惊发得之。师曰：奔豚病从少腹起，上冲咽喉，发作欲死，复还止，皆从惊恐得之。

Shī yuē: Bìng yǒu bēn tún, yǒu tù nóng, yǒu jīng bù, yǒu huǒ xié, cǐ sì bù bìng, jiē cóng jīng fā dé zhī. Shī yuē: Bēn tún bìng cóng shào fù qǐ, shàng chōng yān hóu, fā zuò yù sǐ, fù huán zhǐ, jiē cóng jīng kǒng dé zhī.

The Master says: "Running piglet, ejection of pus, fright-scare, and fire evil are four diseases that all come from fright." The Master says: "Running piglet disease refers to a surging from the lesser abdomen to the throat. During attacks, [the patient seems as if] about to die; then [the qì] returns and the disease stops. This all comes from fright."

Synopsis, Line 8.1

This line discusses the cause and symptoms of running piglet qì disease.

Commentary, Line 8.1

The present line starts by stating that running piglet, ejection of pus, fright-scare, and fire evil are all the result of fright. Since the text does not give information concerning any other disease besides running piglet, commentators have suggested that the relevant text must have gone missing. According to the chapter, "Greater Yáng Disease" in the *Shāng Hán Lùn* ("On Cold Damage"), fright patterns may occur as a result of fire evil, but not the other way round. Similarly, it is doubtful that ejection of pus is caused by fright. Hence, the first statement of the Master in this line is not considered reliable.

Running piglet is characterized by episodes that begin with pain in the lesser abdomen followed by a subjective feeling of qì surging from the lesser abdomen to the heart, chest, and throat.

Although the text does not mention this, the pathway of the qì surge corresponds to the pathway of the thoroughfare vessel. During these episodes, the patient suffers extreme discomfort, but as the signs disappear the patient returns to normal. Hence, we are told, "During attacks, [the patient seems as if] about to die; then [the qì] returns and the disease stops."

Regarding the pathomechanism of running piglet, the line tells us that it is the result of fright. However, the disease is now in fact associated with the liver and kidney and with the thoroughfare vessel, which starts in the lower burner and ascends into the throat. When there is insufficiency in the heart and kidney, cold qì in the lower burner can surge up along the thoroughfare vessel and cause running piglet. Nevertheless, the disease can also arise because fright, fear, or anger cause depressed liver qì to ascend counterflow along the thoroughfare vessel. Thus, running piglet is related to affect-mind, but can also be caused by other factors.

Line 8.2

奔豚，气上冲胸，腹痛，往来寒热，奔豚汤主之。

甘草　芎藭　当归各二两　半夏四两　黄芩二两　生葛五两　芍药二两　生姜四两　甘李根白皮一升

右九味，以水二斗，煮取五升，温服一升，日三夜一服。

Bēn tún, qì shàng chōng xiōng, fù tòng, wǎng lái hán rè, bēn tún tāng zhǔ zhī.

Gān cǎo, xiōng qióng, dāng guī gè èr liǎng; bàn xià sì liǎng; huáng qín èr liǎng; shēng gé wǔ liǎng; sháo yào èr liǎng; shēng jiāng sì liǎng; gān lǐ gēn bái pí yī shēng

Yòu jiǔ wèi, yǐ shuǐ èr dǒu, zhǔ qǔ wǔ shēng, wēn fú yī shēng, rì sān yè yī fú.

For running piglet with qì surging up into the chest, abdominal pain, and alternating [aversion to] cold and heat [effusion], Running Piglet Decoction (奔豚汤 *bēn tún tāng*) governs.

Running Piglet Decoction
(奔豚汤 *bēn tún tāng*)

licorice (甘草 *gān cǎo*, Glycyrrhizae Radix) 2 *liǎng*
chuanxiong (芎藭 *xiōng qióng*, Chuanxiong Rhizoma) 2 *liǎng*
Chinese angelica (当归 *dāng guī*, Angelicae Sinensis Radix) 2 *liǎng*
pinellia (半夏 *bàn xià*, Pinelliae Rhizoma) 4 *liǎng*
scutellaria (黄芩 *huáng qín*, Scutellariae Radix) 2 *liǎng*
raw pueraria (生葛 *shēng gé*, Puerariae Radix Cruda) 5 *liǎng*
peony (芍药 *sháo yào*, Paeoniae Radix) 2 *liǎng*
fresh ginger (生姜 *shēng jiāng*, Zingiberis Rhizoma Recens) 4 *liǎng*
plum root bark (甘李根白皮 *gān lǐ gēn bái pí*, Pruni Salicinae Radicis Cortex) 1 *shēng*

Boil the above nine ingredients in two *dǒu* of water to get five *shēng*. Take one *shēng* [per dose] warm, three times a day and once at night.

SYNOPSIS, LINE 8.2

This line discusses the signs and treatment of running piglet originating in the liver.

COMMENTARY, LINE 8.2

Fright, fear, and anger can cause liver qì to become depressed and bound. As a result, depressed liver qì transforms into heat and rises counterflow along the thoroughfare vessel. When liver qì is depressed, the stagnation of qì inhibits the movement of blood; hence there is abdominal pain.

The liver stands in exterior-interior relationship with the gallbladder, whose associated channel is the foot lesser yáng channel. When liver qì is depressed, the qì of the lesser yáng channel is disharmonious, so there is alternating aversion to cold and heat effusion. Alternating heat and cold is observed only in running piglet patterns that are associated with liver depression; it is not a basic characteristic of running piglet.

The formula prescribed to treat running piglet originating in the liver is Running Piglet Decoction (*bēn tún tāng*). This formula nourishes the blood and calms the liver, and harmonizes the stomach and downbearsqì. Plum root bark (*lǐ gēn pí*) is bitter in flavor and cold in nature. It is used here to downbear running piglet qì and is the chief medicinal of the formula. Chinese angelica (*dāng guī*), chuanxiong (*chuān xiōng*), and peony (*sháo yào*) nourish the blood and emolliate the liver, as well as moving blood and relieving pain. Pinellia (*bàn xià*) and fresh ginger (*shēng jiāng*) downbear turbidity and check counterflow. Scutellaria (*huáng qín*) clears liver and gallbladder heat. Scutellaria (*huáng qín*) combined with pinellia (*bàn xià*) and fresh ginger (*shēng jiāng*) further has the effect of "draining the heart"; it regulates heat and cold, disperses glomus and binds, and downbears the counterflow surging. Pueraria (*gé gēn*) engenders liquid and clears heat. Licorice (*gān cǎo*) relaxes tension and relieves pain; in combination with white peony (*bái shao*), its strength is even greater. The formula as a whole tends toward cold and is therefore suitable for treating heat-type running piglet.

Line 8.3

发汗后，烧针令其汗，针处被寒，核起而赤者，必发奔豚，气从少腹上至心，灸其核上各一壮，与桂枝加桂汤主之。

桂枝五两　芍药三两　甘草（炙）二两　生姜三两　大枣十二枚

右五味，以水七升，微火煮取三升，去滓，温服一升。

Fā hàn hòu, shāo zhēn lìng qí hàn, zhēn chù bèi hán, hé qǐ ér chì zhě, bì fā bēn tún, qì cóng shào fù shàng zhì xīn, jiǔ qí hé shàng gè yī zhuàng, yǔ guì zhī jiā guì tāng zhǔ zhī.

Guì zhī wǔ liǎng; sháo yào sān liǎng; gān cǎo (zhì) èr liǎng; shēng jiāng sān liǎng; dà zǎo shí èr méi

Yòu wǔ wèi, yǐ shuǐ qī shēng, wēi huǒ zhǔ qǔ sān shēng, qù zǐ, wēn fú yī shēng.

If, after promoting sweating, red-hot needling is used to further cause the patient to sweat, the needling site can contract cold, [as a result of which] a lump rises and becomes red. This invariably means that running piglet will ensue, with qì [surging] from the lesser abdomen to the heart. Burn two cones of moxa on top of the lump. Cinnamon Twig Decoction Plus Extra Cinnamon (桂枝加桂汤 *guì zhī jiā guì tāng*) governs.

Cinnamon Twig Decoction Plus Extra Cinnamon (桂枝加桂汤 *guì zhī jiā guì tāng*)
cinnamon twig (桂枝 *guì zhī*, Cinnamomi Ramulus) 5 *liǎng*
peony (芍药 *sháo yào*, Paeoniae Radix) 3 *liǎng*
licorice (甘草 *gān cǎo*, Glycyrrhizae Radix) 2 *liǎng* (mix-fry)
fresh ginger (*shēng jiāng*) 3 *liǎng*
jujube (大枣 *dà zǎo*, Jujubae Fructus) 12 pieces

Boil the above five ingredients in seven *sheng* of water over a small flame to get three *shēng*. Remove the dregs and take one *shēng* [per dose] warm.

SYNOPSIS, LINE 8.3

This line discusses the signs and treatment of running piglet resulting from inappropriate sweating.

COMMENTARY, LINE 8.3

When red-hot needling (燒針 *shāo zhēn*) is inappropriately used after a patient has sweated, this can make the patient sweat more profusely and thereby cause damage to yáng. When this happens, cold evil can enter the body at the needling site. From there, it can give rise to internally exuberant yīn cold, which ascends to intimidate heart yáng and causes qì to surge up from the lesser abdomen to the region below the heart.

This pathomechanism involves the heart and kidney channels and requires external as well as internal treatment. Thus, this line recommends to apply moxibustion externally to warm the channels and disperse cold, and to give Cinnamon Twig Decoction Plus Extra Cinnamon (*guì zhī jiā guì tāng*) internally to harmonize yīn and yáng and to downbear counterflow qì.

Line 8.4

发汗后，脐下悸者，欲作奔豚，茯苓桂枝甘草大枣汤主之。

茯苓半斤　桂枝四两　甘草（炙）二两　大枣十五枚

右四味，以甘澜水一斗，先煮茯苓，减二升，内诸药，煮取三升，去滓，温服一升，日三服。

Fā hàn hòu, qí xià jì zhě, yù zuò bēn tún, fú líng guì zhī gān cǎo dà zǎo tāng zhǔ zhī.

Fú líng bàn jīn; guì zhī sì liǎng; gān cǎo (zhì) èr liǎng; dà zǎo shí wǔ méi

Yòu sì wèi, yǐ gān lán shuǐ yī dǒu, xiān zhǔ fú líng, jiǎn èr shēng, nà zhū yào, zhǔ qǔ sān shēng, qù zǐ, wēn fú yī shēng, rì sān fú.

If sweating is followed by palpitation below the umbilicus, running piglet is about to occur. Poria, Cinnamon Twig, Licorice, and Jujube Decoction (茯苓桂枝甘草大枣汤 *fú líng guì zhī gān cǎo dà zào tāng*) governs.

Poria, Cinnamon Twig, Licorice, and Jujube Decoction (茯苓桂枝甘草大枣汤 *fú líng guì zhī gān cǎo dà zào tāng*)
poria (茯苓 *fú líng*, Poria) ½ *jīn* cinnamon twig (桂枝 *guì zhī*, Cinnamomi Ramulus) 4 *liǎng* licorice (甘草 *gān cǎo*, Glycyrrhizae Radix) 2 *liǎng* (mix-fry) jujube (大枣 *dà zǎo*, Jujubae Fructus) 15 fruits

Of the above four ingredients, first boil the poria (*fú líng*) in one *dǒu* of worked water[1] until reduced to two *shēng*. Add all the [other] ingredients and boil to get three *shēng*. Remove the dregs. Take one *shēng* [per dose] warm, three times a day.

TEXT NOTE, LINE 8.4

[1] Worked water 甘澜水 *gān lán shuǐ*: Water that has been lifted with a ladle and poured over and over. This is explained in a note at the end of the paragraph: "Method for making worked water: Pour two *dǒu* of water into a large basin, and lift it [continuously] with a ladle. When there are five or six thousand globules on the water, all joined together, it is ready for use."

SYNOPSIS, LINE 8.4

This line describes the signs and treatment of running piglet due to water-rheum.

COMMENTARY, LINE 8.4

This line discusses running piglet that arises in patients with a pre-existing condition where water-rheum has collected in the lower burner because inhibited qì transformation prevented it from being eliminated. If such patients are treated with inappropriate promotion of sweating, detriment to heart yáng can result. If yáng becomes so vacuous that it is insufficient for restraining kidney water, the qì of water-cold can exploit the vacuity and stir, causing the patient to subjectively experience a pounding below the umbilicus. Since running piglet begins with discomfort in the lesser abdomen, the pounding below the umbilicus can be taken to mean that running piglet is about to occur.

The formula proposed for this condition is Poria, Cinnamon Twig, Licorice, and Jujube Decoction (*fú líng guì zhī gān cǎo dà zào tāng*), which frees yáng, downbears counterflow, and banks up earth to dam water (培土制水 *péi tǔ zhì shuǐ*). The individual actions of the medicinals in the formula are as follows: Poria (*fú líng*) and cinnamon twig (*guì zhī*) are the chief medicinals; they free yáng and transform water, thereby checking qì counterflow. Licorice (*gān cǎo*) and jujube (*dà zǎo*) bank up earth and restrain water, thereby also helping to restrain the upsurge of qì. At the same time, poria (*fú líng*) combined with cinnamon twig (*guì zhī*) promotes heart-kidney interaction, helping to treat the stirring palpitation.

胸痹心痛短气病脉证治第九

CHAPTER 9

Chest Impediment, Heart Pain, and Shortness of Breath

Pulses, Signs, Treatments

‡ OVERVIEW

Although the title mentions three disease categories—chest impediment, heart pain, and shortness of breath—this chapter deals essentially with chest impediment and heart pain. Shortness of breath is in fact not a separate category, but rather a symptom of the two other diseases, especially chest impediment.

CHEST IMPEDIMENT

The earliest extant text in which the term "chest impediment" (胸痹 *xiōng bì*) appears is the *Líng Shū* ("Magic Pivot"), in the chapter, "Viscera" (本藏 *běn zàng*). However, the *Jīn Guì Yào Lüè* is the first text to provide comprehensive details for pattern identification and treatment. The Chinese disease name as well as its literal English translation imply both a locus and a pathomechanism. Impediment means stoppage, and "when there is stoppage there is pain" (不通則痛 *bù tòng zé tòng*). Hence, the term indirectly alludes to the main sign, namely glomus blockage and pain in the anterior chest. Chest impediment is caused by devitalization of chest yáng, which is exploited by water-rheum and cold evil, thereby impeding the movement of clear yáng.

It is important to note that the character 痹 *bì* ("impede" or "block") is otherwise used to denote diseases that are caused by a combination of wind, cold, and dampness and are characterized by pain and numbness (classically including arthritis and sciatica (see Chapter 5, "Wind-Stroke and Joint-Running"). However, chest impediment is unrelated to wind-cold-damp impediment and shares with wind-cold-damp impediment only the notion of blockage represented by the same character 痹 *bì*.

Heart Pain

The term "heart pain" (心痛 *xīn tòng*) suggests a symptom of a specific location. In practice, it has denoted different conditions in the works of different writers. The *Líng Shū* chapter, "Five Evils" (五邪 *wǔ xié*) states: "When the evil is in the heart, [the person] ails by heart pain." The *Líng Shū* chapter, "Visiting of Evil" (邪客 *xié kè*) makes the distinction between "true heart pain" (真心痛 *zhēn xīn tòng*) and "reversal heart pain" (厥心痛 *jué xīn tòng*). "True heart pain" refers to precordial pain that is caused by disease of the heart viscus itself. "Reversal heart pain," a concept further developed in the *Nàn Jīng* ("Classic of Difficult Issues"), refers to heart pain that is caused by disease of one of the other four viscera moving counterflow to affect the heart. Much later, Zhū Dān-Xī categorically stated, "Heart pain is pain in the stomach duct."

In the *Jīn Guì Yào Lüè,* heart pain can carry an even broader meaning, chiefly referring to pain in the pit of the stomach spreading into the precordial region, poststernal region, or to the back. This corresponds to the reversal heart pain described in the *Líng Shū* ("The Magic Pivot") and what Yáng Xuán-Cāo 杨玄操 called "pain caused by counterflow surging of the qì of the five viscera, not pain of the heart itself."

Whenever there is great vacuity of chest yáng, internal exuberance of yīn cold, and evil qì attacking the heart, this can cause true heart pain. When external cold enters through the mouth and nose, and internal and external cold evil attack the stomach duct, the result is heart and stomach pain. Thus, yīn overwhelming yáng and a root vacuity with tip repletion is the general pathomechanism of heart pain.

Common Points

Chest impediment and heart pain are both characterized by pain and occur in adjacent areas. Both may be attended by shortness of breath. Both are essentially due to upper burner yáng vacuity with center and lower burner yīn cold, but may also involve factors such as external evils and dampness or phlegm-rheum arising internally. Since their causes and pathomechanisms are similar, they are mutually conducive, can occur together, and may be poorly distinguishable from each other.

Schematic Overview

Chest Impediment, Heart Pain, and Shortness of Breath

1. Chest impediment and heart pain can be divided into three kinds on the basis of vacuity and repletion, degree of severity, and degree of urgency.

   a) Vacuity and repletion

   Vacuity: Center yáng failing to move is treated by supplementing the center and assisting yáng with Ginseng Decoction (*rén shēn tāng*).

Repletion: Impeded chest yáng with phlegm-rheum rising can be treated by freeing yáng and dispersing binds and by sweeping phlegm and precipating qì, using formulas such as with Trichosanthes, Long-Stamen Onion, and Pinellia Decoction (*guā lóu xiè bái bàn xià tāng*).

b) Severity

Mild cases: Mild chest impediment due to water-rheum can be treated with Poria, Apricot Kernel and Licorice Decoction (*fú líng xìng rén gān cǎo tāng*) to diffuse the lung and transform rheum. When due to qì stagnation, it can be treated with Tangerine Peel, Unripe Bitter Orange, and Ginger Decoction (*jú zhǐ jiāng tāng*) to move qì and dowbear counterflow. Mild heart pain due to cold rheum can be treated with Cinnamon Twig, Fresh Ginger, and Unripe Bitter Orange (*guì zhī shēng jiāng zhǐ shí tāng*) to transform rheum and downbear counterflow, while discharging glomus and relieving pain.

Severe cases: Severe chest impediment can be treated with Unripe Bitter Orange, Long-Stamen Onion, and Cinnamon Twig Decoction (*zhǐ shí xiè bái guì zhī tāng*), Trichosanthes, Long-Stamen Onion, and Pinellia Decoction (*guā lóu xiè bái bàn xià tāng*), or Coix and Aconite Powder (*yì yǐ fù zǐ sǎn*), depending on the condition of the patient. Severe heart pain due to exuberant yīn cold and debilitated yáng qì. with pain stretching into the back, can be treated with Aconite Main Root and Halloysite Pill (*wū tóu chì shí zhī wán*) to dispel cold and assist yáng. Pain in the chest and abdomen due to binding yīn cold can be treated with Nine Pains Pill (*jiǔ tòng wán*) to break yīn, dispel cold, and relieve pain.

c) Urgency

Great urgency: Treat the root—support the right and supplement vacuity, e.g., Ginseng Decoction (*rén shēn tāng*) to warm and supplement yáng qì.

Lesser urgency: Treat the tip—dispel evil and relieve pain, e.g., episodes of chest impediment treated with Coix and Aconite Powder (*yì yǐ fù zǐ sǎn*).

2. Different treatment when the pattern changes: Trichosanthes, Long-Stamen Onion, and White Wine Decoction (*guā lóu xiè bái bái jiǔ tāng*) is a standard formula for classical chest impediment patterns. If phlegm-rheum ascending counterflow becomes more serious, preventing the patient from lying down and causing heart pain that goes through to the back, then Trichosanthes, Long-Stamen Onion, and Pinellia Decoction (*guā lóu xiè bái bàn xià tāng*) should be used instead because of the stronger phlegm-dispelling counterflow-downbearing action of pinellia (*bàn xià*). If yīn cold binds with water-rheum and surges upward to cause glomus in the heart region, chest fullness, and counterflow under the rib-side prodding the heart, Unripe Bitter Orange, Long-Stamen Onion, and Cinnamon Twig Decoction (*zhǐ shí xiè bái guì zhī tāng*) can be used to discharge fullness and downbear counterflow.

Line 9.1

师曰：夫脉当取太过不及，阳微阴弦，即胸痹而痛，所以然者，责其极虚也。今阳虚知在上焦，所以胸痹心痛者，以其阴弦故也。

Shī yuē: Fū mài dāng qǔ tài guò bù jí, yáng wēi yīn xián, jí xiōng bì ér tòng, suǒ yǐ rán zhě, zé qí jí xū yě. Jīn yáng xū zhī zài shàng jiāo, suǒ yǐ xiōng bì xīn tòng zhě, yǐ qí yīn xián gù yě.

The Master says: "In pulse [diagnosis], take excess and deficiency[1] [as the measure]. When the yáng [pulses] are faint, and the yīn [pulses][2] are stringlike, this means chest impediment and pain. The reason for this can be attributed to extreme vacuity there. We now know that the yáng vacuity is in the upper burner, causing chest impediment and heart pain, because the yīn pulses are stringlike.

TEXT NOTES, LINE 9.1

[1] Excess and deficiency 太过不及 *tài guò bù jí*: Excess means more exuberant than normal; deficiency means less exuberant than normal. For example, a pulse that is floating, large, stringlike, slippery, rapid, or forceful is excessive and indicates evil repletion. A pulse that is sunken, slow, faint, weak, rough, or forceless is deficient and indicates right vacuity.

[2] Yáng [pulses], yīn [pulses] 阳、阴 *yáng, yīn*: Here, yáng means distal to the bar, while yīn means proximal to the bar.

SYNOPSIS, LINE 9.1

This line describes the causes and basic pathomechanism of chest impediment and heart pain in terms of the pulse.

COMMENTARY, LINE 9.1

Zhāng Jī here emphasizes the significance of noting excesses and deficiencies when taking the pulse, because all diseases involve either evil exuberance or right vacuity. In heart impediment and heart pain, "the yáng [pulses] are slight, and the yīn [pulses] are stringlike." Thus these conditions too are characterized by excess and deficiency. The faint yáng pulse reflects an insufficiency of yáng qì in the upper burner and chest. The stringlike yīn pulse indicates excessive exuberance of yīn cold. The simultaneous appearance of slight yáng and stringlike yīn means that chest impediment and heart pain are attributable to yáng vacuity in the upper burner, which is being exploited by yīn evil, and to contention between right and evil. Yáng vacuity and evil exuberance are necessary conditions for chest impediment and heart pain.

Line 9.2

平人, 无寒热, 短气不足以息者, 实也。

Píng rén, wú hán rè, duǎn qì bù zú yǐ xī zhě, shí yě.

When an [otherwise] healthy person presents with no cold or heat, but with shortness of breath insufficient to breathe[1], this means repletion.

TEXT NOTE, LINE 9.2

[1] Shortness of breath insufficient to breathe 短气不足以息 *duǎn qì bù zú yǐ xī*: Severe shortness of breath.

SYNOPSIS, LINE 9.2

Continuing from the preceding line, this line describes shortness of breath due to interior repletion.

COMMENTARY, LINE 9.2

This line carries on from the first line in explaining the pathomechanism of chest impediment and heart pain. Some chest impediment and heart pain patients appear to be in normal health between attacks. They do not manifest signs of external contraction like heat effusion and aversion to cold, or the pulses described in the previous line. However, they suddenly experience glomus and blockage in the chest and diaphragm with shortness of breath, or in serious cases labored breathing. This condition is caused by phlegm-rheum and food congealing and gathering in the chest, diaphragm, stomach, and stomach duct and impeding the upbearing and downbearing action of the qì dynamic. This line therefore describes the repletion aspect of chest impediment and heart pain, in contrast to the previous line, which emphasizes "extreme vacuity" as the root of the condition discussed there.

Line 9.3

胸痹之病，喘息咳唾，胸背痛，短气，寸口脉沉而迟，关上小紧数，栝蒌薤白白酒汤主之。

栝蒌实一枚（捣）　薤白半斤　白酒七升

右三味，同煮取二升，分温再服。

Xiōng bì zhī bìng, chuǎn xī ké tuò, xiōng bèi tòng, duǎn qì, cùn kǒu mài chén ér chí, guān shàng xiǎo jǐn shuò, guā lóu xiè bái bái jiǔ tāng zhǔ zhī.

Guā lóu shí (dǎo) yī méi; xiè bái bàn jīn; bái jiǔ qī shēng

Yòu sān wèi, tóng zhǔ qǔ èr shēng, fēn wēn zài fú.

For chest impediment disease with panting, coughing, and spitting, pain in the chest and back, shortness of breath, a sunken and slow inch opening pulse, and a small,[1] tight, and rapid bar [pulse], Trichosanthes, Long-Stamen Onion, and White Wine Decoction (栝楼薤白白酒汤 *guā lóu xiè bái bái jiǔ tāng*) governs.

White Wine Decoction (栝楼薤白白酒汤 *guā lóu xiè bái bái jiǔ tāng*)
trichosanthes fruit (栝蒌实 *guā lóu shí*, Trichosanthis Fructus) 1 piece (crush) long-stamen onion (薤白 *xiè bái*, Allii Macrostemonis Bulbus) ½ *jīn* white wine (白酒 *bái jiǔ*, vino alba) 7 *shēng*[2]

Boil the above three ingredients all together to get two *shēng*. Divide into two [doses] and take warm.

TEXT NOTES, LINE 9.3

[1] Small 小 *xiǎo*: Same as 细 *xì*, fine.

[2] White wine 白酒 *bái jiǔ*: There are four possible interpretations of this term:

(1) *Bái jiǔ* is what is now also called 白干 *bái gān* or 烧酒 *shāo jiǔ*, i.e., a distilled liquor of high alcohol content. This interpretation seems unlikely since the text suggests seven *shēng*, which is equal to 1,400 ml. This would be far too much alcohol. Furthermore, distillation was not yet in practice at the time of the *Jīn Guì Yào Lüè*.

(2) *Bai jiǔ* is the same as 苦酒 *kǔ jiǔ*, literally "bitter wine," a term used in the *Jīn Guì Yào Lüè* to refer to vinegar. This seems unlikely since Zhāng Jī uses the term *bái jiǔ* systematically in the discussion of his treatment of chest impediment and the term *kǔ jiǔ* in the discussion of yellow sweat, suggesting that the terms represent two different things.

(3) *Bái jiǔ* is regular rice wine of the Shàoxīng 紹興 kind. This is unlikely, because rice wine of this kind is yellow.

(4) *Bái jiǔ* means new wine with dregs, i.e., what is now called 醪糟酒 *láo zāo jiǔ*. This appears to be the most likely meaning of the term in this text.

SYNOPSIS, LINE 9.3

This line describes the classic signs and treatment of chest impediment.

COMMENTARY, LINE 9.3

As we have mentioned above, chest impediment and heart pain are attributable to devitalized yáng in the chest and to yīn qì counterflow ascent from the center and lower burner. Disturbing the qì dynamic in terms of the spleen's upbearing and the lung's downbearing functions, this pathomechanism gives rise to cough, shortness of breath, and panting. Yīn turbidity stagnating and blocking the chest causes pain that radiates through to the back. All these are classic signs of chest impediment.

The description of "a sunken and slow inch opening pulse and a small, tight, and rapid bar pulse" has been a matter of dispute. The primary point of contention regards the simultaneous appearance of a slow and rapid pulse. The main opinions are as follows:

(1) A "rapid" pulse does not fit with the picture of yáng vacuity and exuberant cold, and hence is a redundancy probably introduced by mistranscription.

(2) "Rapid" hints at a complex pattern of cold combined with dryness fire.

(3) "Rapid" suggests not speed, but an agitated, staccato quality.

(4) The word 数 *shuò* in the original text does not belong to the pulse description, but to the description of the treatment that follows it, and should therefore be translated as "frequently" instead of "rapid." According to this interpretation, the last part of the line reads: "…small and tight bar pulse. Frequent [use of] Trichosanthes, Long-Stamen Onion, and White Wine Decoction (*guā lóu xiè bái bái jiǔ tāng*) governs." (5) Lastly, Táo Bǎo-Sūn 陶葆荪 has argued that "rapid" and "slow" pulses can appear at the same time.

Contemporary scholars tend to favor explanations 1 and 3 as the most likely explanation of this line.

The formula suggested is Trichosanthes, Long-Stamen Onion, and White Wine Decoction (*guā lóu xiè bái bái jiǔ tāng*), which frees yáng, disperses binds, sweeps phlegm, and precipitates qì. In the formula, trichosanthes (*guā lóu*) opens the chest and flushes phlegm; long-stamen onion (*xiè bái*) courses stagnation and disperses binds; white wine (*bái jiǔ*) frees yáng and diffuses impediment.

Line 9.4

胸痹，不得卧，心痛彻背者，栝蒌薤白半夏汤主之。

栝蒌实一枚（捣） 薤白三两 半夏半斤 白酒一斗

右四味，同煮取四升，温服一升，日三服。

Xiōng bì, bù dé wò, xīn tòng chè bèi zhě, guā lóu xiè bái bàn xià tāng zhǔ zhī.

Guā lóu shí yī méi (dǎo); xiè bái sān liǎng; bàn xià bàn jīn; bái jiǔ yī dǒu

Yòu sì wèi, tóng zhǔ qǔ sì shēng, wēn fú yī shēng, rì sān fú.

For chest impediment with inability to lie down and heart pain going through to the back, Trichosanthes, Long-Stamen Onion, and Pinellia Decoction (栝楼薤白半夏汤 *guā lóu xiè bái bàn xià tāng*) governs.

Trichosanthes, Long-Stamen Onion, and Pinellia Decoction (栝楼薤白半夏汤 *guā lóu xiè bái bàn xià tāng*)
trichosanthes fruit (栝蒌实 *guā lóu shí*, Trichosanthis Fructus) I piece (crush) long-stamen onion (薤白 *xiè bái*, Allii Macrostemonis Bulbus) 3 *liǎng* pinellia (半夏 *bàn xià*, Pinelliae Rhizoma) ½ *shēng* white wine (白酒 *bái jiǔ*, vino alba) 1 *dǒu*

Boil the above four ingredients together to get four *shēng*. Take one *shēng* [per dose] warm, three times a day.

SYNOPSIS, LINE 9.4

This line discusses chest impediment caused by severe counterflow ascent of phlegm-rheum.

COMMENTARY, LINE 9.4

According to the previous line, the main signs of chest impediment are "panting, coughing and spitting, pain in the chest and back, shortness of breath." Since the list of indications begins with "chest impediment," we can presume that the signs associated with chest impediment are all present. The additional mention of "inability to lie down and heart pain going through to the back" suggests a severe form of chest impediment that is caused by phlegm-drool congestion. The formula suggested is Trichosanthes, Long-Stamen Onion, and Pinellia Decoction (*guā lóu xiè bái bàn xià tāng*), which is identical to the formula from the previous line, namely Trichosanthes, Long-Stamen Onion, and White Wine Decoction (*guā lóu xiè bái bái jiǔ tāng*), with the addition of pinellia (*bàn xià*) to expel rheum and downbear counterflow.

Line 9.5

胸痹，心中痞，留气结在胸，胸满，胁下逆抢心，枳实薤白桂枝汤主之，人参汤亦主之。

枳实四枚　厚朴四两　薤白半斤　桂枝一两　栝蒌实（捣）一枚

右五味, 以水五升, 先煮枳实, 厚朴, 取二升, 去滓, 内诸药, 煮数沸, 分温三服。

人参 甘草 干姜 白术各三两

右四味，以水八升，煮取三升，温服三升，日三服。

Xiōng bì, xīn zhōng pǐ, liú qì jié zài xiōng, xiōng mǎn, xié xià nì qiāng xīn, zhǐ shí xiè bái guì zhī tāng zhǔ zhī, rén shēn tāng yì zhǔ zhī.

Zhǐ shí sì méi; hòu pò sì liǎng; xiè bái bàn jīn; guì zhī yī liǎng; guā lóu shí (dǎo) yī méi

Yòu wǔ wèi, yǐ shuǐ wǔ shēng, xiān zhǔ zhǐ shí, hòu pò, qǔ èr shēng, qù zǐ, nà zhū yào, zhǔ shù fèi, fēn wēn sān fú.

Rén shēn, gān cǎo, gān jiāng, bái zhú gè sān liǎng

Yòu sì wèi, yǐ shuǐ bā shēng, wēn fú sān shēng, rì sān fú.

For chest impendiment with glomus in the heart,[1] abiding qì binding in the chest,[2] fullness in the chest, and counterflow under the rib-side prodding the heart, Unripe Bitter Orange, Long-Stamen Onion, and Cinnamon Twig Decoction (枳实薤白桂枝汤 *zhǐ shí xiè bái guì zhī tāng*) governs.

Unripe Bitter Orange, Long-Stamen Onion, and Cinnamon Twig Decoction (枳实薤白桂枝汤 *zhǐ shí xiè bái guì zhī tāng*)

- unripe bitter orange (枳实 *zhǐ shí*, Aurantii Fructus Immaturus) 4 pieces
- officinal magnolia bark (厚朴 *hòu pò*, Magnoliae Officinalis Cortex) 4 *liǎng*
- long-stamen onion (薤白 *xiè bái*, Allii Macrostemonis Bulbus) ½ *jīn*
- cinnamon twig (桂枝 *guì zhī*, Cinnamomi Ramulus) 1 *liǎng*
- trichosanthes seed (栝蒌实 *guā lóu shí*, Trichosanthis Semen) 1 piece (crushed)

Of the above five ingredients, first boil the unripe bitter orange (*zhǐ shí*) and officinal magnolia bark (*hòu pò*) in five *shēng* of water to get two *shēng*. Remove the dregs, add all the [remaining] medicinals, and bring to a boil several times. Divide into three [doses] and take warm.

Ginseng Decoction (人参汤 *rén shēn tāng*) also governs.

Ginseng Decoction (人参汤 *rén shēn tāng*)

ginseng (人参 *rén shēn*, Ginseng Radix) 3 *liǎng*
licorice (甘草 *gān cǎo*, Glycyrrhizae Radix) 3 *liǎng*
dried ginger (干姜 *gān jiāng*, Zingiberis Rhizoma) 3 *liǎng*
white atractylodes (白朮 *bái zhú*, Atractylodis Macrocephalae Rhizoma) 3 *liǎng*

Boil the above four ingredients in eight *shēng* of water to get three *shēng*. Take three *shēng* [per dose] warm, three times a day.

TEXT NOTES, LINE 9.5

[1] Glomus in the heart 心中痞 *xīn zhōng pǐ*: Here, heart refers to a general area rather than the heart viscus. Glomus in the heart means fullness and oppression in the stomach duct, with a sensation of blockage and with pain.

[2] Abiding qì binding in the chest 留气结在胸 *liú qì jié zài xiōng*: This explains the pathomechanism of glomus in the heart: Cold rheum lodged in the chest obstructs the qì dynamic and causes qì to bind and form glomus.

SYNOPSIS, LINE 9.5

This line discusses the signs and treatment of both vacuity and repletion chest impediment.

COMMENTARY, LINE 9.5

The present line describes a form of chest impediment that affects the stomach and rib-sides. In addition to the basic signs of chest impediment ("panting, coughing and spitting, pain in the chest and back, shortness of breath"), this line mentions "glomus in the heart," which refers to a feeling of blockage in the stomach duct. As the text explains, there is "abiding qì binding in the chest." The "abiding qì," presumably referring to water-rheum or phlegm turbidity, thus causes the fullness in the chest. It also affects, on the one hand, the stomach duct to cause the glomus in the heart and, on the other, the rib-side region, giving rise to "counterflow under the rib-side prodding the heart."

The line proposes two formulas to treat this condition: Unripe Bitter Orange, Long-Stamen Onion, and Cinnamon Twig Decoction (*zhǐ shí xiè bái guì zhī tāng*) and Ginseng Decoction (*rén shēn tāng*). Chest impediment is a vacuity-repletion complex that essentially results from yáng qì vacuity and exuberant yīn cold. The relative severity of vacuity and repletion varies. In the present line, the first formula addresses a condition in which the repletion is more severe, while the latter formula addresses a condition in which the vacuity is more pronounced.

Unripe Bitter Orange, Long-Stamen Onion, and Cinnamon Twig Decoction (*zhǐ shí xiè bái guì zhī tāng*) is Trichosanthes, Long-Stamen Onion, and White Wine Decoction (*guā lóu xiè bái bái jiǔ tāng*) plus unripe bitter orange (*zhǐ shí*), officinal magnolia bark (*hòu pò*), and cinnamon twig (*guì zhī*). It has the effect of freeing yáng and opening binds on the one hand, and of disharging fullness and downbearing counterflow on the other.

In the formula, medicinals that free yáng and open binds are trichosanthes (*guā lóu*), long-stamen onion (*xiè bái*), and cinnamon twig (*guì zhī*). In particular, cinnamon twig (*guì zhī*) diffuses the yáng of the heart and chest in the upper body, and warms and transforms yīn cold in the lower body. The medicinals that discharge fullness and downbear counterflow are unripe bitter orange (*zhǐ shí*), officinal magnolia bark (*hòu pò*), and cinnamon twig (*guì zhī*). Unripe bitter orange (*zhǐ shí*) discharges the stagnant qì in the chest, while officinal magnolia bark (*hòu pò*) frees the stagnant qì of the rib-side.

White wine (*bái jiǔ*) is not included in this formula, because it has an upbearing action that is not suitable for condition with counterflow ascent from the center and lower burners. Unripe bitter orange (*zhǐ shí*) and officinal magnolia bark (*hòu pò*) are boiled for a longer time to increase their capacity to downbear counterflow qì and drain fullness. Trichosanthes (*guā lóu*), long-stamen onion (*xiè bái*), and cinnamon twig (*guì zhī*) are boiled for a shorter time so that their acrid dispersing, buoyant quality is not destroyed.

Ginseng Decoction (*rén shēn tāng*) treats yáng vacuity with cold stagnation. Within the formula, Ginseng (*rén shēn*), white atractylodes (*bái zhú*) and licorice (*gān cǎo*) supplement center qì. Dried ginger (*gān jiāng*) warms the center and assists yáng. The formula as a whole restores yáng qì so that yīn cold naturally disperses.

Line 9.6

胸痹，胸中气塞，短气，茯苓杏仁甘草汤主之；橘枳姜汤亦主之。

茯苓三两　杏仁五十个　甘草一两

右三味，以水一斗，煮取五升，温服一升，日三服，不差更服。

橘皮一斤 枳实三两 生姜半斤

右三味，以水五升，煎取二升，分温再服。(《肘后》、《千金》云：治胸痹，胸中愊愊如满，噎塞习习如痒，喉中涩燥唾沫)

Xiōng bì, xiōng zhōng qì sè, duǎn qì, fú líng xìng rén gān cǎo tāng zhǔ zhī; jú zhǐ jiāng tāng yì zhǔ zhī.

Fú líng sān liǎng; xìng rén wǔ shí ge; gān cǎo yī liǎng

Yòu sān wèi, yǐ shuǐ yī dǒu, zhǔ qǔ wǔ shēng, wēn fú yī shēng, rì sān fú, bù chài gèng fú.

Jú pí yī jīn; zhǐ shí sān liǎng; shēng jiāng bàn jīn

Yòu sān wèi, yǐ shuǐ wǔ shēng, jiān qǔ èr shēng, fēn wēn zài fú.

For chest impediment with qì blockage in the chest and shortness of breath, Poria, Apricot Kernel, and Licorice Decoction (茯苓杏仁甘草汤 *fú líng xìng rén gān cǎo tāng*) governs.

Poria, Apricot Kernel, and Licorice Decoction (茯苓杏仁甘草汤 *fú líng xìng rén gān cǎo tāng*)
poria (茯苓 *fú líng*, Poria) 3 *liǎng* apricot kernel (杏仁 *xìng rén*, Armeniacae Semen) 50 pieces licorice (甘草 *gān cǎo*, Glycyrrhizae Radix) 1 *liǎng*

Boil the above three ingredients in one *dǒu* of water to get five *shēng*. Take one *shēng* [per dose] warm, three times a day. If recovery does not ensue, take more.

Tangerine Peel, Unripe Bitter Orange, and Ginger Decoction (橘皮枳实生姜汤 *jú zhǐ jiāng tāng*) also governs.

Tangerine Peel, Unripe Bitter Orange, and Ginger Decoction (橘皮枳实生姜汤 *jú zhǐ jiāng tāng*)
tangerine peel (橘皮 *jú pí*, Citri Reticulatae Pericarpium) 1 *jīn*
unripe bitter orange (枳实 *zhǐ shí*, Aurantii Fructus Immaturus) 3 *liǎng*
fresh ginger (生姜 *shēng jiāng*, Zingiberis Rhizoma Recens) ½ *jīn*

Boil the above three ingredients in five *shēng* of water to get two *shēng*. Divide into two [doses] and take warm.[1]

TEXT NOTE, LINE 9.6

[1] The commentary adds a note: "The *Zhǒu Hòu Bèi Jí Fāng* ("Emergency Standby Remedies") and *Qiān Jīn Yào Fāng* ("A Thousand Gold Pieces Prescriptions") state that [this formula is used] to treat chest impediment with fullness-like binding depression in the chest, dysphagia with an itch-like flapping sensation (噎塞习习如痒 *yē sāi xí xí rú yǎng*), dry throat, and foamy spittle."

SYNOPSIS, LINE 9.6

This line discusses the signs and treatment of mild chest impediment, offering two treatments depending on the predominance of rheum evil or qì obstruction.

COMMENTARY, LINE 9.6

Chest impediment is normally characterized by chest pain and shortness of breath. This line starts off with "chest impediment" and also lists "shortness of breath," but fails to mention chest pain, only adding "qì blockage." It thus emphasizes the aspect of qì congestion in the chest and resulting shortness of breath. Accordingly, we can explain the condition described in this line by the pathomechanism of rheum obstruction causing qì stagnation.

Just as preceeding line, the present line also offers two formulas, one for conditions in which rheum evil is more severe and the other for conditions in which qì obstruction is predominant.

Poria, Apricot Kernel, and Licorice Decoction (*fú líng xìng rén gān cǎo tāng*) treats predominance of rheum evil with cough and counterflow, ejection of foamy drool, and inhibited urination. It diffuses the lung and transforms rheum. Within the formula, apricot kernel (*xìng rén*) diffuses and disinhibits lung qì; poria (*fú líng*) transforms phlegm and eliminates rheum; licorice (*gān cǎo*) harmonizes the center.

By contrast, Tangerine Peel, Unripe Bitter Orange, and Fresh Ginger Decoction (*jú pí zhǐ shí shēng jiāng tāng*) treats predominance of qì stagnation with qì blockage in the chest and shortness of breath, usually presenting with glomus and fullness below the heart and vomiting. It moves and transforms rheum, while at the same time harmonizing the stomach and downbearing counterflow. Within the formula, tangerine peel (*chén pí*) rectifies qì, harmonizes the stomach, and frees the qì dynamic; unripe bitter orange (*zhǐ shí*) precipitates qì and disperses phlegm; fresh ginger (*shēng jiāng*) transforms rheum, harmonizes the stomach, and downbears counterflow.

Line 9.7

胸痹缓急者，薏苡仁附子散主之。

薏苡仁十五两　大附子（炮）十枚

右二味，杵为散，服方寸匕，日三服。

Xiōng bì huǎn jí zhě, yì yǐ rén fù zǐ sǎn zhǔ zhī.

Yì yǐ rén shí wǔ liǎng; dà fù zǐ (pào) shí méi

Yòu èr wèi, chǔ wéi sǎn, fú fāng cùn bǐ, rì sān fú.

For acute[1] chest impediment, Coix and Aconite Powder (薏苡仁附子散 *yì yǐ rén fù zǐ sǎn*) governs.

Coix and Aconite Powder (薏苡仁附子散 *yì yǐ rén fù zǐ sǎn*)
coix (薏苡仁 *yì yǐ rén*, Coicis Semen) 15 *liǎng* aconite (大附子 *dà fù zǐ*, Aconiti Radix Lateralis Praeparata) 10 pieces (blast-fry)

Pestle the above two ingredients into a powder. Take a square-inch-spoonful, three times a day.

TEXT NOTE, LINE 9.7

[1] Acute 缓急 *huǎn jí*: Although the Chinese literally says "relaxed and acute," this phrase is understood to refer merely to acuteness. This kind of construction, called 偏义复词 *piān yì fù cí* (lit. "biased compound") in which one of the elements of the compound does not contribute to the meaning, is quite prevalent in early Chinese literature. An alternative interpretation of this compound explains this as pain that alternatingly eases up and intensifies. As yet a third alternative, it could refer to the sinews now relaxing, now tensing, as a result of the chest impediment affecting the sinews.

SYNOPSIS, LINE 9.7

This line discusses the treatment of acute chest impediment.

COMMENTARY, LINE 9.7

The present line merely states that Coix and Aconite Powder (*yì yǐ rén fù zǐ sǎn*) is prescribed for acute chest impediment. We know that the basic signs of chest impediment are panting, cough and spitting, chest and back pain, and heart pain going through to the back. However, this line does not give the defining signs of acute chest impediment. In such cases, we can apply the principle of "determining the signs from the medicinals" (以药测证 *yǐ yào cè zhèng*). The indications of the ingredients of the formula (as well as from clinical experience in the treatment of chest impediment), tell us that this formula is given for severe chest pain with a pale glossy tongue fur and a pulse that is sunken or hidden, possibly rough, possibly fine, faint, and slow, or possibly tight, fine, and urgent. In some cases, there may also be hypertonicity of the sinews.

Coix and Aconite Powder (*yì yǐ rén fù zǐ sǎn*) frees yáng qì and eliminates cold-damp. Within the formula, blast-fried aconite (*pào fù zǐ*) warms the interior and dispels cold, and frees yáng and relieves pain. Coix (*yì yǐ rén*) eliminates dampness, diffuses impediment, and can also relax hypertonicity of the sinews and vessels.

Line 9.8

心中痞，诸逆心悬痛，桂枝生姜枳实汤主之。

桂枝三两　生姜三两　枳实五枚

右三味，以水六升，煮取三升，分温三服。

Xīn zhōng pǐ, zhū nì xīn xuán tòng, guì zhī shēng jiāng zhǐ shí tāng zhǔ zhī.

Guì zhī sān liǎng; shēng jiāng sān liǎng; zhǐ shí wǔ méi

Yòu sān wèi, yǐ shuǐ liù shēng, zhǔ qǔ sān shēng, fēn wēn sān fú.

For glomus in the heart with all [types of] counterflow[1] and suspension pain in the heart,[2] Cinnamon Twig, Fresh Ginger, and Unripe Bitter Orange Decoction (桂枝生姜枳实 *guì zhī shēng jiāng zhǐ shí tāng*) governs.

Cinnamon Twig, Fresh Ginger, and Unripe Bitter Orange Decoction (桂枝生姜枳实 *guì zhī shēng jiāng zhǐ shí tāng*)

cinnamon twig (桂枝 *guì zhī*, Cinnamomi Ramulus) 3 *liǎng*
fresh ginger (生姜 *shēng jiāng*, Zingiberis Rhizoma Recens) 3 *liǎng*
unripe bitter orange (枳实 *zhǐ shí*, Aurantii Fructus Immaturus) 5 pieces

Boil the above three ingredients in six *shēng* of water to get three *shēng*. Divide into three [doses] and take warm.

Text Notes, Line 9.8

[1] All [types of] counterflow 诸逆 *zhū nì*: Water-rheum or cold evil ascending counterflow from beneath the heart and rib-sides into the heart and chest.

[2] Suspension pain in the heart 心悬痛 *xīn xuán tòng*: A sensation of upward pulling in the pit of the heart.

Synopsis, Line 9.8

This line discusses the signs and treatment of heart pain due to phlegm-rheum and qì counterflow.

Commentary, Line 9.8

When phlegm-rheum and cold evil collect below the heart, the result is glomus and oppression with a sensation of blockage in the stomach-duct; hence the text says "glomus in the heart." Here the term "heart" apparently refers not to the heart viscus, but to the region below the heart (the pit of the stomach). When stomach qì is normal, harmonious downbearing occurs. However, when stomach yáng is devitalized, fluid is retained instead of being transformed, and water-rheum exploits the insufficiency of heart yáng to cause counterflow in the heart vessel, hypertonicity of the channels and network vessels, and non-diffusion of heart yáng. The result is stifling oppression in the heart and chest, and in severe cases, blockage in the channels and network vessels. Thus, non-diffusion of yáng qì and water-rheum from the diaphragm intruding counterflow into the heart vessel is the main pathomechanism in this condition, to be treated by diffusing heart yáng, harmonizing the stomach and transforming rheum, discharging glomus, and relieving pain.

Line 9.9

心痛彻背，背痛彻心，乌头赤石脂丸主之。

蜀椒一两（一法二分）　乌头（炮）一分　附子（炮）半两（一法一分）　赤石脂一两（一法二分）　干姜一两（一法一分）

右五味，末之，蜜丸如梧子大，先食服一丸，日三服，不知，稍加服。

Xīn tòng chè bèi, bèi tòng chè xīn, wū tóu chì shí zhī wán zhǔ zhī.

Shǔ jiāo yī liǎng (yī fǎ èr fēn); wū tóu (pào) yī fēn; fù zǐ (pào) bàn liǎng (yī fǎ yī fēn); chì shí zhī yī liǎng (yī fǎ èr fēn); gān jiāng yī liǎng (yī fǎ yī fēn)

Yòu wǔ wèi, mò zhī, mì wán rú wú zǐ dà, xiān shí fú yī wán, rì sān fú, bù zhī, shāo jiā fú.

For heart pain going through to the back and back pain going through to the heart, Aconite Main Root and Halloysite Pill (乌头赤石脂丸 *wū tóu chì shí zhī wán*) governs.

Aconite Main Root and Halloysite Pill (乌头赤石脂丸 *wū tóu chì shí zhī wán*)
zanthoxylum (蜀椒 *shǔ jiāo*, Zanthoxyli Pericarpium) 1 *liǎng*[1]
aconite main root (乌头 *wū tóu*, Aconiti Radix Wutou) 1 part (blast-fry)
aconite lateral root (附子 *fù zǐ*, Aconiti Radix Lateralis) ½ *liǎng* (blast-fry)[2]
halloysite (赤石脂 *chì shí zhī*, Halloysitum Rubrum) 1 *liǎng*[3]
dried ginger (干姜 *gān jiāng*, Zingiberis Rhizoma) 1 *liǎng*[4]

Pulverize the above five ingredients and [mix with] honey to form into pills the size of firmiana sees. Before meals, take one pill three times a day. If no [effect] is noticed, increase the dose slightly.

Text Notes, Line 9.9

[1] An alternate version gives "2 parts."
[2] An alternate version gives "1 part."
[3] An alternate version gives "2 parts."
[4] An alternate version gives "1 part."

Synopsis, Line 9.9

This line discusses the signs and treatment of heart pain due to yīn cold binding and debilitation of yáng qì.

Commentary, Line 9.9

The pathomechanism of "heart pain going through to the back and back pain going through to the heart" can take two shapes: When evil is contracted in the pericardium, the evil qì of yīn cold can ascend in reverse counterflow to harass the upper body. Lodging in the heart vessel, it blocks the channels and network vessels and deprives the heart of nourishment; hence we see heart pain. If it further affects the vessels in the chest and back and disorders the normal flow of qì and blood, cold evil can flow into the external transport points of the back. Hence, we see "heart pain going through to the back." On the other hand, cold can invade the transport points on the back and enter the body from there. When it follows the heart transport points on the back to the heart, it causes "back pain going through to the back." When severe, this condition is similar to "true heart pain" and, if not treated promptly, leads to cold in the extremities and then death.

The key pathomechanism in this condition is yīn cold binding and surging into the heart and back, and debilitation of yáng qì. It is therefore treated by expelling yīn evil, warming yáng, dispersing cold, and securing heart yáng. The formula recommended here uses aconite main root (*wū tóu*), aconite (*fù zǐ*), zanthoxylum (*huā jiāo*), and dried ginger (*gān jiāng*), which are all strong acrid and hot ingredients, to expel wind cold and alleviate pain. Aconite main root (*wū tóu*) and aconite (*fù zǐ*) are used together because cold evil in this condition affects the heart and back, inside and outside, bowels and viscera, and channels and network vessels. Halloysite (*chì shí zhī*) is added to settle heart yáng, contain yáng qì, and supplement heart blood, while banking up the stomach and intestines to ensure the absorption of such a large amount of strong acrid and warm medicinals.

[附方] Appended Formulas

Nine Pains Pill (九痛丸 *jiǔ tòng wán*)

治九种心痛

附子（炮）三两 生狼牙(炙香)一两 巴豆(去皮心，熬研如脂)一两 人参 干姜 吴茱萸各一两

右六味，末之，炼蜜丸如梧子大，酒下，强人初服三丸，日三服；弱者二丸。兼治卒中恶，腹胀痛，口不能言。又治连年积冷，流注心胸痛，并冷冲上气，落马坠车血疾等，皆主之。忌口如常法。

Zhì jiǔ zhǒng xīn tòng

Fù zǐ (pào) sān liǎng; shēng láng yá (zhì xiāng) yī liǎng; bā dòu (qù pí xīn, áo yán rú zhī) yī liǎng; rén shēn, gān jiāng, wú zhū yú, gè yī liǎng

Yòu liù wèi, mò zhī, liàn mì wán rú wú zǐ dà, jiǔ xià, qiáng rén chū fú sān wán, rì sān fú; ruò zhě èr wán. Jiān zhì cù zhòng wù, fù zhàng tòng, kǒu bù néng yán. Yòu zhì lián nián jī lěng, liú zhù xīn xiōng tòng, bìng lěng chōng shàng qì, luò mǎ zhuì chē xuè jí děng, jiē zhǔ zhī. Jì kǒu rú cháng fǎ.

For treating the nine kinds of heart pain.

Nine Pains Pill (九痛丸 *jiǔ tòng wán*)
aconite (附子 *fù zǐ*, Aconiti Radix Lateralis Praeparata) 3 *liǎng* (blast-fry) potentilla cryptotaenia root (生狼牙 *shēng láng yá*, Potentillae Cryptotaeniae Radix) 1 *liǎng* (mix-fry until fragrant)

croton (巴豆 *bā dòu*, Crotonis Fructus) 1 *liǎng* (remove the skin and heart, simmer, and grind to a paste)
ginseng (人参 *rén shēn*, Ginseng Radix) 1 *liǎng*
dried ginger (干姜 *gān jiāng*, Zingiberis Rhizoma) 1 *liǎng*
evodia (吴茱萸 *wú zhū yú*, Evodiae Fructus) 1 *liǎng*

Pulverize the above six ingredients and blend with processed honey to form pills the size of firmiana seeds. Drink them down with wine. For strong patients, begin with three pills [per dose], three times a day. For weak patients, take two pills [per dose]. This [formula] also treats sudden malignity strike with abdominal distention and pain, and inability to speak. It furthermore treats accumulated cold having lasted for several years that streams into the heart and chest [causing] pain, as well as cold qì surging upward, falls from horses or carts, and blood disorders. It treats all these [conditions]. Observe the usual dietary contraindications.[2]

FORMULA NOTES, LINE 9.9

[1] Potentillae Cryptotaeniae Radix (生狼牙 *shēng láng yá*): Some scholars believe this could also be agrimonia root sprout (仙鹤草根芽 *xiān hè cǎo gēn yá*, Agrimoniae Rhizoma Pullulatum.

[2] Observe the usual dietary contraindications 忌口如常法 *jì kǒu rú cháng fǎ*: To gain some idea of dietary contraindications for patients suffering from heart pain in the Hàn Dynasty, see 25.34 ("In the tenth month, do not eat raw vegetables that have been exposed to frost, [since it] will cause a dull facial complexion, dry eyes, heart and lumbar pain…"); 25.40 ("Eating raw scallion or garlic chive within four days of eating sugar or honey causes heart pain"); 25.53 ("Eating water pepper fruit in excess makes heart pain erupt"); 25.70 ("Drinking wine and eating fresh xanthium causes heart pain.")

SYNOPSIS, LINE 9.9

This line discusses the preparation of and indications for Nine Pains Pill (*jiǔ tòng wán*).

COMMENTARY, LINE 9.9

"Nine kinds of heart pain" refers to a variety of pains in the heart, chest, stomach, and stomach duct that are rooted in the key pathomechanism of yáng vacuity and yīn exuberance. As many commentators suggest, this formula was not originally composed by Zhāng Jī, but is found in such other classics as the *Qiān Jīn Fāng* ("Thousand Gold Pieces Prescriptions") and *Wài Tái Mì Yào* ("Secrets from the *Wài Tái* Library"). In this formula, aconite (*fù zǐ*), dried ginger (*gān jiāng*), and evodia (*wú zhū yú*) warm the center and open depression, and also free yáng and relieve pain; ginseng (*rén shēn*) supplements the center and boosts qì, croton (*bā dòu*) warms, frees, kills worms, breaks up accumulations, and eliminates phlegm-rheum; and potentilla cryptotaenia root (*láng yá*) kills worms. On the basis of these medicinal actions, we know that the formula has the purpose of expelling cold, dispersing binds, killing worms, and warming and freeing.

腹满寒疝宿食病脉证治第十

CHAPTER 10

Abdominal Fullness, Cold Mounting, and Abiding Food

Pulses, Signs, Treatments

‡ OVERVIEW

This chapter discusses the pulses and signs, causes, and treatment of abdominal fullness (腹满 *fù mǎn*), cold mounting (寒疝 *hán shàn*), and abiding food (宿食 *sù shí*). Because these pathoconditions are similar as regards location, signs, pathomechanisms, pulses, and treatment, Zhāng Zhòng-Jing chose to discuss them together. All three conditions involve the spleen, stomach, and intestines. Abdominal fullness is associated with the spleen and stomach; cold mounting with the liver and spleen; and abiding food with the spleen, stomach, and intestines. All are characterized by abdominal distention, fullness, and pain, as well as by a stringlike tight pulse. Abdominal fullness and cold mounting occur in vacuity cold patterns that share similar pathomechanisms. In addition, abdominal fullness occurs in repletion patterns that are similar to those of abiding food.

ABDOMINAL FULLNESS

Abdominal fullness falls into two categories. One is repletion and heat patterns, which usually involve the stomach and intestine, or sometimes the exterior. The other is vacuity and cold patterns, which involve the spleen and kidney, and sometimes the liver.

COLD MOUNTING

In the *Jīn Guì Yào Lüè*, cold mounting is a condition of yīn-cold pain with tension in the abdomen. It is accompanied by aversion to cold, cold limbs, cold sweating from the head, and in some cases generalized pain. It is attributable to gathering and binding of cold qì. Since antiquity, the term "mounting" (疝 *shàn*) referred not only to cold mounting but also what was later called 疝气 *shàn qì*, i.e., a disease in which the scrotum or testicles become swollen, cold, hard, and painful. This latter category includes conditions that Western medicine identifies as inguinal hernia and hydrocele. In fact, in modern medicine the term 疝气 *shàn qì* is used to refer to inguinal hernia. However the *Jīn Guì Yào Lüè* does not include this latter category and only discusses cold mounting characterized by abdominal pain. In terms of eight principles, cold mounting includes both vacuity or repletion patterns, and may take the form of interior cold or dual cold of the exterior and interior.

ABIDING FOOD

Abiding food, often called food damage or food accumulation, refers to conditions in which food remains in the stomach and intestines overnight without being dispersed. It stems from spleen-stomach dysfunction and is characterized by abdominal distention, glomus and oppression, putrid belching, acid swallowing, vomiting, abdominal pain, and irregularities of stool. Food can collect in different locations (upper stomach duct, center stomach duct, and lower stomach duct), each of which is characterized by different signs. Depending on the location, the *Jīn Guì Yào Lüè* prescribes ejection or precipitation as treatment. Abiding food usually forms a repletion pattern, but can also take the form of repletion complicated by vacuity.

SCHEMATIC OVERVIEW

ABDOMINAL FULLNESS

1. Pathomechanisms, diagnosis, and treatment method

   a) Repletion heat

      Pathomechanism: Repletion heat in the stomach and intestines causing dry stool to collect in the intestinal tract

      Signs: Abdominal fullness with no relief and pain when press; a red tongue with yellow fur; a replete pulse.

      Treatment method: Offensive precipitation.

   b) Vacuity Cold

      Pathomechanism: Spleen and kidney vacuity cold giving rise to qì stagnation.

      Signs: Abdominal fullness with periodic relief and no pain when pressure is applied; pale tongue with white fur: a pulse that is faint and stringlike.

      Treatment method: Warming and supplementing.

   c) Cold repletion

Pathomechanism: Cold evil binding internally depressing yáng qì.

Signs: Pain under the rib-side; heat effusion; difficult defecation; a pulse that is tight and stringlike.

Treatment method: Warm precipitation.

2. Pattern identification and treatment

   a) Repletion heat

      Abdominal fullness; heat effusion; normal intake of food and drink; a pulse that is floating and rapid: Resolve exterior and interior using Officinal Magnolia Bark Seven Agents Decoction (厚朴七物汤 *hòu pò qī wù tāng*).

      Fullness and pain below the heart on palpation: Harmonize the exterior and attack the interior with Major Bupleurum Decoction (*dà chái hú tāng*).

      Pain and constipation: move qì and eliminate fullness using Officinal Magnolia Bark Three Agents Decoction (*hòu pò sān wù tāng*).

      Abdominal fullness without relief or no relief to speak of: Flush repletion heat with Major Qì-Coordinating Decoction (*dà chéng qì tāng*).

   b) Cold repletion: Pain under the rib-side, heat effusion, and a pulse that is tight and stringlike: Warm precipitation using Rhubarb and Aconite Decoction (*dà huáng fù zǐ tāng*).

   c) Vacuity cold

      Thunderous rumbling and cutting pain in the abdomen; counterflow fullness in the chest and rib-side; vomiting: Warm the center and transform dampness with Aconite and Rice Decoction (*fù zǐ jīng mǐ tāng*).

      Great cold pain in the heart and chest; retching with inability to eat; upward surging that lifts the skin with a lump that has a head and foot, together with pain so severe that it cannot be touched: Warm the center and disperse cold with Major Center-Fortifying Decoction (*dà jiàn zhōng tāng*).

Cold Mounting

1. Causes: Yáng vacuity and exuberant cold.
2. Main signs: Severe episodic pain around the umbilicus; sweating; cold limbs; a pulse that is sunken and tight.
3. Patern identification and treatment

   a) Pain around the umbilicus occurring in episodes with white sweating, reversal cold of the extremities, and a pulse that is sunken and stringlike: Disperse cold and relieve pain with Major Aconite Main Root Brew (*dà wū tǒu jiān*).

   b) Pain in the abdomen stretching into the rib-side with abdominal urgency: Nourish the blood and disperse cold using Chinese Angelica, Fresh Ginger, and Goat Meat Decoction (*dāng guī shēng jiāng yáng ròu tāng*).

c) Pain in the abdomen; counterflow cold; insensitivity of the extremities; generalized pain (dual cold of the interior of and exterior): Harmonize construction and defense while dispersing cold and relieving pain using Aconite Main Root and Cinnamon Twig Decoction (*wū tóu guì zhī tāng*).

d) Reversal cold of the extremities; abdominal pain; counterflow retching; dizzy head; heart palpiations: warm cold and flush rheum with Red Pill (*chì wán*).

ABIDING FOOD

1. Cause: Intemperate eating causing food to accumulating in the stomach and intestines overnight.
2. Principles of treatment
   a) Abiding food in the upper body: ejection
   b) Abiding food in the lower body: precipitation
3. Pattern identification and treatment
   a) Inch opening (*cùn*) pulse floating and large, rough under pressure and faint and rough at the cubit: attack the repletion accumulation with Major Qì-Coordinating Decoction (*dà chéng qì tāng*).
   b) A pulse that is rapid and slippery: attack the repletion accumulation with Major Qì-Coordinating Decoction (*dà chéng qì tāng*).
   c) Diarrhea with no desire to eat: attack the repletion accumulation with Major Qì-Coordinating Decoction (*dà chéng qì tāng*).
   d) Abiding food in the upper stomach duct with upwelling and desire to vomit: eject with Melon Stalk Powder (*guā dì sǎn*).

Line 10.1

趺阳脉微弦，法当腹满，不满者必便难，两胠疼痛，此虚寒从下上也。当以温药服之。

Fū yáng mài wēi xián, fǎ dāng fù mǎn, bù mǎn zhě bì biàn nán, liǎng qū téng tòng, cǐ xū hán cóng xià shàng yě. Dāng yǐ wēn yào fú zhī.

When the instep yáng pulsē is faint and stringlike, it should indicate abdominal fullness. If there is no abdominal fullness, there must be difficult defecation and pain in both rib-sides.[2] This is vacuity cold ascending from below. Treat it with warm medicinals.

Text Notes, Line 10.1

[1] Instep yáng pulse 趺阳脉 *fū yáng mài*: The pulsating vessel felt at Surging Yáng (*chōng yáng2*, ST-42) on the dorsum of the foot.

[2] Rib-sides 胠 *qū*: The rib-side region is normally called 胁 *xié* in Chinese. 胠 is an archaic synonym.

Synopsis, Line 10.1

This line discusses the pathomechanism, signs, and treatment of vacuity-cold abdominal fullness.

Commentary, Line 10.1

The instep yáng pulse lies at Surging Yáng (*chōng yáng*, ST-42) on the foot yáng brightness stomach channel. In antiquity, this pulse was palpated so as to diagnose spleen and stomach disease. Hence it corresponded to the right bar on the inch opening. In this line, the instep yáng pulse is faint, which indicates insufficiency of center yáng. In addition, its stringlike quality is associated with the liver, as well as with cold and with pain. The pathomechanism described in this line is spleen-stomach vacuity cold exacerbated by cold qì ascending counterflow from the lower burner and liver. This pathomechanism can account for all the signs mentioned. When evil qì from the liver invades the spleen and stomach, spleen yáng fails to move and transform; hence there is glomus blockage and abdominal fullness. Because this is a vacuity cold pattern, the abdominal fullness likes pressure. Even if there is no abdominal fullness, the evil qì of the liver can still surge upward and collect in the rib-side area, giving rise to local pain. When liver qì ascends counterflow, the spleen loses the free-coursing action of liver qì, giving rise to qì stagnation in the stomach and intestines. This results in difficult defecation.

The recommended treatment for these patterns is to warm and disperse vacuity cold. Even though the condition is one of fullness, the line calls for a warming and supplementing rather than a precipitating treatment.

Line 10.2

病者腹满，按之不痛为虚，痛者为实，可下之。舌黄未下者，下之黄自去。

Bìng zhě fù mǎn, àn zhī bù tòng wéi xū, tòng zhě wéi shí, kě xià zhī. Shé huáng wèi xià zhě, xià zhī huáng zì qù.

In a patient with abdominal fullness, absence of pain when pressed indicates vacuity; pain indicates repletion. [In the case of repletion], you may precipitate. If the tongue is yellow before precipitation, the yellowness will naturally disappear when you precipitate.

SYNOPSIS, LINE 10.2

This line describes the identification of vacuity and repletion in patients with abdominal fullness, as well as the treatment of repletion patterns.

COMMENTARY, LINE 10.2

Abdominal fullness can be ascribed to either repletion or vacuity. Repletion fullness generally arises as a result of abiding food in the stomach or of dry stool accumulating in the intestines. It is characterized by persistent fullness without letup and by pain when pressure is applied. Vacuity fullness is the result of spleen vacuity cold with impaired movement and transformation and with qì stagnation. It is characterized by periods of relief and by no pain when pressure is applied.

Tongue examination also helps to distinguish between repletion fullness and vacuity fullness. A tongue fur that is thick, yellow, and dry indicates a condition of repletion heat, for which precipitation is appropriate. The text at this point alerts us that the yellow tongue fur will naturally disappear when repletion fullness is treated by precipitation. The wording of the text hints at the fact that further precipitation may not be appropriate for a patient who has already been treated with precipitation and still has a yellow tongue, or that such a patient may have had a condition that should have not been treated with precipitation in the first place.

Line 10.3

腹满时减，复如故，此为寒，当与温药。

Fù mǎn shí jiǎn, fù rú fù, cǐ wéi hán, dāng yǔ wēn yào.

When abdominal fullness lessens periodically and then returns as before, this indicates cold. Treat it by giving warm medicinals.

SYNOPSIS, LINE 10.3

This line describes the identification and treatment of vacuity cold abdominal fullness.

COMMENTARY, LINE 10.3

This line provides information that is complementary to the preceeding line. Abdominal fullness that periodically abates completely is due to cold. We know that "cold" here means vacuity cold because only vacuity cold is characterized by periodic relief from abdominal fullness. The condition discussed in this line thus refers to vacuity cold in the spleen and stomach, which causes impaired movement and transformation. Related to this, we can deduce that the treatment with warm medicinals refers to warming the interior rather than to warm precipitation. Hence Center-Rectifying Decoction (*lǐ zhōng tāng*) or Aconite Center-Rectifying Decoction (*fù zǐ lǐ zhōng tāng*) is indicated.

Line 10.4

病者痿黄，躁而不渴，胸中寒实，而利不止者，死。

Bìng zhě wěi huáng, zào ér bù kě, xiōng zhōng hán shí, ér lì bù zhǐ zhě, sǐ.

When a patient presents with a withered yellow [complexion] and with agitation[1] but no thirst, [this is] cold repletion in the chest. In such a patient, incessant diarrhea means death.

TEXT NOTE, LINE 10.4

[1] Agitation 躁 *zào*: The meaning of this character is subject to scholarly debate. While some editors interpret it literally (as we have done above), others suggest that this is a textual mistake and should be read as 燥 *zào*, "dry." See the commentary below.

SYNOPSIS, LINE 10.4

This line describes a critical pattern of cold repletion binding internally, with debilitation of yáng qì.

COMMENTARY, LINE 10.4

Debilitation of spleen qì manifests in a withered-yellow facial complexion. The fact that the patient experiences no thirst suggests that there is no heat in the interior. The presence of agitation despite the absence of heat indicates a pattern of cold repletion binding in the chest as a result of exuberant yīn and debilitated yáng. This type of agitation is called "yīn agitation." If the patient in addition to these signs suffers from incessant diarrhea, this means that yáng qì is vanquished and expiring, that visceral qì is deserting downward, and that the patient is in a critical condition of right vacuity and evil repletion. This may result in death.

The symptom "agitation but no thirst" has been the subject of disagreement. The *Jīn Jiàn* ("The Golden Mirror") suggests that 躁 *zào* (agitated) should be interpreted as 燥 *zào* (dry), referring to dryness in the mouth. The argument in favor of "agitated" is supported by line 298 of the *Shāng Hán Lùn*, where a similar condition that may also result in death is characterized by "agitation without vexation." This kind of agitation is due to yáng qì being on the verge of expiration. It is not associated with heart vexation because it is caused by yīn-cold congealing in the chest (which cannot cause vexation).

Line 10.5

寸口脉弦，即胁下拘急而痛，其人啬啬恶寒也。

Cùn kǒu mài xián, jí xié xià jū jí ér tòng, qí rén sè sè wù hán yě.

[In patients with abdominal fullness], if the inch opening pulse is stringlike, there will [also] be hypertonicity and pain below the rib-side, and the person will have huddled aversion to cold.[1]

TEXT NOTE, LINE 10.5

[1] Huddled aversion to cold 啬啬恶寒 *sè sè wù hán*: Aversion to cold that causes patients to curl up or draw themselves together.

SYNOPSIS, LINE 10.5

This line describes abdominal fullness that is caused by dual cold of the interior and exterior.

COMMENTARY, LINE 10.5

The inch (*cùn*) position of the wrist pulse indicates the exterior. A stringlike pulse means cold and and pain; it also points to the liver. A stringlike pulse at the inch position accompanied by huddled aversion to cold indicates cold in the exterior. The rib-side belongs to the liver. Hypertonicity and pain below the rib-side combined with a stringlike pulse indicate liver qì with cold evil. Hence, the condition described here is one of both exterior and interior cold. This can be treated with Bupleurum and Cinnamon Twig Decoction (*chái hú guì zhī tāng*) minus scutellaria (*huáng qín*) and plus peony (*sháo yào*).

Line 10.6

夫中寒家喜欠，其人清涕出，发热色和者，善嚏。

Fū zhōng hán jiā xǐ qiàn, qí rén qīng tì chū, fā rè sè hé zhě, shàn tì.

Patients with center cold have a tendency to yawn. If such persons present with clear snivel, heat effusion, and a harmonious complexion,[1] they will also have a tendency to sneeze.

TEXT NOTE, LINE 10.6

[1] Harmonious complexion 色和 *sè hé*: Normal complexion, as in healthy persons.

SYNOPSIS, LINE 10.6

This line discusses patients with habitual vacuity cold who have recently contracted cold evil.

COMMENTARY, LINE 10.6

The present line opens with an ambiguity. The term 中寒 can be read as *zhōng hán*, "center cold" (as we have done above), or as *zhòng hán*, "cold strike" (i.e., contraction of cold evil). It should be noted that this ambiguity is found also in the next line 10.7. Both these lines include interior and exterior signs. Most scholars nowadays read the term as "center cold." This refers to conditions of yáng vacuity and exuberant yīn cold in the center burner, which makes the patient prone to catching cold.

A person with a weak constitution that is characterized by insufficiency of center yáng is usually prone to yawning. If such a person has a runny nose and heat effusion, but a normal complexion, this is attributable to an external contraction. In this case, the condition will also be characterized by sneezing.

Line 10.7

中寒，其人下利，以里虚也，欲嚏不能，此人肚中寒。

Zhōng hán, qí rén xià lì, yǐ lǐ xū yě, yù tì bù néng, cǐ rén dǔ zhōng hán.

In center cold, if the patient has diarrhea, [this is] because of interior vacuity. [If the patient] desires to sneeze but is unable to, this person has cold in the stomach.[1]

TEXT NOTE, LINE 10.7

[1] Cold in the stomach 肚中寒 *dǔ zhōng hán*: An alternative version of the text has "pain in the stomach."

SYNOPSIS, LINE 10.7

This line describes a disease pattern of interior vacuity with contraction of cold.

COMMENTARY, LINE 10.7

This line continues the train of thought from the preceeding line, describing a similar but more serious condition in which the patient's resistance is weakened to the point where they are unable to sneeze. If patients with center cold due to insufficiency of center yáng contract cold evil, they will often quickly develop diarrhea. The reason for this is as follows: Externally contracted cold exacerbates the interior vacuity and thereby impairs splenic movement and transformation. This manifests in diarrhea. Because the diarrhea causes further detriment to yáng qì, yáng qì is unable to expel the evil. Hence we see a desire but inability to sneeze.

Line 10.8

夫瘦人绕脐痛，必有风冷，谷气不行，而反下之，其气必冲，不冲者，心下则痞也。

Fū sòu rén rào qí tòng, bì yǒu fēng lěng, gǔ qì bù xíng, ér fǎn xià zhī, qí qì bì chōng, bù chōng zhě, xīn xià zé pǐ yě.

If thin people present with pain around the umbilicus, they must have [contracted] wind-cold, [as a result of which] grain qì fails to move. If [such patients] are inappropriately treated with precipitation, their qì will invariably surge;[1] if it does not surge, there will be glomus below the heart.

TEXT NOTE, LINE 10.8

[1] Their qì will invariably surge 其气必冲 *qí qì bì chōng*: The qì in the abdomen will surge upward.

SYNOPSIS, LINE 10.8

This line describes a transmuted condition that is caused by inappropriate precipitation in cold patterns.

COMMENTARY, LINE 10.8

When weak, emaciated patients with insufficiency of right qì suffer from pain around the umbilicus and grain qì failing to move, this is mostly due to contraction of wind-cold. The pain is caused by wind-cold entering the interior and congealing in the abdomen. Impairing splenic movement and transformation, it also causes fecal stoppage. Fecal stoppage due to wind-cold, often referred to as "cold bind" (寒结 *hán jié*), is usually accompanied by a liking for heat, harmony of mouth (e.g., normal taste in the mouth and absence of dryness and thirst or sliminess), and long voidings of clear urine. It is treated by warming and transforming (温化 *wēn huà*) or warming and freeing (温通 *wēn tōng*).

Physicians may mistake this condition for dryness repletion. One reason for this is the notion in Chinese medicine that "thin people tend to have copious fire" (瘦人多火 *shòu rén duō huǒ*). Another reason is that yáng bind is more common than yīn bind. If the physician mistakes the above condition for dryness repletion and gives the patient cold, bitter medicinals, these will indeed move the grain qì and free the stool, but the wind-cold will still be present and yáng qì will have sustained further damage.

If the damage to yáng qì affects the lower burner and fails to restrain the yīn-cold evil, it will inevitably surge upward. If the damage to yáng qì affects the center burner, yīn cold will fail to transform and give rise to glomus below the heart, in which case there will be no upward surging of qì.

Line 10.9

病腹满，发热十日，脉浮而数，饮食如故，厚朴七物汤主之。

厚朴半斤　甘草三两　大黄三两　大枣十枚　枳实五枚　桂枝二两　生姜五两

右七味，以水一斗，煮取四升，温服八合，日三服。呕者加半夏五合，下利去大黄，寒多者加生姜至半斤。

Bìng fù mǎn, fā rè shí rì, mài fú ér shuò, yǐn shí rú fù, hòu pò qī wù tāng zhǔ zhī.

Hòu pò bàn jīn; gān cǎo sān liǎng; dà huáng sān liǎng; dà zǎo shí méi; zhǐ shí wǔ méi; guì zhī èr liǎng; shēng jiāng wǔ liǎng

Yòu qī wèi, yǐ shuǐ yī dǒu, zhǔ qǔ sì shēng, wēn fú bā gě, rì sān fú. Ǒu zhě jiā bàn xià wǔ gě, xià lì qù dà huáng, hán duō zhě jiā shēng jiāng zhì bàn jīn.

When a patient presents with abdominal fullness, heat effusion [that has lasted] for ten days, and a floating and rapid pulse, but eats and drinks like a healthy person, Officinal Magnolia Bark Seven Agents Decoction (厚朴七物汤 *hòu pò qī wù tāng*) governs.

Officinal Magnolia Bark Seven Agents Decoction (厚朴七物汤 *hòu pò qī wù tāng*)
officinal magnolia bark (厚朴 *hòu pò*, Magnoliae Officinalis Cortex) ½ *jīn*

licorice (甘草 *gān cǎo*, Glycyrrhizae Radix) 3 *liǎng*
rhubarb (大黄 *dà huáng*, Rhei Radix et Rhizoma) 3 *liǎng*
jujube (大枣 *dà zǎo*, Jujubae Fructus) 10 pieces
unripe bitter orange (枳实 *zhǐ shí*, Aurantii Fructus Immaturus) 5 fruits
cinnamon twig (桂枝 *guì zhī*, Cinnamomi Ramulus) 2 *liǎng*
fresh ginger (生姜 *shēng jiāng*, Zingiberis Rhizoma Recens) 5 *liǎng*

Boil the above seven ingredients in one *dǒu* of water, boil to get four *shēng*. Take eight *gě* [per dose] warm, three times a day. For cases with retching, add five *gě* of pinellia (*bàn xià*). For cases with diarrhea, remove the rhubarb (*dà huáng*). For cases with copious cold, add up to half a *jīn* of fresh ginger (*shēng jiāng*).

SYNOPSIS, LINE 10.9

This line describes the signs and treatment of abdominal fullness with exterior signs.

COMMENTARY, LINE 10.9

The present line discusses abdominal fullness with exterior signs, and prescribes Officinal Magnolia Bark Seven Agents Decoction (*hòu pò qī wù tāng*) to treat it. On the basis of the formula, we know that the abdominal fullness is due to qì stagnation and heat congestion. Because the patient has suffered from heat effusion for longer than from abdominal fullness, the condition is one of external contraction of wind-cold that has transformed into heat and entered the interior. The rapid and floating pulse indicates that the exterior signs remain present. The fact that the evil qì has transformed into heat, entered the interior, damaged fluids, and caused repletion heat to bind in the intestines is reflected in the abdominal fullness. The simultaneous presence of heat effusion and abdominal fullness means that there must also be signs such as dry stool, dry mouth, and bitter taste in the mouth.

The recommended formula, Officinal Magnolia Bark Seven Agents Decoction (*hòu pò qī wù tāng*), combines Officinal Magnolia Bark Three Agents Decoction (*hòu pò sān wù tāng*) for moving qì, eliminating fullness, and draining interior repletion heat, with Cinnamon Twig Decoction (*guì zhī tāng*) for resolving the exterior evil and harmonizing construction and defense, thereby treating the interior and exterior simultaneously.

Line 10.10

腹中寒气，雷鸣切痛，胸胁逆满，呕吐，附子粳米汤主之。

附子（炮）一枚　半夏半升　甘草一两　大枣十枚　粳米半升

右五味，以水八升，煮米熟汤成，去滓，温服一升，日三服。

Fù zhōng hán qì, léi míng qiē tòng, xiōng xié nì mǎn, ǒu tù, fù zǐ jīng mǐ tāng zhǔ zhī.

fù zǐ (pào) yī méi; bàn xià bàn shēng; gān cǎo yī liǎng; dà zǎo shí méi; jīng mǐ bàn shēng

Yòu wǔ wèi, yǐ shuǐ bā shēng, zhǔ mǐ shóu tāng chéng, qù zǐ, wēn fú yī shēng, rì sān fú.

For cold qì in the abdomen with thunderous rumbling and cutting pain,[1] counterflow fullness in the chest and rib-side, and retching and vomiting, Aconite and Rice Decoction (附子粳米汤 *fù zǐ jīng mǐ tāng*) governs.

Aconite and Rice Decoction (附子粳米汤 *fù zǐ jīng mǐ tāng*)

aconite (附子 *fù zǐ*, Aconiti Radix Lateralis Praeparata) 1 piece
pinellia (半夏 *bàn xià*, Pinelliae Rhizoma) ½ *shēng*
licorice (甘草 *gān cǎo*, Glycyrrhizae Radix) 1 *liǎng*
jujube (大枣 *dà zǎo*, Jujubae Fructus) 10 pieces
non-glutinous rice (粳米 *jīng mǐ*, Oryzae Semen) ½ *shēng*

Boil the above five ingredients in eight *shēng* of water until the rice is cooked and the decoction is done. Remove the dregs. Take one *shēng* [per dose] warm, three times a day.

TEXT NOTE, LINE 10.10

[1] Cutting pain 切痛 *qiē tòng*: Pain as if being cut by a knife.

SYNOPSIS, LINE 10.10

This line discusses the signs and treatment of abdominal fullness caused by spleen-stomach vacuity cold and water-damp collecting internally.

COMMENTARY, LINE 10.10

"Cold qì in the abdomen" refers to a condition where yáng qì in the spleen-stomach is vacuous and yīn-cold exuberates internally. It is caused by vacuity cold in the spleen-stomach and by accumulating water-damp. When cold qì and water-damp flow into the stomach and intestines, they give rise to rumbling intestines and cutting pain. When cold qì moves cross counterflow, it invades the chest and rib-side, giving rise to counterflow fullness there. When it affects the stomach, it impairs the harmonious downbearing of the stomach and causes vomiting.

The recommended formula is Aconite and Rice Decoction (*fù zǐ jīng mǐ tāng*), which disperses cold and downbears counterflow, as well as warming the center and relieving pain. Aconite (*fù zǐ*) warms the center and disperses cold, thereby relieving pain. Pinellia (*bàn xià*) transforms dampness and downbears counterflow, thereby checking vomiting. Non-glutinous rice (*jīng mǐ*), licorice (*gān cǎo*), and jujube (*dà zǎo*) support the spleen and stomach in order to relax tension. In cases of pronounced spleen-stomach cold, you may add zanthoxylum (*huā jiāo*) and dried ginger (*gān jiāng*) to enhance the cold-expelling and counterflow-downbearing action.

Line 10.11

痛而闭者，厚朴三物汤主之。

厚朴八两　大黄四两　枳实五枚

右三味，以水一斗二升，先煮二味，取五升，内大黄煮取三升，温服一升，以利为度。

Tòng ér bì zhě, hòu pò sān wù tāng zhǔ zhī.

Hòu pò bā liǎng; dà huáng sì liǎng; zhǐ shí wǔ méi

Yòu sān wèi, yǐ shuǐ yī dǒu èr shēng, xiān zhǔ èr wèi, qǔ wǔ shēng, nà dà huáng zhǔ qǔ sān shēng, wēn fú yī shēng, yǐ lì wéi duò.

For pain[1] with constipation, Officinal Magnolia Bark Three Agents Decoction (厚朴三物汤 *hòu pò sān wù tāng*) governs.

Officinal Magnolia Bark Three Agents Decoction (厚朴三物汤 *hòu pò sān wù tāng*)

officinal magnolia bark (厚朴 *hòu pò*, Magnoliae Officinalis Cortex) 8 *liǎng*
rhubarb (大黄 *dà huáng*, Rhei Radix et Rhizoma) 4 *liǎng*
unripe bitter orange (枳实 *zhǐ shí*, Aurantii Fructus Immaturus) 5 pieces

Of the above three ingredients, first boil the two ingredients [officinal magnolia bark (*hòu pò*) and unripe bitter orange (*zhǐ shí*)] in one *dǒu* and two *shēng* of water to get five *shēng*. Add the rhubarb (*dà huáng*) and boil to get 3 *shēng*. Take one *shēng* [per dose] warm until [the stool] is disinhibited.

TEXT NOTE, LINE 10.11

[1] Pain 痛 *tòng*: As will be apparent from the commentary below, "pain" refers to abdominal pain.

SYNOPSIS, LINE 10.11

This line describes the signs and treatment of abdominal fullness with distention that is more pronounced than accumulation.

COMMENTARY, LINE 10.11

Pain and constipation are the only two signs given in this line. In themselves, they only minimally constitute a basis for prescribing Officinal Magnolia Bark Three Agents Decoction (*hòu pò sān wù tāng*). Nevertheless, we can determine the condition more precisely from the formula. Officinal Magnolia Bark Three Agents Decoction has exactly the same three ingredients as Minor Qì-Coordinating Decoction (*xiǎo chéng qì tāng*), which is an offensive precipitating formula that is used to treat yáng bind (heat constipation). The difference lies in the quantities of the individual ingredients, which affects the overall action of the formula. While Minor Qì-Coordinating Decoction places the emphasis on rhubarb (*dà huáng*) and is therefore an offensive precipitating formula used to treat yáng bind (heat constipation), the present formula emphasizes officinal magnolia bark (*hòu pò*), making it principally a formula that moves qì and eliminates fullness.

Therefore we take "pain and constiptation" to mean abdominal pain with distention and fullness as well as constipation, forming a repletion heat pattern in which qì stagnation is more severe than heat accumulation.

Line 10.12

按之心下满痛者，此为实也，当下之，宜大柴胡汤。

柴胡半斤　黄芩三两　芍药三两　半夏（洗）半斤　枳实（炙）四枚 大黄二两　大枣十二枚　生姜五两

右八味，以水一斗二升，煮取六升，去滓，再煎温服一升，日三服。

Àn zhī xīn xià mǎn tòng zhě, cǐ wéi shí yě, dāng xià zhī, yí dà chái hú tāng.

Chái hú bàn jīn; huáng qín sān liǎng; sháo yào sān liǎng; bàn xià (xǐ) bàn jīn; zhǐ shí (zhì) sì méi; dà huáng èr liǎng; dà zǎo shí èr méi; shēng jiāng wǔ liǎng

Yòu bā wèi, yǐ shuǐ yī dǒu èr shēng, zhǔ qǔ liù shēng, qù zǐ, zài jiān wēn fú yī shēng, rì sān fú.

When on pressing there is fullness and pain below the heart, this is repletion. One should precipitate this. Major Bupleurum Decoction (大柴胡汤 *dà chái hú tāng*) is appropriate.

Major Bupleurum Decoction (大柴胡汤 *dà chái hú tāng*)

- bupleurum (柴胡 *chái hú*, Bupleuri Radix) ½ *jīn*
- scutellaria (黄芩 *huáng qín*, Scutellariae Radix) 3 *liǎng*
- peony (芍药 *sháo yào*, Paeoniae Radix) 3 *liang*
- pinellia (半夏 *bàn xià*, Pinelliae Rhizoma) ½ *shēng* (wash)
- unripe bitter orange (枳实 *zhǐ shí*, Aurantii Fructus Immaturus) 4 fruits (mix-fry)
- rhubarb (大黄 *dà huáng*, Rhei Radix et Rhizoma) 2 *liǎng*
- jujube (大枣 *dà zǎo*, Jujubae Fructus) 12 pieces
- fresh ginger (生姜 *shēng jiāng*, Zingiberis Rhizoma Recens) 5 *liǎng*

Boil the above eight ingredients in one *dǒu* and two *shēng* of water to get six *shēng*. Remove the dregs and decoct again. Take one *shēng* [per dose] warm, three times a day.

Synopsis, Line 10.12

This line describes the signs and treatment of fullness and pain below the heart.

Commentary, Line 10.12

The present line discusses a pattern of fullness and pain below the heart, for which it recommends Major Bupleurum Decoction (*dà chái hú tāng*). As we know from the *Shāng Hán Lùn*, this formula is used to treat lesser yáng and yáng brightness combination disease, characterized by pain in the stomach duct and in the lesser yáng rib-side regions on either side of the body. We can therefore presume that the present line describes a comparable pattern that is characterized by slight vexation, alternating aversion to cold and heat effusion, a yellow tongue fur, and a stringlike and forceful pulse.

Line 10.2 states, "…absence of pain when pressed indicates vacuity; pain indicates repletion." The present line and line 10.2 both describe repletion patterns, but the place at which the repletion evil is gathering differs. While in line 10.2 the evil is gathering in the abdomen, in the present line it is below the heart. Repletion that is centered in the abdomen is treated with Major Qì-Coordinating Decoction (*dà chéng qì tāng*), which classically addresses yáng brightness bowel repletion patterns. The condition described in the present line, by contrast, affects a higher location and is therefore treated with a different formula, namely Major Bupleurum Decoction (*dà chái hú tāng*).

This formula is derived from Minor Bupleurum Decoction (*xiǎo chái hú tāng*), which contains bupleurum (*chái hú*), scutellaria (*huáng qín*), pinellia (*bàn xià*), ginseng (*rén shēn*), licorice (*gān cǎo*), fresh ginger (*shēng jiāng*), and jujube (*dà zǎo*). Major Bupleurum Decoction differs in that it lacks ginseng (*rén shēn*) and licorice (*gān cǎo*), but contains a greater quantity of fresh ginger (*shēng jiāng*), and adds peony (*sháo yào*), rhubarb (*dà huáng*), and unripe bitter orange (*zhǐ shí*). The chief medicinal is bupleurum (*chái hú*). In combination with pinellia (*bàn xià*) and fresh ginger (*shēng jiāng*), these medicinals function to resolve lesser yáng evil. Peony (*sháo yào*), rhubarb (*dà huáng*), and unripe bitter orange (*zhǐ shí*) are added to precipitate heat bind repletion in yáng brightness. Jujube (*dà zǎo*) is included to quiet the center. Thus the formula addresses fullness and pain under the heart when pressure is applied.

Ever since Zhāng Jī's time, physicians have used Major Bupleurum Decoction (*dà chái hú tāng*) to treat a much wider scope of conditions than lesser yáng and yáng brightness combination disease. For example, with the addition of mirabilite (*máng xiāo*), we use it to drain fire and free stool in conditions that manifest with constipation that has lasted for several days, exuberant heat, vexation and agitation, dry tongue and thirst, red face, and a surging and replete pulse. For repletion pain below the heart connecting to the left rib-side, difficulty turning sides, and replete stool, we add trichosanthes seed (*guā lóu*) and tangerine peel (*qīng pí*) to clear heat and precipitate qì. To treat yellowing, we add virgate wormwood (*yīn chén*) and phellodendron (*huáng bǎi*). And to treat patterns of mania caused by liver fire attacking upward, we add such heat-clearing, downward-draining substances as indigo (*qīng dài*), gardenia (*zhī zǐ*), moutan (*mǔ dān pí*), and mirabilite (*máng xiāo*).

Line 10.13

腹满不减，减不足言，当须下之，宜大承气汤。

Fù mǎn bù jiǎn, jiǎn bù zú yán, dāng xū xià zhī, yí dà chéng qì tāng.

Abdominal fullness that fails to lessen [or] lessens to no degree to speak of should be treated by precipitation. Major Qì-Coordinating Decoction (大承气汤 *dà chéng qì tāng*) is appropriate.[1]

TEXT NOTE, LINE 10.13

[1] For the formula, see Chapter 2, "Tetanic Disease," Line 2.13.

SYNOPSIS, LINE 10.13

This line describes the signs and treatment of interior repletion patterns in which accumulation and distention are equally severe.

COMMENTARY, LINE 10.13

Fullness that fails to lessen periodically is a sign of serious interior repletion caused by qì stagnation and dry stool binding internally. By contrast, fullness with periodic relief is a vacuity pattern of the kind described in line 10.3 above. The pattern described in this line is thus one of pronounced repletion. Hence the text instructs us to use precipitation and recommends prescribing Major Qì-Coordinating Decoction (*dà chéng qì tāng*).

Line 10.14

心胸中大寒痛，呕不能饮食，腹中寒，上冲皮起，出见有头足，上下痛而不可触近，大建中汤主之。

蜀椒（去汗）二合　干姜四两　人参二两

右三味，以水四升，煮取二升，去滓，内胶饴一升，微火煎取一升半，分温再服，如一炊顷，可饮粥二升，后更服，当一日食糜，温覆之。

Xīn xiōng zhōng dà hán tòng, ǒu bù néng yǐn shí, fù zhōng hán, shàng chōng pí qǐ, chū jiàn yǒu tóu zú, shàng xià tòng ér bù kě chù jìn, dà jiàn zhōng tāng zhǔ zhī.

Shǔ jiāo (qù hàn) èr gě; gān jiāng sì liǎng; rén shēn èr liǎng

Yòu sān wèi, yǐ shuǐ sì shēng, zhǔ qǔ èr shēng, qù zǐ, nà jiāo yí yī shēng, wēi huǒ jiān qǔ yī shēng bàn, fēn wēn zài fú, rú yī chuī qǐng, kě yǐn zhōu èr shēng, hòu gèng fú, dāng yī rì shí mí, wēn fù zhī.

For great cold pain in the heart and chest, retching and inability to eat or drink, and cold in the abdomen that surges upward, lifts the skin,[1] and protrudes as if with head and feet, with pain above and below [so severe that] you cannot touch it, Major Center-Fortifying Decoction (大建中汤 *dà jiàn zhōng tāng*) governs.

Major Center-Fortifying Decoction (大建中汤 *dà jiàn zhōng tāng*)
zanthoxylum (蜀椒 *shǔ jiāo*, Zanthoxyli Pericarpium) 2 *gě* (remove sweat)[2] dried ginger (干姜 *gān jiāng*, Zingiberis Rhizoma) 4 *liǎng* ginseng (人参 *rén shēn*, Ginseng Radix) 2 *liǎng*

Boil the above three ingredients in four *shēng* of water to get two *shēng*. Remove the dregs, add 1 *shēng* of malt sugar (*jiāo yí*), and decoct over a low flame to get one-and-a-half *shēng*. Divide into two doses and take warm. After about the time it takes to cook a meal, [the patient] may eat two *shēng* of gruel and then take another dose. [The patient] should eat gruel all day long, cover [up, and keep] warm.

TEXT NOTES, LINE 10.14

[1] Skin 皮 *pí*: This refers to the skin and muscle of the abdomen.

[2] Remove sweat 去汗 *qù hàn*: to remove the water and oil.

SYNOPSIS, LINE 10.14

This line describes the signs and treatment of vacuity cold abdominal fullness.

COMMENTARY, LINE 10.14

The cause of the condition described in the present line is "cold in the abdomen." This is caused by spleen-stomach yáng vacuity giving rise to severe center burner cold. The cold evil can be judged to be exuberant because it affects a broad area stretching from the chest to the abdomen and because the signs are severe ("great cold pain," "pain above and below [so severe that] you cannot touch it").

When cold evil invades the stomach, it disturbs the harmonious downbearing of stomach qì and causes vomiting and inability to eat or drink. Ascending counterflow with stomach qì into the chest, it furthermore causes fullness and pain in the chest. The abdominal lump that protrudes as if it had a head and feet can be interpreted as the result of either yīn cold or of the presence of roundworm.

The condition is thus one of yáng vacuity causing exuberant internal yīn cold, which ascends counterflow to the stomach and chest. The suggested formula is Major Center-Fortifying Decoction (*dà jiàn zhōng tāng*). Its intended effect is to warm the center and promote movement and transformation, as well as to dispel cold and eliminate pain. Amongst the ingredients, zanthoxylum (*huā jiāo*) and dried ginger (*gān jiāng*) warm the center and disperse cold. Together with ginseng (*rén shēn*) and malt sugar (*yí táng*), they warm and supplement the stomach and spleen. Furthermore, zanthoxylum (*huā jiāo*) has a worm-killing effect. When movement and transformation are restored, the yīn cold naturally disappears.

The formula uses two gě (about 10 g) of zanthoxylum (*huā jiāo*), which is quite a large quantity. This is dry-fried to "remove the sweat," i.e., to remove moisture and oil. This is done by heating it until it crackles and then leaving it to cool. This method of processing reduces the toxicity. The present formula is often used for vacuity cold pain with vomiting, vacuity cold worm accumulations, and mounting-conglomerations (疝瘕 *shàn jiǎ*). When abdominal distention and fullness are severe, you can add officinal magnolia bark (*hòu pò*) and amomum (*shā rén*). For pronounced cold or headache and dizzy vision, evodia (*wú zhū yú*) can be added. For severe vomiting, add pinellia (*bàn xià*) and fresh ginger (*shēng jiāng*). For severe spleen vacuity, add white atractylodes (*bái zhú*). For blood vacuity, add Chinese angelica (*dāng guī*). For dry mouth, add white peony (*bái sháo*). For numbness of the extremities, add cinnamon twig (*guì zhī*).

Line 10.15

胁下偏痛，发热，其脉紧弦，此寒也，以温药下之，宜大黄附子汤。

大黄三两 附子（炮）三枚 细辛二两

右三味，以水五升，煮取二升，分温三服，若强人煮取二升半，分温三服，服后如人行四五里，进一服。

Xié xià piān tòng, fā rè, qí mài jǐn xián, cǐ hán yě, yǐ wēn yào xià zhī, yí dà huáng fù zǐ tāng.

Dà huáng sān liǎng; fù zǐ (pào) sān méi; xì xīn èr liǎng

Yòu sān wèi, yǐ shuǐ wǔ shēng, zhǔ qǔ èr shēng, fēn wēn sān fú, ruò qiáng rén zhǔ qǔ èr shēng bàn, fēn wēn sān fú, fú hòu rú rén xíng sì wǔ lǐ, jìn yī fú.

One-sided pain below the rib-side, heat effusion, and a tight and stringlike pulse means cold. Use warm medicinals to precipitate it. Rhubarb and Aconite Decoction (大黄附子汤 *dà huáng fù zǐ tāng*) is appropriate.

Rhubarb and Aconite Decoction (大黄附子汤 *dà huáng fù zǐ tāng*)
rhubarb (大黄 *dà huáng*, Rhei Radix et Rhizoma) 3 *liǎng* aconite (附子 *fù zǐ*, Aconiti Radix Lateralis Praeparata) 3 pieces (blast-fry) asarum (细辛 *xì xīn*, Asari Radix et Rhizoma) 2 *liǎng*

Boil the three above ingredients in five *shēng* of water to get 2 *shēng*. Divide into three doses and take warm. If the patient is strong, boil to get two-and-a-half *shēng*, divide into three and take warm. After the [first] dose, wait for the time it takes to walk four or five *lǐ*[1] and then take another dose.

TEXT NOTE, LINE 10.15

[1] The time it takes to walk four or five *lǐ* 如人行四五里 *rú rén xíng sì wǔ lǐ*: *Lǐ* is a unit of distance roughly half a kilometer or a third of a mile. Accordingly, walking four to five *lǐ* takes about 30 minutes. Here it means that the patient should wait about 30 minutes in between doses.

SYNOPSIS, LINE 10.15

This line describes the signs and treatment of abdominal fullness and pain due to cold repletion binding internally.

COMMENTARY, LINE 10.15

This line clearly states that the condition it describes is attributable to cold. A tight and stringlike pulse indicates cold and pain; hence we know that cold repletion is binding internally. The suggested treatment is warm precipitation.

The presence of heat effusion in a cold pattern is perplexing. Some scholars have tried to explain it away by saying the condition described in the present line is a cold-heat complex. However, this does not conform with the treatment, which is a warm precipitation formula that does not address heat. Furthermore, heat effusion most commonly occurs in exterior patterns, in yáng brightness bowel repletion patterns, and in yīn vacuity patterns. None of these is associated with a pulse that is tight and stringlike. In exterior wind-heat, the pulse is floating; in yáng brightness patterns, the pulse is rapid and slippery; in yīn vacuity patterns, the pulse is fine and rapid. The present pattern is marked by a tight and stringlike pulse that conforms with none of these patterns. The pattern described in the present line is thus a rare instance of heat effusion occurring in a cold pattern. We can explain it here as a depression of yáng qì that is disturbing construction and defense. It is important to note that heat effusion may arise when yáng qì is depressed, but does not always.

"One-sided pain below the rib-side" has also attracted scrutiny. It is generally interpreted as pain that affects either the left or the right side of the body, associated with abdominal pain. Commentators explain this as being the manifestation of yīn cold complicated by repletion evil, which is lying depressed in a single location, unable to stretch out.

Finally, because the treatment offered is warm precipitation, we can presume that constipation, though not actually mentioned in the line, is among the signs. The constipation in the present condition has to be differentiated from the cold-type difficult defecation described in line 10.1, which is associated with fullness and pain with periodic relief and attributed to spleen-stomach vacuity cold preventing normal movement and transformation. The constipation mentioned in the present line is associated with abdominal fullness that refuses pressure and a pulse that tight and stringlike. It is attributed to cold repletion binding internally. Accordingly, while the pattern described in line 10.1 is treated by warm supplementation, the one described here is treated by warm precipitation.

The formula offered is Rhubarb and Aconite Decoction (*dà huáng fù zǐ tāng*), which warms yáng and dispels cold on the one hand and frees the stool and moves stagnation on the other. Aconite (*fù zǐ*) is an acrid and hot warming medicinal that dispels deep cold in the bowels and viscera. Asarum (*xì xīn*) disperses cold and relieves pain. These two medicinals together make a hot acrid cold-dispersing combination that provides effective pain relief. Rhubarb (*dà huáng*) is cold in nature and frees the stool in order to drain the internal cold repletion bind.

This formula can be modified according to need. For severe abdominal pain that likes warmth, add cinnamon twig (*guì zhī*) and peony (*sháo yào*) to harmonize construction and relieve pain. For severe abdominal distention and fullness, add officinal magnolia bark (*hòu pò*) and costusroot (*mù xiāng*) to move qì and abduct stagnation. For patients with constitutional vacuity or with mild accumulation and stagation, use processed rhubarb (*zhì dà huáng*) to mitigate the draining precipitation effect. For serious constitutional vacuity, add codonopsis (*dǎng shēn*) and Chinese angelica (*dāng guī*) to boost qì and nourish the blood.

Line 10.16

寒气厥逆，赤丸主之。

茯苓四两　半夏（洗）　四两 乌头（炮）二两　细辛一两

右四味，末之，内真朱为色，炼蜜丸

如麻子大，先食酒饮下三丸，日再夜一服，不知，稍增之，以知为度。

Hán qì jué nì, chì wán zhǔ zhī.

Fú líng sì liǎng; bàn xià (xǐ) sì liǎng; wū tóu (pào) èr liǎng; xì xīn yī liǎng

Yòu sì wèi, mò zhī, nà zhēn zhū wéi sè, liàn mì wán rú má zǐ dà, xiān shí jiǔ yǐn xià sān wán, rì zài yè yī fú, bù zhī, shāo zēng zhī, yǐ zhī wéi dù.

For cold qì reverse flow,[1] Red Pill (赤丸 *chì wán*) governs.

Red Pill (赤丸 *chì wán*)
poria (茯苓 *fú líng*, Poria) 4 *liǎng*
pinellia (半夏 *bàn xià*, Pinelliae Rhizoma) 4 *liǎng* (wash)[2]
aconite main root (乌头 *wū tóu*, Aconiti Radix) 2 *liǎng* (blast-fry)[3]
asarum (细辛 *xì xīn*, Asari Radix et Rhizoma) 1 *liǎng*[4]

Pulverize the above four ingredients. Add cinnabar (真朱 *zhēn zhū*, Cinnabaris) for color. Blend with processed honey (炼蜜 *liàn mì*, Mel Praeparatum) and form into pills the size of hemp seed. Before meals, take three pills with wine, twice a day and once at night. If no effect is felt, increase the dose gradually until you can feel an effect.

TEXT NOTES, LINE 10.16

[1] Reverse flow 厥逆 *jué nì*: The term connotes both a pathomechanism of qì flowing in an abnormal direction and as well the symptom counterflow cold of the extremities.

[2] The commentary adds: "Another formula uses cinnamon twig (*guì zhī*) [instead]."

[3] Aconite main root (乌头 *wū tóu*, Aconiti Radix): In modern times, the name *wū tóu* can refer to either *chuān wū* (Aconiti Radix) or *cǎo wū* (Aconiti Kusnezoffii Radix). The use of *cǎo wū* was not yet documented in Chinese medicine at the time of the *Jīn Guì*, so the item used here is believed to be *chuān wū*.

[4] The commentary adds: "The *Qiān Jīn Fāng* ("Thousand Gold Pieces Prescriptions") uses ginseng (*rén shēn*) [instead]."

SYNOPSIS, LINE 10.16

This line describes the signs and treatment of cold rheum reverse flow.

COMMENTARY, LINE 10.16

Despite the tersity of the present line, modern scholars tend to agree that the pattern described is one of spleen-stomach yáng vacuity that causes exuberant water-rheum to ascend counterflow with cold qì and prevents yáng qì from fully reaching the limbs, causing reversal cold of the extremities. Consequently, it is generally agreed that in addition to reversal cold of the extremities, there is also abdominal pain and possibly vomiting and palpitation below the heart.

The formula offered is Red Pill (*chì wán*), which disperses cold and relieves pain on the one hand, and transforms rheum and downbears counterflow on the other. Aconite (*wū tóu*) is a hot and acrid medicinal that assists spleen and kidney yáng. It is combined with warm and acrid cold-dispersing asarum (*xì xīn*) to disperse the intractable cold in the abdomen, relieve pain, and stem reversal. Poria (*fú líng*) and pinellia (*bàn xià*) are used to transform rheum and downbear counterflow, making the water-rheum flow downward and checking vomiting. The coating of cinnabar (*zhū shā*), the red colorof which incidentally accounts for the name of the formula, helps the downbearing action.

The preparation form is of significance here since pills are generally used for chronic conditions. While Counterflow Cold Decoction (*sì nì tāng*) and Vessel-Freeing Counterflow Cold Decoction (*tōng mài sì nì tāng*) are suitable for fulminant yáng vacuity with cold reversal of sudden onset, Red Pill is suitable for conditions that develop slowly.

Finally, one must pay attention to the medicinal preparation of aconite (*wū tóu*). Because of its toxity, it should be either appropriately processed before decocting, or taken with wine.

Line 10.17

(1)腹痛，脉弦而紧，弦则卫气不行，即恶寒；紧则不欲食，邪正相搏，即为寒疝。

(2)寒疝绕脐痛，若发则白津出，手足厥冷，其脉沉紧者，大乌头煎主之。

乌头大者五枚（熬去皮，不□咀）

右以水三升，煮取一升，去滓，内蜜二升，煎令水气尽，取二升，强人服七合，弱人服五合。不差，明日更服，不可一日再服。

(1) Fù tòng, mài xián ér jǐn, xián zé wèi qì bù xíng, jí wù hán; jǐn zé bù yù shí, xié zhèng xiāng bó, jí wéi hán shàn.

(2) Hán shàn rào qí tòng, ruò fā zé bái jīn chū, shǒu zú jué lěng, qí mài chén jǐn zhě, dà wū tóu jiān zhǔ zhī.

Wū tóu dà zhě wǔ méi (áo qù pí, bù fǔ jǔ)

Yòu yǐ shuǐ sān shēng, zhǔ qǔ yī shēng, qù zǐ, nà mì èr shēng, jiān lìng shuǐ qì jìn, qǔ èr shēng, qiáng rén fú qī gě, ruò rén fú wǔ gě. Bù chài, míng rì gèng fú, bù kě yī rì zài fú.

(1) In abdominal pain, when the pulse is stringlike and tight, stringlike indicates defense qì failing to move, and hence aversion to cold; tight indicates lack of appetite, and contention between evil and right, and hence cold mounting.

(2) If cold mounting with pain around the umbilicus manifests with discharge of white liquid[1] at the onset of the condition, reversal cold of the extremities, and a sunken and tight pulse, [use] Major Aconite Main Root Brew (乌头煎 *dà wū tóu jiān*).

Major Aconite Main Root Brew (乌头煎 *dà wū tóu jiān*).
aconite (乌头 *wū tóu*, Aconiti Radix) 5 large pieces (simmer and remove skin; do not chew)

Boil the above ingredient in three *shēng* of water to get one *shēng*. Remove the dregs, add two *shēng* of honey, and boil until the water qì has disappeared, to get two *shēng*. Strong patients should take seven *gě* [per dose]; weak patients should take five *gě*. If [the patient] does not recover, take [another dose] the next day. You may not take two doses in one day.

Text Note, Line 10.17

[1] Discharge of white liquid 白津出 *bái jīn chū*: Numerous alternative versions of this text instead have "discharge of white sweat" (白汗出 *bái hàn chū*), which is certainly the intented meaning of the phrase. In addition, the character 白 bái ("white") may be a mistranscription of 自 *zì*, "spontaneous." In this way, the phrase is interpreted to mean spontaneous discharge of cold sweat, as a result of the pain and severity of the attack.

Synopsis, Line 10.17

This line describes the pathomechanism, pattern, and treatment of cold mounting.

Commentary, Line 10.17

The line begins by describing a pattern with abdominal pain and a stringlike and tight pulse. As we have already learned, this type of pulse indicates exuberant cold. When exuberant cold arises because interior yáng is vacuous and defense qì cannot move in the outer body, the result is aversion to cold. When yáng qì is debilitated internally, movement and transformation are impaired and the patient therefore has no desire to eat or drink. Cold qì binding in the interior and preventing yáng qì from moving results in severe pain around the umbilicus. This is the pathomechanism of cold mounting.

The second section of the line describes what happens in episodes of cold mounting. Episodes are mainly characterized by pain around the umbilicus. As the pain gradually worsens, sweat issues and the limbs become cold. At this point the pulse changes from stringlike and tight to sunken and tight. This change reflects the severity of the pain.

The formula proposed is Major Aconite Main Root Brew (*dà wū tǒu jiān*), which breaks accumulations, disperses cold, and relieves pain. Aconite main root (*wū tóu*) is greatly hot and is therefore in clinical practice used primarily to treat deep, intractable cold. It dispels cold and assists yáng, helping to relieve the abdominal pain, cold limbs, and the sunken, stringlike pulse, all of which mark episodes of cold mounting. The formula is made with honey to reduce the toxicity of aconite (*wū tóu*) as well as to prolong the effect of the medicine. The suggestion of different doses for strong and weak patients draws attention to the fact that the formula is drastic in its action and therefore must be used with care.

Line 10.18

寒疝，腹中痛，及胁痛里急者，当归生姜羊肉汤主之。

当归三两　生姜五两　羊肉一斤

上三味，以水八升，煮取三升，温服七合，日三服。若寒多者，加生姜成一斤；痛多呕者，白朮一两。加生姜者，亦加水五升，煮取三升二合，服之。

Hán shàn, fù zhōng tòng, jí xié tòng lǐ jí zhě, dāng guī shēng jiāng yáng ròu tāng zhǔ zhī.

Dāng guī sān liǎng; shēng jiāng wǔ liǎng; yáng ròu yī jīn

Shàng sān wèi, yǐ shuǐ bā shēng, zhǔ qǔ sān shēng, wēn fú qī gě, rì sān fú. Ruò hán duō zhě, jiā shēng jiāng chéng yī jīn; tòng duō ǒu zhě, bái zhú yī liǎng. Jiā shēng jiāng zhě, yì jiā shuǐ wǔ shēng, zhǔ qǔ sān shēng èr gě, fú zhī.

In cold mounting, when there is pain in the abdomen and pain and tension in the rib-sides, Chinese Angelica, Fresh Ginger, and Goat Meat Decoction (当归生姜羊肉汤 *dāng guī shēng jiāng yáng ròu tāng*) governs.

Chinese Angelica, Fresh Ginger, and Goat Meat Decoction (当归生姜羊肉汤 *dāng guī shēng jiāng yáng ròu tāng*)

Chinese angelica (当归 *dāng guī*, Angelicae Sinensis Radix) three *liǎng*
fresh ginger (生姜 *shēng jiāng*, Zingiberis Rhizoma Recens) five *liǎng*
goat/lamb meat (羊肉 *yáng ròu*, Caprae seu Ovis Caro) 1 *jīn*

Boil the three above ingredients in eight *shēng* of water boil to get three *shēng*. Take seven *gě* warm, three times a day. For pronounced cold, add one *jīn* of fresh ginger (*shēng jiāng*). For pronounced pain and retching, [add] one *liǎng* of white atractylodes (*bái zhú*). If fresh ginger (*shēng jiāng*) is added, also add five *shēng* of water, boil to get three *shēng* and two *gě*, and take it.

SYNOPSIS, LINE 10.18

This line describes the signs and treatment of blood vacuity cold mounting.

COMMENTARY, LINE 10.18

Cold mounting is usually due to exuberant cold. However, the condition discussed in this line is due to blood vacuity and is therefore characterized by abdominal pain and rib-side pain and tension. The two rib-sides belong to the liver, which stores blood. Because blood is the mother of qì, vacuity of blood can result in vacuity of qì. When qì is vacuous, cold can arise internally. As a result, the rib-sides and abdomen lose the warming effect of qì and the nourishment of blood. Hypertonicity of the sinews then causes "pain in the abdomen and pain and tension in the rib-sides." This kind of pain is normally mild and relieved by pressure. It is accompanied by a pulse that is stringlike and slightly rough or slightly tight and forceless.

The formula sugested is Chinese Angelica, Fresh Ginger, and Goat/Lamb Meat Decoction (*dāng guī shēng jiāng yáng ròu tāng*) for its blood-nourishing and cold-dispersing effect. If the cold evil is abnormally exuberant, you may increase the amount of fresh ginger to increase the warming and dispersing effect of the formula. For cases with retching and vomiting, add white atractylodes (*bái zhú*) and tangerine peel (*chén pí*) to fortify the spleen and rectify qì.

Line 10.19

寒疝腹中痛，逆冷，手足不仁，若身疼痛，灸刺諸药不能治，抵當乌头桂枝汤主之。

乌头

上一味，以蜜二斤，煎减半，去滓，以桂枝汤五合解之，得一升后，初服二合，不知，即服三合；又不知，复加至五合。其知者，如醉狀，得吐者，爲中病。

桂枝三两（去皮） 芍药三两 甘草二两（炙） 生薑三两 大枣十二枚

上五味，剉，以水七升，微火煮取三升，去滓。

桂枝汤

Hán shàn fù zhōng tong, nì lěng, shǒu zú bù rén, ruò shēn téng tòng, jiǔ cì zhū yào bù néng zhì, dǐ dāng wū tóu guì zhī tāng zhǔ zhī.

Wū tóu

Shàng yī wèi, yǐ mì èr jīn, jiān jiǎn bàn, qù zǐ, yǐ guì zhī tāng wǔ gě jiě zhī, dé yī shēng hòu, chū fú èr gě, bù zhī, jí fú sān hé;yòu bù zhī, fù jiā zhì wǔ gě. Qí zhī zhě, rú zuì zhuàng, dé tù zhě, wéi zhòng bìng.

Guì zhī tāng

Guī zhī sān liǎng; (qù pí) sháo yào sān liǎng; gān cǎo èr liǎng; (zhì) shēng jiāng sān liǎng; dà zǎo shí èr méi

Shàng wǔ wèi, cuò, yǐ shuǐ qī shēng, wēi huǒ zhǔ qǔ sān shēng, qù zǐ.

In cold mounting with pain in the abdomen, counterflow cold, insensitivity of the extremities, and generalized pain [that neither] moxibustion, needling, nor other medicinals can cure, Dead-On Aconite Main Root and Cinnamon Twig Decoction (抵當乌头桂枝汤 *dǐ dàng wū tóu guì zhī tāng*) governs.

Dead-On Aconite Main Root and Cinnamon Twig Decoction (抵當乌头桂枝汤 *dǐ dàng wū tóu guì zhī tāng*)
aconite (乌头 wū tóu, Aconiti Radix Wutou)

Decoct the above ingredient in two *jīn* of honey (*mì*) until reduced to half. Remove the dregs. Use five *gě* of Cinnamon Twig Decoction (*guì zhī tāng*) to dissolve it.[1] Having obtained one *shēng*, for the first dose take two *gě*. If no effect is felt, take three *gě* [for the second dose]. If still no effect is felt, further increase [the dose], up to five *gě*. You will know the effect when [the patient] has the appearance of being drunk. When [the patient] vomits, this means that [the treatment has] struck the disease.[2]

Cinnamon Twig Decoction (桂枝汤 *guì zhī tāng*)
cinnamon twig (桂枝 *guì zhī*, Cinnamomi Ramulus) 3 *liǎng* (remove skin) peony (芍药 *sháo yào*, Paeoniae Radix) 3 *liǎng* licorice (甘草 *gān cǎo*, Glycyrrhizae Radix) 2 *liǎng* (processed) fresh ginger (生姜 *shēng jiāng*, Zingiberis Rhizoma Recens) 3 *liǎng* jujube (大枣 *dà zǎo*, Jujubae Fructus) 12 pieces

Grate the above five ingredients and boil in seven *shēng* of water over a low flame to get three *shēng*. Remove the dregs.

TEXT NOTES, LINE 10.19

[1] Dissolve it 解之 *jiě zhī*: Honey is viscous and needs to be diluted.

[2] The disease is stricken 中病 *zhòng bìng*: The treatment has been effective.

SYNOPSIS, LINE 10.19

This line describes the signs and treatment of cold mounting in exterior patterns.

COMMENTARY, LINE 10.19

Cold mounting is caused by cold evil. The fact that it is here accompanied by counterflow cold and insensitivity of the extremities tells us that yáng qì is greatly debilitated and that internal yīn cold is exuberant. The abdominal pain is caused by stagnating cold evil, while the counterflow cold and the numbness of the extremities arises when yáng qì lacks strength to propel and blood stagnates. The generalized pain is due to the presence of external cold obstructing the fleshy exterior because yáng qì is unable to resist the evil, and causing construction-defense disharmony. This pain is attributable to cold, but the invasion of external cold is encouraged by internal yáng qì vacuity. This is what the phrase from the *Nèi Jīng* ("The Inner Canon") "when yáng is vacuous there is external cold" refers to. In short, the pattern described in the present line is one of major debilitation of yáng qì with cold in both the interior and exterior. In such cases, the sole use of moxibustion or acupuncture to warm the interior or dispel the external cold will be to no avail. The recommended treatment is Dead-On Aconite Main Root and Cinnamon Twig Decoction (*dǐ dàng wū tóu guì zhī tāng*), which resolves both interior and exterior cold.

The formula consists of aconite main root (*wū tóu*), which dispels cold and relieves pain, in combination with Cinnamon Twig Decoction (*guì zhī tāng*), which harmonizes construction and defense and disperses exterior cold.

Aconite main root (*wū tóu*) is toxic. Here it is boiled with honey to reduce the toxicity (and prolong the effect of the formula) and then melted in the Cinnamon Twig Decoction. Regardless, one must carefully determine the dosage of aconite main root (*wū tóu*) according to need.

Line 10.20

其脉数而紧乃弦，状如弓弦，按之不移。脉数弦者，当下其寒；脉紧大而迟者，必心下坚；脉大而紧者，阳中有阴，可下之。

Qí mài shuò ér jǐn nǎi xuán, zhuàng rú gōng xián, àn zhī bù yí. Mai shuò xián zhě, dāng xià qí hán; mai jǐn dà ér chí zhě, bì xīn xià jiān; mài dà ér jǐn zhě, yáng zhōng yǒu yīn, kě xià zhī.

A pulse that is rapid and tight at the same time is stringlike. It resembles the string of a bow and does not change when pressed. When the pulse is rapid and stringlike, you should precipitate the cold. When the pulse is tight, large, and slow, there must be hardness below the heart. When the pulse is large and tight, this means that there is yīn within yáng, in which case you may precipitate.

SYNOPSIS, LINE 10.20

This line describes the pulses and treatment of cold repletion patterns that can be treated by precipitation.

COMMENTARY, LINE 10.20

Pulses that are stringlike or tight are yīn pulses. They indicate cold and pain. The text tells us that a stringlike pulse is a pulse that is tight and rapid; it feels like the string of a bow and when pressed, remains unchanged. We can infer from this that the pulse is forceful. Generally speaking, a pulse that is large and rapid is yáng, while a pulse that is stringlike, tight, or slow is yīn. In a patient suffering from hardness below the heart, the pulse may be rapid and stringlike, or tight, large, and slow, or large and tight. In such cases, the rapid and large qualities reflect evil repletion, while the stringlike, tight, and slow qualities indicate internal cold. Rapid and large pulses are yáng pulses, while a tight pulse is yīn. The significance of a large and tight pulse in the present pattern is therefore to indicate "yīn within yáng."

附方 APPENDED FORMULAS, LINE 10.20

ACONITE MAIN ROOT DECOCTION (乌头汤 *wū tóu tāng*)
from the *Wài Tái Mì Yào* ("Secrets from the *Wài Tái* Library")

治寒疝腹中绞痛，贼风入攻五脏，拘急不得转侧，发作有时，使人阴缩，手足厥逆。方见上

Zhì hán shàn fù zhōng jiǎo tòng, zéi fēng rù gōng wǔ zàng, jū jiw bù dé zhuǎn cè, fā zuò yǒu shí, shǐ rén yīn suō, shǒu zú jué nì. Fāng jiàn shàng.

For treating cold mounting with gripping pain in the abdomen, bandit wind entering and attacking the five viscera, and hypertonicity that prevents [the patient from] turning sides, in episodes that occur at [set] times and cause the person [to suffer from] retraction of the genitals and reverse-flow of the extremities. For the formula, see above.

GALLOPING HORSE DECOCTION (走马汤 *zǒu mǎ tāng*)[1]
from the *Wài Tái Mì Yào* ("Secrets from the *Wài Tái* Library")

治中恶心痛腹胀，大便不通。

杏仁二枚 巴豆二枚(去皮心，熬)

上二味，以绵缠搥令碎，热汤二合，捻取白汁，饮之，当下。老小量之。通治飞尸鬼击病。

Zhì zhòng è xīn tòng fù zhàng, dà biàn bù tōng.

Xìng rén èr méi; bā dòu èr méi (qù pí xīn, áo).

Shàng èr wèi, yǐ mián chán chī lìng suì, rè tāng èr gě, niǎn qǔ bái hàn, yǐn zhī, dāng xià. Lǎo xiǎo liáng zhī. Tōng fēi zhì shī guǐ jī bìng.

To treat malignity strike with heart pain, abdominal distention, and fecal stoppage.

Galloping Horse Decoction (走马汤 *zǒu mǎ tāng*)
apricot kernel (*xìng rén*) 2 pieces croton (*bā dòu*) 2 pieces (remove skin and core; simmer)

Wrap the above two ingredients in gauze, pound to pieces, place in two *gě* of hot water, and wring out the white sweat.[2] Drink this. This should precipitate. Modify the dose according to [the patient's] age. It also treats flying corpse and attacks by demons.

FORMULA NOTES, LINE 10.20

[1] The formula derives its name from the fast-acting nature of the condition as well as for the effectiveness of its medicinals, which act with the speed of galloping horses.

[2] White sweat 白汗 *bái hàn*: A white oily liquid.

Line 10.21

问曰：人病有宿食，何以别之？师曰：寸口脉浮而大，按之反涩，尺中亦微而涩，故知有宿食，大承气汤主之。

Wèn yuē: rén bìng you sù shí, hé yǐ bié zhī? Shī yuē: cùn dǒu mài fú ér dà, àn zhī fǎn sè, chǐ zhōng yī wēi ér sè, gù zhī yǒu sù shí, dà chéng qì tāng zhǔ zhī.

Question: "One human disease [categories] is abiding food. How do you identify it?" The Master says: "When the inch opening pulse is floating and large, but rough when pressed, and the cubit [pulse] is also faint and rough, thereby you know the presence of abiding food. Major Qì-Coordinating Decoction (大承气汤 *dà chéng qì tāng*) governs."

SYNOPSIS, LINE 10.21

This line describes the pulse and treatment of abiding food.

COMMENTARY, LINE 10.21

Abiding food is a condition in which dietary irregularities (overeating, eating unclean food, etc.) cause food to stagnate and fail to transform. It is characterized by abdominal distention, glomus, oppression, putrid belching, and acid swallowing. In some cases, there may also be abdominal pain or stool irregularities.

The text tells us that we can identify this disease by an inch opening pulse (i.e., the pulse at the inch position) that is floating and large, but rough when pressed. The floating and large quality reflects the upward congestion of qì that occurs when abiding food binds internally. This pulse is forceful. When the accumulation and stagnation have lasted for days, qì stagnates and hampers the movement of blood. As a result the pulse feels rough and forceful when you apply pressure. A rough pulse is often caused by scant qì and blood or by scant blood and blood stasis. The condition described in the present line, however, it is the result of food evil obstructing the qì dynamic. The text also tells us that the cubit pulse is faint and rough. Commentators generally agree that "faint" and "rough" here are not the forceless qualities associated with interior vacuity patterns, but that they reflect a stoppage of qì and blood in the lower burner. This is caused by enduring stagnation impairing spleen-stomach movement and transformation and causing waste to collect in the large intestine.

Regardless of the pulse, you should urgently flush abiding food using Major Qì-Coodinating Decoction (*dà chéng qì tāng*). If you do not precipitate swiftly, the patient's right qì may weaken, in which case you may no longer use offensive treatment effectively.

Line 10.22

脉数而滑者，实也，此有宿食，下之愈，宜大承气汤。

Mài shuò ér huá zhě, shí yě. Cǐ you sù shí, xià zhī yù, yí dà chéng qì tāng.

A rapid and slippery pulse [indicates] repletion. This [means] that there is abiding food. Precipitate it, and recovery will ensue. Major Qì-Coordinating Decoction (*dà chéng qì tāng*) is appropriate.

Synopsis, Line 10.22

This line continues the discussion of the pulses and treatment of abiding food.

Commentary, Line 10.22

As stated in the commentary to the preceding line, abiding food is characterized by abdominal distention, glomus, oppression, putrid belching, acid swallowing, and in some cases by abdominal pain or stool irregularities as well. When these signs are present, a rapid pulse means heat in the stomach and intestines, while a slippery pulse means abiding food that has collected recently. Both these pulses together reflect evil repletion. While some commentaries suggest that the slippery pulse may indicate the presence of phlegm, most scholars agree that abiding food at its onset may be characterized by a slippery pulse.

As in the previous line, the suggested treatment is to flush the food stagnation and accumulated heat from the stomach and intestines using Major Qì-Coordinating Decoction (*dà chéng qì tāng*).

Line 10.23

下利不欲食者，有宿食也，当下之，宜大承气汤。

大承气汤方，见前痉病中。

Xià lì bù yù shí zhě, you sù shí, dāng xià zhī, yí dà chéng qì tang.

Dà chéng qì tāng fāng, jiàn qián jìng bìng zhōng.

Diarrhea with no desire to eat means the presence of abiding food. You should precipitate. Major Qì-Coordinating Decoction (大承气汤 *dà chéng qì tāng*) is appropriate.

See the chapter on Tetanic Disease for the formula for Major Qì-Coordinating Decoction.

SYNOPSIS, LINE 10.23

This line describes the signs and treatment of abiding food with diarrrhea.

COMMENTARY, LINE 10.23

Thin stool or diarrhea can occur in abiding food when accumulation and stagntion impair the qì dynamic, disturb the normal upbearing and downbearing of the spleen and stomach, and prevent the digestion of grain and water. As the previous lines have described, preciptiation is the standard treatment for abiding food, and the spontaneous appearance of diarrhea can therefore bring about resolution. However, if diarrhea is accompanied by lack of appetite, this means that the abiding food is still present and that the function of the stomach and intestine has not yet recovered. The text tells us that under such circumstances it is still appropriate to use Major Qì-Coordinating Decoction (*dà chéng qì tāng*).

Line 10.24

宿食在上脘，当吐之，宜瓜蒂散。

瓜帝一分（熬） 赤小豆一分（煮）

上二味，杵为散，以香豉七合煮取汁，和散一钱匕，温服之，不吐者，少加之，以快吐为度而止。亡血及虚者不可与之。

Sù shí zài shàng wǎn, dāng tǔ zhī, yí guā dì sǎn.

Guā dì yī fèn (áo); chì xiǎo dòu yī fèn (zhǔ)

Shàng èr wèi, zhǔ wéi sǎn, yǐ xiāng chǐ qī gě zhǔ qǔ zhī, huó sǎn yī qián bǐ, wēn fú zhī, bù tù zhě, shào jiā zhī, yǐ kuài tù wéi dù ér zhǐ. Wáng xuè jí xū zhě bù kě yǔ zhī.

When abiding food is in the upper stomach duct,[1] you should eject it. Melon Stalk Powder (瓜蒂散 *guā dì sǎn*) is appropriate.

Melon Stalk Powder (瓜蒂散 *guā dì sǎn*)
melon stalk (瓜帝 *guā dì*, Melonis Pedicellus) 1 part (simmer)

rice bean (赤小豆 *chì xiǎo dòu*, Phaseoli Semen) 1 part (boil)

Pestle the above two ingredients into powder. Boil seven *gě* of fermented soybean (*xiāng chǐ*) [in water] and take the juice. Mix one qián-spoon of the powder into this and take it warm. If there is no vomiting, take a little more. When there is gratifying vomiting, stop. You may not give this to patients with blood collapse or vacuity.

TEXT NOTE, LINE 10.24

[1] Upper stomach duct 上脘 *shàng wǎn*: The Chinese for "stomach duct" (胃脘 *wèi wǎn*) has two meanings: (1) the stomach as a tube-like organ (note that in the *Mài Jīng* ("The Pulse Canon") and *Qiān Jīn Yào Fāng* ("A Thousand Gold Pieces Prescriptions"), the word 脘 is also written as 管 *guǎn*, literally "tube."); (2) the part of the abdomen beneath the surface of which lies the stomach. The stomach duct in the first meaning is divided into three sections, upper, middle, and lower. The upper section is mentioned here as the location of abiding food. Other texts speak of abiding food in the middle and lower stomach ducts.

SYNOPSIS, LINE 10.24

This line describes the treatment of abiding food in the upper stomach duct.

COMMENTARY, LINE 10.24

Although the upper stomach duct is regarded as an anatomical location, strictly speaking it is not physically possible for food to stagnate in the upper part of the stomach. Commentators therefore interpret "abiding food in the upper stomach duct" to mean abiding food with glomus and oppression in the chest and stomach duct, putrid belching, acid swallowing, and vomiting or desire to vomit with upflow, which reflects the effort of right qì to expel the evil out of the body. In accord with the principle stated in the *Sù Wèn* to "bring up and out what is high," this condition is treated with Melon Stalk Powder (*guā dì sǎn*), which causes the patient to vomit. Of course, if the patient vomits spontaneously, there is usually no need for this treatment.

As for abiding food in the middle stomach and lower stomach ducts, Wú Qiān (吴谦) tells us in the *Jīn Jiàn* ("Golden Mirror"): "The stomach has three ducts. Abiding food in the upper duct is characterized by pain in the diaphragm and vomiting; it may be ejected but not precipitated. Abiding food in the middle stomach duct is characterized by pain below the heart and vomiting, or pain and no vomiting; it may be ejected but not precipitated. Abiding food in the lower burner is characterized by pain above the umbilicus and no vomiting; this may not be ejected, but can be precipiated." From this we can see clearly that the distinction between the three stomach ducts is a matter of symptoms, which then determine the choice of treatment.

Line 10.25

脉紧如转索无常者，有宿食也。

Mài jǐn rǔ zhuǎn suǒ wú cháng zhě, yǒu sù shí yě.

A pulse that is tight, like a twisting rope without constancy,[1] means the presence of abiding food.

TEXT NOTE, LINE 10.25

[1] Tight, like a twisting rope without constancy 紧如转索无常 *jǐn rú zhuǎn suǒ wú cháng*: The pulse is like a rope that it is being twisted, sometimes tight and sometimes loose.

SYNOPSIS, LINE 10.25

This line describes the pulse of abiding food.

COMMENTARY, LINE 10.25

A tight pulse not only indicates exterior cold, but may also occur in abiding food. A pulse that is tight like a twisting rope reflects congestion and stagnation of the qì dynamic, which is caused by abiding food.

Line 10.26

脉紧，头痛风寒，腹中有宿食不化也。

Mài jǐn, tóu tòng fēng hán, fù zhōng yǒu sù shí bù huà yě.

A tight pulse [can mean either] headache wind-cold [or] abiding food in the abdomen that fails to transform.[1]

TEXT NOTE, LINE 10.26

[1] A textual variation has "tight inch opening pulse" instead.

SYNOPSIS, LINE 10.26

This line discusses the occurrence of a tight pulse in abiding food and in wind-cold.

COMMENTARY, LINE 10.26

A tight pulse most commonly appears in external contraction of wind-cold, but it can also appear when abiding food fails to transform. Furthermore, both diseases may also manifest with aversion to cold and heat effusion. Nevertheless, there are differences. In external contraction of wind-cold, the tightness is constant and combined with a floating characteristic. In patients with such a pulse, aversion to cold with heat effusion is due to wind-cold directly damaging construction and defense, causing construction-defense disharmony. Normally, these symptoms are accompanied by headache and generalized pain. In abiding food that fails to transform, a tight pulse is due to food accumulation that is causing qì congestion and thereby tightening the vessels. The disturbance in the qì dynamic causes a tight pulse that is not constant: sometimes it is tight and sometimes not. The spleen-stomach disturbance causes defense-construction disharmony, which in turn gives rise to heat effusion and aversion to cold. The food accumulation also affects the upbearing of the clear and thereby makes turbid qì ascend and cause headache. In addition, these symptoms are accompanied by signs of abiding food such as acid swallowing and putrid belching.

五脏风寒积聚病脉证治第十一

CHAPTER 11

Wind and Cold in the Five Viscera and Accumulations and Gatherings

Pulses, Signs, Treatments

‡ OVERVIEW

This chapter deals with the diseases of wind or cold striking the five viscera as well as with accumulations and gatherings in the bowels and viscera.

This is the most incomplete chapter of the *Jīn Guì Yào Lüè*, both in terms of conditions covered as well as treatments recommended. Although the title suggests that it deals with the five viscera being struck by wind and cold, there is no mention of "wind-strike" or "cold strike" in the kidney, or of "cold strike" in the spleen. There is no mention of "damage" to the liver, spleen, lung, or kidney. There is no mention of "evil qì settling" in the heart, spleen, or lung, or of depletion of the center burner. Specific formulas for treatment are included only in the discussions on liver fixity, kidney fixity, and straitened spleen, but not for any other conditions. In the schematic overview below, apparently missing elements found in other surviving sources have been added to complete the picture.

Wind-strike and cold strike in the five viscera refers to symptoms in the five viscera that are caused by either wind or cold strike internally affecting the viscera, but that are not necessarily caused by externally contracted wind and cold. These conditions are difficult to treat and have a poor prognosis, because they involve wind or cold evil passing through the channels and network vessels into the viscera in the inner body. As the *Sù Wèn* ("Plain Questions") states:

> *"At the onset of evil wind, the disease is like rain or wind. Thus, when you need treat [only] the skin and body hair, the condition is the easiest to address... After this, you treat the viscera. When you must treat the viscera, half of the patients die, half live."*

Zhāng Zhòng-Jǐng includes in this chapter descriptions of the "true visceral pulses," which are the pulses associated with each viscera that indicate imminent death.

Wind-strike and cold strike in the five viscera refers to conditions of internal damage and hence differs from the diseases of wind-strike and cold damage as discussed in the chapter on Greater Yáng Disease in the *Shāng Hán Lùn,* as well as from the conditions treated in Chapter 5 of the *Jīn Guì Yào Lüè,* "Wind-stroke and Joint Running."

The discussion on accumulations and gatherings accords with the definition of these diseases in Chapter 50 of the *Nàn Jīng.* Accordingly, "accumulation" refers to an accumulation of qì that is characterized by pain of fixed location, and is a disease of the viscera; "gathering" refers to a gathering of qì that is characterized by pain of unfixed location, and is a disease of the bowels.

‡ Schematic Overview

Wind-strike of the Five Viscera

1. Lung wind-stroke: Dry mouth and panting; body movements and heaviness; veiling and swelling and distention.
2. Liver wind-stroke: Twitching of the head and eyes; pain in the two rib-sides; often walking in a hunched [posture]; liking for sweet food.
3. Heart wind-stroke: Feather-warm heat effusion; inability to get up; hunger in the heart region; immediate vomiting after eating.
4. Spleen wind-stroke: Feather-warm heat effusion; appearance like a drunkard; vexation and heaviness in the abdomen; twitching of the skin and eyes; shortness of breath.
5. Kidney wind-stroke: The *Sān Yīn Fāng* ("Three Causes Prescriptions") states, "Profuse sweating; aversion to cold; complexion like soot, large face like puffy swelling; pain in the lumbar spine stretching into the smaller abdomen; inhibited bending and stretching, clouded sleeping with increased sweating; anxious and confused mind."

Cold Strike of the Five Viscera

1. Lung cold strike: Turbid snivel.
2. Liver cold strike: Inability to lift the arms; dry tongue root; sighing; pain in the chest with inability to turn sides; vomiting after eating; sweating.
3. Heart cold strike: sucking garlic; in severe cases heart pain reaching through to the back or back pain reaching through to the heart; gǔ infixation; floating pulse; recovery after vomiting.

4. Spleen cold strike: The *Sān Yīn Fāng* ("Three Causes Prescriptions") states, "Distention in the heart and abdomen; hypertonicity of the limbs; belches that fail to escape; visceral qì that fails to pass; constipation or diarrhea."
5. Kidney cold strike: The *Sān Yīn Fāng* states, "A pulse that is sunken, tight, and slippery; black helices; spiritless eyes; weak breathing; shortage of qì; deafness; lumbar pain; cold, hypertonicity, and pain below the knees; clouding (of the spirit) with inability to recognize people.

Death Pulses of the Five Viscera

1. Death pulse of the lung: Vacuous when floating, weak like scallion leaves when pressed, with no root below.
2. Death pulse of the liver: Weak when floated, like a rope failing to come when pressed, possibly sinuous like a snake moving.
3. Death pulse of the heart: Replete like hemp seeds when floated, even more agitated and racing when pressed.
4. Death pulse of the spleen: Large and hard when floated, clean [of contents] like an upturned cup when pressed.
5. Death pulse of the kidney: Hard when floating, chaotic like a spinning pill when pressed.

Disease Patterns of the Five Viscera and Their Treatment

1. Lung: The *Mài Jīng* ("Pulse Canon") states, "In damage to the lung, when the person suffers from taxation fatigue, there is coughing and spitting of blood, and when the pulse is fine, tight, floating, and rapid, there is spitting of blood. This comes from agitation and anger causing damage to the lung and congestion of qì."
2. Liver
   a) Damage to the liver: The *Mài Jīng* ("Pulse Canon") states, "In damage to liver, the person sheds flesh and [stays] reclined, the mouth wants to open, the hands and feet are blue-green, the eyes are heavy and pupils are painful. This is caused by damage to the liver viscus."
   b) Liver fixity:

      Signs: Liver fixity [manifests in] the patient's constant desire for stamping on their chest (see text note, line 11.17) and desiring only hot fluids prior to onset of the condition. Inula Decoction (*xuán fù huā tāng*) governs.

      Pathomechanism: Qì depression and blood stagnation, with yáng qì binding.

      Treatment: Inula Decoction (*xuán fù huā tāng*) (to move qi and quicken the blood and to free yáng and disperse binds).
3. Heart
   a) Damage to the heart: In damage to the heart, when the person suffers from taxation fatigue, there is immediately redness of the head and face and heaviness of

the lower [body], pain in the heart and subjectively felt vexation, heat effusion, beating at the umbilicus, and in a stringlike pulse. These signs are caused by damage to the heart.

b) Heart vacuity: When evil crying makes the ethereal and corporeal souls disquieted, [this means that] blood and qì are scant. Scantiness of blood and qì is associated with the heart. A patient with heart qì vacuity [experiences] fear, closed eyes and desire to sleep, dreams of traveling afar, separated and dispersed essence and spirit, and frenetic wandering of the ethereal and corporeal souls. Debilitation of yīn qì causes withdrawal; debilitation of yáng qì causes mania.

4. Spleen: Straitened spleen

Signs: When the instep yáng pulse is floating and rough, floating means that stomach qì is strong, [while] rough means that urination is frequent. The floating and rough [pulse qualities] contend with each other, [which means that] the stool is hard, and the spleen is straitened.

Pathomechanism: Strong stomach qì and weak spleen yīn.

Treatment: Cannabis Seed Pill (*má zǐ rén wán*) to drain heat and moisten dryness and to gently free the stool.

5. Kidney: Kidney fixity

Signs: The disease of kidney fixity [manifests in] heaviness of the patient's body, cold in the lumbus as if sitting in water, and an appearance like water [qì disease], but no thirst, uninhibited urination, and eating and drinking like normal. This disease is associated with the lower burner. Upon physical taxation, the patient sweats so that the clothing becomes cold and damp on the inside. When [this condition] has persisted for a long time, there will be cold and pain below the lumbus and heaviness in the abdomen as if [the patient] carried five thousand cash in the belt.

Pathomechanism: Yáng qì failing to move and cold-damp lodged in the lumbus.

Treatment: Licorice, Dried Ginger, Poria, and White Atractylodes Decoction (*gān jiāng fú líng bái zhú tāng*) to warm the center and disperse cold and to fortify the spleen and eliminate dampness.

Accumulations, Gatherings, and Grain Qì Disease

1. Accumulations: Disease among the viscera characterized by masses that do not move.

a) Pulse: Pulse comes quick and is fixed to the bone.

b) Section

Inch: Accumulation in the chest

Just out of the inch: Accumulation in the throat.

Above the bar: Accumulation at the umbilicus.

Slightly below the bar: Accumulation in the lesser abdomen.

Cubit: Accumulation in the qì thoroughfare.

Pulse to the left: Accumulation on the left side of the body.

Pulse on the right: Accumulation on the right side of the body.

Pulse on both sides: Accumulation in the center.

2. Gatherings:

   Disease of the bowels characterized by episodes with pain that moves around.

   Gatherings are curable.

3. Grain qì: Pain under the rib-side that is relieved by pressure and that is recurrent.

Line 11.1

肺中风者，口燥而喘，身运而重，冒而肿胀。

Fèi zhòng fēng zhě, kǒu zào ér chuǎn, shēn yùn ér zhòng, mào ér zhǒng zhàng.

Wind-strike in the lung [manifests in] dry mouth and panting, bodily movements[1] and heaviness, and veiling[2] with swelling and distention.

Text Notes, Line 11.1

[1] Bodily movements 身运 *shēn yùn*: The body shakes uncontrollably.

[2] Veiling 冒 *mào*: The head is clouded and unclear, as if covered by cloth.

Synopsis, Line 11.1

This line describes the signs of wind-strike in the lung.

Commentary, Line 11.1

The lung governs qì, and qì governs the transformation of liquid. When wind, a yáng evil and dry by nature, strikes the lung, it scorches the fluids and prevents qì from distributing liquid. Because the fluids fail to moisten the mouth, we see dryness of the mouth. When the lung and the airways are deprived of moisture, breath becomes congested and fails to downbear; hence there is panting. The lung is in charge of regulating the whole body, and when ancestral qì is damaged, the qì dynamic is impaired and defensive yáng is prevented from reaching the outer body. Hence the body shakes and is heavy. The lung also governs the regulation of the waterways. When lung qì is inhibited, the waterways are therefore unregulated; clear yáng does not upbear and turbid yīn does not bear downward. Water qì seeps into the fleshy exterior, giving rise to swelling as well as clouding and veiling.

Wú Qiān 吴谦 suggests that 身运而重 *shēn yùn ér zhòng* is a textual mistake for 头运而身重 *tóu yùn ér shēn zhòng*, "moving head [dizziness] and heavy body."

Line 11.2

肺中寒，吐浊涕。

Fèi zhòng hán, tù zhuó tì.

Cold strike in the lung [manifests in] ejection of turbid snivel.[1]

TEXT NOTE, LINE 11.2

[1] Ejection of turbid snivel 吐浊涕 *tù zhuó tì*: Most commentators interpret "ejection" here as discharge through the mouth, owing to blockage of the nasal orifices. Another explanation is that "ejection of turbid snivel" refers to nasal discharge of turbid spittle and foamy drool as in lung wilting, rather than actual mucus produced in the nose. Neither explanation is in conflict with clinical reality.

SYNOPSIS, LINE 11.2

This line describes the signs of cold strike in the lung.

COMMENTARY, LINE 11.2

Snivel is the humor of the lung. When the lung is struck by cold, chest yáng is unable to spread out, and the fluids congeal, gather, and form turbid nasal mucus. Because the nasal orifices are blocked as a result of lung qì failing to diffuse, the snivel cannot come out of the nose and is discharged through the mouth instead.

Line 11.3

肺死藏，浮之虚，按之弱如葱叶，下无根者死。

Fèi sǐ zàng, fú zhī xū, àn zhī ruò rú cōng yè, xià wú gēn zhě sǐ.

The dying viscus [pulse][1] of the lung is vacuous when floated,[2] and weak like a scallion leaf when pressed, with no root below. [This is the sign of imminent] death.

TEXT NOTES, LINE 11.3

[1] Dying viscus [pulse] 死藏 *sǐ zàng*: A type of true viscus pulse that appears when the visceral qì is about to expire. The manifestation of such a pulse conveys an unfavorable prognosis, and it is therefore called "dying viscus."

[2] Floated 浮 *fú*: Pressed lightly, i.e., felt at the superficial level.

SYNOPSIS, LINE 11.3

This line describes the dying viscus pulse of the lung.

COMMENTARY, LINE 11.3

When the true qì of the lung is dissipated and yáng floats upward, yīn is weak in the lower body. Accordingly when you feel the pulse lightly, it appears vacuous, and when you press down, it feels week like a scallion stalk, i.e., it is empty in the middle. In addition, it is rootless at the deepest level, which signifies the expiration of lung qì and consequently the impending death of the patient.

Line 11.4

肝中风者，头目瞤，两胁痛，行常伛，令人嗜甘。

Gān zhòng fēng zhě, tóu mù shùn, liǎng xié tòng, xíng cháng yǔ, lìng rén shì gān.

Wind-strike in the liver [manifests in] twitching head and eyes, pain in both rib-sides, often walking in a hunched [posture], and a predilection for sweets.

Synopsis, Line 11.4

This line describes the signs of wind-strike in the liver.

Commentary, Line 11.4

The liver is the viscus of wind and wood. It opens at the eyes; its channel ascends to the vertex. Prevalent wind causes stirring, and when the liver is struck by wind, the head and eyes twitch. This conforms with the statement in the *Nèi Jīng* ("Inner Canon"), "All wind with shaking and dizzy vision is ascribed to the liver." The liver governs the sinews. When wind prevails, the sinews become hypertonic; hence the two rib-sides are painful and may cause the patient to assume a hunched posture. Lastly, the patient may have a craving for sweet foods because this can relax possible tension in the liver.

Line 11.5

肝中寒者，两臂不举，舌本燥，喜太息，胸中痛，不得转侧，食则吐而汗出也。

Gān zhòng hán zhě, liǎng bèi bù jǔ, shé běn zào, xǐ tài xī, xiōng zhōng tòng, bù dé zhuǎn cè, shí zé tù ér hàn chū yě.

Cold strike in the liver [manifests in] inability to lift both arms, dryness at the root of the tongue, tendency to sigh, pain in the chest preventing [the patient] from turning sides, and vomiting with sweating upon eating.[1]

Text Note, Line 11.5

[1] The *Mài Jīng* ("Pulse Canon") and *Qiān Jīn Fāng* ("Thousand Gold Pieces Prescriptions") quote this passage as follows: "…periodic night sweating and cough, and vomiting the juice upon eating."

Synopsis, Line 11.5

This line describes the signs of cold strike in the liver.

COMMENTARY, LINE 11.5

The liver governs the sinews and is in charge of movement. When it is struck by cold evil, this causes hypertonicity in the reverting yīn sinews in the inner face of the arm, which prevents the patient from lifting the arms. The liver channel passes along the throat and nets around the root of the tongue. In cases of liver cold, the fluids are not distributed along its channel, so that the tongue and pharynx are deprived of moisture, hence the root of the tongue is dry. The liver likes orderly reaching, and when liver qì is depressed, there is sighing. The liver channel passes through the diaphragm. When depressed cold in the liver channel prevents chest yáng from spreading, the result is pain in the chest to the point where it prevents the patient from turning sides. When liver cold invades the stomach and affects the intake of food, the fluids are forced outward, hence there is vomiting and sweating.

Throughout history, commentators have debated the meaning of this line. Wú Qiān 吴谦 believes that "inability to lift both arms," "dryness at the root of the tongue," and "sweating" do not belong in the present line on liver cold strike. Cáo Yǐng-Fǔ 曹颖甫 suggests that these three phrases belong in line 11.4 and therefore describe clinical manifestations of liver wind strike instead. Tán Rì-Qiáng 谭日强 states that the symptoms described in the present line may in fact be a description of cold strike in the spleen, which is entirely missing from the current version of the text. He further believes that the preceding line on liver wind-strike might contain text that originally belonged to the line on liver cold strike, because the symptoms there closely resemble the symptoms of liver cold strike as described in the sixth chapter of the *Mài Jīng* ("Pulse Canon"). In his opinion, the symptoms of liver wind-strike are described by lines that are now associated with heart wind-strike and spleen wind-strike.

As we can see, this issue is difficult to resolved and continues to demand further research.

Line 11.6

肝死藏，浮之弱，按之如索不来，或曲如蛇行者死。

Gān sǐ zàng, fú zhī ruò, àn zhī rú suǒ bù lái, huò qū rú shé xíng zhě sǐ.

The dying viscus [pulse] of the liver is weak when floated; like a rope failing to come when pressed; and possibly sinuous like a snake moving.[1] [This is the sign of imminent] death.

TEXT NOTES, LINE 11.6

[1] Like a rope failing to come 如索不来 *rú suǒ bù lai*: Like a rope hanging in mid-air, drifting around, disappearing as soon as the hand feels it, and not returning.

[2] Sinuous like a snake moving 曲如蛇行 *qǔ rú shé xíng*: Like the wavy motion of a snake moving along the ground.

SYNOPSIS, LINE 11.6

This line describes the dying viscus pulse of the liver.

COMMENTARY, LINE 11.6

The true visceral pulse of the liver is forceless at the superficial level, and soft, weak, and spiritless when lightly pressed. In other words, it is scattered and completely unable to straighten out. Alternatively, it is "sinuous like a snake moving," i.e., wavy like a snake moving along the ground, turning and shifting, but unable to reach, as if trying but failing to become stringlike, with no gentleness at all. This kind of pulse arises when stomach qì is insufficient to nourish the liver, and liver blood is therefore depleted to point that vital qì is lost, which is to say, all signs of vitality have disappeared.

Line 11.7

肝着，其人常欲蹈其胸上，先未苦时，但欲饮热，旋覆花汤主之。

旋覆花三两 葱十四茎 新绛少许

右三味，以水三升，煮取一升，顿服之。

Gān zhuó, qí rén cháng yù dǎo qí xiōng shàng, xiān wèi kǔ shí, dàn yù yǐn rè, xuán fù huā tāng zhǔ zhī.

Xuán fù huā sān liǎng; cōng shí sì jīng; xīn jiàng shǎo xǔ

Yòu sān wèi, yǐ shuǐ sān shēng, zhǔ qǔ yī shēng, dùn fú zhī.

Liver fixity [manifests in] the patient's constant desire for stamping on their chest[1] and desiring only hot fluids prior to onset of the condition.[1] Inula Decoction (旋覆花汤 *xuán fù huā tāng*) governs.[2]

Inula Decoction (旋覆花汤 *xuán fù huā tāng*)

- inula flower (旋覆花 *xuán fù huā*, Inulae Flos) 3 *liǎng*
- scallion (葱 *cōng*, Allii Fistulosi Herba) 14 stems
- fresh madder (新绛 *xīn jiàng*, Rubiae Radix Recens)[3] a small amount

Boil the above three ingredients in three *shēng* of water to get one *shēng*. Quaff.

TEXT NOTES, LINE 11.7

[1] Constant desire for stamping on their chest 常欲蹈其胸上 *cháng yù dǎo qí xiōng shàng*: While somewhat awkward, this is a literal translation of the Chinese. Most commentators interpret this metaphorically to mean that the patient often likes to beat his/her chest, although some adopt the view held by Táng Zōng-Hǎi 唐宗海 that it means that the patient literally likes to have someone stamp on his/her chest. The difference between the metaphorical and literal interpretations affects only the intensity of the stimulus that brings relief to the discomfort.

[2] The commentary adds: "Chén Yì and colleagues have checked all versions of Inula Decoction (*xuán fù huā tāng*) [and found them] all to be identical."

[3] Fresh madder 新绛 *xīn jiàng*: This term, literally meaning "new crimson," has been the subject of much debate. One view is that this refers to newly dyed crimson silk cloth, as was used for hats and pouches. Commentators identify the dye variously as madder (茜草 *qiàn cǎo*), saffron (藏红花 *zàng hóng huā*), sappan (苏木 *sū mù*) or even gorilla's blood (猩猩血 *xīng xīng xuè*).

Another view, which is held most prominently by Táo Hóng-Jǐng 陶宏景 and is followed in the translation here, is that 绛 *jiàng* refers to the plant madder (*qiàn cǎo gēn*), and that 新绛 *xīn jiàng* means fresh madder. Táo Hóng-Jǐng 陶宏景 specifically states that this medicinal is effective for liver fixity and late miscarriage due to blood stasis. Its blood-moving, vessel-freeing qualities are also mentioned in the *Běn Cǎo Gāng Mù* ("Herbal Foundation Compendium"). In clinical practice, the use of madder in this formula has proven effective.

Synopsis, Line 11.7

This line describes the pattern and treatment of liver fixity.

Commentary, Line 11.7

Liver fixity arises when the liver loses its function of orderly reaching and free coursing, and qì and blood of the liver channel become depressed and stagnant. Because the liver vessel spreads over the rib-side and nets around the chest, signs associated with the liver vessel include glomus and oppression in the chest and rib-side, and in severe cases distending pain or stabbing pain, which may be relieved by rubbing, patting, or pummeling with the hands.

The phrase, "desiring only hot fluids prior to onset of the condition" refers to the fact that the qì aspect is affected by contraction of liver fixity; hence hot drinks can help to free the qì dynamic. As the disease progresses, hot drinks are no longer of avail, and only patting and rubbing provide relief. It is for this more advanced stage that Inula Decoction (*xuán fù huā tāng*) is prescribed.

Commentators over the ages have disagreed about the locus, causes, and pathomechanisms of liver fixity. Some have identified it as liver depression overwhelming the spleen; some state that it is the liver overwhelming the lung. Some have explained it as yáng vacuity with congealing cold, others as blood becoming fixed in the diaphragm. Some have identified the chest as the locus; others, the rib-side. The authors of the 1984 *Jīn Guì Yào Lüè Jiǎng Yì* ("Lecture Notes on Essential Prescriptions of the Golden Cabinet") believe that it is depression and stagnation of qì and blood in the liver channel.

Inula Decoction (*xuán fù huā tāng*) moves qì and quickens the blood, and frees yáng and dissipates binds. Inula flower (*xuán fù huā*) frees the network vessels of the liver and moves qì. Madder (*qiàn cǎo gēn*) quickens blood and transforms stasis. Scallion (*cōng*) warms and frees yáng qì and dissipates binds.

Line 11.8

心中风者，翕翕发热，不能起，心中饥，食即呕吐。

Xīn zhòng fēng zhě, xī xī fā rè, bù néng qǐ, xīn zhōng jī, shí jí ǒu tù.

Wind-strike in the heart [manifests in] feather-warm heat effusion,[1] inability to get up, hunger in the heart,[2] and vomiting immediately upon eating.

Text Notes, Line 11.8

[1] Feather-warm heat effusion 翕翕发热 *xī xī fā rè*: Gentle heat effusion that is felt in the skin and fleshy exterior, as if the body were wrapped in feathers.

[2] Heart 心 *xīn*: The area around or just below the heart.

Synopsis, Line 11.8

This line describes the signs of wind-strike in the heart.

Commentary, Line 11.8

The heart is associated with fire heat and is a yáng viscus. Wind is a yáng evil. When wind strikes the heart, fire heat steams inside the heart and strays outward. Hence there is feather-like heat effusion. Exuberant internal heat causes fire to consume qì. Thus, the patient is unable to get up. When fire is stirring in the center, there is hunger in the region of the heart. The stomach and heart are interconnected, so wind heat in the heart also harasses the stomach, damaging liquid, depriving it of moisture, and preventing harmonious downbearing. Hence we see vomiting immediately after eating.

Line 11.9

心中寒者，其人苦病心如啖蒜状，剧者心痛彻背，背痛彻心，譬如蛊注，其脉浮者，自吐乃愈。

Xīn zhòng hán zhě, qí rén kǔ bìng xīn rú dàn suàn zhuàng, jù zhě xīn tòng chè bèi, bèi tòng chè xīn, pì rú gǔ zhù, qí mài fú zhě, zì tù nǎi yù.

Cold strike in the heart [manifests in] suffering in the heart as if from eating garlic, and in severe cases, in heart pain stretching through to the back and back pain stretching through to the heart, as in gǔ influx.[1] If the pulse is floating, spontaneous vomiting will bring about recovery.

Text Note, Line 11.9

[1] Gǔ influx 蛊注 *gǔ zhù*: An ancient disease name denoting a condition that occurs in bouts characterized by vexation pain in the heart and abdomen and in severe cases is transmissible and fatal. Gǔ refers to poisonous insects that in ancient times were intentionally and furtively added to the food of others to harm them. Note that 注 *zhù* (influx) is similar to the modern notion of "infection."

Synopsis, Line 11.9

This line describes the signs and prognosis of cold strike in the heart.

Commentary, Line 11.9

Cold is a yīn evil. When there is cold evil stagnating in the heart, yáng qì becomes depressed and binds, and heart fire becomes blocked and contained within. This gives rise to a sensation in the region of the heart like pain but not pain and like heat but not heat, which the text compares to the experience of eating raw garlic. When the condition is severe, yīn cold becomes exuberant in the upper body and obstructs heart yáng, thereby preventing it from moving qì and blood. This results in pain in the heart stretching through to the back and back pain stretching through to the heart. The pain is difficult to endure; hence the text compares it to the sensation of "gǔ influx." The fact that vomiting can cause recovery in patients with a floating pulse tells us that the disease is located in the upper burner and that the evil has not yet penetrated deeply. Therefore, a gradual recovery of heart yáng will allow yīn cold to move outward. If the patient spontaneously vomits without taking medicine, yáng qì will be able to stretch out and bring the evil up and out of the body, so that the patient recovers naturally.

Line 11.10

心伤者，其人劳倦，即头面赤而下重，心中痛而自烦，发热，当脐跳，其脉弦，此为心脏伤所致也。

Xīn shāng zhě, qí rén láo juàn, jí tóu miàn chì ér xià zhòng, xīn zhōng tòng ér zì fán, fā rè, dāng qí tiào, qí mài xián, cǐ wéi xīn zàng shāng suǒ zhì yě.

In damage to the heart, when the person suffers from taxation fatigue,[1] there is immediate redness of the head and face and heaviness of the lower [body], pain in the heart and subjectively felt vexation, heat effusion, beating at the umbilicus, and in a stringlike pulse. These signs are caused by damage to the heart.

Text Note, Line 11.10

[1] Taxation fatigue 劳倦 *láo juàn*: Fatigue as a result of taxing the body (hard work or strenuous exercise).

SYNOPSIS, LINE 11.10

This line describes the signs of heart damage.

COMMENTARY, LINE 11.10

The meaning of the term "heart damage" has been the subject of much debate. Yóu Yí 尤怡 suggests it means heart vacuity; Cáo Jiā-Dá 曹家达 explains it as construction vacuity; and Gāo Xué-Shān 高学山 interprets it as damage to both heart qì and blood. The general view amongst today's scholars is that the term refers to vacuity of heart blood, giving rise to dual vacuity of heart qì and blood. In vacuity of heart qì and blood, patients easily suffer from taxation fatigue. When blood is insufficient, vacuous yáng floats upward; hence we see redness of the head and face. Exuberance in the upper body is followed by vacuity in the lower body. When center qì is insufficient, the lumbus and lower limbs are heavy and powerless. When spleen qì falls, there is sagging in the anus and prolapse of the rectum. When the heart is vacuous and deprived of nourishment, vacuity heat harasses the center, so there is vacuity vexation, heat effusion, and pain in the heart. When heart qì is vacuous in the upper body, and kidney qì stirs in the lower body, there is beating at the umbilicus. The healthy pulse of the heart can be described as "one beat after the other like threaded pearls" (累累如贯珠 *lěi lěi rú guàn zhū*), but when blood is vacuous and fails to nourish the vessels, the pulse is stringlike.

Line 11.11

心死藏，浮之实，如丸豆，按之益躁疾者死。

Xīn sǐ zàng, fú zhī shí, rú wán dòu, àn zhī yì zào jí zhě sǐ.

The dying viscus [pulse] of the heart is replete when floated, like a pellet or bean,[1] and in addition agitated and racing [when] pressed. [This is the sign of imminent] death.

TEXT NOTE, LINE 11.11

[1] Like a pellet or bean 丸豆 *wán dòu*: In the Zhào block-printed edition (赵刻本 *zhào kè běn*), this was originally written as 麻豆 *má dòu*, which can be interpreted to mean either sesame seeds (芝麻 *zhī mā*) or hemp seeds (麻子仁 *mā zǐ rén*).

SYNOPSIS, LINE 11.11

This line describes the dying viscus pulse of the heart.

COMMENTARY, LINE 11.11

A healthy heart pulse should be round and smooth, coming quickly and departing slowly (see *Nàn Jīng* Chapter 15). By contrast, the true visceral pulse of the heart is hard and replete at the superficial level, wobbling like a sling pellet or bean, and with no gentleness at all. Furthermore, when pressed heavily it is agitated, disquieted and disordered. This pulse reflects the desiccation of heart blood and the dissipation of heart qì.

Line 11.12

邪哭使魂魄不安者，血气少也。血气少者，属于心，心气虚者，其人则畏，合目欲眠，梦远行而精神离散，魂魄妄行。阴气衰者为癫，阳气衰者为狂。

Xié kū shǐ hún pò bù ān zhě, xuè qì shǎo yě. Xuè qì shǎo zhě, shǔ yú xīn, xīn qì xū zhě, qí rén zé wèi, gě mù yù mián, mèng yuǎn xíng ér jīng shén lí sàn, hún pò wàng xíng. Yīn qì shuāi zhě wéi diān, yáng qì shuāi zhě wéi kuáng.

When evil crying[1] disquiets the ethereal and corporeal souls, [this means that] blood and qì are scant. Scantiness of blood and qì is associated with the heart. A patient with heart qì vacuity [experiences] fear, closed eyes and desire to sleep, dreams of traveling afar, separated and dispersed essence and spirit, and frenetic wandering of the ethereal and corporeal souls.[2] Debilitation of yīn qì causes withdrawal; debilitation of yáng qì causes mania.[3]

TEXT NOTES, LINE 11.12

[1] Evil crying 邪哭 *xié kū*: Explanations of this phrase differ. It can either refer to crying and emotional disturbance that is caused by or appears as if caused by possession by evil spirits. Alternatively, we can read it as crying due to an invasion of external evil. A third explanation is that 哭 *kū* is used in an abstract sense of affliction, so that the phrase reads "evil affliction."

[2] Ethereal and corporeal souls 魂魄 *hún pò*: Two elements of psychic life. The ethereal soul is stored by the liver and is closely related to the blood, while the corporeal soul is stored by the lung and is closely related to qì.

[3] Withdrawal…mania 癫 … 狂 *diān... kuáng*: Two forms of mental derangement. Withdrawal is characterized by emotional depression, indifference, deranged speech, taciturnity, and obliviousness to hunger or satiety. Mania is a state of mental excitement characterized by noisy, unruly, and even aggressive behavior, offensive speech, constant singing and laughter, irascibility, springing up walls and climbing roofs, and inability to remain tidily dressed.

SYNOPSIS, LINE 11.12

This line describes mental derangement due to heart blood and qì vacuity.

COMMENTARY, LINE 11.12

According to most commentaries, "evil crying" refers to emotional disturbance that occurs for no apparent reason, as if the patient were possessed by ghosts or demons. It causes disquietude of the ethereal and corporeal souls, thus giving rise to signs of mental derangement. The text suggests that the root cause of such a condition is not evil spirits, but "scant blood and qì." The ethereal soul is stored by the liver, which also stores the blood; the corporeal soul is stored by the lung, which governs qì. When blood is scant, the liver has nothing to store. This affects liver function in general and hence disquiets the ethereal soul. When qì is scant, this affects the lung function in general and hence disquiets the corporeal soul.

The text tells us that scant qì and blood is a problem of the heart. Although the blood belongs to the liver and qì belongs to the lung, the heart is master of both. Furthermore, the heart stores the spirit. When the heart is vacuous, the spirit experiences fear. Insufficiency of spirit qì causes the patient to close their eyes and to want to sleep. Because the spirit fails to remain contained within its abode, the patient dreams of traveling afar. When the heart spirit is not contained, essential qì is dissipated. As a result, the ethereal and corporeal souls are deprived of control and hence move frenetically. If the condition develops any further, yīn qì vacuity can give rise to withdrawal, while yáng qì vacuity can give rise to mania.

Line 11.13

脾中风者，翕翕发热，形如醉人，腹中烦重，皮目瞤而短气。

Pí zhòng fēng zhě, xī xī fā rè, xing rú zuì rén, fù zhōng fán zhòng, pí mù shùn ér duǎn qì.

Wind-strike in the spleen [manifests in] feather-warm heat effusion, an appearance as if inebriated, vexation and heaviness in the abdomen, twitching of the skin and eyes,[1] and shortness of breath.

TEXT NOTE, LINE 11.13

[1] Skin and eyes 皮目 *pí mù*: The *Mài Jīng* ("The Pulse Canon") and *Qiān Jīn Fāng* ("Thousand Gold Pieces Prescriptions") have 皮肉 *pí ròu*, skin and flesh.

SYNOPSIS, LINE 11.13

This line describes the signs of wind-strike in the spleen.

COMMENTARY, LINE 11.13

The spleen governs the limbs and the flesh. It is closely connected with the stomach, and construction and defense originate in the spleen and stomach. Wind is a yáng evil. When the spleen is struck by wind, there is feather-warm heat effusion. When wind evil strikes and impedes spleen qì, yáng qì is unable to reach the extremities. As a result, the patient loses the use of the limbs and hence has the appearance of being drunk. The spleen resides in the abdomen and governs dampness. When it is invaded by wind evil, wind and dampness contend with each other; hence there is vexation and heaviness in the abdomen. The phrase "twitching of the skin and eyes" may be a mistake for "twitching of the skin and flesh." Both interpretations are possible since the flesh is governed by the spleen, and the upper and lower eyelids also belong to the spleen. When wind prevails, there is stirring, and this manifests in twitching. Lastly, when the spleen fails to move dampness, the qì dynamic is impeded. As a result, breathing is inhibited, and we see shortness of breath.

Line 11.14

脾死藏，浮之大坚，按之如覆杯洁洁，状如摇者死。

Pí sǐ zàng, fú zhī dà jiān, àn zhī rú fù bei jié jié, zhuàng rú yáo zhě sǐ.

The dying viscus [pulse] of the spleen is large and hard when floated, clean [of contents][1] like an upturned cup when pressed, and feels as if wobbling. [This is the sign of imminent] death.[2]

TEXT NOTES, LINE 11.14

[1] Clean [of contents] 洁洁 *jié jié*: Empty.

[2] The commentary adds: "Chén Yì and colleagues explain that the five viscera are all affected by wind-strike and cold strike. However, the present [discussion on] the spleen only mentions wind-strike. Wind-strike in the kidney and cold strike are not mentioned either. This is because the text is corrupted in numerous places and comes from such a remote age that there are no other texts that we can use to reconstruct it."

SYNOPSIS, LINE 11.14

This line describes the dying viscus pulse of the spleen.

COMMENTARY, LINE 11.14

A healthy spleen pulse moves at a calm and leisurely pace. It is harmonious, moderate, and spirited. If the pulse is large and hard when you apply light pressure, this means that vessel qì is no longer gentle and harmonious. When you increase pressure, this type of pulse feels like a cup turned upside-down, hard on the outside and empty on the inside. "Feeling as if wobbling" suggests that the pulse is erratic, irregular, agitated, and urgent, and without root. These pulse qualities are all signs that spleen qì is vanquished and dissipated and that stomach qì is depleted, strong on the outside and dry in the middle. This kind of true visceral pulse indicates that the bowels and viscera, the channels and network vessels are deprived of nourishment. The descriptions of this pulse are similar to "dead spleen pulse" (死脾脉 *sǐ pí mài*) and "true spleen pulse" (真脾脉 *zhēn pí mài*) as described in the *Nèi Jīng*. Different commentators have put forth different views: Gāo Xué-Shān 高学山, for example, explains the pulse described here as fine and faint, while Cáo Jiā-Dá 曹家达 describes it as a "pecking sparrow pulse" (雀啄脉 *què zhuó mài*).

Line 11.15

趺阳脉浮而涩，浮则胃气强，涩则小便数，浮涩相搏，大便则坚，其脾为约，麻子仁丸主之。

麻子仁二升　芍药半斤　枳实一斤
大黄一斤　厚朴一尺　杏仁一升

右六味，末之，炼蜜和丸梧子大，饮服十丸，日三，以知为度。

Fū yáng mài fú ér sè, fú zé wèi qì qiáng, sè zé xiǎo biàn shuò, fú sè xiāng bó, dà biàn zé jiān, qí pí wéi yuē, má zǐ rén wán zhǔ zhī.

Má zǐ rén èr shēng; sháo yào bàn jīn; zhǐ shí yī jīn; dà huáng yī jīn; hòu pò yī chǐ xìng rén yī shēng

Yòu liù wèi, mò zhī, liàn mì huò wán wú zǐ dà, yǐn fú shí wán, rì sān, yǐ zhī wéi dù.

When the instep yáng pulse is floating and rough, floating means that stomach qì is strong, [while] rough means that urination is frequent. The floating and rough [pulse qualities] contend with each other, [which means that] the stool is hard and the spleen is straitened.[1] Cannabis Seed Pill (麻子仁丸 *má zǐ rén wán*) governs.

Cannabis Seed Pill
(麻子仁丸 *má zǐ rén wán*)

- cannabis seed (麻子仁 *má zǐ rén*, Cannabis Semen) 2 *shēng*
- peony (芍药 *sháo yào*, Paeoniae Radix) ½ *jīn*
- unripe bitter orange (枳实 *zhǐ shí*, Aurantii Fructus Immaturus) 1 *jīn*
- rhubarb (大黄 *dà huáng*, Rhei Radix et Rhizoma) 1 *jīn*
- officinal magnolia bark (厚朴 *hòu pò*, Magnoliae Officinalis Cortex) 1 *chǐ*[2]
- apricot kernel (杏仁 *xìng rén*, Armeniacae Semen) 1 *shēng*

Grind the above six ingredients and blend with processed honey (*liàn mì*) to form into pills the size of firmiana seeds. Take ten pills in fluid three times a day, until the effect is noticed.

TEXT NOTES, LINE 11.15

[1] Straitened spleen 脾约 *pí yuē*: A disease characterized by constipation that arises because splenic movement and transformation are impaired and the stool becomes dry.

[2] *Chǐ* 尺 *chǐ*: In the Han Dynasty, 1 *chǐ* was equivalent to 23 cm.

SYNOPSIS, LINE 11.15

This line describes the pathomechanism, signs, and treatment of straitened spleen on the basis of the instep yáng pulse.

COMMENTARY, LINE 11.15

The instep yáng pulse indicates disease of the spleen and stomach. As this line tells us, the key sign of straitened spleen is a floating and rough instep yáng pulse. A floating pulse is one that is superabundant when lifted (i.e., when pressure is released so that only the superficial level is felt). It is a yáng pulse that signifies exuberant stomach heat. A rough pulse is one that feels stagnant and disfluent when pressed. This is a yīn pulse, indicating insufficiency of the spleen fluids.

When spleen yīn is insufficient, it cannot move the fluids of the stomach and thus deprives the intestinal tract of moisture. When stomach heat is exuberant, it damages stomach yīn. As a result, the stool becomes dry and bound, urination becomes frequent, and the stream of urine becomes long and fine. This condition is called straitened spleen, because the stomach is strong and the spleen is weak, and the spleen is fettered by stomach heat. It is treated by discharging heat, moistening dryness, and gently freeing the stool with Cannabis Seed Pill (*má zǐ rén wán*).

Cannabis seed (*huǒ má rén*) and apricot kernel (*xìng rén*) moisten dryness and lubricate the intestines. Peony (*sháo yào*) nourishes yīn and harmonizes the spleen. Rhubarb (*dà huáng*), unripe bitter orange (*zhǐ shí*), and officinal magnolia bark (*hòu pò*) discharge heat and abduct stagnation. Honey is used to form the powdered ingredients into pills for two reasons: one is that it provides sweet, mild moist precipitation to discharge yáng brightness dryness heat; the other is that it enriches greater yīn fluids.

The formula's intended action is offensive precipitation combined with enriching and moistening. This combination provided impetus to the development of warm disease theory. Humor-Increasing Decoction (*zēng yè tāng*) devised by Wú Jú-Tōng 吴菊通 is essentially derived from this formula.

Line 11.16

肾著之病，其人身体重，腰中冷，如坐水中，形如水状，反不渴，小便自利，饮食如故，病属下焦，身劳汗出，衣里冷湿，久久得之，腰以下冷痛，腹重如带五千钱，甘姜苓术汤主之。

甘草二两　白朮二两　干姜四两　茯苓四两

右四味，以水五升，煮取三升，分温三服，腰中即温。

Shèn zhuò zhī bìng, qí rén shēn tǐ zhòng, yāo zhōng lěng, rú zuò shuǐ zhōng, xing rú shuǐ zhuàng, fǎn bù kě, xiǎo biàn zì lì, yǐn shí rú gù, bìng shǔ xià jiāo, shēn láo hàn chū, yī lǐ lěng shī, jiǔ jiǔ dé zhī, yāo yǐ xià lěng tòng, fù zhòng rú dài wǔ qiān qián, gān jiāng líng zhú tāng zhǔ zhī.

Gān cǎo èr liǎng; bái zhú èr liǎng; gān jiāng sì liǎng; fú líng sì liǎng

Yòu sì wèi, yǐ shuǐ wǔ shēng, zhǔ qǔ sān shēng, fēn wēn sān fú, yāo zhōng jí wēn.

The disease of kidney fixity[1] [manifests in] heaviness of the patient's body, cold in the lumbus as if sitting in water, and an appearance like water [qì disease], but no thirst, uninhibited urination,[2] and normal eating and drinking. This disease is associated with the lower burner. Upon physical taxation, the patient sweats so that the clothing becomes cold and damp on the inside.[3] When [this condition] has persisted for a long time, there will be cold and pain below the lumbus and heaviness in the abdomen as if [the patient] carried five thousand cash in the belt. Licorice, Dried Ginger, Poria, and White Atractylodes Decoction (甘草干姜茯苓白朮汤 *gān cǎo gān jiāng fú líng bái zhú tāng*) governs.

Licorice, Dried Ginger, Poria, and White Atractylodes Decoction (甘草干姜茯苓白朮汤 *gān cǎo gān jiāng fú líng bái zhú tāng*)

- licorice (甘草 *gān cǎo*, Glycyrrhizae Radix) 2 *liǎng*
- white atractylodes (白朮 *bái zhú*, Atractylodis Macrocephalae Rhizoma) 2 *liǎng*
- dried ginger (干姜 *gān jiāng*, Zingiberis Rhizoma) 4 *liǎng*
- poria (茯苓 *fú líng*, Poria) 4 *liǎng*

Boil the above four ingredients in five *shēng* water to get 3 *shēng*. Divide into three doses and take warm. [The patient will feel] immediate warmth in the lumbus.

TEXT NOTES, LINE 11.16

[1] Kidney fixity 肾著 *shèn zhuó*: Cold pain and heaviness in the lumbar region that prevents normal turning and is exacerbated by yīn-type (overcast and wet) weather. It is attributed to kidney vacuity and to cold-damp becoming "fixed" in the inner body. In modern texts, the character 著 *zhuó* is more commonly written as 着, which is pronounced identically and used interchangeably.

[2] Uninhibited urination 小便自利 *xiǎo biàn zì lì*: normal free urination.

[3] So that the clothing becomes cold and damp on the inside 衣里冷湿 *yī lǐ lěng shī*: An alternative version has: "so that there is cold and dampness in the exterior and interior" (表里冷湿 *biǎo lǐ lěng shī*).

SYNOPSIS, LINE 11.16

This line describes the causes, signs, and treatment of kidney fixity.

COMMENTARY, LINE 11.16

Kidney fixity is a technical term referring to a condition of cold-damp impediment in the lumbus with local cold pain and heaviness that prevents normal turning and is exacerbated by yīn-type (overcast, wet) weather. It is called "kidney fixity," because the lumbus is the house of the kidney and because there is difficulty of movement due to discomfort in that area. It usually arises after sweating from strenuous physical labor and is the result of the lumbar region contracting cold-damp and of yáng qì becoming impeded. In spite of the fact that the disease is located in the lower part of the body, the bowels and viscera are not yet affected, and the patient therefore does not suffer from thirst, inhibited urination, or eating and drinking disorders. As regards treatment, there is no need to warm the kidney, since kidney fixity disappears as soon as the cold and dampness are eliminated from the channels and network vessels.

The suggested formula is Licorice, Dried Ginger, Poria, and White Atractylodes Decoction (*gān cǎo gān jiāng fú líng bái zhú tāng*). This formula makes heavy use of dried ginger (*gān jiāng*) combined with licorice (*gān cǎo*), to warm the center and dissipate cold. In addition, poria (*fú líng*) and white atractylodes (*bái zhú*) fortify the spleen and eliminate dampness. Since the formula specifically addresses kidney fixity, it is also called Kidney Fixity Decoction (*shèn zhuó tāng*).

Line 11.17

肾死藏，浮之坚，按之乱如转丸，益下入尺中者死。

Shèn sǐ zàng, fú zhī jiān, àn zhī luàn rú zhuǎn wán, yì xià rù chǐ zhōng zhě sǐ.

The dying viscus [pulse] of the kidney is hard when floated, chaotic like spinning pellets when pressed, and spills downward into the cubit,[1] [This is the sign of imminent] death.

Text Note, Line 11.17

[1] Spilling into the cubit 益下入尺中 *yì xià rù chǐ zhōng*: The character 益 *yì*, which normally means "more" or "increase," is here read as 溢 *yì*, meaning "to spill." The phrase as a whole then refers to what later texts call "falling into the cubit marsh" (垂入尺泽 *chuí rù chǐ zé*). Both expressions describe the shifting of the inch opening pulse into the region of the Cubit Marsh (*chǐ zé*, LU-5).

Synopsis, Line 11.17

This line describes the dying viscus pulse of the kidney.

Commentary, Line 11.17

A healthy kidney pulse is sunken, replete, and forceful. If the pulse instead is hard and replete when lightly pressed, this means that the pulse is not deep and is beating on the outside. This signifies that the kidney has lost the support of stomach qì, and the pulse has therefore lost its gentle and harmonious quality. When you apply pressure, this pulse feels like pellets spinning chaotically. Thus instead of the sunken replete pulse, you detect an agitated, stirred pulse, which "spills down into the cubit," i.e., is even more conspicuous at the cubit position. This signifies insecurity of true qì and heralds outward desertion.

Line 11.18

问曰：三焦竭部，上焦竭善噫，何谓也？师曰：上焦受中焦，气未和，不能消谷，故能噫耳；下焦竭，即遗溺失便，其气不和，不能自禁制，不须治，久则愈。

Wèn yuē: Sān jiāo jié bù, shàng jiāo jié shàn yì, hé wèi yě? Shī yuē: Shàng jiāo shòu zhōng jiāo, qì wèi hé, bù néng xiāo gǔ, fù néng yì ěr; xià jiāo jié, jí yí niào shī biàn, qí qì bù hé, bù néng zì jìn zhì, bù xū zhì, jiǔ zé yú.

Question: "[Regarding] exhaustion of the triple burner in [its different] sections, exhaustion in the upper burner causes a tendency to belching. Why is that?" The Master says: "The upper burner receives [qì from] the center burner. If qì is not in harmony, it cannot disperse grain,[1] hence there is belching. Exhaustion in the lower burner causes enuresis and fecal incontinence. [The reason for this is that] if qì is not in harmony, it cannot by itself ensure continence. You do not need to treat this condition; [the patient] will recover over time."

TEXT NOTE, LINE 11.18

[1] Disperse grain 消谷 *xiāo gǔ*: Digest food.

SYNOPSIS, LINE 11.18

This line describes the functional decline in the upper, center, and lower sections of the triple burner, giving rise to disease in that section or another section.

COMMENTARY, LINE 11.18

The three burners are all interrelated. For example, the upper burner receives qì from the center burner. When the functions of the spleen and stomach in the center burner are impaired so that the center burner cannot digest gain and water, the upper burner receives the putrid qì of the stomach. The result is frequent belching with the smell of food. The lower burner is associated with the kidney, bladder, small intestine, and large intestine. If the functions of these organs decline, there is enuresis or fecal incontinence. In this case, the lower burner is directly giving rise to disease.

The functions of each of the three burners are interdependent and mutually complementary. When certain functions temporarily decline, it is not always necessary to give the patient medicines. As soon as the qì of the triple burner regains its harmony and right qì is restored, the disease will naturally disappear.

Line 11.19

师曰：热在上焦者，因咳为肺痿；热在中焦者，则为坚；热在下焦者，则尿血，亦令淋秘不通。大肠有寒者，多鹜溏；有热者，便肠垢；小肠有寒者，其人下重便血，有热者必痔。

Shī yuē: Rè zài shàng jiāo zhě, yīn ké wéi fèi wěi; rè zài zhōng jiāo zhě, zé wéi jiān; rè zài xià jiāo zhě, zé niào xuè, yì lìng lín bì bù tōng. Dà cháng yǒu hán zhě, duō wù táng; yǒu rè zhě, biàn cháng gòu; xiǎo cháng yǒu hán zhě, qí rén xià zhòng biàn xuè, yǒu rè zhě bì zhì.

The Master says: "Heat in the upper burner results in coughing and because of this, lung wilting.[1] Heat in the center burner results in hardness. Heat in the lower burner results in bloody urine and also causes strangury and stoppage. Cold in the large intestine causes profuse duck's slop[2]; heat there causes intestinal grime[3] in the stool. Cold in the small intestine causes heaviness in the lower [body][4] and bloody stool; heat there invariably causes hemorrhoids."

TEXT NOTES, LINE 11.19

[1] Lung wilting 肺痿 *fèi wěi*: A condition characterized by a dull-sounding cough, ejection of thick turbid foamy drool, panting at the slightest exertion, dry mouth and pharynx, emaciation, red dry tongue, and a vacuous rapid pulse. It is attributed to dryness heat and enduring cough damaging the lung, or to damage to fluid from another disease depriving the lung of moisturization.

[2] Duck's slop 鹜溏 *wù táng*: 鹜 *wù* is an archaic word for duck, corresponding to the modern 鸭 *yā*, hence 鹜溏 *wù táng* means what is nowadays called 鸭溏 *yā táng*, i.e., a condition in which stool and water are passed together.

[2] Intestinal grime 肠垢 *cháng gòu*: This expression refers to mucus in the stool, as well as to the condition it characterizes. It is observed in heat-related dysentery.

[4] Heaviness in lower [body] 下重 *xià zhòng*: A feeling of heaviness in the anus.

SYNOPSIS, LINE 11.19

This line describes the signs of heat in the triple burner and of heat and cold in the large and small intestines.

COMMENTARY, LINE 11.19

Heat in the upper burner impairs the depurative downbearing of the spleen. The result is qì counterflow with cough. Enduring cough causes damage to both liquid and qì, which can lead to the development of lung wilting. Heat in the center burner scorches the yīn liquid of the spleen and stomach and thereby deprives the intestinal tract of moisture and makes the stool dry, bound, and hard. Heat in the lower burner affects the kidney and the bladder. When the network vessels are damaged, there is bloody urine. When heat binds in the qì aspect, it affects qì transformation, which results in dribbling urination with pain in the urethra or else dribbling urinary block.

The large intestine holds the office of conveyance. When it is affected by disease, we need to differentiate between cold and heat. As a result of cold, stool and water descend mixed, which the text refers to as "duck's slop." The result of heat is called "intestinal grime." The small intestine holds the office of receiving plenitude. When this function is impaired, we again need to differentiate between cold and heat. As a result of cold, yáng is vacuous and qì falls and fails to control the blood so that there is blood in the stool. Heat in the small intestine, on the other hand, moves to the rectum and thereby gives rise to hemorrhoids.

Line 11.20

(1)问曰：病有积、有聚、有䅽气，何谓也？师曰：积者藏病也，终不移。聚者腑病也；发作有时，辗转痛移，为可治。䅽气者胁下痛，按之则愈，复发，为䅽气。

(2)诸积大法：脉来细而附骨者，乃积也。寸口，积在胸中；微出寸口，积在喉中；关上积在脐傍；上关上，积在心下；微下关，积在少腹。尺中，积在气冲；脉出左，积在左；脉出右，积在右；脉两出，积在中央，各以其部处之。

(1) Wèn yuē: Bìng yǒu jī, yǒu jù, yǒu gǔ qì, hé wèi yě? Shī yuē: Jī zhě zàng bìng yě, zhōng bù yí; jù zhě fǔ bìng yě; fā zuò yǒu shí, zhǎn zhuǎn tòng yí, wéi kě zhì; gǔ qì zhě xié xià tòng, àn zhī zé yú, fù fā, wéi gǔ qì.

(2) Zhū jī dà fǎ: mài lái xì ér fù gǔ zhě, nǎi jī yě. Cùn kǒu, jī zài xiōng zhōng; wēi chū cùn kǒu, jī zài hóu zhōng; guān shàng jī zài qí páng; shàng guān shàng, jī zài xīn xià; wēi xià guān, jī zài shào fù. Chǐ zhōng, jī zài qì chōng; mài chū zuǒ, jī zài zuǒ; mài chū yòu, jī zài yòu; mài liǎng chū, jī zài zhōng yāng, gè yǐ qí bù chù zhī.

(1) Question: "What do the diseases accumulations, gatherings, and grain qì[1] refer to?" The Master says: "Accumulations are a disease of the viscera; they never move. Gatherings are a disease of the bowels; they erupt intermittently, spread from place to place, and manifest with mobile pain; they can be treated. Grain qì is pain under the rib-side that is relieved by pressure; when it is recurrent, it is grain qì.

(2) The general method for diagnosing the various accumulations:[2] A pulse that is fine on arrival and is fixed to the bone indicates accumulations. When [this type of pulse occurs] at the inch opening, the accumulation is in the chest; when it is slightly outside the inch opening, the accumulation is in the throat; when it is on the bar, the accumulation is beside the umbilicus; when it is above the bar,[3] the accumulation is below the heart; when it is slightly below the bar,[4] the accumulation is in the lesser abdomen; when it is in the cubit, the accumulation is in the qì thoroughfare.[5] When [this type of] pulse appears on the left, the accumulation is on the left; when [this type of] pulse appears on the right, the accumulation is on the right; when it appears on both sides, the accumulation is in the middle. You can locate each according to the position [of this pulse]."

Text Notes, Line 11.20

[1] Grain qì 槃气 *gŭ qì*: The character 槃 is an archaic alternative form of 穀, which is now written as 谷.

[2] Various accumulations 诸积 *zhū jī*: This includes the accumulations of the five viscera described in the *Nàn Jīng* ("Classic of Difficult Issues"), Chapter 56: Deep-lying beam (伏梁 *fú liáng*), the accumulation of the heart; fat qì (肥气 *féi qì*), the accumulation of the liver; glomus qì (痞气 *pĭ qì*), the accumulation of the spleen; rushing respiration (息贲 *xī bēn*), the accumulation of the lung; and running piglet (奔豚 *bēn tún*), the accumulation of the kidney. All these can be caused by accumulation and stagnation of qì, blood, food, phlegm, and worms.

[3] Above the bar 上关上 *shàng guān shàng*: Distal to the bar position.

[4] Slightly below the bar 下关 *xià guān*: Proximal to the bar position.

[5] Qì thoroughfare 气冲 *qì chōng*: Name of an acupuncture point on the foot yáng brightness stomach channel, also known as Qì Street (*qì jiē*, ST-30), located on either side below the umbilicus.

Synopsis, Line 11.20

This line describes how to identify accumulations, gatherings, and grain qì, and how to determine their location by the pulse.

Commentary, Line 11.20

Accumulations and gatherings are both lumps in the body. Accumulations are a disease in the viscera; they do not move when pushed. Accordingly they are associated with pain of fixed location. Gatherings are a disease of the bowels; they are of unfixed location, and come and go. Accumulations are more severe and harder to treat than gatherings. Grain qì refers to conditions that combine blockage of grain qì with binding depression of liver qì. In grain qì, we see pain beneath the rib-side that is relieved by pressure. However, the relief is only temporary and the pain returns. The grain qì has to be dispersed in order to eliminate the pain definitively.

The second section presents the pulse diagnosis of accumulations. The first statement points out that the pulse that indicates accumulations is fine and stuck to the bone, i.e., fine and sunken or hidden. The rest of this section proposes correspondences between the pulse and locations of the accumulation. In terms of clinical application, these are of dubious value.

痰饮咳嗽病脉证治第十二

CHAPTER 12

Phlegm-Rheum and Cough

Pulses, Signs, Treatments

‡ OVERVIEW

According to the title, this chapter appears to discuss phlegm-rheum and cough as two disease categories. In actuality, the subject of this section is phlegm-rheum, and cough is merely dealt with as one symptom of it. Cough due to other causes is not discussed.

"Phlegm-rheum" (痰饮 *tán yǐn*) is a general term for pathological phlegm-like and drool-like fluids. The Chinese 饮 *yǐn* literally means "drink," and in other contexts refers to ingested fluids. Its medical use as a term meaning pathological fluid seems to be derived from this. In its sense as pathological fluid, we translate 饮 *yǐn* as "rheum," which is a term derived from the Greek word denoting pathological fluid, because a literal translation could be confusing to the reader. Early medical texts like the *Mài Jīng* and *Qiān Jīn Fāng* refer to phlegm-rheum as 淡饮 *dàn yǐn*, a compound of 饮 *yǐn* with the word 淡 *dàn*, which in other contexts means "bland" or "flavorless," but in pre-Sòng medical literature is used also in the sense of pathological fluid. The word 痰 *tán*, phlegm, does not appear in the *Nèi Jīng* or in China's earliest dictionary, the *Shuō Wén Jiě Zì* ("Explanation of Simple Graphs and Complex Characters"). It is first found in the present chapter of the *Jīn Guì Yào Lüè*. It was most likely derived from 淡 *dàn* as a way to distinguish the latter character's more recent association of pathological fluid. Medical literature from the Sòng period onward uses 痰 *tán* ("phlegm") to denote a thick turbid substance, and 饮 *yǐn* ("rheum") to denote a thinner, clearer form of pathological fluid. Although the present chapter is titled 痰饮 *tán yǐn*, it primarily focuses on conditions associated with thin pathological fluid, 饮 *yǐn*, particularly in the context of cold-rheum.

In this chapter, phlegm-rheum is used as a generic term to denote a disease that takes four specific forms: phlegm-rheum, suspended rheum, spillage rheum, and propping rheum. Thus, use of the term "phlegm-rheum" is not only generic, but also denotes one of the four specific forms. The four kinds of phlegm-rheum are distinguished by location. "Phlegm-rheum" (in the narrow sense) is water-rheum collecting in the stomach and intestines, which is identified by rumbling intestines. "Suspended rheum" is water-rheum collecting in the rib-side, which is identified by cough associated with pain in the rib-side. Spillage rheum is water-rheum flowing out into the flesh of the four limbs, which is identified by pain in the limbs and a subjective feeling of heaviness. "Propping rheum" is water-rheum collecting in the chest and diaphragm, which is identified by shortness of breath preventing the patient from lying down.

In addition to the four above-mentioned specific forms, the present chapter furthermore discusses the diseases of lodged rheum and deep-lying rheum.

‡ Schematic Overview

Patterns

1. Phlegm-rheum patterns (narrow meaning)
   a) *Location*: Stomach and intestines.
   b) *Pathomechanism:* Impairment of splenic movement and transformation.
   c) *Main signs*: Water moving in the intestines, producing a gurgling sound and causing abdominal fullness; dry mouth and tongue.
      Rheum collecting below the heart: cold in the back [an area] the size of a hand; propping rheum in the chest and rib-side; dizzy vision; shortness of breath.
      Phegm-rheum in the stomach: vomiting of phlegm-drool.
      Water below the heart due to insufficiency of kidney yáng: urinary abnormalities; shortness of breath; heart palpitation.
      Rheum collecting in the lower burnering affecting the center and upper burners: palpitation below the umbilicius, ejection of foamy drool, and dizziness.
      Rheum that fails to go: hidden pulse, urge to spontaneously defecate, relief after diarrhea, and continuing hardness and fullness below the heart despite diarrhea.
2. Suspended rheum patterns
   a) *Location*: rib-side.
   b) *Pathomechanism*: Phlegm rheum accumulating in the triple burner and disharmony of the liver and gallbladder vessel networks.
   c) *Main signs*: Fullness and distention in the chest and rib-side; cough and spitting that causes pain; dry retching; shortness of breath; and a pulse that is stringlike.
3. Spillage rheum patterns
   a) *Location*: Flesh and skin.

b) *Pathomechanism*: Absence of sweating when there should have been sweating; impairment of the lung's diffusion and depurative downbearing; impairment of the spleen's movement and transformation.

c) *Main signs*: Aversion to cold; absence of sweating; generalized pain and heavy-headedness; pain in the joints; cough, panting, and vomiting of phlegm-drool; a pulse that is floating and tight or stringlike and tight.

4. Propping rheum patterns

a) *Location*: Propping rheum in the heart, lung, chest, and diaphragm.

b) *Pathomechanism*: Insufficiency of chest yáng causing rheum to collect in the chest and diaphragm, affecting both heart and lung.

c) *Main signs*: Cough counterflow; propped breathing, shortness of breath, and inability to lie flat; panting and fullness; hard glomus below the heart; veiling dizziness; heart palpitation; pain in the chest; vomiting and retching; absence of thirst; soot-black facial complexion; swollen appearance of the body; stringlike pulse.

Treatment

1. Main treatment principle: harmonize with warm medicinals.

a) Warming yáng and transforming rheum:

Mild spleen-stomach yáng vacuity with propping rheum: Disinhibit water and supplement the spleen with Alisma Decoction (*zé xiè tāng*).

Severe spleen-stomach yáng vacuity with phlegm-rheum or propping rheum: Warm the center and downbear counterflow using Poria, Cinnamon Twig, White Atractylodes, and Licorice Decoction (*líng guì zhú gān tāng*).

Spleen yáng vacuity with cold rheum gathering and impairment of triple burner and bladder qì transformation with phlegm-rheum: Promote qì transformation and move water using Poria Five Powder (*wǔ líng sǎn*).

Propping rheum or phlegm-rheum of recent onset due to stomach yáng vacuity and counterflow ascent of water-rheum: Warm the stomach and downbear counterflow with Minor Pinellia Decoction (*xiǎo bàn xià tāng*).

Propping rheum or phlegm-rheum of older onset due to stomach yáng vacuity and counterflow ascent of water-rheum: Abduct rheum downwards with Minor Pinellia Decoction Plus Poria (*xiǎo bàn xià jiā fú líng tāng*).

Propping rheum due to insufficiency of kidney qì preventing qì transformation and the movement of water, with water qì intimidating the heart manifesting in palpitation below the heart, shortness of breath, and urinary irregularities: warm the kidney and promote qì transformation with Kidney Qì Pill (*shèn qì wán*).

Phlegm-rheum or propping rheum due to phlegm and water in the heart and chest, which after being ejected leaves the vacuity in the heart and chest, qì fullness, and inability to eat: Supplement the spleen, disperse phlegm qì and eliminate distention and fullness using Poria Beverage (*fú líng yǐn*) from the *Wài Tái Mì Yào* ("Secrets from the *Wài Tái* Library").

Kidney yáng vacuity with persistent rheum, affecting the lung, spleen, and kidney and giving rise to cough, panting, and fullness in the chest: Cinnamon, Poria, Schisandra, and Licorice Decoction (*guì líng wǔ wèi gān cǎo tāng*); Poria, Licorice, Schisandra, Ginger, and Asarum Decoction (*líng gān wǔ wèi jiāng xīn tāng*); Poria, Licorice, Schisandra, Ginger, Asarum, Pinellia Decoction (*líng gān wǔ wèi jiāng xīn bàn xià tāng*); Poria, Licorice, Schisandra, Ginger, Asarum, Pinellia and Apricot Kernel Decoction (*líng gān wǔ wèi jiāng xīn bàn xià xìng rén tāng*); or Poria, Licorice, Schisandra, Ginger, Asarum, Pinellia, Apricot Kernel and Rhubarb Decoction (*líng gān wǔ wèi jiāng xīn bàn xià xìng dà huáng tāng*).

b) Dual resolution of the exterior and interior: This applies when there is internal rheum with external cold disturbing the lung.

Propping rheum or spillage rheum: Transform rheum and resolve the exterior using Minor Black Dragon Decoction (*xiǎo qīng lóng tāng*).

External wind cold with rheum evil lying depressed and transforming into heat: promote sweating, clear heat, and dispel rheum using Major Black Dragon Decoction (*dà qīng lóng tāng*).

c) Coursing the stomach and intestines:

Phlegm-rheum lying depressed in the stomach and intestines, transforming into heat, affecting splenic movement and transformation, and giving rise to abdominal fullness and and dry tongue and mouth: Fangji, Zanthoxylum, Lepidium/Descurainiae, and Rhubarb Pill (*jǐ jiāo lì huáng wán*).

Heat and rheum binding in the chest and stomach to create propping rheum with distention and fullness in the chest and abdomen: Expel rheum, flush heat, move qì, and resolve depression with Officinal Magnolia Bark and Rhubarb Decoction (*hòu pò dà huáng tāng*).

d) Drain water and expel rheum:

Phlegm-rheum due to water-rheum shooting into the lung, giving rise to panting and inability to lie down: Discharge the lung and expel water using Lepidium/Descurainiae and Jujube Lung-Draining Decoction (*tíng lì dà zǎo xiè fèi tāng*).

Phlegm-rheum: Expel water-rheum through the stool and urine using Kansui and Pinellia Decoction (*gān suì bàn xià tāng*).

e) Supporting right and dispelling rheum:

Propping rheum with vacuity of right and rheum and heat binding together that fails to respond to ejection or precipitation: Free yáng, disinhibit water, supplement vacuity and clear heat using Woody Fangji Decoction (*mù fáng jǐ tāng*).

Peristent hard glomus below the heart: Free yáng, disinhibit water, soften hardness, and supplement vacuity using Woody Fangji Decoction Minus Gypsum Plus Poria and Mirabilite (*mù fáng jǐ qù shí gāo jiā fú líng máng xiāo tāng*).

Line 12.1

问曰：夫饮有四，何谓也？师曰：有痰饮，有悬饮，有溢饮，有支饮。

Wèn yuē: Fū yǐn yǒu sì, hé wèi yě? Shī yuē: Yǒu tán yǐn, yǒu xuán yǐn, yǒu yì yǐn, yǒu zhī yǐn.

Question: "There are four [kinds of] rheum. What are they?" The Master says: "There is phlegm-rheum, suspended rheum, spillage rheum, and propping rheum."

Synopsis, Line 12.1

This line lists the four specific forms of phlegm-rheum.

Commentary, Line 12.1

The present chapter uses the term "rheum" (饮 *yǐn*) as a generic concept to refer to drool-like pathological fluid (see the chapter introduction). In this line, it carries the same meaning as the compound term "phlegm-rheum" (痰饮 *tán yǐn*) appearing in the chapter title. The present line mentions four kinds of rheum, which later physicians refer to as the "four rheums." Note that one of the four types of rheum is called "phlegm-rheum." This is a particular kind of rheum, which is different from "phlegm-rheum," as it is used in the general sense. The following lines discuss the four kinds of rheum in detail.

Line 12.2

问曰：四饮何以为异？师曰：其人素盛今瘦，水走肠间，沥沥有声，谓之痰饮；饮后水流在胁下，咳唾引痛，谓之悬饮；饮水流行，归于四肢，当汗出而不汗出，身体疼重，谓之溢饮；咳逆倚息，气短不得卧，其形如肿，谓之支饮。

Wèn yuē: Sì yǐn hé yǐ wéi yì? Shī yuē: Qí rén sù shèng jīn shòu, shuǐ zǒu cháng jiān, lì lì yǒu shēng, wèi zhī tán yǐn; yǐn hòu shuǐ liú zài xié xià, ké tuò yǐn tòng, wèi zhī xuán yǐn; yǐn shuǐ liú xíng, guī yú sì zhī, dāng hàn chū ér bù hàn chū, shēn tǐ téng zhòng, wèi zhī yì yǐn; ké nì yǐ xī, qì duǎn bù dé wò, qí xíng rú zhǒng, wèi zhī zhī yǐn.

Question: "How do you differentiate between the four rheums?" The Master says: "When a person with a plentiful constitution becomes emaciated[1] and has water running into the intestines with gurgling sounds, [this] means phlegm-rheum. When drinking and the water afterwards flows under the rib-side, resulting in coughing and spitting that induces pain, [this] means suspended rheum. When [a person] drinks water and this water homes to the limbs, resulting in absence of sweating when the person should sweat, and in generalized pain and heaviness, [this] means spillage rheum. Cough counterflow and propped breathing,[2] with shortness of breath and inability to lie down, and an appearance as if swollen means propping rheum."

Text Notes, Line 12.2

[1] Plentiful constitution…becomes emaciated 素盛今瘦 *sù shèng jīn shòu*: Well-built or adequately fleshed before the illness developed, but now emaciated as a result of the illness.

[2] Cough counterflow and propped breathing 咳逆倚息 *ké nì yǐ xī*: Cough counterflow means cough and counterflow qì ascent that manifests as panting. Propped breathing denotes a condition in which the patient can only breathe comfortably when propped up.

Synopsis, Line 12.2

This line describes the signs and pathomechanisms of the four rheums.

Commentary, Line 12.2

The present line lucidly describes the four kinds of rheum, and we can add little to make the content clearer. The first kind of rheum, "phlegm-rheum," refers to water-rheum that collects in the stomach and intestines. Because it is fluid in nature, it causes a gurgling sound in the intestinal tract, which is the key sign of this condition. Under normal circumstances, the spleen moves and transforms grain and water (the solid and liquid foods ingested into the body). When this function is disturbed, water can collect and gather to form phlegm-rheum. At the same time, the impaired function of the spleen can deprive the flesh of nourishment. Hence, phlegm-rheum is often accompanied by emaciation.

"Suspended rheum" means water-rheum collecting in the rib-side. It gives rise to cough with copious phlegm, and resulting pain in the rib-side.

"Spillage rheum" refers to a condition of excessive water-rheum soaking into the skin and spilling outward into the four limbs. Failing to be discharged through sweating, it collects and hence causes generalized pain and heaviness.

"Propping rheum" means water-rheum collecting in the chest and diaphragm and obstructing the diffusion and downbearing of the lung. The main sign is cough and counterflow with propped breathing, i.e., cough with counterflow ascent of qì that manifests in shortness of breath so severe that it prevents the patient from breathing comfortably in a fully reclined posture and forces him/her to rest propped up with pillows.

Line 12.3

水在心，心下坚筑，短气，恶水，不欲饮。

Shuǐ zài xīn, xīn xià jiān zhù, duǎn qì, wù shuǐ, bù yù yǐn.

Water in the heart [manifests in] hardness and pounding below the heart,[1] shortness of breath, aversion to water, and no desire to drink.

TEXT NOTE, LINE 12.3

[1] Hardness and pounding below the heart 心下坚筑 *xīn xià jiān zhù*: The character 筑 *zhù* presently means to construct (buildings), but an earlier meaning was "to pound earth to make it solid." Hardness and pounding below the heart means hard glomus below the heart with fullness, oppression, and palpitation like the pounding of earth.

SYNOPSIS, LINE 12.3

This line describes the signs of water-rheum in the heart.

COMMENTARY, LINE 12.3

Water-rheum not only collects in the intestines, rib-side, chest and diaphragm, and limbs, but can also affect the five viscera. Note, however, that water-rheum does not actually collect in the viscus itself, but rather outside the viscus, and merely affects its function.

When water-rheum intimidates the heart, the result is hard glomus beneath the heart and palpitation. When water-rheum obstructs heart yáng, we also see shortness of breath and aversion to water, as a result of which the patient has no desire to drink.

Line 12.4

水在肺，吐涎沫，欲饮水。

Shuǐ zài fèi, tǔ xián mò, yù yǐn shuǐ.

Water in the lung [manifests as] ejection of drool and foam, and desire to drink water.

SYNOPSIS, LINE 12.4

This line describes the signs of water-rheum in the lung.

COMMENTARY, LINE 12.4

The lung governs qì, moves construction and defense, regulates the waterways, and distributes fluid. When water-rheum shoots into the lung, it disinhibits lung qì, collects in the lung, and transforms into drool and foam. Water-rheum and qì dash against each other, and water floods upwards with qì, giving rise to ejection of drool and foam. Because qì fails to transform liquid, there is an excess of liquid, which is not dispersed around the body, but ejected outward. Since the lung and stomach are deprived of moistening, the patient desires to drink water.

Line 12.5

水在脾，少气身重。

Shuǐ zài pí, shǎo qì shēn zhòng.

Water in the spleen [manifests in] shortage of qì[1] and generalized heaviness.

TEXT NOTE, LINE 12.5

[1] Shortage of qì 少气 *shǎo qì*: Shortness of breath; mild breathing difficulty.

SYNOPSIS, LINE 12.5

This line describes the signs of water-rheum in the spleen.

COMMENTARY, LINE 12.5

The spleen is averse to dampness. When water-rheum invades and encumbers the spleen, it causes insufficiency of center qì, which results in shortage of qì. Since the spleen governs the flesh, water-rheum invading the spleen can affect the flesh, giving rise to generalized heaviness.

Line 12.6

水在肝，胁下支满，嚏而痛。

Shuǐ zài gān, xié xià zhī mǎn, tì ér tòng.

Water in the liver [manifests in] propping fullness under the rib-side[1] and pain on sneezing.

TEXT NOTE, LINE 12.6

[1] Propping fullness under the rib-side 胁下支满 *xié xià zhī mǎn*: Distention and fullness inside the body at the lower end of the ribs that makes the patient feel as if the area was propped up.

SYNOPSIS, LINE 12.6

This line describes the signs of water-rheum in the liver.

COMMENTARY, LINE 12.6

When water-rheum invades the liver, it can cause depression of liver qì and disharmony in the liver network vessels. As a result, there is propping distention and fullness beneath the rib-side. Water-rheum follows the liver channel upward into the lung and prevents lung qì from perfusing, which results in sneezing. Because this sneezing is not due to a contraction of external evil but to water-rheum in the liver network vessels, sneezing is followed by pain below the rib-side.

Line 12.7

水在肾，心下悸。

Shuǐ zài shèn, xīn xià jì.

Water in the kidney [manifests in] palpitation below the heart.

Synopsis, Line 12.7

This line describes the signs of water-rheum in the kidney.

Commentary, Line 12.7

Water-rheum that invades the kidney debilitates the life gate fire and prevents kidney qì from properly transforming qì and moving the fluids. As a result, water amasses below the umbilicus and surges counterflow, causing stirring palpitation.

Line 12.8

夫心下有留饮，其人背寒冷如手大。

Fū xīn xià yǒu liú yǐn, qí rén bèi hán lěng rú shǒu dà.

Lodged rheum below the heart manifests in cold in the back [over an area] as large as a hand.

Synopsis, Line 12.8

This line describes the signs of lodged rheum below the heart.

Commentary, Line 12.8

Lodged rheum means water-rheum that collects instead of dispersing. Apart from the accumulation of fluid itself, lodged rheum also obstructs yáng qì. When cold rheum floods into the heart transport points, which are located on the back, yáng qì is unable to outthrust, which impairs the warming function of the governing vessel. Thus, lodged rheum below the heart results in coldness in a palm-sized area on the back.

Line 12.9

留饮者，胁下痛引缺盆，咳嗽则辄已。

Liú yǐn zhě, xié xià tòng yǐn quē pén, ké sòu zé zhé yǐ.

Lodged rheum [manifests in] pain under the rib-side stretching into the supraclavicular fossa that is exacerbated by coughing.[1]

TEXT NOTE, LINE 12.9

[1] Exacerbated by coughing 咳嗽则辄已 *ké sòu zé zhé yǐ*: There are two antithetical interpretations of the phrase 辄已 *zhé yǐ*. One is that the pain stops immediately on coughing; the other is that it intensifies on coughing. The latter interpretation, which most modern editions as well as the present translation follow, is supported by an alternative version that is found in a citation of this line in the *Qiān Jīn Fāng* ("Thousand Gold Pieces Prescriptions"). There, the phrase is replaced with the characters 转甚 *zhuǎn shèn*, which means "turns more severe." The problem hinges on the translation of the character 辄 *zhé*, which has two different meanings. It can either mean "immediately" or "resolute/ruthless." To complicate matters further, the character 已 *yǐ* means to stop, but can also serve as simply a final particle.

SYNOPSIS, LINE 12.9

This line describes the signs of lodged rheum beneath the rib-side.

COMMENTARY, LINE 12.9

Lodged rheum beneath the rib-side causes disharmony of the network vessels of the liver, which is a suspended rheum pattern. Water-rheum lodging below the rib-side not only impairs the upward and downward bearing action of the qì dynamic in the liver and lung, but also inhibits the flow in the liver and gallbladder channel. The result is pain beneath the rib-side stretching into the supraclavicular fossa that is exacerbated by coughing.

Line 12.10

胸中有留饮，其人短气而渴，四肢历节痛，脉沉者，有留饮。

Xiōng zhōng yǒu liú yǐn, qí rén duǎn qì ér kě, sì zhī lì jié tòng, mài chén zhě, yǒu liú yǐn.

Lodged rheum in the chest [manifests in] shortness of breath and thirst, joint-running pain in the four limbs,[1] and a sunken pulse. [This indicates] the presence of lodged rheum.

TEXT NOTE, LINE 12.10

[1] Joint-running pain in the four limbs 四肢历节痛 *sì zhī lì jié tòng*: Pain pervading the joints of the limbs.

SYNOPSIS, LINE 12.10

This line describes the signs and pulse of lodged rheum in the chest or limbs.

COMMENTARY, LINE 12.10

When rheum lodges in the chest, it prevents lung qì from downbearing and inhibits breathing; hence we see shortness of breath. Because the fluids are not transformed, the diaphragm dries out; hence there is thirst.

Lodged rheum is similar in nature to the disease evil dampness in how it affects the joints. Since the lung governs qì, rheum evil can follow lung qì and stream into the joints in the limbs. There, it impedes the joints and causes stoppage of yáng qì, as a result of which we see joint-running pain and a sunken pulse. Since internal blockage of yáng qì is a necessary component of all conditions of lodged rheum, they should all manifest with a sunken pulse, regardless of the location of the disease. Sunken pulse is therefore an important sign for diagnosing lodged rheum (see line 14.10).

Line 12.11

膈上病痰，满喘咳吐，发则寒热，背痛腰疼，目泣自出，其人振振身瞤剧，必有伏饮。

Gé shàng bìng tán, mǎn chuǎn ké tù, fā zé hán rè, bèi tòng yāo téng, mù qì zì chū, qí rén zhèn zhèn shēn shùn jù, bì yǒu fú yǐn.

[A patient] suffering from phlegm above the diaphragm [will have] fullness, panting, cough, and vomiting, [aversion to] cold and heat [effusion] during episodes, back and lumbar pain, spontaneous tearing, and severe quivering twitching of the body.[1] These invariably [indicate] the presence of deep-lying rheum.

TEXT NOTE, LINE 12.11

[1] Severe quivering and twitching of the body 振振身瞤剧 *zhèn zhèn shēn rún jù*: Severe tremor.

SYNOPSIS, LINE 12.11

This line describes the signs of phlegm-rheum lying hidden above the diaphragm, during and between episodes.

COMMENTARY, LINE 12.11

Deep-lying rheum means rheum lodged in the inner body that erupts in episodes and is difficult to eliminate. When there is deep-lying rheum above the diaphragm, it obstructs lung qì. The result is fullness in the chest, panting, and cough, as well as vomiting of phlegm-drool. If the patient contracts wind-cold, this will stir deep-lying rheum. Externally contracted wind-cold damages greater yáng, and this gives rise to aversion to cold and heat effusion, pain in the lumbar and back, and generalized discomfort. When the cold fetters the exterior and stirs the rheum internally, the combination of the external and internal evils distresses the lung, giving rise to cough that is so severe as to cause spontaneous tearing. When the external evil stirs the deep-lying rheum and obstructs the diffusion of yáng qì, the whole body trembles uncontrollably.

Commentators have differed in their interpretation of the nature and scope of deep-lying rheum. Some scholars such as a Chén Xiū-Yuán 陈修园 believe that it refers to "wheezing and panting" (asthma). Others such as Táng Róng-Chuān 唐容川 claim that the scope is larger than this. Xú Zhōng-Kě 徐忠可 and Lù Yuān-Léi 陆渊雷 suggest that deep-lying rheum falls within the scope of propping rheum. Liáng Yùn-Tōng 梁运通 lastly has identified deep-lying rheum as a recurrent condition associated with enduring illness.

Line 12.12

夫病人饮水多，必暴喘满，凡食少饮多，水停心下，甚者则悸，微者短气。脉双弦者寒也，皆大下后喜虚。脉偏弦者饮也。

Fū bìng rén yǐn shuǐ duō, bì bào chuǎn mǎn, fán shí shǎo yǐn duō, shuǐ tíng xīn xià, shèn zhě zé jì, wēi zhě duǎn qì. Mài shuāng xián zhě hán yě, jiē dà xià hòu xǐ xū. Mài piān xián zhě yǐn yě.

When a patient drinks much water, there will inevitably be fulminant panting and fullness. Whenever [a patient] eats little and drinks much, water collects below the heart. In severe cases, [this results in] palpitation; in mild cases, in shortness of breath. When the pulses on both sides are stringlike, [this means] cold, which is always [due to] a tendency toward vacuity after major precipitation. When the pulse on one side is stringlike,[1] [this means] rheum.

TEXT NOTE, LINE 12.12

[1] The pulse on one side is stringlike 脉偏弦者 *mài piān xián zhě*: One of the wrist pulses is stringlike.

SYNOPSIS, LINE 12.12

This line describes the cause, pathomechanism, signs, and pulses of phlegm-rheum in the broad sense.

COMMENTARY, LINE 12.12

Although the line only mentions "water collecting below the heart" and "rheum," commentators generally agree that it describes the causes, signs, and pulses of phlegm-rheum in general. Excessive consumption of fluid can cause fulminant panting and fullness. This may be an isolated event. If a patient with a weak spleen and stomach eats little and drinks much, water can collect below the heart. In severe cases, this hampers breathing, resulting in shortness of breath. It is also possible that water qì intimidates the heart, giving rise to palpitation.

Phlegm-rheum is mostly characterized by a stringlike pulse, which is also characteristic of vacuity cold. However, there may be a difference. After major precipitation, when the interior is vacuous and yáng is debilitated, the patient suffers from generalized vacuity cold, so the pulse is stringlike, and usually moderate and forceless, on both wrists. In phlegm-rheum, however, the water-rheum often pours into one side of the body or the other. Thus, the pulse of only one wrist is stringlike. This is particularly true in the case of suspended rheum when there may also be pain in one rib-side. Nevertheless, as the following line 12.13 states, lung rheum does not have to manifest with a stringlike pulse, while line 12.14 suggests that in propping rheum the pulse may be normal.

Line 12.13

肺饮不弦，但苦喘短气。

Fèi yǐn bù xián, dàn kǔ chuǎn duǎn qì.

In lung rheum,[1] [the pulse is] not stringlike, and [the patient] only suffers from panting and shortness of breath.

TEXT NOTE, LINE 12.13

[1] Lung rheum 肺饮 *fèi yǐn*: Water-rheum invading the lung; propping rheum.

SYNOPSIS, LINE 12.13

This line describes the pulse and signs of water-rheum in the lung.

COMMENTARY, LINE 12.13

Lung rheum refers to propping rheum in the area of the heart and lung. The lung governs breathing and qì. When water-rheum invades the lung, lung qì ascends counterflow and causes panting characterized by short, hasty breathing that prevents the patient from lying flat.

In cases of rheum in the lung, we do not necessarily see the stringlike pulse that the text has previously identified as a key symptom of rheum disease in general. Commentators have interpreted the absence of a stringlike pulse as indicating a) that the disease has not yet progressed to a deep level, b) that this emphasizes the fact that the disease is located in the lung and does not affect the vessels, and c) that this is a special characteristic of propping rheum, in contrast to suspended rheum, which manifests in a stringlike pulse. Regardless of the particular reasoning, in clinical application we need to apply all four methods of diagnosis together, instead of relying solely on pulse diagnosis, to identify rheum disease.

Line 12.14

支饮亦喘而不能卧，加短气，其脉平也。

Zhī yǐn yì chuǎn ér bù néng wò, jiā duǎn qì, qí mài píng yě.

Propping rheum [may] also [manifest in] panting and inability to lie down, plus[1] shortness of breath; [in such cases,] the pulse is normal.

TEXT NOTE, LINE 12.14

[1] Plus 加 *jiā*: The character 加 *jiā* is quite possibly a redundant addition to the original text.

SYNOPSIS, LINE 12.14

This line describes the signs and pulse of propping rheum.

COMMENTARY, LINE 12.14

This line repeats some of the information about propping rheum contained in line 2, which described the symptoms of propping rheum this way: "Cough counterflow and propped breathing, with shortness of breath and inability to lie down, and an appearance as if swollen means propping rheum." The present line describes a condition of panting characterized by short, hasty breathing that prevents the patient from lying flat. It does not mention swelling, but draws attention to the patient's "normal," that is, healthy, pulse.

As to the "normal" pulse, commentators have interpreted this in two slightly different ways. One is that it refers to the pulse being like that of a normal, healthy person. It thus indicates that the rheum evil has not yet penetrated deeply enough into the body to be reflected in a stringlike pulse. The second interpretation is that "normal" means not stringlike, thus suggesting that propping rheum does not necessarily manifest with a stringlike pulse. Hence, the discerning physician must beware not to misdiagnose this disease on the basis of the pulse.

Line 12.15

病痰饮者，当以温药和之。

Bìng tán yǐn zhě, dāng yǐ wēn yào hé zhī.

[When a patient] is sick with phlegm-rheum, harmonize with warm medicinals.

Synopsis, Line 12.15

This line presents the general principle for treating phlegm-rheum.

Commentary, Line 12.14

Rheum is a yīn evil and damages yáng qì. Hence, rheum disease usually takes the form of a combined vacuity and repletion pattern. When yáng qì is able to perform movement and transformation, rheum will spontaneously disappear. For this reason, the main principle of treatment is to restore the harmony of the body with warm medicinals to vitalize yáng qì, open the interstices, and free the waterways.

The medicinals Zhāng Jī uses in the treatment of phlegm-rheum include cinnamon twig (*guì zhī*), white atractylodes (*bái zhú*), aconite (*fù zǐ*), asarum (*xì xīn*), dried ginger (*gān jiāng*), fresh ginger (*shēng jiāng*), pinellia (*bàn xià*), and zanthoxylum seed (*jiāo mù*). The formula most representative of the principle of harmonizing with warm medicines is Poria, Cinnamon Twig, White Atractylodes, and Licorice Decoction (*líng guì zhú gān tāng*). Other major formulas are Kidney Qì Pill (*shèn qì wán*), Minor Black Dragon Decoction (*xiǎo qīng lóng tāng*), and True Warrior Decoction (*zhēn wǔ tāng*). All these formulas exemplify the principle of harmonizing with warm medicinals.

Contemporary scholars generally agree on this interpretation of the present line. In the past, however, different interpretations have been proposed. Some scholars have said that "harmonizing with warm medicines" refers to a method of adjustment after the water-rheum has been eliminated, or to a method of adjustment that should be combined with sweating, disinhibiting urine, and expelling rheum. Still others have argued that harmonizing with warm medicinals is not the method of treatment appropriate for phlegm-rheum, proposing that "harmonize" (和 *hé*) is a mistake for "disinhibit" (利 *lì*).

Line 12.16

心下有痰饮，胸胁支满，目眩，苓桂术甘汤主之。

茯苓四两 桂枝 白术各三两 甘草二两

右四味，以水六升，煮取三升，分温三服，小便则利。

Xīn xià yǒu tán yǐn, xiōng xié zhī mǎn, mù xuàn, líng guì zhú gān tāng zhǔ zhī.

Fú líng sì liǎng; guì zhī; bái zhú gè sān liǎng; gān cǎo èr liǎng

Yòu sì wèi, yǐ shuǐ liù shēng, zhǔ qǔ sān shēng, fēn wēn sān fú, xiǎo biàn zé lì.

For phlegm-rheum below the heart [manifesting in] propping fullness[1] in the chest and rib-side, and dizzy vision, Poria, Cinnamon Twig, White Atractylodes, and Licorice Decoction (苓桂术甘汤 *líng guì zhú gān tāng*) governs.

Poria, Cinnamon Twig, White Atractylodes, and Licorice Decoction (苓桂术甘汤 *líng guì zhú gān tāng*)

poria (茯苓 *fú líng*, Poria) 4 *liǎng*
cinnamon twig (桂枝 *guì* zhī, Cinnamomi Ramulus) 3 *liǎng*
white atractylodes (白术 *bái zhú*, Atractylodis Macrocephalae Rhizoma) 3 *liǎng*
licorice (甘草 *gān cǎo*, Glycyrrhizae Radix) 2 *liǎng*

Boil the above four ingredients in six *shēng* of water to get three *shēng*. Divide into three doses and take warm. This will disinhibit urine.

TEXT NOTE, LINE 12.16

[1] Propping fullness 支满 *zhī mǎn*: A feeling of fullness that the patient subjectively feels is propping them up.

SYNOPSIS, LINE 12.16

This line describes the signs and treatment of phlegm-rheum in the narrow sense.

COMMENTARY, LINE 12.16

The region below the heart refers to the stomach. When rheum collects in the stomach, the result is propping fullness in the chest and rib-side. When rheum is obstructing the center, clear yáng fails to bear upward; hence there is dizzy head and vision.

Treat this condition with Poria, Cinnamon Twig, White Atractylodes, and Licorice Decoction (*líng guì zhú gān tāng*), which has the effect of warming yáng and eliminating rheum, as well as fortifying the spleen and disinhibiting water. Poria (*fú líng*) disinhibits water by bland percolation, while cinnamon twig (*guì zhī*) frees yáng with warmth and acridity. These two medicinals in combination warm yáng and transform water. White atractylodes (*bái zhú*) fortifies the spleen and dries dampness, while licorice (*gān cǎo*) harmonizes the center and boosts qì. These two medicinals assist each other to supplement earth and dam water.

Line 12.17

夫短气有微饮，当从小便去之，苓桂朮甘汤主之。肾气丸亦主之。

Fū duǎn qì yǒu wēi yǐn, dāng cóng xiǎo biàn qù zhī, líng guì zhú gān tāng zhǔ zhī. shèn qì wán yì zhǔ zhī.

In shortness of breath with mild rheum, eliminate [the rheum] through the urine. Poria, Cinnamon Twig, White Atractylodes, and Licorice Decoction (*líng guì zhú gān tāng*) governs.[1] Kidney Qì Pill (*shèn qì wán*) also governs.[2]

Text Notes, Line 12.17

[1] The commentary adds: "For the formula, see above." This refers to the previous line.

[2] The commentary adds: "For the formula, see the chapter, "Miscellaneous Women's Diseases." This refers to 22.19 below.

Synopsis, Line 12.17

This line describes the signs and treatment of mild rheum.

Commentary, Line 12.17

In cases of mild rheum, the outward signs are not marked and can be limited to shortness of breath. However, the water-rheum causes internal obstruction and prevents yáng qì from performing transformation. The root of this condition lies in the spleen and kidney, and should be treated as early as possible. When water-rheum gathers, it hampers the upbearing and downbearing of qì; hence there is shortness of breath. When yáng qì fails to perform transformation, urination is inhibited; hence the text advises to eliminate the rheum through the urine, i.e., by promoting qì transformation and disinhibiting urine. When qì transformation is restored, water moves and rheum has a way out, so that the shortness of breath also disappears spontaneously.

The line offers two formulas. This is because the problem may lie in either the spleen or the kidney, which each require their own treatment. When the problem lies in the spleen, water collects and forms into rheum as a result of center yáng failing to move. In such cases, the signs include counterflow fullness below the heart and dizziness upon rising. For the reasons outlined in the commentary on the previous line, which also apply in this case, we treat this condition with Poria, Cinnamon Twig, White Atractylodes, and Licorice Decoction (*líng guì zhú gān tāng*). However, if the problem is rooted in the kidney, yáng vacuity in the lower burner impairs the transformation of water and hence causes the development of rheum. Consequently, water floods up to the region below the heart. In such cases, the signs include fear of cold, cold in the lower extremities, and tension in the smaller abdomen. In such cases, the recommended treatment is Kidney Qì Pill (*shèn qì wán*).

Line 12.18

病者脉伏，其人欲自利，利反快，虽利，心下续坚满，此为留饮欲去故也。甘遂半夏汤主之。

甘遂大者三枚 半夏（以水一升煮取半升，去滓）十二枚 芍药五枚 甘草

右四味，以水二升，煮取半升，去滓，以蜜半升，和药汁煎取八合，顿服之。

Bìng zhě mài fú, qí rén yù zì lì, lì fǎn kuài, suī lì, xīn xià xù jiān mǎn, cǐ wéi liú yǐn yù qù gù yě. Gān suì bàn xià tāng zhǔ zhī.

Gān suì dà zhě sān méi; bàn xià (yǐ shuǐ yī shēng zhǔ qǔ bàn shēng, qù zǐ) shí èr méi; sháo yào wǔ méi; gān cǎo

Yòu sì wèi, yǐ shuǐ èr shēng, zhǔ qǔ bàn shēng, qù zǐ, yǐ mì bàn shēng, huó yào zhī jiān qǔ bā gě, dùn fú zhī.

When a patient has a hidden pulse, is on the verge of spontaneous diarrhea, and experiences gratification after diarrhea, but despite the diarrhea continues [to suffer from] hardness and fullness below the heart, this is caused by lodged rheum that is about to disappear.[1] Kansui and Pinellia Decoction (甘遂半夏汤 *gān suì bàn xià tāng*) governs.

Kansui and Pinellia Decoction (甘遂半夏汤 *gān suì bàn xià tāng*)

kansui (甘遂 *gān suì*, Kansui Radix) 3 large pieces
pinellia (半夏 *bàn xià*, Pinelliae Rhizoma) (boil in 1 *shēng* of water to get ½ *shēng*, and remove the dregs) 12 pieces
peony (芍药 *sháo yào*, Paeoniae Radix) 5 pieces
licorice (甘草 *gān cǎo*, Glycyrrhizae Radix)[2]

Boil the above four ingredients in two *shēng* of water to get half a *shēng*. Remove the dregs. Mix half a *shēng* of honey into the medicinal liquid and decoct to get eight *gě*. Quaff.

Text Notes, Line 12.18

[1] Lodged rheum that is about to disappear 留饮欲去 *liú yǐn yù qù*: The patient is about to recover from lodged rheum.

[2] The commentary adds: "One finger-sized piece, mix-fried. One version [of this formula] lacks this ingredient."

Synopsis, Line 12.18

This line describes the pulse, signs, and treatment of lodged rheum that is about to disappear but fails to do so.

Commentary, Line 12.18

Collecting water-rheum stops the flow of yáng qì, which is reflected in a hidden pulse. If a patient with lodged rheum and a hidden pulse suddenly feels diarrhea coming on and relief after the diarrhea, but this is not the result of being treated by offensive precipitation to expel the evil, it indicates that the lodged rheum is beginning to disappear. Nevertheless, if the water-rheum persists after diarrhea, this means that although it was about to disappear, it was not, and new rheum is continuing to accumulate daily, so that the patient continues to suffer from hard glomus associated with distention and fullness.

We treat this condition with medicines that have an offensive downbearing, phlegm-eliminating, disinhibiting, and abducting action such as Kansui and Pinellia Decoction (*gān suì bàn xià tāng*). Within this formula, kansui (*gān suì*) attacks and dispels water-rheum, pinellia (*bàn xià*) dissipates binds and eliminates phlegm, while peony (*sháo yào*), licorice (*gān cǎo*), and honey (*mì*) quiet the center by sour contraction and sweet relaxation.

Line 12.19

脉浮而细滑，伤饮。

Mài fú ér xì huá, shāng yǐn.

A floating, fine, and slippery pulse [means] damage by rheum.

SYNOPSIS, LINE 12.19

This line describes the pulse of sudden damage by external rheum.

COMMENTARY, LINE 12.19

In rheum disease, the pulse tends to be stringlike. In this line, however, the pulse is described as floating and at the same time fine and slippery. This pulse is associated with sudden damage by external rheum, that is, imbibed fluids. In this condition, fluid has not yet accumulated internally to form pathological rheum. It is therefore still a relatively shallow condition. Because lung qì is still able to outthrust the evil to the exterior, the pulse is floating. The sunken, stringlike pulse of water-rheum lying deep in the body has not yet appeared. A pulse that is fine and slippery is clinically associated with water-rheum beginning to gather. As a whole, the pulse qualities mentioned in this line therefore suggest that the evil is still shallow.

Line 12.20

脉弦数，有寒饮，冬夏难治。

Mài xián shuò, yǒu hán yǐn, dōng xià nán zhì.

A stringlike and rapid pulse [in a patient] with cold rheum is hard to treat, whether in winter or summer.

SYNOPSIS, LINE 12.20

This line describes an incongruent pulse in cold rheum, which results in a poor prognosis both in winter and summer.

COMMENTARY, LINE 12.20

If a pulse that is stringlike and rapid appears in cold rheum, the pulse and pattern are incongruent. While cold rheum has a tendency to damage yáng qì and therefore manifests in a stringlike pulse, it should not be rapid, since a rapid pulse indicates that collecting rheum has transformed into heat and damaged yīn. Thus, when we see cold rheum appearing with a stringlike and rapid pulse that indicates phlegm-heat, pulse and pattern are incongruent.

From the point of view of the seasons, the cold of winter is favorable to eliminating heat, but is unfavorable to treating rheum. The heat of summer is favorable to eliminating rheum, but unfavorable to treating heat. Similarly, from the point of view of use of medicinals, using hot medicinals to treat rheum is unfavorable to the elimination of heat, while using cold medicinals to treat heat is unfavorable as regards eliminating cold rheum. Hence, in both winter and summer, cold rheum and heat are difficult to treat simultaneously. Treatment therefore always requires a blend of warm and cold medicinals.

Line 12.21

脉沉而弦者，悬饮内痛。

Mài chén ér xián zhě, xuán yǐn nèi tòng.

When the pulse is sunken and stringlike, suspended rheum [is causing] pain in the inner body.[1]

TEXT NOTE, LINE 12.21

[1] Pain in the inner body 内痛 *nèi tòng*: In this case, specifically pain in the chest and rib-side.

SYNOPSIS, LINE 12.21

This line describes the signs and pulse of suspended rheum.

COMMENTARY, LINE 12.21

A sunken pulse means that the disease is in the interior; a stringlike pulse indicates rheum and pain, and is also the main pulse of liver disease. A pulse that is sunken and stringlike at the same time means that water-rheum is binding internally and accumulating in the chest and rib-side, obstructing the qì dynamic of the liver, lung, and triple burner. Qì stagnation in the chest and rib-side manifests in local pain in the inner body.

Line 12.22

病悬饮者，十枣汤主之。

芫花（熬） 甘遂 大戟各等分

右三味，捣筛，以水一升五合，先煮肥大枣十枚，取八合，去滓，内药末，强人服一钱匕，羸人服半钱，平旦温服之，不下者，明日更加半钱，得快之后，糜粥自养。

Bìng xuán yǐn zhě, shí zǎo tāng zhǔ zhī.

Yuán huā (áo); gān suì; dà jǐ gè děng fèn

Yòu sān wèi, dǎo shāi, yǐ shuǐ yī shēng wǔ gě, xiān zhǔ féi dà zǎo shí méi, qǔ bā gě, qù zǐ, nà yào mò, qiáng rén fú yī qián bǐ, léi rén fú bàn qián, píng dàn wēn fú zhī, bù xià zhě, míng rì gèng jiā bàn qián, dé kuài zhī hòu, mí zhōu zì yǎng.

For the disease of suspended rheum, Ten Jujubes Decoction (十枣汤 *shí zǎo tāng*) governs.

Ten Jujubes Decoction (十枣汤 *shí zǎo tāng*)

genkwa (芫花 *yuán huā*, Genkwa Flos) (simmer)
kansui (甘遂 *gān suì*, Kansui Radix)
euphorbia/knoxia (大戟 *dà jǐ*, Euphorbiae seu Knoxiae Radix)

Crush and sift equal amounts of the above three ingredients. Then first boil ten plump jujubes in one *shēng* and five *gě* of water to get eight *gě*, and remove the dregs. Add the powdered medicinals. Strong patients should take one qián-spoonful [per dose]; markedly emaciated patients should take half a *qián*. Take it warm at daybreak. If there is no precipitation, take a further half *qián* on the next day. After you have achieved gratification, take gruel for nourishment.

SYNOPSIS, LINE 12.22

This line describes the treatment of suspended rheum.

COMMENTARY, LINE 12.22

Suspended rheum (also described in line 12.2, 12.21, 12.32, 12.33) arises when water-rheum flows beneath the rib-side, giving rise to cough that induces pain. When rheum evil has bound to form suspended rheum, we treat it by breaking the accumulation and expelling water, using Ten Jujubes Decoction (*shí zǎo tāng*).

Kansui (*gān suì*) is cold in nature and bitter in flavor, and is able to drain water-damp from the channels and outthrust with speed. Euphorbia/knoxia (*dà jǐ*) is cold in nature and bitter and acrid in flavor; it drains water-damp from the bowls and viscera. Genkwa (*yuán huā*) is warm in nature and bitter in flavor; it breaks the water-rheum accumulation. These three medicines together form a rheum-attacking combination. To prevent them from damaging right qì, the formula adds ten jujubes as an assistant to harmonize and quiet the center and resolve the toxin of the other medicinals.

In modern clinical practice, we grind all the agents into a powder and pack it into capsules. The usual dose is 5 fēn to 1 qián, once a day, on an empty stomach, swallowed with a decoction of jujubes. One course of treatment is 4—6 days.

We recommend consulting the relevant parts of the *Shāng Hán Lùn* when studying the treatment of suspended rheum. Note that if there is an exterior pattern, it must be resolved first before treating the suspended rheum.

Line 12.23

病溢饮者，当发其汗，大青龙汤主之，小青龙汤亦主之。

麻黄（去节）六两　桂枝（去皮）二两　甘草（炙）二两　杏仁（去皮尖）四十个　生姜三两　大枣十二枚　石膏（如鸡子大，碎）

右七味，以水九升，先煮麻黄，减二升，去上沫，内诸药，煮取三升，去滓，温服一升，取微似汗，汗多者温粉粉之。

麻黄(去节)三两 芍药三两 五味子半升 干姜三两 甘草（炙）三两 细辛三两 桂枝（去皮）三两 半夏(洗)半升

右八味，以水一斗，先煮麻黄，减二升，去上沫，内诸药，煮取三升，去滓，温服一升。

Bìng yì yǐn zhě, dāng fā qí hàn, dà qīng lóng tāng zhǔ zhī, xiǎo qīng lóng tāng yì zhǔ zhī.

Má huáng (qù jié) liù liǎng; guì zhī (qù pí) èr liǎng; gān cǎo (zhì) èr liǎng; xìng rén (qù pí jiān) sì shí gè; shēng jiāng sān liǎng; dà zǎo shí èr méi; shí gāo (rú jī zǐ dà, suì)

Yòu qī wèi, yǐ shuǐ jiǔ shēng, xiān zhǔ má huáng, jiǎn èr shēng, qù shàng mò, nà zhū yào, zhǔ qǔ sān shēng, qù zǐ, wēn fú yī shēng, qǔ wēi sì hàn, hàn duō zhě wēn fěn fěn zhī.

Má huáng (qù jié) sān liǎng; sháo yào sān liǎng; wǔ wèi zǐ bàn shēng; gān jiāng sān liǎng; gān cǎo (zhì) sān liǎng; xì xīn sān liǎng; guì zhī (qù pí) sān liǎng; bàn xià (xǐ) bàn shēng

Yòu bā wèi, yǐ shuǐ yī dǒu, xiān zhǔ má huáng, jiǎn èr shēng, qù shàng mò, nà zhū yào, zhǔ qǔ sān shēng, qù zǐ, wēn fú yī shēng.

In a patient with spillage rheum, effuse sweat. Major Black Dragon Decoction (大青龙汤 *dà qīng lóng tāng*) governs. Minor Black Dragon Decoction (小青龙汤 *xiǎo qīng lóng tāng*) also governs.

Major Black Dragon Decoction (大青龙汤 *dà qīng lóng tāng*)

ephedra (麻黄 *má huáng*, Ephedrae Herba) (remove nodes) 6 *liǎng*
cinnamon twig (桂枝 *guì zhī*, Cinnamomi Ramulus) (remove skin) 2 *liǎng*
licorice (甘草 *gān cǎo*, Glycyrrhizae Radix) (mix-fry) 2 *liǎng*
apricot kernel (杏仁 *xìng rén*, Armeniacae Semen) (remove skin and tips) 40 pieces
fresh ginger (生姜 *shēng jiāng*, Zingiberis Rhizoma Recens) 3 *liǎng*
jujube (大枣 *dà zǎo*, Jujubae Fructus) 20 pieces
gypsum (石膏 *shí gāo*, Gypsum Fibrosum) (a piece the size of a chicken egg, crush)

Of the above seven ingredients, first boil the ephedra (*má huáng*) in nine *shēng* of water until [the liquid] is reduced by two *shēng*. Remove the scum on top, add all [the other] ingredients, and boil to get three *shēng*. Take one *shēng* [per dose] warm, to achieve an appearance like slight sweating. If [the patient] sweats profusely, apply warm rice powder.[1]

Minor Black Dragon Decoction (小青龙汤 *xiǎo qīng lóng tāng*)

ephedra (麻黄 *má huáng*, Ephedrae Herba) (remove nodes) 3 *liǎng*
peony (芍药 *sháo yào*, Paeoniae Radix) 3 *liǎng*
schisandra (五味子 *wǔ wèi zǐ*, Schisandrae Fructus) ½ *shēng*
dried ginger (干姜 *gān jiāng*, Zingiberis Rhizoma) 3 *liǎng*
licorice (甘草 *gān cǎo*, Glycyrrhizae Radix) (mix-fry) 3 *liǎng*
asarum (细辛 *xì xīn*, Asari Radix et Rhizoma) 3 *liǎng*
cinnamon twig (桂枝 *guì zhī*, Cinnamomi Ramulus) (remove skin) 3 *liǎng*
pinellia (半夏 bàn xià, Pinelliae Rhizoma) (wash) ½ *shēng*

Of the above eight ingredients, first boil the ephedra (*má huáng*) in one *dǒu* of water until reduced by two *shēng*. Remove the scum on top, add all [other] ingredients, and boil to get three *shēng*. Remove the dregs. Take one *shēng* [per dose] warm.

TEXT NOTE, LINE 12.23

[1] Apply warm rice powder 温粉粉之 *wēn fěn fěn zhī*: The application of warm rice powder is a method used to check copious sweating. Commentators disagree as to the exact ingredients of the powder and method of application.

SYNOPSIS, LINE 12.23

This line describes two different treatments for spillage rheum.

COMMENTARY, LINE 12.23

Spillage rheum refers to water-rheum that is spilling into the fleshy exterior instead of flowing out with the sweat. It is characterized by generalized heaviness. Spillage rheum arises when lung qì becomes depressed and blocked, usually owing to contraction of external evils or voracious drinking (drinking of large quantities of fluid at one time). This affects both diffusion and depurative downbearing, in particular the ability to regulate the waterways. As a result, ingested fluid does not flow down to the bladder, but is forced outward to the four limbs, where it stagnates in the fleshy exterior. Owing to non-diffusion of lung qì, the interstices are tightly closed, preventing sweating and the discharge of the rheum through it.

Since spillage rheum under certain conditions can be naturally discharged through sweating, we treat it by promoting sweating to help it on its way. The text suggests two formulas as treatment: Major Black Dragon Decoction (*dà qīng lóng tāng*) and Minor Black Dragon Decoction (*xiǎo qīng lóng tāng*). These formulas resolve both the exterior and interior and are used to treat spillage rheum.

The major formula promotes sweating, dissipates water, and clears heat; it is suitable for spillage rheum with exuberant evil in the exterior due to external contraction of wind-cold, with depressed heat in the interior. It is therefore appropriate when there is an exterior pattern of heat effusion and aversion to cold, generalized pain, absence of sweating, and a tight pulse, combined with an interior pattern of panting with vexation and agitation.

The minor formula moves water, warms the lung, and downbears qì; it is suitable for spillage rheum due to external contraction of wind-cold, with cold rheum in the interior. It is appropriate when there is an external pattern of aversion to cold and heat effusion and an internal pattern of glomus in the chest, dry retching, cough, and panting.

Note that spillage rheum is similar to, but different from, wind water. Spillage rheum is marked by generalized pain, heaviness, and absence of sweating, while wind water is characterized by pain in the joints and swelling. However, spillage rheum can develop into wind swelling, which is a more severe condition.

Line 12.24

膈间支饮，其人喘满，心下痞坚，面色黧黑，其脉沉紧，得之数十日，医吐下之不愈，木防己汤主之；虚者即愈，实者三日复发，复与不愈者，宜木防己汤去石膏加茯苓芒硝汤主之。

木防己三两　石膏十二枚　鸡子大 桂枝二两　人参四两

右四味，以水六升，煮取二升，分温再服。

木防己 桂枝各二两 人参 茯苓各四两 芒硝三合

右五味，以水六升，煮取二升，去滓，内芒硝，再微煎，分温再服，微利则愈。

Gé jiān zhī yǐn, qí rén chuǎn mǎn, xīn xià pǐ jiān, miàn sè lí hēi, qí mài chén jǐn, dé zhī shù shí rì, yī tù xià zhī bù yù, mù fáng jǐ tāng zhǔ zhī; xū zhě jí yú, shí zhě sān rì fù fā, fù yǔ bù yù zhě, yí mù fáng jǐ tāng qù shí gāo jiā fú líng máng xiāo tāng zhǔ zhī.

Mù fáng jǐ sān liǎng; shí gāo shí èr méi; jī zǐ dà guì zhī èr liǎng; rén shēn sì liǎng

Yòu sì wèi, yǐ shuǐ liù shēng, zhǔ qǔ èr shēng, fēn wen zài fú.

Mù fáng jǐ guì zhī gè èr liǎng rén shēn fú líng gè sì liǎng máng xiāo sān gě

Yòu wǔ wèi, yǐ shuǐ liù shēng, zhǔ qǔ èr shēng, qù zǐ, nà máng xiāo, zài wēi jiān, fēn wēn zài fú, wēi lì zé yú.

Propping rheum in the region of the diaphragm [manifests in] panting and fullness, hard glomus below the heart, a soot-black facial complexion, and a sunken and tight pulse. When [the condition] has persisted for several tens of days, and the physican has treated it with ejection and precipitation without bringing about recovery, Woody Fangji Decoction (木防己汤 *mù fáng jǐ tāng*) governs. [Patients with] vacuity [in the region below the heart] will recover immediately; [those with] repletion [in the region below the heart] will relapse in three days. If you give another preparation and they still fail to recover, Woody Fangji Decoction Minus Gypsum Plus Poria and Mirabilite (防已去石膏加茯苓芒硝汤 *mù fáng jǐ tāng qù shí gāo jiā fú líng máng xiāo tāng*)[1] governs.

Woody Fangji Decoction (木防已汤 *mù fáng jǐ tāng*)
woody fangji (木防己 *mù fáng jǐ*, Cocculi Radix) 3 *liǎng*
gypsum (石膏 *shí gāo*, Gypsum Fibrosum) 12 pieces (the size of chicken's eggs)
cinnamon twig (桂枝 *guì zhī*, Cinnamomi Ramulus) 2 *liǎng*
ginseng (人参 *rén shēn*, Ginseng Radix) 4 *liǎng*

Boil the above four ingredients in six *shēng* of water to get two *shēng*. Divide into two [doses] and take warm.

Woody Fangji Decoction Minus Gypsum Plus Poria and Mirabilite (防已去石膏加茯苓芒硝汤 *mù fáng jǐ qù shí gāo jiā fú líng máng xiāo tāng*)

woody fangji (木防已 *mù fáng jǐ*, Cocculi Radix)
cinnamon twig (桂枝 *guì zhī*, Cinnamomi Ramulus) 2 *liǎng* each
ginseng (人参 *rén shēn*, Ginseng Radix)
poria (茯苓 *fú líng*, Poria) 4 *liǎng* each
mirabilite (芒硝 *máng xiāo*, Natrii Sulfas) 3 *gě* each

Of the above five ingredients, boil [the first four] in six *shēng* of water to get two *shēng*. Remove the dregs, add the mirabilite (*máng xiāo*), and decoct a little more. Divide into two [doses] and take warm. Slight diarrhea will result in recovery.

TEXT NOTE, LINE 12.24

[1] Woody Fangji Decoction Minus Gypsum Plus Poria and Mirabilite 木防已汤去石膏加茯苓芒硝汤 *mù fáng jǐ tāng qù shí gāo jiā fú líng máng xiāo tāng*: The character 汤 *tāng* is repeated in the Chinese formula name, presumably by error.

SYNOPSIS, LINE 12.24

This line describes the signs, pulse, and treatment of severe cases of propping rheum in the region of the diaphragm, taking into account both vacuity and repletion patterns.

COMMENTARY, LINE 12.24

Propping rheum in the region of the diaphragm arises when water-rheum collects below the heart and distresses lung qì and heart yáng. As a result, we see panting and fullness. Water-rheum binding internally prevents the spleen from distributing liquid, and causes depressed heat which manifests in hard glomus below the heart. When cold rheum gathers, binds, and becomes lodged in the interior, the pulse is sunken and tight. When it gathers in the diaphragm and floats upward, the movement of construction and defense is inhibited, yīn overwhelms yáng, and rheum and depressed heat steam upward into the face; hence we see a soot-black complexion.

When these symptoms have persisted for several tens of days, which is a relatively long time, right qì has a tendency to become vacous. Treating this condition with ejection or precipitation is inappropriate because it is not related to food accumulation and interior repletion, and the disease is not centered in the spleen and stomach. Such treatment will not expel the propping rheum but will damage liquid and qì. In this situation, the patient suffers from a severe propping rheum pattern with qì vacuity and rheum and heat binding. The appropriate treatment consists of supplementing vacuity, clearing heat, freeing yáng and disinhibiting water, and resolving propping rheum through urination.

Under these circumstances, the appropriate formula is Woody Fangji Decoction (*mù fáng jǐ tāng*). Woody fangji (*mù fáng jǐ*) is bitter while cinnamon twig (*guì zhī*) is acrid. Together they move water-rheum and disspiate binding qì, to eliminate the hard glomus below the heart. Gypsum (*shí gāo*) is a cool, acrid downsinking medicinal. It clears depressed heat and can settle counterflow ascending evils. Ginseng (*rén shēn*) restores right and supplements vacuity, addressing the damage to right qì resulting from a disease that has lasted for several tens of days and from inappropriate treatment by ejection and precipitation.

If the hard glomus becomes vacuous and soft after the patient has taken the formula, this is a sign that the water is leaving and qì is moving. If the glomus remains hard, this means that water is still collecting and qì is still obstructed. If a second preparation of the same formula still fails to bring about recovery, remove cool acrid gypsum (*shí gāo*) and add poria (*fú líng*) to abduct the water downward, and mirabilite (*máng xiāo*) to soften hardness and break the bind.

Line 12.25

心下有支饮，其人苦冒眩，泽泻汤主之。

泽泻五两　白朮二两

右二味，以水二升，煮取一升，分温再服。

Xīn xià yǒu zhī yǐn, qí rén kǔ mào xuàn, zé xiè tāng zhǔ zhī.

Zé xiè wǔ liǎng; bái zhú èr liǎng

Yòu èr wèi, yǐ shuǐ èr shēng, zhǔ qǔ yī shēng, fēn wēn zài fú.

Propping rheum below the heart [manifests in] veiling dizziness.[1] Alisma Decoction (*zé xiè tāng*) governs.

Alisma Decoction (*zé xiè tāng*)
alisma (泽泻 *zé xiè*, Alismatis Rhizoma) 5 *liǎng* white atractylodes (白朮 *bái zhú*, Atractylodis Macrocephalae Rhizoma) 2 *liǎng*

Boil the above two ingredients in two *shēng* of water to get one *shēng*. Divide into two [doses] and take warm.

TEXT NOTE, LINE 12.25

[1] Veiling dizziness 冒眩 *mào xuàn*: clouded head and dizzy vision. "Veiling" means clouded head as if the head were covered.

SYNOPSIS, LINE 12.25

This line describes the signs and treatment of veiling dizziness due to propping rheum.

COMMENTARY, LINE 12.25

When water collects below the heat and clear yáng fails to bear upwards, turbid yīn ascends to cause clouding dizziness of the head and eyes. This is a commonly observed symptom of phlegm-rheum. We treat this condition with Alisma Decoction (*zé xiè tāng*). This formula is composed of two ingredients only: alisma (*zé xiè*), which disinhibits water and eliminates rheum, and white atractylodes (*bái zhú*), which supplements the spleen, dries dampness, and restrains water.

Line 12.26

支饮胸满者，厚朴大黄汤主之。

厚朴一尺　大黄六两　枳实四枚

右三味，以水五升，煮取二升，分温再。

Zhī yǐn xiōng mǎn zhě, hòu pò dà huáng tāng zhǔ zhī.

Hòu pò yī chǐ; dà huáng liù liǎng; zhǐ shí sì méi

Yòu sān wèi, yǐ shuǐ wǔ shēng, zhǔ qǔ èr shēng, fēn wēn zài fú.

For propping rheum with fullness in the chest, Officinal Magnolia Bark and Rhubarb Decoction (厚朴大黄汤 *hòu pò dà huáng tāng*) governs.

Officinal Magnolia Bark and Rhubarb Decoction (厚朴大黄汤 *hòu pò dà huáng tāng*)

officinal magnolia bark (厚朴 *hòu pò*, Magnoliae Officinalis Cortex) 1 *chǐ*

rhubarb (大黄 *dà huáng*, Rhei Radix et Rhizoma) 6 *liǎng*

unripe bitter orange (枳实 *zhǐ shí*, Aurantii Fructus Immaturus) 4 pieces

Boil the above three ingredients in five *shēng* of water to get two *shēng*. Divide into two [doses] and take warm.

Synopsis, Line 12.26

This line describes the signs and treatment of propping rheum with abdominal fullness.

Commentary, Line 12.26

Propping rheum with abdominal fullness refers to propping rheum with "stomach domain repletion" (repletion in the stomach and intestines). The disease of propping rheum is originally located in the chest and diaphragm and affects the upper burner. However, the heart and lung stand in an exterior-interior relationship with the large and small intestines, and if rheum and heat become overly exuberant in the upper burner, this can affect the movement of the qì dynamic in the stomach and intestines. Thus, we see constipation.

The text recommends Officinal Magnolia Bark and Rhubarb Decoction (*hòu pò dà huáng tāng*) as a treatment for this condition because it expels rheum, flushes out heat, moves qì, and opens depression.

Line 12.27

支饮不得息，葶苈大枣泻肺汤主之。

Zhī yǐn bù dé xī, tíng lì dà zǎo xiè fèi tāng zhǔ zhī.

For propping rheum with inability to breathe, Lepidium/Descurainiae and Jujube Lung-Draining Decoction (*tíng lì dà zǎo xiè fèi tāng*) governs.[1]

TEXT NOTE, LINE 12.27

[1] The commentary adds: "For the formula, see the chapter on Pulmonary Abscess (肺痈 *fèi yōng*)."

SYNOPSIS, LINE 12.27

This line describes the signs and treatment of propping rheum congesting the lung and transforming into heat.

COMMENTARY, LINE 12.27

This line discusses a repletion pattern of water-rheum congesting the lung. When propping rheum obstructs the chest and diaphragm, phlegm-drool causes congestion that inhibits lung qì; hence there is oppression in the chest, panting, and cough. These symptoms are identical to the panting and inability to lie down that appear in patterns of damp-heat congesting the lung, in the initial stage of pulmonary abscess.

Treat this condition with Lepidium/Descurainiae and Jujube Lung-Draining Decoction (*tíng lì dà zǎo xiè fèi tāng*), which drains the lung qì block and expels phlegm-rheum, while also supplementing the spleen and harmonizing the center. In this formula, lepidium/descurainiae (*tíng lì zǐ*) drains the lung, open the bind, and calms panting. It is assisted by jujube (*dà zǎo*), which supports the spleen and moderates the strong nature of *tíng lì zǐ*, so as to eliminate the evil without damaging right qì.

Line 12.28

呕家本渴，渴者为欲解，今反不渴，心下有支饮故也。小半夏汤主之。

半夏一升　生姜半斤

右二味，以水七升，煮取一升半，分温再服。

Ǒu jiā běn kě, kě zhě wéi yù jiě, jīn fǎn bù kě, xīn xià yǒu zhī yǐn gù yě. Xiǎo bàn xià tāng zhǔ zhī.

Bàn xià yī shēng; shēng jiāng bàn jīn

Yòu èr wèi, yǐ shuǐ qī shēng, zhǔ qǔ yī shēng bàn, fēn wēn zài fú.

Patients with habitual vomiting are generally thirsty. Thirst means that [the condition] is about to resolve. However, if the patient presently has no thirst, this is because there is propping rheum below the heart. Minor Pinellia Decoction (小半夏汤 *xiǎo bàn xià tāng*) governs.[1]

Minor Pinellia Decoction
(小半夏汤 *xiǎo bàn xià tāng*)

pinellia (半夏 *bàn xià*, Pinelliae Rhizoma) *1 shēng*
fresh ginger (生姜 *shēng jiāng*, Zingiberis Rhizoma Recens) ½ *jīn*

Boil the above two ingredients in seven *shēng* of water to get one-and-one-half *shēng*. Divide into two [doses] and take warm.

TEXT NOTE, LINE 12.28

[1] The commentary adds: "The *Qiān Jīn Fāng* ("Thousand Gold Pieces Prescriptions") has Minor Pinellia Decoction Plus Poria (*xiǎo bàn xià jiā fú líng tāng*)."

SYNOPSIS, LINE 12.28

This line describes the signs, treatment, and prognosis of propping rheum with simultaneous vomiting.

COMMENTARY, LINE 12.28

Retching and vomiting usually damage liquid and humor and hence tend to cause thirst. In patients with phlegm rheum, vomiting with thirst indicates that the rheum is being eliminated through vomiting, and that the disease is about to resolve. However if there is no thirst after vomiting, you know that water-rheum is continuing to collect below the heart, and that the vomiting is failing to remove it.

The treatment for this condition is Minor Pinellia Decoction (*xiǎo bàn xià tāng*), which harmonizes the stomach and checks vomiting, disperses rheum, and downbears counterflow. Pinellia (*bàn xià*) and fresh ginger (*shēng jiāng*) eliminate rheum, dissipate bind, and open the glomus. They also downbear counterflow and check vomiting, diffuse the yáng of the upper and center burners, and dispel cold and abiding rheum.

The formula method stipulates that seven shēng of water be boiled down to one-and-a-half shēng. This long boiling process is used to reduce the toxicity of the fresh pinellia.

Line 12.29

腹满口舌干燥，此肠间有水气，已椒苈黄丸主之。

防已　椒目　葶苈（熬）　大黄各一两

右四味，末之，蜜丸如梧子大，先食饮服一丸，日三服，稍增，口中有津液，渴者加芒硝半两。

Fù mǎn kǒu shé gān zào, cǐ cháng jiān yǒu shuǐ qì, jǐ jiāo lì huáng wán zhǔ zhī.

Fáng jǐ, jiāo mù, tíng lì (áo), dà huáng gè yī liǎng

Yòu sì wèi, mò zhī, mì wán rú wú zǐ dà, xiān shí yǐn fú yī wán, rì sān fú, shāo zēng, kǒu zhōng yǒu jīn yè, kě zhě jiā máng xiāo bàn liǎng.

Abdominal fullness and dry throat and mouth [indicates that] there is water qì in the intestines. Fangji, Zanthoxylum, Lepidium /Descurainiae, and Rhubarb Pill (已椒苈黄丸 *jǐ jiāo lì huáng wán*) governs.

Fangji, Zanthoxylum, Lepidium/Descurainiae, and Rhubarb Pill (已椒苈黄丸 *jǐ jiāo lì huáng wán*)

- fangji (防已 *fáng jǐ*, Stephaniae Tetrandrae Radix) 1 *liǎng*
- zanthoxylum seed (椒目 *jiāo mù*, Zanthoxyli Semen) 1 *liǎng*
- lepidium/descurainiae (葶苈 *tíng lì*, Lepidii/Descurainiae Semen) 1 *liǎng* (simmer)
- rhubarb (大黄 *dà huáng*, Rhei Radix et Rhizoma) 1 *liǎng*

Pulverize the above four ingredients and blend them with honey to form pills the size of firmiana seeds. Take one pill [per dose] with fluid before meals, three times a day, increasing the dose bit by bit until there is fluid in [the patient's] mouth. If [the patient] suffers from thirst, add half a *liǎng* of mirabilite (*máng xiāo*).

SYNOPSIS, LINE 12.29

This line describes the signs and treatment of phlegm-rheum in the intestines.

COMMENTARY, LINE 12.29

When water runs into the intestines, and rheum evil binds internally, there is abdominal fullness due to water qì in the intestines. As the second line of this chapter states, "When a person with a plentiful constitution becomes emaciated and has water running into the intestines with gurgling sounds, [this] means phlegm-rheum." This condition is caused by a breakdown of conveyance in the intestines and stomach, as a result of which the fluids are not completely passed downwards to the bladder, but stagnate in the intestines instead. When water qì fails to transform, and spleen qì fails to bear liquid upward, there is dry mouth and tongue. The dry mouth should not be mistaken for a simple sign of heat. Heat may be binding with rheum in the intestines, but the main disease-causing element in this condition is rheum, not heat.

The formula suggested is Fangji, Zanthoxylum, Lepidium/Descurainiae, and Rhubarb Pill (*jǐ jiāo lì huáng wán*), which disperses the water-rheum and abducts the evil downward, so that abdominal fullness and dry mouth naturally disappear. The actions of the ingredients are as follows: Fangji (*fáng jǐ*) and zanthoxylum seed (*jiāo mù*) are acrid diffusing and bitter discharging medicines; they abduct water through the urine. Lepidium/Descurainiae (*tíng lì zǐ*) and rhubarb (*dà huáng*) attack hardness and drain congestion, expelling water through the stool. As a result of these actions, lung qì should be able to downbear and spleen qì should be able to upbear, as a result of which phlegm is eliminated and the fluids are able to ascend. Hence, "there is fluid in [the patient's] mouth."

Line 12.30

卒呕吐，心下痞，膈间有水，眩悸者，小半夏加茯苓汤主之。

半夏一升　生姜半斤　茯苓三两

右三味，以水七升，煮取一升五合，分温再服。

Cù ǒu tù, xīn xià pǐ, gé jiān yǒu shuǐ, xuàn jì zhě, xiǎo bàn xià jiā fú líng tāng zhǔ zhī.

Bàn xià yī shēng; shēng jiāng bàn jīn; fú líng sān liǎng

Yòu sān wèi, yǐ shuǐ qī shēng, zhǔ qǔ yī shēng wǔ gě, fēn wēn zài fú.

For sudden retching and vomiting accompanied by glomus below the heart, water in the diaphragm, dizziness, and palpitation, Minor Pinellia Decoction Plus Poria (小半夏加茯苓汤 *xiǎo bàn xià jiā fú líng tāng*) governs.

Minor Pinellia Decoction Plus Poria (小半夏加茯苓汤 *xiǎo bàn xià jiā fú líng tāng*)

pinellia (半夏 *bàn xià*, Pinelliae Rhizoma) 1 *shēng*
fresh ginger (生姜 *shēng jiāng*, Zingiberis Rhizoma Recens) ½ *jīn*
poria (茯苓 *fú líng*, Poria) 3 *liǎng*[1]

Boil the above three ingredients in seven *shēng* of water to get one *shēng* and five *gě*. Divide into two [doses] and take warm.

Text Note, Line 12.30

[1] The commentary adds: "According to another method, 4 liǎng."

Synopsis, Line 12.30

This line describes the signs and treatment of propping rheum with retching and vomiting, dizziness, and palpitation.

Commentary, Line 12.30

When rheum collects in the stomach, it impairs the harmonious downbearing of the stomach, giving rise to counterflow ascent that manifests in sudden vomiting. Because the water-rheum is accumulating, there is glomus and fullness beneath the heart. Clear yáng fails to rise, hence there is clouding dizziness of the head and eyes. As water ascends to intimidate the heart, we see palpitation. All these symptoms, among which vomiting is foremost, are traceable to water in the region of the diaphragm.

The suggested formula is Minor Pinellia Decoction Plus Poria (*xiǎo bàn xià jiā fú líng tāng*), which harmonizes the stomach and checks vomiting, while also conducting water downward.

Line 12.31

假令瘦人，脐下有悸，吐涎沫而癫眩，此水也。五苓散主之。

泽泻一两一分　猪苓三分（去皮）　茯苓三分　白朮三分　桂二分（去皮）

右五味，为末，白饮服方寸匕，日三服，多饮暖水，汗出愈。

Jiǎ lìng shòu rén, qí xià you jì, tù xián mò ér diān xuàn, cǐ shuǐ yě. Wǔ líng sǎn zhǔ zhī.

Zé xiè yī liǎng yī fēn; zhū líng sān fēn (qù pí); fú líng sān fēn; bái zhú sān fēn; guì èr fēn (qù pí)

Yòu wǔ wèi, wéi mò, bái yǐn fú fāng cùn bǐ, rì sān fú, duō yǐn nuǎn shuǐ, hàn chū yú.

If an emaciated person[1] suffers from palpitation below the umbilicus, foaming drool at the mouth, and dizziness,[2] this [indicates] water. Poria Five Powder (五苓散 *wǔ líng sǎn*) governs.

Poria Five Powder (五苓散 *wǔ líng sǎn*)

alisma (泽泻 *zé xiè*, Alismatis Rhizoma) 1 *liǎng* and 1 part
polyporus (猪苓 *zhū líng*, Polyporus) 3 parts (remove the skin)
poria (茯苓 *fú líng*, Poria) 3 parts
white atractylodes (白术 *bái zhú*, Atractylodis Macrocephalae Rhizoma) 3 parts
cinnamon twig (桂枝 *guì zhī*, Cinnamomi Ramulus) 2 parts (skin removed)

Pulverize the above five ingredients. Take a square-inch-spoonful in thin rice gruel,[3] three times a day. Drink large amounts of warm water. When sweating occurs, recovery will ensue.

TEXT NOTES, LINE 12.31

[1] Emaciated person 瘦人 *shòu rén*: According to most commentators, this refers to a common symptom of phlegm-rheum as described in line 12.2 above, "when a person with a plentiful constitution becomes emaciated"; in other words, this is a patient who has become emaciated as a result of the present illness.

[2] Dizziness 癫眩 *diān xuàn*: 癫 *diān* should be read as 颠 *diān* meaning the top of the body, i.e., the head.

[3] Thin rice gruel 白饮 *bái yǐn*: Literally "white fluid," it is an alternative name for 米汤 *mǐ tāng* ("rice decoction") and refers to a thin decoction of rice that is used as a medium for taking medicines in order to assist stomach qì.

SYNOPSIS, LINE 12.31

This line describes the signs and treatment of counterflow ascent of water-rheum from the center and lower burners.

COMMENTARY, LINE 12.31

Generally speaking, emaciated persons tend to have a superabundance of yáng and an insufficiency of yīn; hence they rarely suffer from internally collecting water-rheum. However, in the present condition, the emaciation is a result of phlegm-rheum accumulating and depriving the flesh of fullness. When water-rheum binds in the lower burner, its quickest way out of the body is through the urine. However, when bladder qì transformation has broken down, rheum is deprived of its way out and instead ascends counterflow, causing ejection of drool and foam on the one hand and dizziness on the other. Water may also stir in the lower region, causing stirring palpitation below the umbilicus and counterflow surging.

The suggested formula is Poria Five Powder (*wǔ líng sǎn*), which promotes qì transformation and disinhibits water. Once water qì descends, all the abovementioned symptoms disappear. Polyporus (*zhū líng*), poria (*fú líng*), and alisma (*zé xiè*) disinhibit water. White atractylodes (*bái zhú*) banks up earth to dam water. Cinnamon twig (*guì zhī*) warms yáng and promotes qì transformation to assist in the movement of water. The formula recommends that the patient drink lots of warm water to promote sweating.

Poria Five Powder (*wŭ líng săn*) has a mild sweating action that helps to prevent the rheum from spilling out into the skin and flesh and thereby creating water swelling.

Poria Five Powder (*wŭ líng săn*) has broad applications in clinical practice. It is used to treat amassment of water-damp, water swelling with inhibited urination, dribbling urinary block, water-rheum surging upward to cause dizziness, clouding reversal, and epilepsy. In modern practice, it is also used to treat hydrocephalus, acute glaucoma, allergic rhinitis, and acute vomiting and diarrhea.

附方 Appended Formula, Line 12.31

Poria Beverage (茯苓饮 *fú líng yǐn*)
from the *Wài Tái Mì Yào* ("Secrets from the *Wài Tái* Library")

治心胸中有停痰宿水，自吐出水后，心胸间虚，气满不能食，消痰气，令能食。

茯苓　人参　白朮各三两　枳实二两　橘皮二两半　生姜四两

右六味，水六升，煮取一升八合，分温三服，如人行八九里进之。

Zhì xīn xiōng zhōng yǒu tíng tán sù shuǐ, zì tù chū shuǐ hòu, xīn xiōng jiān xū, qì măn bù néng shí, xiāo tán qì, lìng néng shí.

Fú ling, rén shēn, bái zhú gè sān liǎng; zhǐ shí èr liǎng; jú pí èr liǎng; bàn shēng jiāng sì liǎng

Yòu liù wèi, shuǐ liù shēng, zhǔ qǔ yī shēng bā gě, fēn wēn sān fú, rú rén xíng bā jiǔ lǐ jìn zhī.

Treats collecting phlegm and abiding water in the heart and chest, which after spontaneous vomiting of water, [manifests in] vacuity in the heart and chest, qì fullness, and inability to eat. It disperses phlegm qì and enables [the person] to eat.

Poria Beverage (茯苓饮 *fú líng yǐn*)

- poria (茯苓 *fú líng*, Poria) 3 *liǎng*
- ginseng (人参 *rén shēn*, Ginseng Radix) 3 *liǎng*
- white atractylodes (白朮 *bái zhú*, Atractylodis Macrocephalae Rhizoma) 3 *liǎng*
- unripe bitter orange (枳实 *zhǐ shí*, Aurantii Fructus Immaturus) 2 *liǎng*
- tangerine peel (橘皮 *jú pí*, Citri Reticulatae Pericarpium) 2.5 *liǎng*
- fresh ginger (生姜 *shēng jiāng*, Zingiberis Rhizoma Recens) 4 *liǎng*

Boil the above six ingredients in six *shēng* of water to get one *shēng* and eight *gě*. Divide into three [doses] and take warm. Separate the doses by the time it takes to walk eight or nine *lǐ*,[1] then take the formula again.

Formula Note, Line 12.31

[1] By the time it takes to walk eight or nine lǐ 如人行八九里 *rú rén xíng bā jiǔ lǐ*: About 30 minutes. One lǐ is a unit of distance roughly equal to a third of a kilometer or half a mile. Accordingly, walking eight or nine lǐ takes about an hour. Here it means that the patient should wait this long in between doses.

Line 12.32

咳家其脉弦，为有水，十枣汤主之。

Ké jiā qí mài xián, wéi yǒu shuǐ, shí zǎo tāng zhǔ zhī.

If a patient with cough has a stringlike pulse, [this] indicates the presence of water. Ten Jujubes Decoction (*shí zǎo tāng*) governs.[1]

TEXT NOTE, LINE 12.32

[1] The commentary adds: "For the formula, see above." The formula is found in line 12.11 above.

SYNOPSIS, LINE 12.32

This line describes the pulse diagnosis and treatment of chronic cough with water.

COMMENTARY, LINE 12.32

Beginning with this line, the remainder of this chapter deals with cough due to phlegm-rheum. There are many causes of cough, all with different accompanying signs and prognoses. In the present case, water-rheum is caused by ingested fluids accumulating in the chest and causing water qì to shoot upward into the lung. The text tells us that cough with a stringlike pulse is due to water-rheum. We can distinguish this from a floating pulse, which indicates external contraction of evil, or a rapid pulse, which indicates lung wilting. According to this line, cough with water-rheum should be treated with Ten Jujubes Decoction (*shí zǎo tāng*). This formula is discussed in the commentary to line 12.22 above.

Line 12.33

夫有支饮家，咳烦，胸中痛者，不卒死，至一百日或一岁，宜十枣汤。

Fū yǒu zhī yǐn jiā, ké fán, xiōng zhōng tòng zhě, bù cù sǐ, zhì yī bǎi rì huò yī suì. Yí shí zǎo tāng.

If a patient suffering from propping rheum with cough, vexation, and pain in the chest does not die suddenly [but the condition continues] for a hundred days or a year, Ten Jujubes Decoction (*shí zǎo tāng*) is appropriate.[1]

TEXT NOTE, LINE 12.33

[1] The commentary adds: "For the formula, see above." This formula is found in line 12.22 above.

SYNOPSIS, LINE 12.33

This line describes the treatment of severe propping rheum with enduring cough.

COMMENTARY, LINE 12.33

Propping rheum is not normally associated with chest pain or heart vexation. However, these signs may appear when the condition persists for a long time. In severe propping rheum, sudden death may occur, or the condition can become chronic, persisting for a hundred days or even a year. In that case, cough and pain in the chest are due to rheum evil intimidating the heart and obstructing the airways. These are signs of severe propping rheum in which both the lung and heart are affected and yáng qì is blocked. Provided that right qì has not yet become vacuous, Ten Jujubes Decoction (*shí zǎo tāng*) is the recommended treatment.

Line 12.34

久咳数岁，其脉弱者可治，实大数者死，其脉虚者必苦冒，其人本有支饮在胸中故也，治属饮家。

Jiǔ ké shù suì, qí mài ruò zhě kě zhì, shí dà shuò zhě sǐ, qí mài xū zhě bì kǔ mào, qí rén běn yǒu zhī yǐn zài xiōng zhōng gù yě, zhì shǔ yǐn jiā.

If a patient with cough that has endured for several years has a weak pulse, [the condition] can be treated; if [the pulse] is replete, large, and rapid, [the patient] will die. If the pulse is vacuous, [the patient] invariably also suffers from veiling. This is because such patients originally have propping rheum in the chest. Treat them like rheum patients.

SYNOPSIS, LINE 12.34

This line describes the pulse, signs, and prognosis of enduring cough due to propping rheum.

COMMENTARY, LINE 12.34

In patients who have suffered from cough due to phlegm-rheum for several years, right qì tends to be severely damaged, which manifests in a weak pulse. Here, the pulse and pattern are congruent. While right qì is vacuous, the rheum evil is also slight; hence, we can most likely still treat this condition by simultaneously supporting right and expelling water-rheum. However, if the pulse is replete, large, and fast, this is a sign of exuberance of evil and debilitation of right. Such cases have a poor prognosis because it is difficult to attack the evil without damaging the right. If the pulse is vacuous, this means that not only right qì is vacuous, but the evil is also already debilitated. In such cases, we should also see clouded dizziness of the head and eyes, because phlegm-rheum ascends and clouds clear yáng. Since the root of this condition is propping rheum, we should still treat such cases like other rheum cases.

Line 12.35

咳逆倚息，不得卧，小青龙汤主之。

Ké nì yǐ xī, bù dé wò, xiǎo qīng lóng tāng zhǔ zhī.

For cough and counterflow with propped breathing[1] and inability to lie down, Minor Black Dragon Decoction (*xiǎo qīng lóng tāng*) governs.[2]

Text Notes, Line 12.35

[1] Cough and counterflow with propped breathing 咳逆倚息 *ké nì yǐ xī*: Cough and counterflow means cough and counterflow qì ascent that manifests as panting. Propped breathing denotes a condition in which the patient is unable to breathe comfortably in reclining posture.

[2] The commentary adds: "For the formula, see above." The formula is found in line 12.23 above.

Synopsis, Line 12.35

This line describes the signs and treatment of propping rheum in which internal rheum is stirred by external cold.

Commentary, Line 12.35

Cough and counterflow with propped breathing is the main sign of propping rheum. It arises when externally contracted cold evil fights with water-rheum that has collected in the upper burner. In such cases, we prescribe Minor Black Dragon Decoction (*xiǎo qīng lóng tāng*) to resolve both external cold and internal rheum. The use of this formula is explained in line 12.23 above.

Line 12.36

青龙汤下已，多唾口燥，寸脉沉，尺脉微，手足厥逆，气从小腹上冲胸咽，手足痹，其面翕热如醉状，因复下流阴股，小便难，时复冒者，与茯苓桂枝五味甘草汤，治其气冲。

茯苓四两　桂枝四两（去皮）　甘草三两（炙）　五味子半升

右四味，以水八升，煮取三升，去滓，分温三服。

Qīng lóng tāng xià yǐ, duō tuò kǒu zào, cùn mài chén, chǐ mài wēi, shǒu zú jué nì, qì cóng xiǎo fù shàng chōng xiōng yān, shǒu zú bì, qí miàn xī rè rú zuì zhuàng, yīn fù xià liú yīn gǔ , xiǎo biàn nán, shí fù mào zhě, yǔ fú líng guì zhī wǔ wèi gān cǎo tāng, zhì qí qì chōng.

Fú líng sì liǎng; guì zhī sì liǎng (qù pí); gān cǎo sān liǎng (zhì); wǔ wèi zǐ bàn shēng

Yòu sì wèi, yǐ shuǐ bā shēng, zhǔ qǔ sān shēng, qù zǐ, fēn wēn sān fú.

If after taking Black Dragon Decoction (*qīng lóng tāng*) the patient presents with profuse spittle, dry mouth, a sunken inch pulse and a faint cubit pulse, reverse flow of the extremities, qì surging up from the smaller abdomen to the chest and pharynx, impediment of the extremities, feather-warm heat in the face as if inebriated, difficult urination due to [qì] returning to flow into the inguinal region, and periodically recurring veiling, give Poria, Cinnamon Twig, Schisandra, and Licorice Decoction (桂苓五味甘草汤 *fú líng guì zhī wǔ wèi gān cǎo tāng*) to treat the surging of qì.

Poria, Cinnamon Twig, Schisandra, and Licorice Decoction (桂苓五味甘草汤 *fú líng guì zhī wǔ wèi gān cǎo tāng*)

- poria (茯苓 *fú líng*, Poria) 4 *liǎng*
- cinnamon twig (桂枝 *guì zhī*, Cinnamomi Ramulus) 4 *liǎng* (remove bark)
- licorice (甘草 *gān cǎo*, Glycyrrhizae Radix) 3 *liǎng* (mix-fry)
- schisandra (五味子 *wǔ wèi zǐ*, Schisandrae Fructus) ½ *shēng*

Boil the above four ingredients in eight *shēng* of water to get three *shēng*. Remove the dregs, divide into three [doses], and take warm.

SYNOPSIS, LINE 12.36

This line describes the signs and treatment of propping rheum in patients with yáng vacuity who after taking Minor Black Dragon Decoction (*xiǎo qīng lóng tāng*) develop a transmuted pattern of surging qì.

COMMENTARY, LINE 12.36

Beginning with this line and continuing through the following four lines, the text discusses the changes that Minor Black Dragon Decoction (*xiǎo qīng lóng tāng*) can induce when we treat patients with constitutional vacuity for cough due to propping rheum with this formula.

Minor Black Dragon Decoction (*xiǎo qīng lóng tāng*) is the chief formula for repletion patterns of propping rheum with cough and panting. The present line deals with surging qì (冲气 *chōng qì*) that occurs as a result of taking this formula. When we treat propping rheum with cough and counterflow and inhibited respiration with Minor Black Dragon Decoction (*xiǎo qīng lóng tāng*), we normally observe copious phlegm and spittle with dry mouth. These are signs that the formula is working and cold rheum is being eliminated. However, if a propping rheum patient suffers from yáng vacuity in the lower burner and exuberant propping rheum in the upper body (i.e., lower body vacuity and upper body repletion), the pulse will be sunken at the inch position and faint and week at the cubit position; there will also be reversal counterflow of the limbs.

In such a patient, the normal treatment for cold rheum in the upper burner, which consists of warming and dissipating, is likely to cause over-effusion of yáng qì, and affect the thoroughfare vessel. It is therefore contraindicated, and what is needed is to devise a treatment that addresses the vacuity-repletion complex in its entirety, taking full account of the lower burner vacuity.

If Minor Black Dragon Decoction (*xiǎo qīng lóng tāng*) is given in such cases, it will temporarily resolve the cold rheum, but it will also cause vacuous yáng to stray upward, prompting surging qì and giving rise to a transmuted pattern. When qì surges upward from the smaller abdomen into the chest and throat, we see numbness of the limbs and feather-warm heat effusion in the face, as if the patient were drunk. Because the disease of the thoroughfare vessel comes and goes, qì sometimes surges and sometimes returns to the lower burner. During qì surges, the qì of the of whole body runs counterflow, so there is difficult urination and clouding and veiling.

We treat such transmuted patterns with Cinnamon, Poria, Schisandra, and Licorice Decoction (*guì líng wǔ wèi gān cǎo tāng*), which calms upward surging qì. Within the formula, cinnamon twig (*guì zhī*) and licorice (*gān cǎo*) are sweet acrid medicinals that form yáng and calm the surging qì. Poria (*fú líng*) conducts counterflow qì downward. Schisandra (*wǔ wèi zǐ*) constrains dissipated qì and prevents vacuous yáng from floating upward.

Line 12.37

冲气即低，而反更咳，胸满者，用桂苓五味甘草汤，去桂加干姜、细辛，以治其咳满。

茯苓四两　甘草　干姜　细辛各三两　五味子半升

右五味，以水八升，煮取三升，去滓，温服半升，日三服。

Chōng qì jí dī, ér fǎn gèng ké, xiōng mǎn zhě, yòng guì líng wǔ wèi gān cǎo tāng, qù guì jiā gān jiāng, xì xīn, yǐ zhì qí ké mǎn.

Fú líng sì liǎng; gān cǎo, gān jiāng, xì xīn gè sān liǎng; wǔ wèi zǐ bàn shēng

Yòu wǔ wèi, yǐ shuǐ bā shēng, zhǔ qǔ sān shēng, qù zǐ, wēn fú bàn shēng, rì sān fú.

When you have lowered the surging qì, but [the patient] again suffers from cough and fullness in the chest, use Cinnamon, Poria, Schisandra, and Licorice Decoction (*guì líng wǔ wèi gān cǎo tāng*), but leave out the cinnamon twig (*guì zhī*) and add dried ginger (*gān jiāng*) and asarum (*xì xīn*) [to the formula] to treat the cough and fullness.

Poria, Licorice, Schisandra, Dried Ginger, and Asarum Decoction (苓甘五味姜辛汤 *líng gān wǔ wèi jiāng xīn tāng*)

- poria (茯苓 *fú líng*, Poria) 4 *liǎng*
- licorice (甘草 *gān cǎo*, Glycyrrhizae Radix) 3 *liǎng*
- dried ginger (干姜 *gān jiāng*, Zingiberis Rhizoma) 3 *liǎng*
- asarum (细辛 *xì xīn*, Asari Radix et Rhizoma) 3 *liǎng*
- schisandra (五味子 *wǔ wèi zǐ*, Schisandrae Fructus) ½ *shēng*

Boil the above five ingredients in eight *shēng* of water to get three *shēng*. Remove the dregs. Take half a *shēng* [per dose] warm, three times a day.

Synopsis, Line 12.37

This line describes the signs and treatment of propping rheum restirring after surging qì has been calmed.

COMMENTARY, LINE 12.37

If Cinnamon, Poria, Schisandra, and Licorice Decoction (*guì líng wǔ wèi gān cǎo tāng*) succeeds in calming the surging qì, but the symptoms of cough and fullness in the chest reoccur, this means that the propping rheum is arising again. This requires further treatment to eliminate rheum and relieve cough.

The formula suggested here is Poria, Licorice, Schisandra, Dried Ginger, and Asarum Decoction (*líng gān wǔ wèi jiāng xīn tang*). Because the surging counterflow has already been calmed, we do not need cinnamon twig (*guì zhī*) any longer. However, because there is cough and fullness, we add dried ginger (*gān jiāng*) and asarum (*xì xīn*) to dissipate cold and discharge fullness. Thus the formula as a whole eliminates rheum and relieves cough.

Line 12.38

咳满即止，而更复渴，冲气复发者，以细辛、干姜为热药也；服之当遂渴，而渴反止者，为支饮也。支饮者，法当冒，冒者必呕，呕者复内半夏，以去其水。

茯苓四两　甘草 细辛　干姜各二两

五味子　半夏各半升

右六味，以水八升，煮取三升，去滓，温服半升，日三。

Ké mǎn jí zhǐ, ér gèng fù kě, chōng qì fù fā zhě, yǐ xì xīn, gān jiāng wéi rè yào yě; fú zhī dāng suì kě, ér kě fǎn zhǐ zhě, wéi zhī yǐn yě. Zhī yǐn zhě, fǎ dāng mào, mào zhě bì ǒu, ǒu zhě fù nà bàn xià, yǐ qù qí shuǐ.

Fú líng sì liǎng; gān cǎo, xì xīn, gān jiāng gè èr liǎng; wǔ wèi zǐ, bàn xià gè bàn shēng

Yòu liù wèi, yǐ shuǐ bā shēng, zhǔ qǔ sān shēng, qù zǐ, wēn fú bàn shēng, rì sān.

After you have stopped the cough and fullness, if thirst and surging qì arise again, this is because asarum (*xì xīn*) and dried ginger (*gān jiāng*) are hot medicinals, and thirst is likely to ensue after taking them. However, if the thirst stops, this means propping rheum. Propping rheum patients should experience veiling, and veiling is invariably accompanied by retching. When there is retching, add pinellia (*bàn xià*) to eliminate the water.

Cinnamon Twig, Poria, Schisandra, and Licorice Decoction Minus Cinnamon Twig Plus Dried Ginger, Asarum, and Pinellia (桂苓五味甘草去桂加干姜细辛半夏汤 *guì líng wǔ wèi gān cǎo qù guī jiā gān jiāng xì xīn bàn xià tāng*)[1]

- poria (茯苓 *fú líng*, Poria) 4 *liǎng*
- licorice (甘草 *gān cǎo*, Glycyrrhizae Radix) 2 *liǎng*
- asarum (细辛 *xì xīn*, Asari Radix et Rhizoma) 2 *liǎng*
- dried ginger (干姜 *gān jiāng*, Zingiberis Rhizoma) 2 *liǎng*
- schisandra (五味子 *wǔ wèi zǐ*, Schisandrae Fructus) ½ *shēng*
- pinellia (半夏 *bàn xià*, Pinelliae Rhizoma) ½ *shēng*

Boil the above six ingredients in eight *shēng* of water to get three *shēng*. Remove the dregs. Take half a *shēng* [per dose] warm, three times a day.

TEXT NOTE, LINE 12.38

[1] Cinnamon Twig, Poria, Schisandra, and Licorice Decoction Minus Cinnamon Twig Plus Dried Ginger, Asarum, and Pinellia (*guì líng wǔ wèi gān cǎo qù guī jiā gān jiāng xì xīn bàn xià tāng*): Also called Poria, Licorice, Schisandra, and Dried Ginger, Asarum, and Pinellia Decoction (*líng gān wǔ wèi jiāng xīn bàn xià tāng*).

SYNOPSIS, LINE 12.38

This line explains how to differentiate between surging qì and propping rheum, and explains the treatment of retching and veiling after taking Poria, Licorice, Schisandra, Dried Ginger, and Asarum Decoction (*líng gān wǔ wèi jiāng xīn tang*).

COMMENTARY, LINE 12.38

Poria, Licorice, Schisandra, Dried Ginger, and Asarum Decoction (*líng gān wǔ wèi jiāng xīn tang*) should alleviate the symptoms of cough and fullness, because it warms and dissipates cold rheum and prevents it from shooting into the lung. This is a sign that the condition is improving. Nevertheless, dried ginger (*gān jiāng*) and asarum (*xì xīn*) can be overly acrid and heating, causing dryness to form and damage liquid. The result is thirst. Furthermore, these two medicinals can stir surging qì and thereby cause the symptom of upward surging qì (originally caused by heart and kidney yang vacuity) to recur. In this case, we should repeat the treatment with Cinnamon, Poria, Schisandra, and Licorice Decoction (*guì líng wǔ wèi gān cǎo tāng*), discussed in line 12.36 above as the treatment to eliminate surging qì.

It is also possible, however, that the addition of dried ginger (*gān jiāng*) and asarum (*xì xīn*) does not result in thirst, in which case the disease cause is propping rheum. This is identical to the statement in line 12.28 above: "Thirst means [the condition] is about to resolve. However, if the patient presently has no thirst, this is because there is propping rheum below the heart." In that case, the condition is one in which the old rheum evil has not been eliminated yet and has been further aggravated by new rheum. Together, they ascend counterflow and cause qì to surge into the chest and diaphragm, causing cough and fullness.

Surging qì and propping rheum are both associated with counterflow ascent with clouding and veiling. The difference is that propping rheum is characterized by retching and vomiting, while surging qì is not. When propping rheum causes veiling and retching, pinellia (*bàn xià*) can be added to the original formula to help eliminate water in the stomach, downbear the counterflow, and check vomiting.

Line 12.39

水去呕止，其人形肿者，加杏仁主之。其证应内麻黄，以其人遂痹，故不内之。若逆而内之者，必厥。所以然者，以其人血虚，麻黄发其阳故也。

茯苓四两　甘草三两　五味子半升
干姜三两　细辛三两　半夏半升　杏

仁半升（去皮尖）

右七味，以水一斗，煮取三升，去滓。温服半升，日三。

Shuǐ qù ǒu zhǐ, qí rén xíng zhǒng zhě, jiā xìng rén zhǔ zhī. Qí zhèng yīng nà má huáng, yǐ qí rén suì bì, fù bù nà zhī. Ruò nì ér nà zhī zhě, bì jué. Suǒ yǐ rán zhě, yǐ qí rén xuè xū, má huáng fā qí yáng gù yě.

Fú líng sì liǎng; gān cǎo sān liǎng; wǔ wèi zǐ bàn shēng; gān jiāng sān liǎng; xì xīn sān liǎng; bàn xià bàn shēng; xìng rén bàn shēng (qù pí jiān)

Yòu qī wèi, yǐ shuǐ yī dǒu, zhǔ qǔ sān shēng, qù zǐ. wēn fú bàn shēng, rì sān.

When the water has gone and the retching has stopped, if the patient has the appearance of swelling, add apricot kernel (*xìng rén*) to govern it. For this pattern, you would [normally] include ephedra (*má huáng*) [in the formula], [but] because the patient suffers from impediment of the extremities, you cannot include it. If you include it contrary to this [rule], it will invariably result in reversal. The reason for this is that the patient's blood is vacuous, and ephedra (*má huáng*) will effuse the yáng.

Poria, Licorice, and Schisandra Decoction Plus Ginger, Asarum, Pinellia, and Apricot Kernel (苓甘五味加姜辛半夏杏仁汤 *líng gān wǔ wèi jiā jiāng xīn bàn xià xìng rén tāng*)

poria (茯苓 *fú líng*, Poria) 4 *liǎng*
licorice (甘草 *gān cǎo*, Glycyrrhizae Radix) 3 *liǎng*
schisandra (五味子 *wǔ wèi zǐ*, Schisandrae Fructus) ½ *shēng*
dried ginger (干姜 *gān jiāng*, Zingiberis Rhizoma) 3 *liǎng*
asarum (细辛 *xì xīn*, Asari Radix et Rhizoma) 3 *liǎng*
pinellia (半夏 *bàn xià*, Pinelliae Rhizoma) ½ *shēng*
apricot kernel (杏仁 *xìng rén*, Armeniacae Semen) ½ *shēng* (remove skin and tips)

Boil the above seven ingredients in one *dǒu* of water to get three *shēng*. Remove the dregs. Take half a *shēng* [per dose] warm, three times as day.

Synopsis, Line 12.39

Carrying on from the preceding line, the present line discusses the treatment of swelling that forms after water-rheum has been eliminated.

Commentary, Line 12.39

After the formula recommended in the previous line, Cinnamon Twig, Poria, Schisandra, and Licorice Decoction Minus Cinnamon Twig Plus Dried Ginger, Asarum, and Pinellia (*guì líng wǔ wèi gān cǎo qù guī jiā gān jiāng xì xīn bàn xià tāng*), has successfully eliminated water and checked retching and vomiting, swelling may appear if lung and defense qì are stagnant. In "vacuity stagnation" of lung qì, exterior qì fails to diffuse, and defense qì is unable to reach the skin and body hair. At the same time, the lung cannot perform its function of depurative downbearing and governing regulation of the waterways, so water floods and spills out into the skin, causing generalized swelling. This development often occurs as a result of repeated cough and panting.

We treat this condition by adding apricot kernel (*xìng rén*) to the previous formula, Cinnamon Twig, Poria, Schisandra, and Licorice Decoction Minus Cinnamon Twig Plus Dried Ginger, Asarum, and

Pinellia (*guì líng wǔ wèi gān cǎo qù guī jiā gān jiāng xì xīn bàn xià tāng*), to make Poria, Licorice, and Schisandra Decoction Plus Ginger, Asarum, Pinellia, and Apricot Kernel (*líng gān wǔ wèi jiā jiāng xīn bàn xià xìng rén tāng*). This new formula warms yáng and dissipates cold, disinhibits the lung and flushes rheum, and disinhibits qì and disperses swelling.

The latter part of this line explains why this pattern should not be treated with ephedra (*má huáng*), which effuses sweat and thereby disperses swelling. This contradicts other lines in the *Jīn Guì Yào Lüè* which recommend the use of promoting sweating to eliminate swelling and spillage rheum. Line 14.18, for example, states, "For swelling from the lumbus up, effuse sweat to bring about recovery." Line 14.26 states, "[To treat] water, effuse sweat, and it will cease." Line 12.23 describes the use of Black Dragon Decoction (*qīng lóng tāng*) to treat spillage rheum with water in the fleshy exterior.

By contrast, the present line states that we would normally use ephedra (*má huáng*) to treat swelling, but in this case, we would not. The reason for this is that this condition is related to qì and blood vacuity, which manifests in "impediment of the extremities" (numbness of the hands and feet). This is similar to the transmutation of propping rheum that occurs after taking Minor Black Dragon Decoction (*xiǎo qīng lóng tāng*), as was described in line 12.36 above: "…a sunken inch pulse and a faint cubit pulse, reverse flow of the extremities, qì surging up from the smaller abdomen to the chest and pharynx, impediment of the extremities," where the numbness is due to the sweat-effusing action of the formula.

If we give ephedra (*má huáng*), a strong sweat-effusing medicinal, to patients with such vacuity signs, it will cause damage to yáng, consume fluid, and possibly damage yīn-blood. Since qì is the leader of blood and blood is engendered by qì, blood vacuity will lead to dual vacuity of yīn and yáng and qì and blood. This manifests in reverse-flow.

Line 12.40

若面热如醉，此为胃热，上冲熏其面，加大黄以利之。

茯苓四两　半夏半升　甘草三两　五味子半升　干姜三两　细辛三两　杏仁半升（去皮尖）　大黄三两

右八味，以水一斗，煮取三升，去滓，温服半升，日三。

Ruò miàn rè rú zuì, cǐ wéi wèi rè, shàng chōng xūn qí miàn, jiā dà huáng yǐ lì zhī.

Fú líng sì liǎng; bàn xià bàn shēng; gān cǎo sān liǎng; wǔ wèi zǐ bàn shēng; gān jiāng sān liǎng; xì xīn sān liǎng; xìng rén bàn shēng (qù pí jiān); dà huáng sān liǎng

Yòu bā wèi, yǐ shuǐ yī dǒu, zhǔ qǔ sān shēng, qù zǐ, wēn fú bàn shēng, rì sān.

If the face is hot as if [the person were] drunk, this is stomach heat surging upward to smoke the face. [In such cases], add rhubarb (*dà huáng*) to disinhibit it.

Poria, Licorice, and Schisandra Decoction Plus Dried Ginger, Asarum, Pinellia, Apricot Kernel and Rhubarb (苓甘五味加姜辛半杏大黄汤 *líng gān wǔ wèi jiāng xīn bàn xià tāng*)

poria (茯苓 *fú líng*, Poria) 4 *liǎng*
pinellia (半夏 *bàn xià*, Pinelliae Rhizoma) ½ *shēng*
licorice (甘草 *gān cǎo*, Glycyrrhizae Radix) 3 *liǎng*
schisandra (五味子 *wǔ wèi zǐ*, Schisandrae Fructus) ½ *shēng*
dried ginger (干姜 *gān jiāng*, Zingiberis Rhizoma) 3 *liǎng*
asarum (细辛 *xì xīn*, Asari Radix et Rhizoma) 3 *liǎng*
apricot kernel (杏仁 *xìng rén*, Armeniacae Semen) ½ *shēng* (remove skin and tips)
rhubarb (大黄 *dà huáng*, Rhei Radix et Rhizoma) 3 *liǎng*

Boil the above ingredients in one *dǒu* of water to get three *shēng*. Remove the dregs. Take half a *shēng* [per dose] warm, three times a day.

SYNOPSIS, LINE 12.40

This line describes the appearance and treatment of stomach heat surging upward in propping rheum that has not resolved.

COMMENTARY, LINE 12.40

This line continues the discussion of transmutations in propping rheum patterns. The word "if" (若 *ruò*), which begins the line, is normally only used by Zhāng Jī to introduce secondary conditions after the main conditions have already been described. Assuming that this line follows line 12.39, the phrase "if the face is hot as if [the person were] drunk" adds another condition to the signs previously noted, namely, cough, fullness in the chest, dizziness and veiling, retching and vomiting, and swelling of the body. The symptom of heat in the face is caused by stomach heat surging upward. Since this is thus a pattern of water-rheum complicated by heat, the formula suggested here is a warming transforming rheum-eliminating formula with the addition of bitter cold heat-discharging rhubarb (*dà huáng*).

Line 12.41

先渴后呕，为水停心下，此属饮家，小半夏茯苓汤主之。

Xiān kě hòu ǒu, wéi shuǐ tíng xīn xià, cǐ shǔ yǐn jiā, xiǎo bàn xià fú líng tāng zhǔ zhī.

Thirst first and retching afterwards [indicates] water collecting below the heart. This [symptom] is associated with rheum patients. Minor Pinellia Poria Decoction (*xiǎo bàn xià fú líng tāng*) governs.[1]

TEXT NOTE, LINE 12.41

[1] Here the commentary adds: "For the formula, see above." This refers to line 12.28 above, where it is called Minor Pinellia Decoction Plus Poria (*xiǎo bàn xià jiā fú líng tāng*).

SYNOPSIS, LINE 12.41

This line describes the signs and treatment of retching caused by new rheum in patients with chronic rheum.

COMMENTARY, LINE 12.41

This line emphasizes the need to distinguish between old and new rheum patterns. The present line describes a case of new rheum, in which thirst appears first and is followed by retching. The thirst is preexisting, not a result of retching or of stomach heat. The change in the condition probably arose when the patient tried to allay thirst by drinking large amounts of water, which then collected below the heart and ascended counterflow because of impaired downbearing by the stomach, giving rise to vomiting and retching. As the line states, this condition is to be treated like conditions of chronic rheum.

The treatment for this condition is Minor Pinellia Decoction Plus Poria (*xiǎo bàn xià jiā fú líng tāng*). Because the rheum evil is relatively severe, the action of Minor Pinellia Decoction (*xiǎo bàn xià tāng*) is not enough to completely dissipate water. Hence, the effect of the formula is strengthened with the addition of poria (*fú líng*), which disinhibits water and thereby eliminates the old rheum, frees spleen yáng, and prevents new rheum from being engendered.

‡ SUMMARY REVIEW OF CHAPTER 12

This chapter ostensibly deals with phlegm-rheum and cough as separate disease entities, but in reality, it only discusses phlegm-rheum and cough that is caused by phlegm-rheum.

Phlegm-rheum is a generic term for conditions attributable to a pathological fluid, often referred to as water-rheum, that arises when the body fails to deal with ingested fluids effectively. The problem may be spleen yáng failing to move and transform, the lung failing to perform its functions of diffusion and depurative downbearing, or a vacuous kidney failing to govern water. We can make a fourfold distinction, based on the locus of the phlegm-rheum. Phlegm-rheum (in the narrow sense) is a phlegm-rheum pattern in which water-rheum collects in the intestines and stomach; it is characterized by gurgling sounds in the intestines. Suspended rheum refers to water-rheum collecting in the rib-side; it is marked by cough and spitting that induces rib-side pain. Spillage rheum is water-rheum collecting in the exterior; it is characterized by absence of sweating and by pain and heaviness of the limbs. Lastly, propping rheum is water-rheum collecting in the chest and diaphragm; it is characterized by cough and counterflow with propped breathing. These four kinds are not always clearly demarcable and are mutually conducive. Phlegm-rheum (in the narrow sense) in particular is related to the other three. In addition, the text also mentions lodged rheum and deep-lying rheum.

Phlegm-rheum patterns are treated mainly by warming and transforming, but also by sweating, offensive precipitation, and disinhibiting urine. Poria, Cinnamon Twig, White Atractylodes, and Licorice Decoction (*líng guì zhú gān tāng*) and Kidney Qì Pill (*shèn qì wán*) fortify the spleen and warm the kidney, thus treating the root. When rheum evil invades the upper body, Minor Pinellia Decoction (*xiǎo bàn xià tāng*), Minor Pinellia Decoction Plus Poria (*xiǎo bàn xià jiā fú líng tāng*), or Lepidium/Descurainiae and Jujube Lung-Draining Decoction (*tíng lì dà zǎo xiè fèi tāng*) can be used to treat the root. When there is a dual exterior-interior pattern, we can use Major or Minor Black Dragon Decoction (*dà/xiǎo qīng lóng tāng*). When the rheum is in the middle or lower burner, Alisma Decoction (*zé xiè tāng*) or Poria Five Powder (*wǔ líng sǎn*) can be used to disinhibit urine. For deep-seated intractable rheum evil, we can use Ten Jujubes Decoction (*shí zǎo tāng*) or Kansui and Pinellia Decoction (*gān suì bàn xià tāng*) to expel water, and Officinal Magnolia Bark and Rhubarb Decoction (*hòu pò dà huáng tāng*) or Fangji, Zanthoxylum, Lepidium/Descurainiae, and Rhubarb Pill (*jǐ jiāo lì huáng wán*) to eliminate the repletion. Persistent phlegm-rheum invariably manifests as a vacuity-repletion complex that can be treated with Woody Fangji Decoction (*mù fáng jǐ tāng*) or with Woody Fangji Decoction Minus Gypsum Plus Poria and Mirabilite (*mù fáng jǐ qù shí gāo jiā fú líng máng xiāo tāng*).

消渴小便利淋病脉证治第十三

CHAPTER 13

Dispersion-Thirst, Inhibited Urination, and Strangury

Pulses, Signs, Treatments

‡ OVERVIEW

This chapter discusses the pulses, signs, and treatments of the three diseases dispersion-thirst, inhibited urination, and strangury. Note that the Chinese title does not list "inhibited urination" (小便不利 *xiào biàn bù lì*), but rather "uninhibited urination" (小便利 *xiǎo biàn lì*). However the content clearly proves that this is merely a mistranscription of "inhibited urination."

DISPERSION-THIRST

Dispersion-thirst, inhibited urination, and strangury disease are all characterized by changes in thirst and urination. In addition, the main pathological changes in all three diseases relate to the kidney and bladder. Therefore, the formulas used to treat them are broadly similar in nature and these three conditions are placed together in one chapter. Altogether, this chapter offers such a short treatment of an important area of disease that most scholars believe that some of the text has been lost.

The name dispersion-thirst is first mentioned in the "Treatise on Strange Diseases" in the *Sù Wèn* ("Plain Questions"): "Fatty [foods] cause internal heat in a person. Sweet [foods] cause center fullness in a person. Because of this, their qì spills upward and transforms into dispersion-thirst." Dispersion-thirst is a chronic disease of internal damage that is mainly characterized by thirst with immoderate fluid intake. It can take the form of upper, center, or lower dispersion, depending on the focus of the disease.

Inhibited Urination

Inhibited urination is a symptom that can manifest as a result of a number of diseases. It refers to short and scant voidings of urine and inhibition in the flow of urine. According to the *Nèi Jīng* ("Inner Canon"), it is caused by kidney vacuity and inhibited qì transformation by the bladder.

Strangury

Strangury is a condition whose main symptom is dribbling, rough, and painful urination. It is first described in the *Sù Wèn* ("Plain Questions") in the "Great Treatise on the Regular Principles of the Six Origins" in this way: "When the spleen contracts the qì of accumulated dampness, urine will be yellow or reddish, and in severe cases there will be strangury." The pathomechanism of strangury is also quite complex, but generally related to kidney vacuity and heat bind in the bladder. Based on the clinical manifestations, contemporary medicine distinguishes between stone strangury, qì strangury, unctuous strangury, taxation strangury, and blood strangury. The present chapter, however, is not comprehensive and only refers to blood strangury and stone strangury.

‡ Schematic Overview

Dispersion-Thirst

1. Upper dispersion-thirst
   a) *Signs*: Thirst with desire to drink water; dry mouth and tongue.
   b) *Treatment*: Clear heat, boost qì, engender liquid, and allay thirst using White Tiger Decoction Plus Ginseng (*bái hǔ jiā rén shēn tāng*).
2. Center dispersion-thirst
   Signs: Hard stool, frequent urination, swift digestion, and thirst with intake of fluids.
   Treatment: Free the bowels and discharge heat using Stomach-Regulating Qì-Coordinating Decoction (*tiáo wèi chéng qì tāng*). This is not mentioned in the original text, but is the general opinion of later scholars.
3. Lower dispersion-thist (kidney vacuity)
   Signs: Passing of as much fluid as is drunk.
   Treatment: Warm yáng and promote qì to steam liquid and retain water.

Inhibited Urination

1. Water and cold binding together (greater yáng water amassment pattern)
   Signs: Floating pulse; inhibited urination; slight heat effusion; dispersion-thirst
   Treatment: Promote qì transformation and move water, while freeing yáng and resolving the exterior with Poria Five Powder (*wǔ líng sǎn*).
2. Water and heat binding together, with depressed heat damaging yīn
   Signs: Floating pulse, heat effusion; thirst with desire to drink; inhibited urination.

Treatment: Disnihibit water and clear heat, while enriching yīn and moistening dryness using Polyporus Decoction (*zhū líng tāng*).

3. Insufficiency of kidney yáng with lower body cold and upper body dryness:

   Signs: Inhibted urination; water qì; bitter taste in the mouth; thirst.

   Treatment: Warm yáng and promote qì transformation, while engendering liquid and moistening dryness using Trichosanthes and Dianthus Pill (*guā lóu qū mài wán*).

4. Lower-burner damp-heat binding with blood stasis impeding bladder qì transformation:

   Signs: Inhibited urination in some cases with short voidings of reddish urine or bloody urine, pain on urination, tension in the lesser abdomen.

   Treatment: Clear heat and disinhibit dampness, while cooling the blood and transforming stasis with Charred Dandelion Powder (*pú huī sǎn*).

5. Lower-burner damp-heat with blood stasis damaging the network vessels:

   Signs: Inhibited urination with bloody urine, pain on urination, tension in the lesser abdomen.

   Treatment: Clear heat and disinhibit dampness, transforming stasis and stanching bleeding with Talcum and Silverfish Powder (*huá shí bái yú sǎn*).

6. Spleen vacuity in the center burner with damp congealing in the lower burner: Fortify the spleen and percolate dampness with Poria and Halite Decoction (*fú líng róng yán tāng*).

7. Stone strangury: Described as urine with millet-like particles, accompanied by inhibited urination with difficult voiding, tension in the smaller abdomen, and pain stretching into the umbilicus.

Line 13.1

厥阴之为病，消渴，气上冲心，心中疼热，饥而不欲食，食即吐蚘，下之不肯止。

Jué yīn zhī wéi bìng, xiāo kě, qì shàng chōng xīn, xīn zhōng téng rè, jī ér bù yù shí, shí jí tù huí, xià zhī bù kěn zhǐ.

Disease of reverting yīn [manifests in] dispersion-thirst, qì surging upward into the heart, pain and heat in the heart, hunger but no desire to eat, and vomiting of roundworm upon eating. If you precipitate, [the resulting diarrhea] will not stop.

Synopsis, Line 13.1

This line describes a reverting yīn pattern of upper body heat and lower body cold, giving a contraindication for its treatment.

Commentary, Line 13.1

Reverting yīn disease falls into two kinds. One is alternating reversal and heat effusion; the other is a cold-heat complex. The condition described in this line appears to be upper body heat and lower body cold, with dispersion-thirst being caused by internal heat scorching the fluids. The foot reverting yīn channel reaches the smaller abdomen and clasps the stomach; hence counterflow ascent of liver qì causes qì to surge into the heart. When heat evil is in the upper body, there is pain and heat in the heart. Because the stomach is cold, it cannot digest food. The result is hunger but no desire to eat, and vomiting after eating. If a patient with this condition is treated inappropriately with precipitation, this will severely damage the spleen and stomach without eliminating the upper body heat. Furthermore, it will exacerbate the lower body cold. The result will be incessant diarrhea.

Line 13.2

(1)寸口脉浮而迟，浮即为虚，迟即为劳，虚则卫气不足，劳则荣气竭。

(2)趺阳脉浮而数，浮即为气，数即消谷而大坚。气盛则溲数，溲数即坚，坚数相搏，即为消渴。

(1) Cùn kǒu mài fú ér chí, fú jí wéi xū, chí jí wéi láo, xū zé wèi qì bù zú, láo zé róng qì jié.

(2) Fū yáng mài fú ér shuò, fú jí wéi qì, shù jí xiāo gǔ ér dà jiān. Qì shèng zé sōu shù, sōu shuò jí jiān, jiān shuò xiāng bó, jí wéi xiāo kě.

(1) When the inch opening pulse is floating and slow, floating means vacuity and slow means taxation. Vacuity results in insufficiency of defense qì, while taxation results in depletion of construction qì.

(2) When the instep yáng pulse is floating and rapid, floating means qì, while rapid means dispersion of grain[1] and great hardness.[2] Exuberance of qì results in frequent urination, and frequent urination results in hard stool. Hard [stool] and frequent [urination] contend with each other, and this constitutes dispersion-thirst.

TEXT NOTES, LINE 13.2

[1] Dispersion of grain 消谷 *xiāo gǔ*: That is, swift digestion.

[2] Hardness 坚 *jiān*: An alternative version of this text has "tightness" (紧 *jǐn*) instead.

SYNOPSIS, LINE 13.2

This line describes the key pathomechanisms and signs of upper disipation and center dispersion.

COMMENTARY, LINE 13.2

Dispersion-thirst disease develops gradually. The inch position of the pulse is the indicator of the heart and lung. The heart governs blood and is associated with construction, while the lung governs qì and is associated with defense. When the inch pulse is at the same time slow and floating, the floating quality indicates yáng vacuity and floating qì, which is a sign that defense qì is insufficient. The slowness of the pulse indicates that the vessels are not full and is therefore evidence of construction qì vacuity. As reflected in this pulse, dual vacuity of construction and defense is the cause of the disease described in the first line. When construction qì is insufficient, dryness-heat arises in the inner body, whereupon dispersion-thirst begins to develop.

When the instep yáng pulse is floating and rapid, the floating quality indicates a superabundance of stomach qì, while the rapidness means exuberant stomach heat. When stomach heat and qì are exuberant, the result is swift digestion, rapid hungering, and thirst with desire to drink water. Superandant qì becomes fire, which distresses water. As a result, water percolates quickly down to the bladder, giving rise to frequent urination. Exuberant heat consumes liquid and exacerbates the vacuity of fluids that results from increased urination. Hence, the intestinal tract is deprived of moisture and the stool is hard. When stomach heat with hard stool, and exuberant qì with frequent urination exacerbate each other, dispersion-thirst arises. This kind of dispersion-thirst is now referred to as center dispersion.

Line 13.3

男子消渴，小便反多，以饮一斗，小便一斗，肾气丸主之。

Nán zǐ xiāo kě, xiǎo biàn fǎn duō, yǐ yǐn yī dǒu, xiǎo biàn yī dǒu, shèn qì wán zhǔ zhī.

Dispersion-thirst in male [patients manifests in] exceptionally profuse urine, so that drinking one *dǒu* results in urinating one *dǒu*. Kidney Qì Pill (*shèn qì wán*) governs.[1]

TEXT NOTE, LINE 13.3

[1] The commentary adds here: "For the formula, see the chapter on Women's Miscellaneous Diseases." The formula is found in Chapter 22, line 22.19.

SYNOPSIS, LINE 13.3

This line describes lower dispersion due to debilitation of kidney qì.

COMMENTARY, LINE 13.3

As mentioned in the chapter introduction, dispersion-thirst can be divided into upper, center, and lower dispersion. Upper dispersion is focused in the lung, center dispersion in the stomach, and lower dispersion in the kidney. While upper and center dispersion are always due to dryness-heat, lower dispersion can be caused either by cold or heat. The kidney is the viscus of water and fire; it contains true yīn and true yáng. Kidney yáng vacuity, kidney yīn vacuity, and dual vacuity of kidney yīn and kidney yáng may all give rise to lower dispersion. The present line describes a condition of lower dispersion due to kidney yáng vacuity.

The subject of the present line is "males." Although both genders are prone to lower dispersion due to kidney yáng vacuity, males specifically are mentioned here because they are associated with yáng, and male sexual matters are related to the kidney. If a male engages excessively in sexual activity, the consumption of essence will inevitably cause damage to yáng. The specification of male here may be nothing more than the inference of kidney vacuity as the cause of lower dispersion.

Copious urine is the main symptom of dispersion-thirst disease. The extraordinary copiousness that is characteristic of lower dispersion in particular can be emphasized by a rough, subjective quantitative datum: urine is the same in volume as fluids ingested. The kidney governs water, and when kidney yáng is debilitated, it fails to "distill" the fluids and return some of the water that goes to the kidney back to the body; hence there is severe thirst. Because kidney yáng cannot perform qì transformation to contain bodily fluids, imbibed fluids largely descend directly to the bladder to be discharged from the body; hence there is copious urination.

The treatment for this condition is to warm and supplement the yáng qì of the kidney, and to restore normal distillation of liquid and qì transformation, using Kidney Qì Pill (肾气丸 *shèn qì wán*). In this formula, rehmannia (*dì huáng*), dioscorea (*shān yào*), and cornus (*shān zhū yú*) enrich kidney yīn, since when yīn is engendered, yáng can grow. Aconite (*fù zǐ*) and cinnamon twig (*guì zhī*) warm kidney yáng and thereby supplement fire within water to rally kidney qì. The formula encourages water and fire to help each other and to coordinate yīn and yáng. In this way, yáng qì is vitalized and the dispersion-thirst resolved.

Kidney Qì Pill (*shèn qì wán*) also contains blood-quickening moutan (*mǔ dān pí*) and water-disinhibiting alisma (*zé xiè*) and poria (*fú líng*) as assistants, which at first sight is surprising, given that profuse urination is the main symptom of this condition. Nevertheless, the urination-disinhibiting and blood-quickening action of these medicinals assists the yīn-enriching yáng-supplementing action of the other medicinals.

Line 13.4

脉浮小便不利，微热消渴者，宜利小便，发汗，五苓散主之。

Mài fú xiǎo biàn bù lì, wēi rè xiāo kě zhě, yí lì xiǎo biàn, fā hàn, wǔ líng sǎn zhǔ zhī.

For a floating pulse, inhibited urination, slight heat [effusion], and dispersion-thirst,[1] it is appropriate to disinhibit urine and effuse sweat. Poria Five Powder (*wǔ líng sǎn*) governs.[2]

Text Notes, Line 13.4

[1] Dispersion-thirst 消渴 *xiāo kě*: In this context, dispersion-thirst refers to the symptom rather than the disease, i.e., thirst with ingestion of large amounts of fluid.

[2] The commentary adds: "For the formula, see above." This refers to line 12.31 above.

Synopsis, Line 13.4

This line describes the signs and treatment of inhibited urination due to cold and water binding together and obstructing bladder qì transformation.

Commentary, Line 13.4

In the context of the present line, a floating pulse signifies the presence of wind-cold fettering the exterior, which normally gives rise to a tight floating pulse. The triple burner and bladder are related to the insterstices and fine body hair. The bladder is the house of the fluids. When its function of qì transformation is normal, fluid flows down to the bladder, and urination is uninhibited; fluid also reaches upward to keep the body hair and the orifices moist and in harmony. However, when cold evil strikes the greater yáng channel and enters the interior, as in the present line, bladder qì transformation is obstructed, and water collects in the lower body, causing inhibited urination. Since qì fails to transform liquid, the fluids are not distilled, so insufficient fluid is returned to the body; hence there is thirst. This kind of thirst is due to cold and water binding together in the bladder. Thus we see thirst without large intake of water or immediate vomiting of ingested fluids. This is a disease that affects both the greater yáng channel and bowel, with emphasis on the bowel.

The treatment offered is Poria Five Powder (*wǔ líng sǎn*), which disinhibits urine and also promotes sweating. For an explanation of this formula, see the commentary to line 12.31 above.

Line 13.5

渴欲饮水，水入则吐者，名曰水逆，五苓散主之。

Kě yù yǐn shuǐ, shuǐ rù zé tù zhě, míng yuē shuǐ nì, wǔ líng sǎn zhǔ zhī.

Thirst with desire for fluid, and vomiting upon drinking water is called water counterflow.[1] Poria Five Powder (*wǔ líng sǎn*) governs.[2]

TEXT NOTES, LINE 13.5

[1] Water counterflow 水逆 *shuǐ nì*: A severe form of water amassment in the bladder, which is characterized not only by inhibited urination, but also by thirst, large intake of fluids, and immediate vomiting of ingested fluids.

[2] Here the commentary adds: "For the formula, see above." The formula is found in line 12.31.

SYNOPSIS, LINE 13.5

This line continues the discussion of inhibited urindation due to cold and water binding together and obstructing bladder qì transformation.

COMMENTARY, LINE 13.5

The present line continues to describe the process of cold and water binding and causing inhibited urination that gives rise to a pattern of water counterflow. When wind-cold evil passes along the foot greater yáng bladder channel into the greater yáng bowel, cold binds with water, causing inhibited bladder qì transformation. As a result, liquid fails to bear upward, giving rise to thirst. When water amasses in the lower burner in excessive quantities, it ascends to affect the stomach. This impairs the harmonious downbearing of stomach qì and causes ingested fluid to be rejected. Here, there is immediate vomiting of ingested fluid. This pathomechanism is called "water counterflow." Again the text recommends Poria Five Powder (*wǔ líng sǎn*) to treat this condition.

Line 13.6

渴欲饮水不止者，文蛤散主之。
文蛤五两
右一味，杵为散，以沸汤五合，和服方寸匕。

Kě yù yǐn shuǐ bù zhǐ zhě, wén gé sǎn zhǔ zhī.

Wén gé wǔ liǎng

Yòu yī wèi, chǔ wéi sǎn, yǐ fèi tāng wǔ gě, huó fú fāng cùn bǐ.

For thirst and incessant desire to drink water, Meretrix Clam Shell Powder (*wén gé sǎn*) governs.

Meretrix Clam Shell Powder (*wén gé sǎn*)
meretrix clam shell (文蛤 *wén gé*, Meretricis Concha) 5 *liǎng*

Pestle the single above ingredient into a powder and mix into five *gě* of boiling water. Take a square-inch-spoonful [per dose].

SYNOPSIS, LINE 13.6

This line describes the signs and treatment of dispersion-thirst due to kidney heat scorching the fluids.

COMMENTARY, LINE 13.6

Thirst with desire to drink water is a sign of heat. Furthermore, when the thirst is not quenched by drinking but continues unabated, this indicates that the ingested water has failed to disperse the heat but is dispersed by the heat instead. In this case, the heat evil has penetrated deeply into the lower burner and stirred kidney yīn, so that exuberant fire flames upward, to the point where ingested water is only able to moisten the dryness in the stomach, but is not sufficient to alleviate kidney heat. This is the situation described here. The text does not mention retching and vomiting. Nor do we see inhibited urination. This means that there is no problem with water collecting in this condition. Hence the treatment is Meretrix Clam Shell Powder (*wén gé sǎn*), a salty cool moist precipitating formula that clears heat, engenders liquid, and allays thirst.

Line 13.7

淋之为病，小便如粟状，小腹弦急，痛引脐中。

Lín zhī wéi bìng, xiǎo biàn rú sù zhuàng, xiǎo fù xián jí, tòng yǐn qí zhōng.

The disease of strangury [manifests in] urine with millet-like [particles],[1] bowstring tightness in the smaller abdomen,[2] and pain stretching into the umbilicus.

TEXT NOTES, LINE 13.7

[1] Urine with millet-like [particles] 小便如粟状: The urine contains small particles of calculus. Hence the condition described here is stone strangury (石淋 *shí lín*).

[2] Bowstring tightness in the smaller abdomen 小腹弦急 *xiǎo fù xián jí*: Tension and pain in the part of the abdomen below the umbilicus like a tightly stretched bowstring.

SYNOPSIS, LINE 13.7

This line describes the symptoms of stone strangury.

COMMENTARY, LINE 13.7

Strangury is a disease that is mainly characterized by urinary frequency and urgency, difficult short voidings, stabbing pain in the urinary tract, and dribbling incontinence. It takes different forms, as exemplified by the five-fold classification into qì stragury, blood strangury, unctuous strangury, stone strangury, and taxation strangury. The present line describes a kind of strangury that is characterized by urine containing particles like millet seeds. This is commonly called stone strangury, known in Western medicine as urinary calculus. Stone straungury is attributed to exuberant bladder heat that scorches the urine, causing solid matter to bind into particles. The particles cause obstruction, which in turn causes the heat to become depressed and qì to stagnate; hence the inhibited urination with difficult voiding, tension in the smaller abdomen, and pain that stretches into the umbilicus. Stone stangury is the most painful kind of strangury.

Line 13.8

趺阳脉数，胃中有热，即消谷引食，大便必坚，小便即数。

Fū yáng mài shuò, wèi zhōng yǒu rè, jí xiāo gǔ yǐn shí, dà biàn bì jiān, xiǎo biàn jí shuò.

When the instep yáng pulse is rapid, there is heat in the stomach. This causes grain dispersion and [constant] intake of food, inevitable hardness of the stool, and frequent urination.

Synopsis, Line 13.8

This line describes the pathomechanism, pulse, and signs of center dispersion.

Commentary, Line 13.8

The present line elaborates on the description of center dispersion that is found in line 13.2: "When the instep yáng pulse is floating and rapid, floating means qì, while rapid means dispersion of grain and great hardness. Exuberance of qì results in frequent urination, and frequent urination results in hard stool." The instep yáng pulse is an indicator of the stomach. A rapid instep yáng pulse thus means heat in the stomach, which causes swift digestion with rapid hungering and thirst with desire to drink water. Because the fluids do not moisten the intestinal tract, but tend to percolate down into the bladder, stool is hard and urination is frequent. This condition is caused by exuberant stomach heat and qì, and has since come to be called "center dispersion."

Line 13.9

淋家不可发汗，发汗则必便血。

Lín jiā bù kě fā hàn, fā hàn zé bì biàn xuè.

A strangury patient may not [be treated by] effusing sweat. Effusing sweat inevitably results in bloody urine.[1]

TEXT NOTES, LINE 13.9

[1] Bloody urine 便血 *biàn xuè*: 便 *biàn* literally means "convenience." It is a Chinese euphemism for stool and urine, with "greater convenience" (大便 *dà biàn*) being stool, and "smaller convenience" being urine. In most current medical contexts, the term 便血 *biàn xuè* refers to bloody stool. However, in the present line, it clearly refers to blood in the urine.

SYNOPSIS, LINE 13.9

This line discusses the prohibition against sweating treatment in strangury patients, and the transmuted pattern that arises when inappropriate sweating is given.

COMMENTARY, LINE 13.9

Strangury disease is usually due to kidney vacuity with accumulated heat in the bladder. As this tends to be associated with a depletion of yīn humor, the use of yáng medicinals to promote sweating inevitably damages the construction aspect, forcing blood to move frenetically, thereby giving rise to bloody urine.

Line 13.10

小便不利者，有水气，其人苦渴，栝蒌瞿麦丸主之。

栝蒌根二两　茯苓三两　薯蓣三两
附子（炮）一枚　瞿麦一两

右五味，末之，炼蜜丸梧子大，饮服三丸，日三服，不知，增至七八丸，以小便利，腹中温为知。

Xiǎo biàn bù lì zhě, yǒu shuǐ qì, qí rén kǔ kě, guā lóu qú mài wán zhǔ zhī.

Guā lóu gēn èr liǎng; fú líng sān liǎng; shǔ yù sān liǎng; fù zǐ yī méi (pào); qú mài yī liǎng

Yòu wǔ wèi, mò zhī, liàn mì wán wú zǐ dà, yǐn fú sān wán, rì sān fú, bù zhī, zēng zhì qī bā wán, yǐ xiǎo biàn lì, fù zhōng wēn wéi zhī.

Inhibited urination means that there is water qì and that the patient suffers from thirst. Trichosanthes and Dianthus Pill (栝蒌瞿麦丸 *guā lóu qú mài wán*) governs.

Trichosanthes and Dianthus Pill (栝蒌瞿麦丸 *guā lóu qú mài wán*)

trichosanthes root (栝蒌根 *guā lóu gēn*, Trichosanthis Fructus Radix) 2 *liǎng*
poria (茯苓 *fú líng*, Poria) 3 *liǎng*
dioscorea (薯蓣 *shǔ yù*, Dioscoreae Rhizoma) 3 *liǎng*
aconite (附子 *fù zǐ*, Aconiti Radix Lateralis Praeparata) 1 piece (blast-fried)
dianthus (瞿麦 *qú mài*, Dianthi Herba) 1 *liǎng*

Pulverize the above five ingredients and blend with processed honey (*liàn mì*) to form into pills the size of firmiana seeds. Take three pills with fluid, three times a day. If no [effect] is noticed, increase [the dosage] to seven or eight pills. Disinhibition of urine and warmth in the stomach can be taken as indicators [that the formula is working].

SYNOPSIS, LINE 13.10

This line describes the signs and treatment of inhibited urination with upper body dryness and lower body cold.

COMMENTARY, LINE 13.10

The kidney governs water and is in charge of qì transformation. If kidney qì fails to perform transformation, urination can become inhibited, so that water qì collects internally. At the same time, liquid is not borne upward, so the upper burner becomes dry and hot. Hence the patient suffers from thirst.

We treat this condition by promoting qì tranformation, disinhibiting water, and moistening dryness. The formula suggested is Trichosanthes and Dianthus Pill (*guā lóu qú mài wán*). Trichosanthes (*guā lóu*) and dioscorea (*shǔ yù*) engender liquid and moisten dryness, hence addressing the thirst. Dianthus (*qú mài*) and poria (*fú líng*) promote percolation and move water, addressing the inhibited urination. Aconite (*fù zǐ*) warms yáng and promotes qì transformation, making the fluids steam upward and water qì descend.

The main feature of the formula is that it combines cold and cool medicinals with warm and dry ones, and also uses bland percolators together with supplementing medicines. Thus although the formula is cold and cool and dryness-moistening, it does not damage yáng qì; despite its yáng-warming capacity, it does not damage yīn liquid; and despite its bland percolating water-disinhibiting action, it does not damage liquid. Thus the formula embodies the principles "acting in tandem without clashing" (并行而不悖 *bìng xíng ér bù bèi*) and "simultaneous attack and supplementation" (攻补兼施 *gōng bǔ jiān shī*).

Line 13.11

小便不利, 蒲灰散主之, 滑石白鱼散, 茯苓戎盐汤并主之。

蒲灰七分　滑石三分

右二味, 杵为散, 饮服方寸匕, 日三服。

滑石二分 乱发二分（烧）白鱼二分

右三味, 杵为散, 饮服半钱匕, 日三服。

茯苓半斤 白朮二两 戎盐弹丸大一枚

右三味, 以水五升, 煮取三升, 分温三服。

Xiǎo biàn bù lì, pú huī sǎn zhǔ zhī, huá shí bái yú sǎn, fú líng róng yán tāng bìng zhǔ zhī.

Pú huī qī fèn; huá shí sān fèn

Yòu èr wèi, chǔ wéi sǎn, yǐn fú fāng cùn bǐ, rì sān fú.

Huá shí èr fèn; luàn fǎ èr fèn (shāo); bái yú èr fèn

Yòu sān wèi, chǔ wéi sǎn, yǐn fú bàn qián bǐ, rì sān fú.

Fú líng bàn jīn; bái zhú èr liǎng; róng yán dàn wán dà yī méi

Yòu sān wèi, yǐ shuǐ wǔ shēng, zhǔ qǔ sān shēng, fēn wēn sān fú.

For inhibited urination, Charred Dandelion Powder (*pú huī sǎn*) governs. Talcum and Silverfish Powder (*huá shí bái yú sǎn*) and Poria and Halite Decoction (*fú líng róng yán tāng*) also govern.

Charred Dandelion Powder (蒲灰散 *pú huī sǎn*)
charred dandelion (蒲灰 *pú huī*, Taraxaci Herba Carbonisata) 7 parts talcum (滑石 *huá shí*, Talcum) 3 parts

Pestle the above two ingredients into a powder. Take a square-inch-spoonful in fluid, three times a day.

Talcum and Silverfish Powder (滑石白鱼散 *huá shí bái yú sǎn*)
talcum (滑石 *huá shí*, Talcum) 2 parts human hair (亂髮 *luàn fǎ*, Crinis Carbonisatus)[1] 2 *fen* (char) silverfish (白鱼 *bái yú*, Lepisma)[2] 2 parts

Pestle the above three ingredients into a powder. Take half a qián-spoonful in fluid, three times a day.

Poria and Halite Decoction (茯苓戎盐汤 *fú líng róng yán tāng*)
poria (茯苓 *fú líng*, Poria) ½ *jīn* white atractylodes (白朮 *bái zhú*, Atractylodis Macrocephalae Rhizoma) 2 *liǎng* halite (戎盐 *róng yán*, Halitum) one lump the size of a pellet

Boil the above three ingredients in five *shēng* of water to get three *shēng*. Divide into three [doses] and take warm.

Text Notes, Line 13.11

[1] Human hair 乱发 *luàn fǎ*: Lit., "disheveled hair." Mentioned in the *Shén Nóng Běn Cǎo Jīng* ("The Divine Husbandman's Herbal Foundation Canon") as a treatment for inhibited urination.

[2] Silverfish 白鱼 *bái yú*: Also called *yī yú* 衣魚. According to the *Shén Nóng Běn Cǎo Jīng* ("Divine Husbandman's Herbal Foundation Canon"), it treats women's mounting conglomeration and inhibited urination.

Synopsis, Line 13.11

This line describes three treatments for inhibited urination.

Commentary, Line 13.11

Inhibited urination is a symptom that can appear in numerous diseases for many different reasons. This line provides three formulas for inhibited urination.

Based on the individual agents in each formula, we can deduce the specific indications that each formula is intended to treat. Charred Dandelion Powder (*pú huī sǎn*) is composed of charred dandelion (*pú huī*) and talcum (*huá shí*). Charred dandelion cools the blood, transforms stasis, and disperses swelling. Talcum (*huá shí*) disinhibits dampness and clears heat. Combined together, they have the effect of transforming stasis, disinhibiting the orifices, and discharging heat. Thus the formula treats inhibited urination, pain in the urethra, and tension and pain in the smaller abdomen due to damp-heat binding in the lower burner.

Talcum and Silverfish Powder (*huá shí bái yú sǎn*) is composed of talcum (*huá shí*), charred hair (*luàn fǎ*), and silverfish (*bái yú*). Talcum disinhibits dampness and clears heat. Charred hair is nowadays used to disperse stasis and staunch bleeding. The *Míng Yī Bié Lùn* ("Additional Records of Famous Physicians") states that it "governs the five stranguries and urinary and fecal stoppage." According to the *Jīn Guì Yào Luè Xīn Diǎn* ("Heart-Insights Classic of the Essential Prescriptions of the Golden Cabinet"), "human hair treats shifted bladder and inhibited urination."

Both these quotations implicitly suggest that human hair disinhibits urine and frees strangury. According to the *Shén Nóng Běn Cǎo Jīng* ("Divine Husbandman's Herbal Foundation Canon"), silverfish (*bái yú*) "governs women's mounting conglomerations and inhibited urination." According to the *Míng Yī Bié Lùn* ("Additional Records of Famous Physicians"), it is "able to open the stomach and precipitate qì, disinhibit water qì, and treat strangury and miscarriage." These three medicinals combined not only cool the blood and transform stasis, but also clear heat and disinhibit dampness. Hence they are used to treat inhibited urination, bloody urine, and pain in the urethra on urination, which are caused by damp-heat binding in the blood-aspect of the bladder, obstructed bladder qì transformation, and damage to the yīn network vessels, that is, conditions later physicians classed as "blood strangury."

Poria and Halite Decoction (*fú líng róng yán tāng*) is composed of poria (*fú líng*), white atractylodes (*bái zhú*), and halite (*róng yán*). Poria and white atractylodes disinhibit dampness and fortify the spleen. Halite, which in Chinese is also called 青盐 *qīng yán*, is cold in nature and salty in flavor. It treats bloody urine and blood ejection, assists the water viscus, and boosts essential qì. The formula as a whole fortifies the spleen, disinhibits dampness, and boosts the kidney. It treats inhibited urination due to vacuity of the center burner and spleen, with severe dampness in the lower burner. Cáo Yǐng-Fǔ 曹颖甫 has stated that this formula is appropriate for blockage of the waterways due to unctuous strangury and blood stangury.

The three formulas given in this line all address inhibited urination as the key symptom. All treat strangury disease and bloody urine that are conditions related to damp-heat binding in the kidney and bladder. However, they differ in their emphasis on treating vacuity and repletion. Charred Dandelion Powder (*pú huī sǎn*) and Talcum and Silverfish Powder (*huá shí bái yú sǎn*) both cool blood and disperse stasis, and as well clear heat and disinhibit dampness. However, the former has a stronger heat-clearing dampness-disinhibiting action, while the lattter has a stronger blood-cooling stasis-dispersing action and is also effective in stanching bleeding. Both treat repletion patterns. Poria and Halite Decoction (*fú líng róng yán tāng*), on the other hand, fortifies the spleen, percolates dampness, softens hardness, and dissipates binds. It addresses damp-heat patterns with mild heat and severe dampness occuring in vacuity-repletion complexes. It is thus a formula that applies the principle of simultaneous attack and supplementation.

Line 13.12

渴欲饮水，口干舌燥者，白虎加人参汤主之。

Kě yù yǐn shuǐ, kǒu gān shé zào zhě, bái hǔ jiā rén shēn tāng zhǔ zhī.

For thirst with desire to drink water, and dry mouth and tongue, White Tiger Decoction Plus Ginseng (*bái hǔ jiā rén shēn tāng*) governs.[1]

TEXT NOTE, LINE 13.12

[1] For the formula, see Chapter 2, "Thermoplegia" (中暍 *zhòng yē*), line 2.26.

SYNOPSIS, LINE 13.12

This line discusses the treatment of dispersion-thirst due to exuberant heat damaging liquid.

COMMENTARY, LINE 13.12

Dispersion-thirst patients suffer from thirst with desire to drink water. If they still have a dry mouth and tongue after drinking, this is because of damage by exuberant lung-stomach heat. Heat damages not only the fluids of the body, but also qì ("vigorous fire consumes qì," 壯火伤气 *zhuàng huǒ shí qì*), and this has an exacerbating effect on the thirst. The reason for this is that qì, when it is vacuous, cannot transform liquid, i.e., it cannot process the fluids of the body. Liquid is normally borne upward to moisten the upper body. When it is depleted, there is nothing to be borne upward; hence we observe thirst that the patient tries to allay by drinking water. However, imbibed fluids fail to extinguish the vigorous fire. Furthermore, because qì cannot spread the fluids, they tend to flow directly down to the bladder, giving rise to frequent urination. Hence fluid depletion and qì vacuity combine to create a vicious circle.

In the condition described in the present line, the heat is located in the lung and stomach, with emphasis on the latter. The stomach belongs to yáng brightness, and the heat is actually not found in the stomach itself, but rather in the yáng brightness channel. Because the yáng brightness bowel is not yet affected, the treatment is to clear rather than to precipitate. Although clearing heat is the appropriate method of treatment, avoid the use of cold bitter medicines that can form dryness and damage the stomach. The formula suggested is White Tiger Decoction Plus Ginseng (*bái hǔ jiā rén shēn tāng*), which clears heat, safeguards liquid, and boosts qì, in order to engender liquid. When liquid is engendered, then the thirst will cease. Gypsum (*shí gāo*), a cool acrid heat-clearing medicinal, is the chief agent within the formula. Anemarrhena (*zhī mǔ*) is bitter, cold, and moistening. It helps gypsum (*shí gāo*) to clear the yáng brightness channel heat; at the same time, it enriches yīn and moistens dryness. Although anemarrhena is bitter in flavor, it does prevent dryness formation, and hence is the assistant medicinal. Ginseng (*rén shēn*) greatly supplements original qì, and boosts qì to engender liquid. Sweet and moist non-glutinous rice (*jīng mǐ*) and mix-fried licorice (*zhì gān cǎo*) nourish the stomach. They not only engender liquid, but also prevent the cold and cool medicines from damaging the stomach. All the agents combined conjugate to clear heat and boost qì, and to engender liquid and allay thirst.

Line 13.13

脉浮发热，渴欲饮水，小便不利者，猪苓汤主之。

猪苓（去皮）茯苓　阿胶 滑石　泽泻各一两

右五味，以水四升，先煮四味，取二升，去滓，内胶烊消，温服七合，日三服。

Mài fú fā rè, kě yù yǐn shuǐ, xiǎo biàn bù lì zhě, zhū líng tāng zhǔ zhī.

Zhū líng (qù pí); fú líng; ē jiāo huá shí; zé xiè gè yī liǎng

Yòu wǔ wèi, yǐ shuǐ sì shēng, xiān zhǔ sì wèi, qǔ èr shēng, qù zǐ, nà jiāo yáng xiāo, wēn fú qī gě, rì sān fú.

For a floating pulse, heat effusion, thirst with desire to drink water, and inhibited urination, Polyporus Decoction (猪苓汤 *zhū líng tāng*) governs.

Polyporus Decoction
(猪苓汤 *zhū líng tāng*)

polyporus (猪苓 *zhū líng*, Polyporus) (remove skin) 1 *liǎng*
poria (茯苓 *fú líng*, Poria) 1 *liǎng*
ass hide glue (阿胶 *ē jiāo*, Asini Corii Colla) 1 *liǎng*
talcum (滑石 *huá shí*, Talcum) 1 *liǎng*
alisma (泽泻 *zé xiè*, Alismatis Rhizoma) 1 *liǎng*

Of the above five ingredients, first boil the four ingredients [except ass hide glue (*ē jiāo*)] in four *shēng* of water to get two *shēng*. Remove the dregs. Add the ass hide glue (*ē jiāo*) and let it melt. Take seven *gě* [per dose] warm, three times a day.

SYNOPSIS, LINE 13.13

This line describes the signs and treatment of inhibited urination due to water and heat binding together and depressed heat damaging yīn.

COMMENTARY, LINE 13.13

The present line is virtually the same as line 223 of the *Shāng Hán Lùn* ("On Cold Damage"), where it appears in the discussion of yáng brightness disease.

Together the symptoms of floating pulse, heat effusion, thirst with desire to drink water, and inhibited urination indicate a pattern of water and heat binding with depressed heat and damaging yīn. The formula suggested is Polyporus Decoction (*zhū líng tāng*), which disinhibits water and enriches yīn. Polyporus (*zhū líng*), poria (*fú líng*), alisma (*zé xiè*), and talcum (*huá shí*) disinhibit water by bland percolation, while at the same time clearing heat. Ass hide glue (*ē jiāo*) enriches yīn and moistens dryness. The formula as a whole thus eliminates water so that the heat has nothing to attach to, and restores liquid so that the thirst is allayed.

This line shares with line 13.4 above the symptoms of inhibited urination, thirst with desire to drink water, a floating pulse, and heat effusion. Nevertheless, that line lists the symptoms as "a floating pulse, inhibited urination, slight heat [effusion], and dispersion-thirst." The different order of the items reflects a completely different cause and pathomechanism. In line 13.4, the cause was wind-cold fettering the exterior and spreading along the greater yáng channel to affect bladder qì transformation. In that line, inhibited urination reflects the pathomechanism causing thirst, so it appears first. In the present line, however, inhibited urination is the result of "heat effusion," and "thirst with desire to drink water"; hence it is placed after them. In line 13.4, the thirst with desire to drink water is caused by qì failing to transform liquid, so that the fluids are not distilled and returned to the body; in the present line, it is caused by depressed heat damaging yīn. In line 13.4, "a floating pulse" and "heat effusion" are exterior signs; in the present line they are signs of interior heat reaching the exterior. For this reason, the heat effusion is more severe and is not accompanied by aversion to cold. In line 13.4, the floating pulse is described by commentators as floating and tight; in the present line, it is most likely to be rapid instead.

In line 13.4, inhibited urination is due to cold in the kidney. The kidney stands in exterior-interior relationship with the bladder. As a result of cold in the kidney, bladder qì tranformation is impaired, which can give rise to inhibited urination. Heat in the kidney can also impair bladder qì transformation and may similarly manifest in inhibited urination. In the present line, the inhibited urination falls into this latter category.

DISPERSION-THIRST				
Location	**Pathomechanism**	**Signs**	**Treatment Principle**	**Formula**
Upper Dissipation	Exuberant lung-stomach heat; damage to liquid and qì	Thirst with desire to drink water; dry mouth and tongue	Clear heat and boost qì; engender liquid and allay thirst	White Tiger Decoction Plus Ginseng (*bái hǔ jiā rén shēn tāng*)
Center Dissipation	Exuberant stomach heat and qì	Swift digestion and rapid hungering; hard stool; frequent urination	Mild precipitation of accumulated heat in yáng brightness	Stomach-Regulating Qì-Coordinating Decoction (*tiáo wèi chéng qì tāng*)
Lower Dissipation	Kidney qì vacuity with inability to ensure containment and absorption	Copious urine (urine as great as imbibed fluids)	Warm the kidney to contain water	Kidney Qì Pill (*shèn qì wán*)

水气病脉证治第十四

CHAPTER 14

Water Qì

Pulses, Signs, Treatments

‡ OVERVIEW

What this chapter refers to as "water qì" (水气 *shuǐ qì*) refers to a condition in which water qì spills or collects, resulting in generalized swelling of the skin and flesh or distention in the abdominal region. The current chapter includes conditions that are now called "water swelling" (水腫 *shuǐ zhǒng*) as well as those now called "qì distention" (气胀 *qì zhàng*). It roughly corresponds to the Western concept of edema.

This chapter discuss the causes, pathomechanisms, pattern identifications, and treatments of water qì. It distinguishes between five varieties of this disease, based on differences in the disease cause, symptoms, and location: wind water, skin water, regular water, stone water, and yellow sweat. It also categorizes water qì in regards to the viscus that is at the root of a particular condition—heart water, lung water, spleen water, etc.—and furthermore distinguishes among water, qì, and blood aspects. All these are different manifestations of essentially the same disease.

The development of water qì can be associated with three factors: (1) impaired qì transformation in the lung and kidney (the lung and the kidney govern qì and water and the upbearing and downbearing of these substances); (2) loss of regular opening and closing in the kidney. (The kidney governs defecation and urination), and (3) cold binding in the spleen and lung (the spleen is the source of construction and defense, the lung governs their distribution, and inhibition of construction and defense qì causes it to transform into water.) Considering all these causes comprehensively, we can see that water qì is a disease originating in the lung, spleen, and kidney, while also related to the triple burner and bladder. As Zhāng Jǐng-Yuè 张景岳 has pointed out, "All patterns of water swelling are related to the lung, spleen, and kidney interfering with one another. Water is consummate yīn, and its root is therefore in the kidney. Water is a transformation of qì, and its tip is therefore in the lung. Water only fears earth, and is therefore restrained by the spleen."

Because this chapter discusses water qì on the basis of yáng vacuity, treatment takes the form of warming and freeing yáng qì, by effusing sweat, disinhibiting urine, and expelling water. However, these three treatment methods only address repletion patterns. For vacuity patterns, we also need to warm yáng, transform qì, or supplement essence-blood.

‡ Schematic Overview

Water Qì

1. Pathomechanisms

   Debilitation of yáng qì affecting the lung's regulation of the waterways, splenic movement and transformation of water-damp, and kidney and bladder qì transformation. In some cases, wind, heat, and cold are involved.

2. Categorization

   a) Wind water, skin water, regular water, stone water, and yellow sweat.

   Wind water: Disturbance of the lung's regulation of the waterways by external evils, giving rise to a floating pulse, aversion to cold, and pain in the bones and joints.

   Skin water: Disturbance of spleen and lung function, manifesting in a floating pulse, puffy swelling that engulfs the fingers when pressed, and drumlike abdominal distention.

   Regular water: Kidney yáng vacuity with cold water shooting into the lung, charcterized by a pulse that is sunken and slow and by panting.

   Stone water: Kidney yáng vacuity giving rise to a pulse that is sunken and abdominal fullness without panting.

   Yellow sweat: Externally contracted dampness causing construction and defense to become depressed so that damp-heat arises, giving rise to a pulse that is sunken and slow, generalized heat effusion, fullness in the chest, swelling of the limbs, head, and face, and yellow sweat.

   b) Liver water, heart water, spleen water, lung water, and kidney water (classification according to the viscus affected after the water swelling has arisen).

   Heart water: Generalized heaviness, shortage of qì, inability to lie down, vexation and agitation, and swollen genitals.

   Liver water: Abdominal distention with inability to turn sides, pain under the rib-side and in the abdomen.

Lung water: Generalized swelling, difficult urination, periodic duck slop diarrhea.

Spleen water: Abdominal distention, heavy limbs, fluids failing to be engendered, shortage of qì, and difficult urination.

Kidney water: Abdominal distention, painful swelling in the waist and umbilical regions, inability to urinate, genitals that are damp and sweaty like a cow's nose, counterflow cold of the legs, and thin face.

3. Principles of treatment

Disinhibiting urine is used for swelling from the waist downward.

Promotion of sweating is used for swelling from the waist upward.

Precipitation is used for an enlarged abdomen.

Various contraindications.

4. Patterns and treatment

a) Wind water with exterior vacuity: Fangji and Astragalus Decoction (*fáng jǐ huáng qí tāng*).

b) Wind water with depressed heat: Spleen-Effusing Decoction (*yuè bì tāng*)

c) Skin water with depressed yáng qì: Fangji and Poria Decoction (*fáng jǐ fú líng tāng*).

d) Skin water with reversal cold of the extremities: Charred Dandelion Powder (*pú huī sǎn*).

e) Skin water with heat: Spleen-Effusing Decoction Plus White Atractylodes (*yuè bì jiā zhú tāng*).

f) Regular water: Ephedrae and Aconite Decoction (*má huáng fù zǐ tāng*).

g) Yellow sweat due to insecurity of the exterior with dampness trapping heat: Astragalus, Peony, Cinnamon Twig, and Vinegar Decoction (*qí sháo guì jiǔ tāng*).

h) Yellow sweat due to disturbance of construction and defense and depressed water-damp: Cinnamon Twig Decoction Plus Astragalus (*guì zhī jiā huáng qí tāng*).

Line 14.1

师曰：病有风水，有皮水，有正水，有石水，有黄汗。风水其脉自浮，外证骨节疼痛，恶风；皮水其脉亦浮，外证胕肿，按之没指，不恶风，其腹如鼓，不渴，当发其汗；正水其脉沉迟，外证自喘；石水其脉自沉，外证腹满不喘，黄汗其脉沉迟，身发热，胸满，四肢头面肿，久不愈，必致痈脓。

Shī yuē: Bìng yǒu fēng shuǐ, yǒu pí shuǐ, yǒu zhèng shuǐ, yǒu shí shuǐ, yǒu huáng hàn. Fēng shuǐ qí mài zì fú, wài zhèng gǔ jié téng tòng, wù fēng; pí shuǐ qí mài yì fú, wài zhèng fū zhǒng, àn zhī mò zhǐ, bù wù fēng, qí fù rú gǔ, bù kě, dāng fā qí hàn; zhèng shuǐ qí mài chén chí, wài zhèng zì chuǎn; shí shuǐ qí mài zì chén, wài zhèng fù mǎn bù chuǎn, huáng hàn qí mài chén chí, shēn fā rè, xiōng mǎn, sì zhī tóu miàn zhǒng, jiǔ bù yù, bì zhì yōng nóng.

The master says: "In [water qì] disease, we [differentiate between] wind water, skin water, regular water, stone water, and yellow sweat. In wind water, the pulse is naturally floating, and the external signs are joint pain and aversion to wind. In skin water, the pulse is also floating, and the external signs are skin swelling,[1] which when pressed engulfs the fingers; absence of aversion to wind; a drum-like abdomen; and absence of thirst. [For both these conditions,] effuse sweat. In regular water, the pulse is sunken and slow, and the external sign is spontaneous panting. In stone water, the pulse is naturally sunken, and the external sign is abdominal fullness without panting. In yellow sweat, the pulse is sunken and slow, [and the external signs are] generalized heat effusion, fullness in the chest, and swelling of the four limbs, head, and face, which if enduring without recovery, will inevitably cause a welling-abscess and pus.

Text Note, Line 14.1

[1] Skin swelling 胕肿 *fū zhǒng*: 胕 *fū* means both the instep and skin. In the present context it means skin.

Synopsis, Line 14.1

This line describes the five kinds of water qì and their chief characteristics.

Commentary, Line 14.1

The present line discusses five kinds of water qì: wind water, skin water, regular water, stone water, and yellow sweat.

Wind water is closely associated with the lung, which governs the skin and body hair. When wind invades the exterior, it manifests in a floating pulse and aversion to wind. The joint pain is a sign of dampness evil floating into the joints. When the skin and body hair contract evil, lung qì loses its ability to diffuse qì and regulate the waterways. As a result, water-damp accumulates in the skin. This is characterized by puffy swelling of the head and face with heat effusion.

Skin water is closely related to the spleen and lung. The spleen resides in the central region; it governs the limbs and the flesh. When the spleen's function of movement and transformation is impaired, water-damp obstructs the network vessels of the spleen and thereby causes abdominal fullness, to the point where it resembles a drum, and absence of thirst. When water-damp spills out into the skin, there is puffy swelling that engulfs the fingers when pressed. Because wind evil is not involved in this disease, there is no aversion to wind. In skin water patients, the water moves in the skin. Because the skin is connected with the lung, and the locus of the disease is the exterior, the pulse is likely to be floating. Skin water arises when water from the spleen and stomach pours out into the skin and flesh. We treat skin water by resolving it through sweating, so as to help it move along its outward course.

Regular water and stone water are both related to the kidney. Regular water arises when kidney yáng is insufficient and fails to distill the fluids so that water accumulates in the inner body; hence the pulse is sunken and slow. Stone water arises when yīn cold congeals in the lower burner; hence the pulse is sunken. In both cases, the disease is in the interior and therefore characterized by abdominal fullness. However, in regular water the water passes along the foot lesser yīn kidney channel and shoots into the lung, impairing the lung's function of depurative downbearing and hence giving rise to panting. Stone water is water qì binding in the lesser abdomen; hence the lesser abdomen is hard and full like a stone, but there is no panting.

Finally, yellow sweat is a disease that is related to the spleen. When water-damp lies depressed in the inner body and affects construction-blood, the pulse is sunken and slow. The spleen is vacuous and therefore unable to move and transform dampness. Instead, dampness ascends to invade the lung and inhibits lung qì; hence the fullness in the chest. When defense is depressed and there is heat in construction, water-damp accumulates in the skin and flesh. Consequently there is generalized heat, and swelling of the limbs, head, and face. At the same time, yellow sweat issues; hence the name of the disease. When yellow sweat persists for a long time, the depressed heat in construction-blood can become even more exuberant, to the point where it putrefies qì and blood. This causes the formation of pus and the development of swollen welling-abscesses.

Line 14.2

(1)脉浮而洪，浮则为风，洪则为气。风气相搏，风强则为隐疹，身体为痒，痒为泄风，久为痂癞；气强则为水，难以俯仰。风气相击，身体洪肿，汗出乃愈。

(2) 恶风则虚，此为风水；不恶风者，小便通利，上焦有寒，其口多涎，此为黄汗。

(1) Mài fú ér hóng, fú zé wéi fēng, hóng zé wéi qì. Fēng qì xiāng bó, fēng qiáng zé wéi yǐn zhěn, shēn tǐ wéi yǎng, yǎng wéi xiè fēng, jiǔ wéi jiā lài; qì qiáng zé wéi shuǐ, nán yǐ fǔ yǎng. Fēng qì xiāng jī, shēn tǐ hóng zhǒng, hàn chū nǎi yù.

(2) Wù fēng zé xū, cǐ wéi fēng shuǐ; bù wù fēng zhě, xiǎo biàn tōng lì, shàng jiāo yǒu hán, qí kǒu duō xián, cǐ wéi huáng hàn.

(1) When the pulse is floating and surging, floating means wind, and surging means qì.[1] Wind and qì contend with each other. When wind is the stronger, the result is dormant papules and itching of the body,[2] which means the discharge of wind[3] or, in enduring cases, scab-lài.[4] When qì is the stronger, the result is water [swelling] and difficulty in bending forward and backward. When wind and qì strike each other, there is swelling in the body. Sweating will bring recovery.

(2) Aversion to wind indicates vacuity; this is wind water. In cases with no aversion to wind, [the symptoms of] uninhibited urination, cold in the upper burner, and copious drooling from the mouth mean yellow sweat.

TEXT NOTES, LINE 14.2

[1] Qì 气 *qì*: Water qì.

[2] Dormant papules 隐疹 *yǐn zhěn*: This is now written as 瘾疹 *yǐn zhěn*. An itchy papular eruption attributed to outthrust of wind evil. Dormant papules are equated with urticaria in Western medicine.

[3] Discharge of wind 风泄 *fēng xiè*: Expulsion of wind evil by defense qì.

[4] Scab and lài 痂癞 *jiā lài*: When dormant papules fail to heal, they can suppurate and form scabs that look like lài disease. Lài is a term that means either leprosy or scab and lichen that leads to hair loss. Commentators disagree on which is meant in the present context.

SYNOPSIS, LINE 14.2

This line describes several pathologies arising from contending wind evil and water qì, and explains the differentiation of wind water and yellow sweat.

COMMENTARY, LINE 14.2

The line is divided into two sections. The first section deals with wind evil and water qì contending with each other. The second half deals with the differentiation of wind water and yellow sweat.

A floating pulse points to a disease of the exterior. Wind is a yáng evil. When it damages the exterior, and defense qì resists, it mostly results in a floating pulse. Hence, the line tells us, "floating means wind." A surging pulse refers to a pulse that is large and powerful, and usually indicates exuberant qì. Here it means water qì that is exuberant in the exterior. Hence, the text tells us that "surging means qì." Wind evil and water qì contending with each other is reflected in a pulse that is floating and surging.

The text next tells us that wind prevailing over qì results in dormant papules. This is characterized by wheals on the flesh and generalized itching, which is caused by exuberant wind-heat toxin invading construction blood. The text tells us that "itching means the discharge of wind." In other words, when there is itching, this indicates that the wind-heat toxin is already on an outward-discharging course, so there is is no need to provide any specific treatment to check it. However, if wind evil is not discharged, but exploits the vacuity to attack the blood and vessels, it can cause putrefaction of the flesh, giving rise to "scab and lài." This refers to stubborn itching, suppuration, and scabbing, a possible result of dormant papules that fail to resolve.

"When qì is the stronger, the result is water" means that when exuberant water-damp qì is is whipped up by wind, it moves uncontrollably and gives rise to swelling. In severe cases, the swelling will result in panting and cough with qì ascent, difficulty in bending the body forward and backward, and inability to lie flat. Because right qì has not yet been damaged, this condition can be treated by sweating.

The second section of the line describes two distinct conditions that can arise when "[water] qì is the stronger." Wind water is caused by contraction of wind evil, but it is also associated with an internal factor, namely insufficiency of yáng qì and inability of kidney qì to perform qì transformation. Hence the text pinpoints "aversion to wind" as a hint. If aversion to wind fails to abate after the patient has been treated with wind-dispelling exterior-resolving medicinals, we can attribute this to vacuity and resulting insecurity of the exterior, which is usually characterized by spontaneous sweating and a floating pulse. Thus the text tells us that "aversion to wind means vacuity." It is therefore a clear sign for the disease of wind water.

If, by contrast, a patient presents with no aversion to wind, this means that the pattern is not rooted in vacuity. Absence of aversion to wind is associated with a repletion that arises when water-damp invades and depresses construction and defense qì in the heart and lung in the upper burner. In such a condition, the disease has not yet affected bladder qì transformation in the lower burner, so urination is still uninhibited. However, because construction and defense in the upper burner are depressed, qì stagnates and causes liquid to gather; hence we see copious drooling. In conclusion, the initial stage of yellow sweat is mostly related to a pattern of superabundance, in which dampness lies depressed and qì stagnates, but has not yet transformed into heat. Wind water, on the other hand, is caused by an internal vacuity that manifests in the key symptom of aversion to wind.

Line 14.3

寸口脉沉滑者，中有水气，面目肿大，有热，名曰风水；视人之目窠上微拥，如蚕新卧起状，其颈脉动，时时咳，按其手足上，陷而不起者，风水。

Cùn kǒu mài chén huá zhě, zhōng yǒu shuǐ qì, miàn mù zhǒng dà, yǒu rè, míng yuē fēng shuǐ; shì rén zhī mù kē shàng wēi yōng, rú cán xīn wò qǐ zhuàng, qí jǐng mài dòng, shí shí ké, àn qí shǒu zú shàng, xiàn ér bù qǐ zhě, fēng shuǐ.

When the inch opening pulse is sunken and slippery, there is water qì in the center, [which manifests in] a swollen and enlarged head and face, and heat [effusion]. This is called "wind water." You will observe slight swelling of the eye nest[1] as if [the person] had just awoken from sleep, a stirring neck pulse, and frequent coughing. When you press the hands and feet, they pit but do not spring back. This constitutes wind water.

TEXT NOTE, LINE 14.3

[1] Eye nest 目窠 *mù kē*: The flesh surrounding the eyes, i.e., the eyelids.

SYNOPSIS, LINE 14.3

This line describes the pulse and signs of severe wind water.

COMMENTARY, LINE 14.3

The pulse of wind water ought to be floating. However, if the pulse at the inch opening position is sunken and slippery, this is a sign of severe water qì, because a sunken pulse indicates water, and a slippery pulse indicates exuberant qì. So if both pulse types are observed at the inch position, this means that the exterior is affected by exuberant water qì with wind evil. We often see this type of pulse in conditions when water swelling gradually becomes more severe.

The head and face are yáng. Wind is a yáng evil and tends to affect the upper part of the body. When wind and water invade the upper body, water-damp accumulates above the chest and neck; hence the head and face are swollen and enlarged. Furthermore, because defense qì is depressed by the water-damp, there is generalized fever. Thus, the swollen and enlarged face and eyes and the generalized heat effusion, like the pulse that is sunken and slippery, reflect wind and water contending in the fleshy exterior.

Upon close inspection of the face, we will find such a patient to have slightly swollen eyelids as if just wakened from sleep. The vessels on both sides of the neck are beating conspicuously. Because the eyelids belong to the spleen and because Man's Prognosis (*rén yíng*, ST-9), the pulse on the neck through which the stomach vessel passes, indicates the lung and stomach, these signs are not only an indication that water evil qì is growing excessively exuberant, but also that it is gradually affecting the spleen and stomach. When wind water soaks the lung and causes counterflow ascent of lung qì, there is frequent coughing. When water qì spreads and spills into the skin and flesh, and right qì is insufficient, there is swelling that pits when pressed, but does not spring back when pressure is released. Puffy swelling of the limbs that pits when pressed but does not spring back is more severe than puffy swelling of the head and face. Because the limbs are governed by the spleen and are the root of all yáng, this kind of swelling in the limbs signifies that spleen vacuity is allowing dampness to collect and that yáng is failing to form qì.

From the analysis of these signs, it is clear that the present line describes a condition in which not only the lung is affected, but also the spleen, indicating the increasing severity of the disease.

Line 14.4

(1)太阳病，脉浮而紧，法当骨节疼痛，反不疼，身体反重而酸，其人不渴，汗出即愈，此为风水。恶寒者，此为极虚，发汗得之。

(2)渴而不恶寒者，此为皮水。

(3)身肿而冷，状如周痹，胸中窒，不能食，反聚痛，暮躁不得眠，此为黄汗，痛在骨节。

(4)咳而喘，不渴者，此为脾胀，其状如肿，发汗即愈。

(5)然诸病此者，渴而下利，小便数者，皆不可发汗。

(1) Tài yáng bìng, mài fú ér jǐn, fǎ dāng gǔ jié téng tòng, fǎn bù téng, shēn tǐ fǎn zhòng ér suān, qí rén bù kě, hàn chū jí yú, cǐ wéi fēng shuǐ. Wù hán zhě, cǐ wéi jí xū, fā hàn dé zhī.

(2) Kě ér bù wù hán zhě, cǐ wéi pí shuǐ.

(3) Shēn zhǒng ér lěng, zhuàng rú zhōu bì, xiōng zhōng zhì, bù néng shí, fǎn jù tòng, mù zào bù dé mián, cǐ wéi huáng hàn, tòng zài gǔ jié.

(4) Ké ér chuǎn, bù kě zhě, cǐ wéi pí zhàng, qí zhuàng rú zhǒng, fā hàn jí yù.

(5) Rán zhū bìng cǐ zhě, kě ér xià lì, xiǎo biàn shuò zhě, jiē bù kě fā hàn.

(1) In greater yáng disease when [there is] a floating and tight pulse, joints that ought to be painful but are not, generalized heaviness and aching, and no thirst, then sweating will bring recovery. This is wind water. If there is aversion to cold, this means extreme vacuity, which the patient contracted from [being treated by] effusing sweat.

(2) Thirst without aversion to cold means skin water.

(3) Swelling and coldness of the body, an appearance like generalized impediment,[1] stifling in the chest, inability to eat, concentrated pain, and agitation at night with inability to sleep means yellow sweat. The pain is in the joints.

(4) Cough and panting and no thirst means spleen distention.[2] [It manifests in] an appearance like swelling. Effusing sweat will bring on recovery.

(5) However, in all these diseases, thirst with diarrhea and frequent urination always means that you may not promote sweating.

Text Notes, Line 14.4

[1] Generalized impediment 周痹 *zhōu bì*: Impediment characterized by generalized migratory pain.

[2] Spleen distention 脾胀 *pí zhàng*: Commentators generally interpret this as a mistranscription of 肺胀 *fèi zhàng*, lung distention.

Synopsis, Line 14.4

This line describes the pattern identification and principles in the treatment of water qì.

Commentary, Line 14.4

The first section of the present line discusses the signs and treatment of wind water. Greater yáng cold damage disease, which is caused by contraction of wind-cold, is characterized by a floating and tight pulse and by joint pain. If instead of joint pain there is generalized heaviness and aching, we cannot identify the condition as cold damage, in spite of the fact that the pulse is floating and tight.

Rather it is wind water, which arises when internal water-damp accumulates in the skin and flesh and is whipped up by externally contracted wind-evil. Stagnating water-damp results in generalized heaviness, and wind evil lodging in the fleshy exterior results in generalized aching. Since water-damp has not yet flowed into the joints, the joints are not painful.

Wind water is characterized by absence of thirst. Thirst has varying diagnostic significance, the most common pathology being interior heat. It can also arise when in lodged rheum (water-rheum) affects the movement of fluids (see line 12.10). In the present line, there is neither interior heat, nor has water qì yet markedly damaged the body's yáng qì.

The text tells us that we should treat wind water by sweating. When water spills into the fleshy exterior, the way to treat it is to help it on its course by promoting sweating. The wind water in the exterior, however, is only the tip of the disease. The root is insufficiency of kidney yáng. So the last sentence of the section, which reads, "If there is aversion to cold, this means extreme vacuity, which the patient contracted from [being treated by] effusing sweat" is a warning that sweating should not exceed the limits that right qì can withstand. Excessive promotion of sweating can weaken right qì, causing "aversion to wind" to give way to the more severe condition of "aversion to cold."

The second section of the line discusses skin water. The text gives two pieces of information about skin water: that it is associated with thirst and with an absence of aversion to cold. The text does not mention swelling as a symptom, but we can assume this from the name of the disease. The line furthermore fails to offer any detail about the distribution of the swelling or its causes. Thirst arises because water-damp that accumulates in the skin prevents the lung from distributing the fluids. The absence of aversion to cold tells us that there is no external evil present, which is thus a key difference from wind water.

The third section discusses yellow sweat. Again, the text enumerates signs of the disease, but does not include any that relate to sweating. It fails to explicitly state the issue of yellow-colored sweat, but we can assume this to be a key symptom due to the name of the disease. No detail is given about the distribution, nature, or causes of the sweating. The text tells us that yellow sweat is characterized by generalized swelling and cold, with the appearance of generalized impediment. Contrasting these two diseases, yellow sweat manifests with pain in the joints and generalized puffy swelling, while generalized impediment manifests with pain in uncertain locations and no swelling or yellow sweat. The stifling in the chest is a result of dampness evil stagnating, devitalizing chest yáng, and preventing lung qì from diffusing freely. Thus the patient feels oppression and stoppage in the chest. As a result of stomach yáng being devitalized and cold preventing the dispersion of grain, the patient suffers from "inability to eat." Concentrated pain in the joints is caused by cold-damp lodging and pouring into the joints, and by loss of warmth in the sinews. Lastly, agitation at night and insomnia are due to the fact that cold strikes at dusk, because this is the time when yáng qì has difficulty stretching out and hence aggravates the joint pain. All these symptoms are related to water-damp lying depressed and impeding construction and defense qì, and to damp-heat steaming the interstices of the flesh.

The fourth section discusses the signs and treatment of pulmonary distention. Cough and panting are the chief signs of this disease. It arises when external cold and interior rheum contend with each other in the lung, impair diffusion and downbearing of the lung, and cause counterflow ascent. The absence of thirst indicates that there is no heat. "Appearance like swelling" suggests puffy swelling of the face. When cold rheum obstructs lung qì, the "mysterious houses" (sweat pores) fail to open, and regulation of the fluids is inhibited. As a result, qì attacks upward, giving rise to puffy swelling of the face. Because the condition is caused by external cold and internal rheum contending with each other in the lung, it is centered in the upper body and in the exterior. We can therefore treat it by promoting sweating.

The fifth section discusses the contraindication against sweating in patterns with yīn vacuity. "In all diseases [like] this" means in any case of wind water, skin water, yellow sweat, and pulmonary distention. In these conditions, although sweating is often the appropriate treatment, it is important to take account of the state of the fluids within the body, since sweating can damage the yīn humor and yáng qì of the body. Therefore it is contraindicated in cases with yáng vacuity, and is not normally recommended in yīn vacuity. "Thirst with diarrhea" suggests a pattern of internal rheum damaging liquid or spleen vacuity and liquid depletion. "Frequent urination" indicates a vacuous kidney that is unable to contain urine and causes fluids to be lost through urination. These are both conditions in which we may not use sweating.

Line 14.5

里水者，一身面目黄肿，其脉沉，小便不利，故令病水，假如小便自利，此亡津液，故令渴也，越婢加朮汤主之。

Lǐ shuǐ zhě, yī shēn miàn mù huáng zhǒng, qí mài chén, xiǎo biàn bù lì, fù lìng bìng shuǐ, jiǎ rú xiǎo biàn zì lì, cǐ wáng jīn yè, fù lìng kě yě, yuè bì jiā zhú tāng zhǔ zhī.

Interior water[1] [manifests in] yellowing and swelling[2] in the whole body and head and eyes, a sunken pulse, and inhibited urination causing water disease. If urination becomes spontaneously uninhibited, this means fluid collapse, which causes thirst. Spleen-Effusing Decoction Plus White Atractylodes (*yuè bì jiā zhú tāng*)[3] governs.[4]

Text Notes, Line 14.5

[1] Interior water 里水 *lǐ shuǐ*: Commentators generally interpret this as a mistranscription for 皮水 *pí shuǐ* ("skin water").

[2] Yellowing and swelling 黄肿 *huǎng zhǒng*: Commentators generally interpret this as a mistranscription for 洪肿 *hóng zhǒng*, welling.

[3] At the time of the *Jīn Guì*, the two medicinals *bái zhú* (derived from *Atractylodes macrocephala Koidz.)* and *cāng zhú* (derived from *Atractylodes lancea*

Thunb.) were not differentiated from one another. In modern texts, *bái zhú* is generally listed for this formula. Throughout this text, when later sources indicate a specific form of atractylodes (*zhú*) for a given formula, this specific form appears in the English translation of the formula title.

[4] The commentary adds: "For the formula, see the chapter on Wind-Stroke." This formula is found among the appended formulas at the end of Chapter 5.

SYNOPSIS, LINE 14.5

This line describes skin swelling complicated by heat.

COMMENTARY, LINE 14.5

When the spleen is vacous and unable to move and transform water-damp, and lung qì fails to diffuse and is unable to regulate the waterways that carry water down to the bladder, the whole body and head and face become swollen and enlarged. Since water-damp is not discharged outward from the skin (governed by the lung) and is also unable to descend and be discharged via the bladder, it becomes depressed in the spleen and stomach and causes heat formation there.

The treatment for this is Spleen-Effusing Decoction Plus White Atractylodes (*yuè bì jiā zhú tāng*). Spleen-Effusing Decoction (*yuè bì tāng*) promotes sweating and moves water, while also clearing internal heat. White atractylodes (*bái zhú*) is added to eliminate dampness from the fleshy exterior.

The sentence that reads, "If urination becomes spontaneously uninhibited, this means fluid collapse, which causes thirst" is an intercalation that offers a contraindication for the use of Spleen-Effusing Decoction Plus White Atractylodes (*yuè bì jiā zhú tāng*). If urine is uninhibited and there is thirst, this means that the fluids are damaged, in which case we should not use this formula.

Line 14.6

趺阳脉当伏，今反紧，本自有寒，疝瘕、腹中痛，医反下之，下之即胸满短气。

Fū yáng mài dāng fú, jīn fǎn jǐn, běn zì yǒu hán, shànjiǎ, fù zhōng tòng, yī fǎn xià zhī, xià zhī jí xiōng mǎn duǎn qì.

The instep yáng pulse should be hidden, but if it is presently tight instead, this is because there is cold at the root [of the condition, which is causing] mounting-conglomerations[1] and pain in the abdomen. If a physician wrongfully precipitates, there will be fullness in the chest and shortness of breath.

TEXT NOTE, LINE 14.6

[1] Mounting conglomerations 疝瘕 *shàn jiǎ*: Accumulation lumps that are either gathered or diffuse, with pain of unfixed location.

SYNOPSIS, LINE 14.6

This line describes the pathomechanism and symptoms of yáng vacuity cold on the basis of changes in the instep yáng pulse.

COMMENTARY, LINE 14.6

The instep yáng pulse is an indicator of the stomach. It is located between two bones on the dorsum of the foot, and for this reason is normally a hidden pulse. If the instep yáng pulse is not hidden but tight, this indicates cold in the abdomen, as occurs in mounting-conglomerations and abdominal pain. Cold is treated by warming, and if a practitioner in such cases wrongly prescribes cold bitter precipitating medicines, this will severely damage yáng qì. In particular, it can cause non-diffusion of lung qì and the development of fullness in the chest and shortness of breath.

Line 14.7

趺阳脉当伏，今反数，本自有热，消谷，小便数，今反不利，此欲作水。

Fū yáng mài dāng fú, jīn fǎn shuò, běn zì yǒu rè, xiāo gǔ, xiǎo biàn shuò, jīn fǎn bù lì, cǐ yù zuò shuǐ.

The instep yáng pulse should be hidden, but if it is presently rapid instead, this is because there is heat at the root, [which is causing] disperson of grain and frequent urination. But if the urination is inhibited instead, this means that water [qì] is about to arise.

SYNOPSIS, LINE 14.7

This line describes the pathomechanism and symptoms of water qì disease on the basis of changes in the instep yáng pulse.

COMMENTARY, LINE 14.7

The instep yáng pulse is normally hidden. If it is rapid, this means heat. In such cases, we most likely see swift digestion and rapid hungering, as well as frequent urination. If urination is inhibited rather than frequent, this is because water and heat are binding together. As a result, qì transformation in the bladder becomes inhibited and water-heat evil accumulates internally instead of being precipitated. Spilling into the fleshy exterior, it is likely to turn into water swelling and the development of water qì disease. By alerting us to this possibility, the present line gives the attentive practitioner a chance to treat this disease preventively.

Line 14.8

(1)寸口脉浮而迟，浮脉则热，迟脉则潜，热潜相搏，名曰沉。

(2)趺阳脉浮而数，浮脉即热，数脉即止，热止相搏，名曰伏。

(3)沉伏相搏，名曰水。沉则络脉虚，伏则小便难，虚难相搏，水走皮肤，即为水矣。

(1) Cùn kǒu mài fú ér chí, fú mài zé rè, chí mài zé qián, rè qián xiāng bó, míng yuē chén.

(2) Fū yáng mài fú ér shuò, fú mài jí rè, shuò mài jí zhǐ, rè zhǐ xiāng bó, míng yuē fú.

(3) Chén fú xiāng bó, míng yuē shuǐ. Chén zé luò mài xū, fú zé xiǎo biàn nán, xū nán xiāng bó, shuǐ zǒu pí fū, jí wéi shuǐ yǐ.

(1) When the inch opening pulse is floating and slow, a floating pulse means heat, while a slow pulse means submersion.[1] When heat and submersion contend with each other,[2] this is called sunken.

(2) When the instep yáng pulse is floating and rapid, a floating pulse means heat, while a rapid pulse means stand-still.[3] When heat and stand-still contend with each other, this is called hidden.[4]

(3) When sunken and hidden become intertwined, this is called water. Sunken means that the network vessels are vacuous,[5] and hidden means that urination is difficult. When vacuity and difficulty contend with each other, this means that water is running into the skin to cause water [qì].

Text Notes, Line 14.8

[1] Submerged 潜 *qián*: Referring to heat evil passing into and becoming submerged in construction-blood.

[2] Contend with each other 相搏 *xiāng bó*: In the *Mài Jīng* ("Pulse Canon") quotation of this passage, this is written as 相摶 *xiāng tuán* (lit. "roll up in each other"). Whatever the character, the meaning is the same: the intertwining interaction of two distinct entities.

[3] Stand-still 止 *zhǐ*: Non-movement, here, refers to the process of heat evil damaging the bladder and inhibiting qì transformation.

[4] Hidden 伏 *fú*: This refers to heat evil hiding in the lower body, unable to be discharged through the urine.

[5] Vacuity 虚 *xū*: Vacuity of construction-blood.

Synopsis, Line 14.8

This line further describes the pathomechanism of water qì disease resulting from the binding of water and heat.

Commentary, Line 14.8

The first section explains the pathomechanism of visiting heat lying hidden deep in the body. The inch position is a yáng position. It is governed by the heart and lung. A floating pulse indicates the exterior and is yáng. Heat is is also yáng.

Therefore, a pulse that is floating at the inch position means wind-heat invading the exterior; hence the text says, "a floating pulse means heat." A slow pulse is yīn; yīn means "hidden," "inconspicuous." Hence, an inch opening pulse that is slow reflects a pathological state in which something is "submerged."

Concretely, "a slow pulse means submersion" refers to a slow pulse at the inch opening that is caused by heat evil lying deep in the body. The heat is submerged because it has passed from the qì aspect to the construction aspect. When heat enters construction yīn, it has difficulty escaping. When construction and defense are inhibited, the pulse is slow and rough. When heat and submersion combine and bind, the result is submerged internal heat that cannot reach outward. This condition is called "sunken," which in this context refers to heat hidden in the inner body, not to a sunken pulse. Thus the sentence "When heat and submersion contend with each other, this is called sunken" sums up in an abstract way a state of wind-heat invading the exterior, passing into the interior, binding with construction-yīn, and failing to reach out to the exterior.

The second section explains the pathomechanism of interior heat halting in the inner body. The instep yáng pulse is governed by the stomach. When the instep yáng pulse is floating, this indicates exuberant stomach heat and qì; hence "a floating pulse means heat." When the instep yáng pulse is rapid, it means "stand-still," because heat evil has damaged the bladder and inhibited its function of qì transformation. The combination of "heat" and "stand-still" is called "hidden." The interior heat fails to move and be discharged from the body because, as the text explains further ahead, "hidden means inhibited urination." When heat scorches the kidney and inhibits bladder qì transformation, water and heat bind together. When water is inhibited, the heat is unable to discharge downward.

As in the meaning of "sunken" above, "hidden" in this context refers to a pathomechanism, not to a hidden pulse. In short, the sentence "when heat and stand-still contend with each other, this is called hidden," sums up in abstract terms the pathomechanism of interior heat scorching the lower body, combining with water evil, inhibiting movement in the waterways, and thereby causing internal heat to remain deep in the inner body and unable to move.

The third section explains the process by which water and heat bind together to create water swelling. As explained in the previous lines, "sunken" refers to upper burner visiting heat lying hidden deep in the interior, and "hidden" refers to center burner evil heat lying hidden and failing to move. When the two types of heat in the upper and center burner combine, heat must become exuberant. In the upper burner, the heart and lung are scorched, construction and defense are inhibited, the upper source is not clear, regulation and freeing are disabled, and the waterways are inhibited. Exuberant heat in the center burner causes thirst with drinking, disordered movement and transformation, evil heat damaging the kidney, impaired kidney qì transformation, and ultimately water and heat binding together. Water-heat evil collects in the interior, spills into the skin, and forms water swelling and the disease of water qì. Thus, the disease of water qì is indicated by impaired fluid and qì transformation, which can be caused either by externally contracted visiting heat, or by evil heat from internal damage.

The last sentence explains further developments of water swelling disease. When externally contracted heat lies submerged in construction yīn, it will over time damage yīn, thus causing vacuity of the network vessels. Similarly, when interior heat is halted in the lower body, it affects the bladder and inhibits qì transformation, hence causing difficult urination. When this condition persists, it will over time turn into the disease of water qì.

Line 14.9

(1)寸口脉弦而紧，弦则卫气不行，即恶寒，水不沾流，走于肠间。

(2)少阴脉紧而沉，紧则为痛，沉则为水，小便即难。

(1) Cùn kǒu mài xián ér jǐn, xián zé wèi qì bù xíng, jí wù hán, shuǐ bù zhān liú, zǒu yú cháng jiān.

(2) Shào yīn mài jǐn ér chén, jǐn zé wéi tòng, chén zé wéi shuǐ, xiǎo biàn jí nán.

(1) When the inch opening pulse is stringlike and tight, stringlike means that defense qì is not moving. As a result, there is aversion to cold, and water does not moisten and flow,[1] but runs into the intestines.

(2) When the lesser yīn pulse is tight and sunken, tight means that there is pain, while sunken means that there is water [qì] and hence difficult urination.

Text Note, Line 14.9

[1] Water does not moisten and flow 水不沾流 *shuǐ bù zhān liú*: Does not provide nourishing moisture for the body and does not flow down to the bladder. Moistening and flowing thus refers to normal water metabolism.

Synopsis, Line 14.9

This line describes the involvement of the lung and kidney in the development of water qì disease.

Commentary, Line 14.9

The inch opening indicates the lung. Defense qì is diffused by the lung, so an inch opening pulse that is stringlike and tight means that cold qì is fettering the exterior and causing defense qì to become depressed. Thus the text states that there is aversion to cold. If lung qì is inhibited and fails to regulate the waterways that carry water down to the bladder, the fluids from grain and water are not moved by qì; hence water accumulates in the intestines, giving rise to water qì.

In the second part of the line, "the lesser yīn pulse" refers to the pulse at Great Ravine (*tài xī*, KI-3), which reflects the state of the kidney. A tight pulse indicates cold and pain, while a sunken pulse indicates the interior and water. A sunken and tight lesser yīn pulse hence means insufficiency of kidney yáng with cold arising as a result. Because yáng qì is not distributed around the whole body, there is joint pain or generalized pain. When kidney yáng is insufficient and fails to perform qì transformation and move water, the result is difficult urination and the development of water qì disease.

Line 14.10

脉得诸沉，当责有水，身体肿重。水病脉出者死。

Mài dé zhū chén, dāng zé yǒu shuǐ, shēn tǐ zhǒng zhòng, shuǐ bìng mài chū zhě sǐ.

When all the pulses are sunken, this generally is the responsibility of water [qì, in which case it is accompanied by] generalized heaviness and swelling. In water disease, when the pulse bursts out, [1] [the person] dies.

Text Note, Line 14.10

[1] The pulse bursts out 脉出 *shuǐ bìng mài chū*: Commentators explain 出 *chū* as meaning 暴出 *bào chū*, "burst out." In water disease, the pulse is normally sunken or hidden. If it suddenly appears at the superficial level with no root, the pulse is said to have "burst out."

Synopsis, Line 14.10

This line describes the signs, pulse, and prognosis of water qì disease.

Commentary, Line 14.10

In water disease the normal pulse becomes sunken because water is a yīn evil. When yīn evil is exuberant, it hampers yáng qì, affecting its blood-propelling function. Furthermore, when the yīn evil is water that has spilled into the skin and flesh, this adds pressure and obstructs construction and defense. Hence, the pulse is usually sunken in this disease. The presence of water in the skin and flesh not only manifests in outwardly observable swelling, but also in a subjective sensation of heaviness; hence, the text says "generalized swelling and heaviness." Since a pulse that is sunken can occur in numerous diseases and patterns—exterior as a well as interior, heat as well as cold, vacuity as well as repletion—it is important to correlate the pulse with all the signs.

In the second sentence, "the pulse [bursts] out" means that a pulse that was originally sunken or hidden suddenly becomes palpable when only light pressure is applied, and dissipated when heavy pressure is applied. This is a large, exuberant pulse without a root. It is different from a floating pulse which is felt at the superficial level, but is much weaker at the deep level. In water qì disease, under normal circumstances, water obstructs vessel qì and thereby inhibits the flow of construction and defense;

hence the pulse is usually sunken or hidden. If the disease abates and the swelling slowly disperses, the pulse will gradually become floating and regular. If on the other hand the swelling does not decrease, and the pulse suddenly becomes exuberant at the superficial level and dissipated or absolutely absent at the deep level, this is due to internally exuberant yīn with yáng straying outward. As a result, true qì is about to desert, and yīn and yáng are about to separate. Naturally, the prognosis for this is poor; hence "[the person] dies."

Line 14.11

夫水病人，目下有卧蚕，面目鲜泽，脉伏，其人消渴。病水腹大，小便不利，其脉沉绝者，有水，可下之。

Fū shuǐ bìng rén, mù xià yǒu wò cán, ér mù xiān zé, mài fú, qí rén xiāo kě. bìng shuǐ fù dà, xiǎo biàn bù lì, qí mài chén jué zhě, yǒu shuǐ, kě xià zhī.

A patient with water disease has sleeping silkworms below the eyes,[1] a bright sheen in the face and eyes, a hidden pulse, and dispersion-thirst. If water disease manifests with an enlarged abdomen, inhibited urination, and a sunken and expiring pulse,[2] [this indicates] the presence of water. You can precipitate it.

TEXT NOTES, LINE 14.11

[1] Sleeping silkworms below the eyes 目下有卧蚕 *mù xià yǒu wò cán*: Swelling of the lower eyelids that has the appearance of sleeping silkwoms. In English, we often describe this as "bags under the eyes."

[2] A sunken and expiring pulse 其脉沉绝者 *qí mài chén jué*: The pulse is very sunken and on the verge of expiration.

SYNOPSIS, LINE 14.11

This line describes the pulse and manifestations of water qì disease that can be treated by precipitation.

COMMENTARY, LINE 14.11

The eyelids belong to the spleen and are traversed by the stomach channel. When the spleen and stomach are encumbered by water-damp, the water-damp will flood up and spill into the eyelids; hence the phrase "sleeping silkworms below the eyes" is a reference to water disease. Exuberant water qì is often reflected in a moist, glossy complexion; hence the text mentions "a bright sheen in the face and eyes" (see also line 1.3 where the complexion of lodged rheum is described in similar terms). Exuberant internal water qì obstructs construction and defense, hence the pulse is described as hidden. Hidden has the same signficance as sunken, but suggests greater severity. When water qì collects, qì binds. As a result, liquid fails to bear upward. If qì is depressed for a long time, it can tranform into heat and cause damage to liquid. Hence, we may see dispersion-thirst, which here refers to severe thirst rather than to dispersion-thirst disease.

The implication is that the patient is not only thirsty, but also drinks large amounts of water. However, when qì transformation is inhibited, yáng qì is unable to process the water, hence urination is inhibited. Water fails to be discharged from the body and instead collects in the abdomen; thus we see an enlarged abdomen.

Finally, the pulse is said to be "sunken and expiring." In the present context, this most likely describes a sunken and hidden quality. The word "expiring" here does not describe a pulse as severely pathological as the "bursting out" pulse in the preceding line (14.10), where the pulse at the deep level is expiring. Rather, it refers to the hidden quality of the pulse that arises when exuberant water qì is gathering internally and obstructing yáng qì, so that vessel qì fails to manifest itself.

The line as a whole tells us that when a patient suffering from water qì presents with an enlarged abdomen, dispersion-thirst, inhibited urination, puffy swelling of the face and eyes, a shiny complexion, and a deep, sunken pulse that fails to manifest outwardly, this indicates "the presence of water," meaning that water qì is accumulating in the interior to form a repletion-heat pattern. Under such circumstances, disinhibiting urine will be to no avail, and the only effective treatment is offensive precipitation to expel the water.

Line 14.12

问曰：病下利后，渴饮水，小便不利，腹满因肿者，何也？答曰：此法当病水，若小便自利及汗出者，自当愈。

Wèn yuē: bìng xià lì hòu, kě yǐn shuǐ, xiǎo biàn bù lì, fù mǎn yīn zhǒng zhě, hé yě? Dá yuē: Cǐ fǎ dāng bìng shuǐ, ruò xiǎo biàn zì lì jí hàn chū zhě, zì dāng yù.

Question: "What does it mean if a patient presents with thirst following diarrhea in spite of drinking, inhibited urination, abdominal fullness, and yīn swelling?[1] Answer: "This must be water disease. If urine is spontaneously disinhibited and sweat issues, recovery should ensue spontaneously."

TEXT NOTE, LINE 14.12

[1] Yīn swelling 因肿 *yīn zhǒng*: Genital swelling. The literal meaning, "swollen cause" or "because of swelling" makes no sense. A quotation of this passage in the *Mài Jīng* ("Pulse Canon") has 阴肿 *yīn zhǒng* (yīn swelling). Hence 因 is taken to be a mistranscription of 阴, which in this context refers to swelling of the anterior yīn, i.e., the external genitals.

SYNOPSIS, LINE 14.12

This line describes the pathomechanism of water disease that occurs after diarrhea, and its spontaneous recovery.

COMMENTARY, LINE 14.12

This line describes a condition in which a patient after suffering from diarrhea or dysentery experiences thirst with desire to drink, inhibited urination, abdominal fulless, and swelling of the anterior yīn. This is due to enduring diarrhea, which has caused damage to spleen and kidney yáng, so that qì fails to transform water properly. When such signs appear, the patient may be suffering from water qì disease. In such cases, if urine is uninhibited and the patient is able to sweat, this means that the disease has not yet developed into yáng qì vacuity or that yáng qì has already been restored. In either case, water-damp can be passed out through the urine or sweat, and this brings about spontaneous recovery.

Line 14.13

心水者，其身重而少气，不得卧，烦而躁，其人阴肿。

Xīn shuǐ zhě, qí shēn zhòng ér shǎo qì, bù dé wò, fán ér zào, qí rén yīn zhǒng.

Heart water [manifests in] heaviness of the body,[1] shortage of qì, inability to lie down, vexation and agitation,[2] and yīn swelling.

TEXT NOTES, LINE 14.13

[1] The *Qiān Jīn Yào Fāng* ("A Thousand Gold Pieces Prescriptions"), volume 21, has 身肿 *shēn zhǒng*, swollen body.

[2] Agitation 燥 *zào*: Some commentaries consider this a mistranscription of 悸 *jì*, palpitation.

SYNOPSIS, LINE 14.13

This line is the first of five lines to discuss water of the five viscera, i.e., water swelling due to disease of a particular viscus. The present line discusses the manifestations of heart water.

COMMENTARY, LINE 14.13

Water of the five viscera means water swelling associated in particular with disease of one or other of the five viscera. It does not mean water swelling in the viscus itself.

The present line discusses water swelling due to heart disease. The heart is a yáng viscus. It governs the blood and vessels of the whole body. When heart yáng is vacuous, the blood and vessels are inhibited, cold congeals, and water collects. Thus heart yáng vacuity can give rise to generalized swelling and heaviness. In combination with exuberant water qì, it also can result in shortage of qì. When water qì intimidates the heart, the result is heart vexation and heart palpitation. Inability to lie flat is due to the fact that water evil runs counterflow into the lung when the patient lies flat, but flows back downward when the patient sits up. This is similar to the inability to lie down that occurs in propping rheum.

Because the kidney channel passes through the anterior yīn and nets the heart. When heart yáng is vacuous, it fails to interact with the kidney. As a result, kidney water is not restrained but spills into the anterior yīn; hence we see swelling of the anterior yīn.

Line 14.14

肝水者，其腹大不能自转侧，胁下腹痛，时时津液微生，小便续通。

Gān shuǐ zhě, qí fù dà bù néng zì zhuǎn cè, xié xià fù tòng, shí shí jīn yè wēi shēng, xiǎo biàn xù tōng.

Liver water [manifests in] an enlarged abdomen, inability to freely turn sides, pain beneath the rib-side and in the abdomen, periodic slight engenderment of fluids [in the mouth],[1] and intermittent freeing of urination.[2]

Text Notes, Line 14.14

[1] Periodic slight engenderment of fluids 时时津液微生 *shí shí jīn yè wéi shēng*: Periods of moistness in a mouth that is otherwise dry.

[2] Intermittent freeing of urination 小便续通 *xiǎo biàn xù tōng*: Ability to urinate after temporary stoppage, i.e., urination that continually starts and stops.

Synopsis, Line 14.14

This line describes the manifestations of water disease caused by disease of the liver.

Commentary, Line 14.14

The liver governs free coursing. When liver qì overwhelms spleen-earth and prevents the spleen from moving and transforming water-damp, water qì can accumulate in the abdomen, giving rise to swelling there. This condition is equivalent to ascites in Western medicine and in severe cases it can reach the point where it prevents the patient from freely turning sides, and confines him or her to bed. "Pain beneath the rib-side and in the abdomen" is observed because the rib-side is the house of the liver, and the liver vessel passes through the lesser abdomen and rib-side. When water qì intimidates the liver, it obstructs the network vessels of the liver, causing qì and blood in the liver channel to become depressed and stagnant. This qì and blood stasis obstruction gives rise to distending or stabbing pain in the rib-side and abdomen. The phrase "periodic slight engenderment of fluids [in the mouth], and intermittent freeing of urination" is the main point of the present line. When the liver's free coursing is disturbed, this affects upbearing and downbearing: The liver and spleen fail to bear upward, and the lung and stomach fail to bear downward. As a result, the regular supply of fluids to the mouth and the flow of water down to the bladder is affected. The disturbance of free coursing generally causes a dry mouth and inhibited urination. Nevertheless, there are intermittent periods of remission in which the patient experiences reduced dryness in the mouth and relatively uninhibited urination.

Line 14.15

肺水者,其身肿,小便难,时时鸭溏。

Fèi shuǐ zhě, qí shēn zhǒng, xiǎo biàn nán, shí shí yā táng.

Lung water [manifests in] generalized swelling, difficult urination, and periodic duck's slop.[1]

TEXT NOTE, LINE 14.15

[1] Duck's slop 鸭溏 *yā táng*: Stool and water descending mixed. This is the same as 鹜溏 *wù táng* appearing in lines 11.19 and 14.19.

SYNOPSIS, LINE 14.15

This line describes the manifestations of water disease caused by disease of the lung.

COMMENTARY, LINE 14.15

The lung governs qì, is in charge of breathing, regulates the waterways, and is the upper source of water. When the lung is vacuous, qì is ungoverned, the waterways are unregulated, and water spills out to the exterior of the body; hence there is generalized swelling. Because the lung fails to regulate the waterways, water is not transported down to the bladder; hence we see difficult urination. As a result of this, water has no way out, and we see generalized swelling. Because the lung and large intestine stand in exterior-interior relationship, when the waterways are not regulated, water runs into the intestines, so that water and stool descend mixed, i.e., the patient passes water and stool from the anus. This type of stool resembles duck's droppings, with clear fluid and unsolid feces; hence it is called duck's slop diarrhea.

Line 14.16

脾水者，其腹大，四肢苦重，津液不生，但苦少气，小便难。

Pí shuǐ zhě, qí fù dà, sì zhī kǔ zhòng, jīn yè bù shēng, dàn kǔ shǎo qì, xiǎo biàn nán.

Spleen water [manifests in] an enlarged abdomen, the four limbs suffering from heaviness, failure to engender fluids, shortage of qì, and difficult urination.

SYNOPSIS, LINE 14.16

This line describes the manifestations of water disease caused by disease of the spleen.

COMMENTARY, LINE 14.16

The spleen is located in the abdomen; it governs the four limbs, which are the root of yáng. When spleen yáng fails to move and transform water-damp, yáng qì becomes depressed and fails to reach the four extremities, so that the limbs become encumbered with water-damp; hence we see an enlarged abdomen and heaviness in the limbs. The fluids are the essence of grain and water, which is engendered by the spleen and stomach. When spleen yáng is vacuous, water-damp encumbers the abdomen and reduces the absorption of grain. At the same time, the spleen is unable to spread the fluids for the stomach; hence engenderment of fluids is impaired. When the spleen fails to transport essence to the lung, lung qì becomes vacuous, and therefore we see shortage of qì. When the lung is too weak to transport fluids down to the bladder, the result is difficult urination.

Line 14.17

肾水者，其腹大，脐肿，腰痛，不得溺，阴下湿如牛鼻上汗，其足逆冷，面反瘦。

Shèn shuǐ zhě, qí fù dà, qí zhǒng, yāo tòng, bù dé niào, yīn xià shī rú niú bí shàng hàn, qí zú nì lěng, miàn fǎn shòu.

Kidney water [manifests in] an enlarged abdomen, swelling of the umbilicus, lumbar pain, inability to pass urine, dampness in the yīn [region] like the sweat on an ox's nose, [and] counterflow cold in the lower extremities, but emaciation in the face.

SYNOPSIS, LINE 14.17

This line describes the manifestations of water disease caused by disease of the kidney.

COMMENTARY, LINE 14.17

The kidney governs water; it is in charge of opening and closing and is the gate of the stomach. When kidney yáng is vacuous and consequently fails to transform qì and move water, water amasses in the lower burner and invades upward, rebelling against earth. As a result, water gathers in the abdomen.

The umbilicus belongs to the kidney. Exuberant water qì causes it to become swollen and stick out. The lumbus is the external house of the kidney. When kidney yáng is vacuous, water and cold can congeal, gather, and stop the flow in the channels and network vessels. The result is lumbar pain.

"Inability to pass urine" means extremely scant urine or no urine. This is the result of kidney yáng debilitation and yīn cold congealing and binding to severely hamper bladder qì transformation.

The kidney opens into the two yīn (anal and genital orifices). When water and cold accumulate in the abdomen instead of being discharged, they can spread into the lower regions; hence we may see "dampness in the yīn [region] like the sweat on an ox's nose."

When kidney yáng is vacuous and thereby unable to warm the lower burner, water and cold flow downward, inhibiting the movement of construction and defense in the legs; hence, we see "counterflow cold in the lower extremities" up to the knees.

Finally, in severe kidney vacuity, essential qì fails to ascend to give luxuriance to the face, to the point that the face becomes emaciated. This stands in contrast to the swelling of the abdomen, hence the text reads, "*but* emaciation in the face." In clinic, patients with kidney water are often found to have swollen faces.

The five visceral waters differ in their location and signs. The liver, spleen, and kidney are yīn viscera and are located in the abdomen. Liver, spleen, and kidney water are therefore all characterized by an enlarged abdomen. The heart and lung are located in the chest and are yáng viscera. Heart water and lung water are both characterized by generalized heaviness, generalized swelling, vexation, and inability to lie down (cough and panting). The five visceral waters overlap to some extent with the four types of water disease (wind, skin, regular, and stone).

Line 14.18

师曰：诸有水者，腰以下肿，当利小便；腰以上肿，当发汗乃愈。

Shī yuē: Zhū yǒu shuǐ zhě, yāo yǐ xià zhǒng, dāng lì xiǎo biàn; yāo yǐ shàng zhǒng, dāng fā hàn nǎi yù.

The master says: "In all cases of water [disease, for swelling from the lumbus[1] down, disinhibit urine; for swelling from the lumbus up, effuse sweat. Recovery will ensue."

TEXT NOTE, LINE 14.18

[1] Lumbus 腰 *yāo*: The Chinese here means both lumbus and waist.

SYNOPSIS, LINE 14.18

This line describes the general treatment principles for water swelling disease.

COMMENTARY, LINE 14.18

In the present line, "water [disease]" refers to the various types of water qì disease that have been described above, such as wind water, skin water, regular water, stone water, and water of the five viscera. We should always treat water disease in accord with its location in the upper or lower body, or in the interior or exterior, in order to successfully rid the evil without damaging right qì. When water qì is in the upper body, it is often related to the exterior. When water qì is in the lower body, it is often related to the interior. In the treatment of water disease, it is important to "help it along its course." In other words, water swelling in the lower half of the body should be eliminated via the lower body and interior, i.e., by disinhibiting urine. Conversely, water swelling in the upper half of the body should be eliminated via the upper body and exterior, i.e., by sweating. This is the principle of treatment discussed in the *Nèi Jīng* ("Inner Canon") as "opening the ghost gates" (开鬼门 *kāi guǐ mén*) and "cleansing the clean bowel" (洁净腑 *jié jìng fǔ*).

It should be noted that the exterior and interior, upper and lower body can influence each other. Often, prescribing sweat-inducing medicinals will not only produce sweating, but also disinhibit urine. This is referred to as "when exterior qì is freed, interior qì is also freed." Similarly, urine-disinhibiting medicinals will not only free urine, but often also produce a slight sweat. This is referred to as "when interior qì is freed, exterior qì is also freed." If sweating medicinals fail to produce a marked effect, you can add urine-disinhibiting medicinals to the formula. Likewise if urine-disinhibiting medicinals fail to produce a marked effect, you can add effusing-dissipating medicinals or lung-diffusing medicinals to the formula to produce a better effect.

Nevertheless, it is important to note that sweat-effusing and urine-disinhibiting methods should only be used in yáng patterns and repletion patterns, and not in yīn patterns and vacuity patterns. Sweating medicinals can dissipate water, but they can also dissipate yáng qì; urine-disinhibiting medicinals can disinhibit water-damp, but can also damage yīn qì. Vacuity patterns should be treated instead by warming yáng and supporting right. Evil-dispelling treatments should not be used indiscriminately.

Line 14.19

师曰：寸口脉沉而迟，沉则为水，迟则为寒，寒水相搏。趺阳脉伏，水谷不化，脾气衰则鹜溏，胃气衰则身肿；少阳脉卑，少阴脉细，男子则小便不利，妇人则经水不通。经为血，血不利则为水，名曰血分。

Shī yuē: Cùn kǒu mài chén ér chí, chén zé wéi shuǐ, chí zé wéi hán, hán shuǐ xiāng bó, fū yáng mài fú, shuǐ gǔ bù huà, pí qì shuāi zé wù táng, wèi qì shuāi zé shēn zhǒng; shào yáng mài bēi, shào yīn mài xì, nán zǐ zé xiǎo biàn bù lì, fù rén zé jīng shuǐ bù tōng. Jīng wéi xuè, xuè bù lì zé wéi shuǐ, míng yuē xuè fèn.

The Master says: "When the inch opening pulse is sunken and slow, sunken means water, while slow means cold; hence we see cold and water contending with each other. When the instep yáng pulse is hidden, there is non-transformation of water and grain; duck's slop [diarrhea] as a result of debilitation of spleen qì; and generalized swelling as a result of debilitation of stomach qì. When the lesser yáng pulse is low[1] and the lesser yīn pulse is fine, [we see] inhibited urination in men, and stopped menstrual flow in women. The menses consist of blood, and when blood is inhibited, this causes water. [This] is called 'blood aspect.'"

TEXT NOTE, LINE 14.19

[1] When the lesser yáng pulse is low 少阳脉卑 *shào yáng mài bēi*: Commentaries vary in their explanation of the position of the "lesser yáng pulse," but the most likely identification is the pulsating vessel felt at TB-22 (Ear Harmony Bone-Hole).

SYNOPSIS, LINE 14.19

This line explains the pathomechanisms and signs of water qì disease in terms of the inch opening, instep yáng, and lesser yáng and lesser yīn pulses.

COMMENTARY, LINE 14.19

Water swelling has many causes, but the most important ones are dysfunctions of the lung, spleen, and kidney. The inch opening pulse, the instep yáng pulse, and the lesser yīn pulse correspond to the lung, spleen, and kidney respectively. Hence the present line attempts an analysis of water swelling disease through a diagnosis of these pulse positions.

The inch opening pulse is governed by lung qì. An inch opening pulse that is sunken and slow is due to exuberant cold and water qì. When lung qì fails to regulate the waterways, water qì gradually congeals and gathers to form water swelling.

The instep yáng pulse indicates the spleen and stomach. If the instep yáng pulse is sunken and hidden, this indicates yáng debilitation and yīn exuberance in the center burner. Because spleen-stomach yáng is insufficient, food is not properly digested; hence the text says "grain and water are not transformed." Because spleen qì is debilitated and fails to move and transform, the clear and the turbid are not separated, so stool and water descend mixed; hence the text says "duck's slop." The text then tells us that because stomach qì is debilitated, there is generalized swelling.

The last section that describes the manifestations of a low lesser yáng pulse and a fine lesser yīn pulse in fact refers to conditions of the kidney. Lesser yáng is related to the kidney, and according to most commentators, the "low" characteristic of the pulse describes a pulse that is sunken and forceless, thus describing an insufficiency of original yáng in the kidney and aresulting inhibition of qì transformation in the triple burner.

Lastly, regarding the lesser yīn pulse, since lesser yīn also indicates the kidney, a fine quality in this pulse points to a depletion of essence-blood in the kidney. When both kidney yīn and kidney yáng are vacuous, this can result in water qì, which manifests differently in men and women. Since men are rooted in yáng and in qì, kidney qì debilitation means that the bladder lacks warmth to transform by steaming. Inhibited urination is the result. Since women are rooted in yīn and blood, kidney essence depletion results in vacuity in the thoroughfare and controlling vessels and in cold lodging in the uterus. When cold congeals and blood is scant, the menstrual flow stops. Essence-blood is the source of the menses, and when essence-blood is depleted, the menstrual period is blocked. As a result, we see qì stagnation, which can cause water disease. The discussion in this line emphasizes at the end that this type of water qì originates in the blood aspect and therefore needs to be treated accordingly.

Line 14.20

问曰：病有血分水分，何也？师曰：经水前断，后病水，名曰血分，此病难治；先病水，后经水断，名曰水分，此病易治。何以故？去水，其经自下。

Wèn yuē: Bìng yǒu xuè fēn shuǐ fēn, hé yě? Shī yuē: Jīng shuǐ qián duàn, hòu bìng shuǐ, míng yuē xuè fēn, cǐ bìng nán zhì; xiān bìng shuǐ, hòu jīng shuǐ duàn, míng yuē shuǐ fen, cǐ bìng yì zhì. Hé yǐ gù? Qù shuǐ, qí jīng zì xià.

Question: "Diseases are either related to the blood aspect or the water aspect. What does this mean?" The Master says: "When a patient suffers first from interrupted menstrual flow and then from water [disease], this is called blood aspect. Such conditions are difficult to treat. When [the patient] first suffers from water [disease], and then from interrupted menstrual flow, this is called water aspect. Such conditions are easily treated. Why is this so? When you get rid of water, the menses will spontaneously descend."

Synopsis, Line 14.20

This line describes the distinction between conditions of the blood-aspect and water-aspect in water disease in women.

Commentary, Line 14.20

In women, the treatment of water swelling is complicated by the physiology of menstruation. We must pay attention to the development of menstrual block (amenorrhea) just before or after water swelling appears. When menstrual block occurs before water swelling develops, this is due to static blood obstructing the waterways. This is called "blood aspect." The blood aspect lies deep in the body and is difficult to free. At the same time, we cannot move water until the blood has been freed; hence the text tells us that this is difficult to treat. In treating such conditions, it is not sufficient to simply address the water; the blood disease has to be treated first. On the other hand, when water swelling develops before menstrual block, this means that water is obstructing the pathways of blood. This is called "water aspect." The water aspect is shallow and easy to move. As soon as we remove the water, the menses will start flowing on its own. Hence the text says that this is easy treat.

Line 14.21

(1)问曰：病者苦水，面目身体四肢皆肿，小便不利，脉之不言水，反言胸中痛，气上冲咽，状如炙肉，当微咳喘，审如师言，其脉何类？

(2)师曰：寸口脉沉而紧，沉为水，紧为寒，沉紧相搏，结在关元，始时尚微，年盛不觉，阳衰之后，荣卫相干，阳损阴盛，结寒微动，肾气上冲，喉咽塞噎，胁下急痛。医以为流饮而大下之，气击不去，其病不除，后重吐之，胃家虚烦，咽燥欲饮水，小便不利，水谷不化，面目手足浮肿；又与葶苈丸下水，当时如小差，食饮过度，肿复如前，胸胁苦痛，象若奔豚，其水扬溢，则浮咳喘逆。当先攻击冲气令止，乃治咳，咳止，其喘自差。先治新病，病当在后。

(1) Wèn yuē: bìng zhě kǔ shuǐ, miàn mù shēn tǐ sì zhī jiē zhǒng, xiǎo biàn bù lì, mài zhī bù yán shuǐ, fǎn yán xiōng zhōng tòng, qì shàng chōng yān, zhuàng rú zhì ròu, dāng wēi ké chuǎn, shěn rú shī yán, qí mài hé lèi?

(2) Shī yuē: Cùn kǒu mài chén ér jǐn, chén wéi shuǐ, jǐn wéi hán, chén jǐn xiāng bó, jié zài guān yuán, shǐ shí shàng wēi, nián shèng bù jué, yáng shuāi zhī hòu, róng wèi xiāng gàn, yáng sǔn yīn shèng, jié hán wēi dòng, shèn qì shàng chōng, hóu yān sè yē, xié xià jí tòng. Yī yǐ wéi liú yǐn ér dà xià zhī, qì jí bù qù, qí bìng bù chú, hòu zhòng tù zhī, wèi jiā xū fán, yān zào yù yǐn shuǐ, xiǎo biàn bù lì, shuǐ gǔ bù huà, miàn mù shǒu zú fú zhǒng; yòu yǔ tíng lì wán xià shuǐ, dāng shí rú xiǎo chài, shí yǐn guò dù, zhǒng fù rú qián, xiōng xié kǔ tòng, xiàng ruò bēn tún, qí shuǐ yán yi, zé fú ké chuǎn nì. Dāng xiān gōng jí chōng qì lìng zhǐ, nǎi zhì ké, ké zhǐ, qí chuǎn zì chài. Xiān zhì xīn bìng, bìng dāng zài hòu.

(1) Question: "A patient suffering from water disease presented with swelling of the face, eyes, body, and four limbs, and inhibited urination. But when [the Master] diagnosed him,[1] he did not discuss water [qì], but instead spoke of pain in the chest, qì surging up into the throat, the feeling of roast meat [stuck in the throat],[2] and [the fact that] he ought to have slight cough and panting. [If] indeed it is as the Master says, how do you analyze this diagnosis?"[3]

(2) The Master says: "The patient's pulse at the inch opening pulse was sunken and tight. Sunken means water, and tight means cold. When sunken and tight contend with each other, they bind at Origin Pass (*guān yuán*, CV-4). Initially, this was insignificant, and in the plentiful years,[4] [the patient] did not feel it. [It is only] after yáng has become debilitated that construction and defense interfere with each other,[5] that detriment to yáng causes yīn exuberance, and that the bound cold stirs slightly.[6] Consequently kidney qì surges upward, causing blockage in the throat and tension and pain under the rib-side. When a physician [mistakenly] identifies this as flowing rheum and [treats it with] major precipitation, the qì attacks[7] would not go away, and the [patient's] disease was not eliminated. Afterwards, he [treated the patient with] heavy ejection. [This caused] stomach domain vacuity and vexation, dry pharynx with desire to drink water, inhibited urination, non-transformation of grain and water, and puffy swelling of the face, eyes, and extremities. Thereupon, [the physician] administered Lepidium/

Descurainiae Pill (*tíng lì wán*) to precipitate the water, which resulted in minor improvement at the beginning, [but when the patient] ate and drank excessively, the swelling returned as before. [Additionally, the patient now suffered] pain in the chest and rib-side as in running piglet, and puffiness, cough, and panting counterflow [because of] water rising and spilling. [In this situation] you should first attack the surging qì in order to calm it, and then treat the cough. When the cough is suppressed, the panting will spontaneously disappear. First treat the new disease, and leave the [water qì] disease until afterwards.

TEXT NOTES, LINE 14.21

[1] Diagnosed 脉 *mài*: The character 脉 *mài* most commonly means vessel or pulse. It can also be used as a verb, meaning "to take the pulse," and is used here in the wider sense of "to examine and diagnose" the patient.

[2] Feeling of roast meat [stuck in the throat] 状如炙肉 *zhuàn rú zhì ròu*: A manifestation of qì surging upward into the throat.

[3] How do you analyze this diagnosis? 其脉何类? *qí mài hé lèi*: 类 *lèi* means class or category. It is also used as a verb meaning to classify or categorize. Here, it means to analyze. The character 脉 *mài* is used here in the same sense as in the previous sentence, explained in note 1 above.

[4] Plentiful years 年盛 *nián shèng*: The prime of life (30–50 years old).

[5] Construction and defense interfere with each other 荣卫相干 *róng wèi xiān gàn*: Construction and defense have become imbalanced and fallen out of harmony.

[6] Bound cold stirs slightly 结寒微动 *jié hán wēi dòng*: "Bound cold" means cold water qì amassing and binding in the lower burner. "Stirs slightly" means "beginning to manifest itself as it surges into the upper burner."

[7] Qì attacks 气击 *qì jī*: The surging of qì.

SYNOPSIS, LINE 14.21

The present line takes the form of a case study that describes the development of water qì disease due to yáng vacuity, and mutations following inappropriate treatment. It also discusses priorities in the treatment of surging qì and water qì occurring together.

COMMENTARY, LINE 14.21

When the inch opening pulse is sunken and tight, sunken means water and tight means cold evil. Sunken and tight pulse types occurring together signify water and cold binding in the lower burner at the Origin Pass (*guān yuán*, CV-4) position, three body inches (*cùn*) below the umbilicus. In the initial stage, the binding of water and cold is mild, and people in the prime of their health may be unaware of it. As middle age progresses, yáng qì gradually becomes debilitated, and the flow of construction and defense becomes inhibited. At this time, congealing water and cold exploit kidney yáng vacuity and surge upward with kidney qì to cause blockage of the throat and tension and pain beneath the rib-side. This can be treated by warming the kidney and dispelling cold.

The present line describes a situation where a physician mistook this condition for lodged rheum and applied precipitation, as a result of which neither the surging qì nor the water swelling were eliminated. After this, the practitioner mistook the condition for cold rheum in the chest and therefore applied ejection. This treatment not only failed to relieve the surging qì, but in addition damaged qì and yīn in the stomach. Thereby, it caused vacuity vexation and dry pharynx with a desire to drink water. At the same time, because kidney yáng became vacuous and failed to perform qì transformation, urination was inhibited. As the stomach vacuity affected the spleen, grain and water were not transformed, and the water qì became increasingly exuberant. This resulted in puffy swelling of the face and eyes as well as the extremities. However, even at this stage, we must still consider the surging qì as the first priority.

The practitioner, by contrast, observed the puffy swelling and prescribed Lepidium/Descurainiae Pill (*tíng lì wán*) to once again precipitate the water. Although the formula is lost, we at least know from the text and from its main ingredient, lepidium/descurainiae (*tíng lì zǐ*), that it has a precipitating effect. After taking the formula, the puffy swelling abated slightly. Nevertheless, the spleen and stomach had not recovered, and when the patient ate and drank excessively, the swelling returned just as before. Furthermore, the surging qì became even more severe, described in the text as "pain in the chest and rib-side as in running piglet." Due to water qì shooting into the lung, there was also cough and panting counterflow.

To sum up the development of this condition, the first stage was characterized by water accumulation, which led to surging counterflow. Next, puffy swelling, panting, and cough arose following inappropriate use of ejection and precipitation. From clinical experience we know that the correct treament for such a condition is first to use a formula such as Cinnamon Twig, Poria, Schisandra, and Licorice Decoction (*guì líng wǔ wèi gān cǎo tāng*) to treat the surging qì. Once the surging qì has been calmed, the cough can be treated, and then finally the water swelling. The surging qì and the cough and panting are new diseases, and the surging qì is the condition that most urgently requires treatment. Therefore, the surging qì should be treated first. This is the principle summed up as "first treat the sudden disease, then treat the more intractable disease."

Line 14.22

风水，脉浮身重，汗出恶风者，防己黄芪汤主之，腹痛者加芍药。

Fēng shuǐ, mài fú shēn zhòng, hàn chū wù fēng zhě, fáng jǐ huáng qí tāng zhǔ zhī, fù tòng zhě jiā sháo yào.

For wind water [that presents with] a floating pulse, heavy body, sweating, and aversion to wind, Fangji and Astragalus Decoction (*fáng jǐ huáng qí tāng*) governs. For abdominal pain, add peony (*sháo yào*).[1]

TEXT NOTE, LINE 14.22

[1] The commentary adds: "For the formula, see the chapter on Dampness Disease." This refers to line 2.22 in Chapter 2, "Tetany, Dampness, and Thermoplegia."

SYNOPSIS, LINE 14.22

This line describes the signs and treatment of exterior vacuity wind water.

COMMENTARY, LINE 14.22

When wind stimulates water, it can cause the disease of wind water to arise. In this condition, the floating pulse reflects wind in the fleshy exterior, while generalized heaviness is the main sign of water-damp. "Sweating and aversion to wind" describes a condition of spontaneous sweating, as a result of which aversion to wind is aggravated. This is a sign of exterior vacuity and insecurity of defense qì, as a result of which wind evil invades the exterior. This differs from initial-stage exterior-pattern aversion to wind with absence of sweating. The present condition is therefore treated by boosting defense and securing the exterior, and by disinhibiting water and dispelling dampness.

The final phrase suggesting the addition of peony (*sháo yào*) for abdominal pain has been the subject of disagreement among scholars. According to Zhāng Lù 张璐, peony is added to treat a secondary condition of liver depression causing abdominal pain. However, this is unlikely since this condition is not mentioned in the line. A more plausible explanation is that peony is added to relax tension and relieve pain, so as to treat blood impediment that can arise when water obstructs qì and thereby causes qì stagnation.

Line 14.23

风水，恶风，一身悉肿，脉浮，不渴，续自汗出，无大热，越婢汤主之。

麻黄六两　石膏半斤　生姜三两　甘草二两　大枣十五枚。

右五味，以水六升，先煮麻黄，去上沫，内诸药，煮取三升，分温三服。恶风者，加附子一枚，炮。风水，加朮四

Fēng shuǐ, wù fēng, yī shēn xī zhǒng, mài fú, bù kě, xù zì hàn chū, wú dà rè, yuè bì tāng zhǔ zhī.

Má huáng liù liǎng; shí gāo bàn jīn; shēng jiāng sān liǎng; gān cǎo èr liǎng; dà zǎo shí wǔ méi

Yòu wǔ wèi, yǐ shuǐ liù shēng, xiān zhǔ má huáng, qù shàng mò, nà zhū yào, zhǔ qǔ sān shēng, fēn wēn sān fú. Wù fēng zhě, jiā fù zǐ yī méi, pào. Fēng shuǐ, jiā zhú sì liǎng.

For wind water [that presents with] aversion to wind, swelling of the whole body, a floating pulse, absence of thirst, intermittent spontaneous sweating, and absence of great heat, Spleen-Effusing Decoction (越婢汤 *yuè bì tāng*[1]) governs.

Spleen-Effusing Decoction (越婢汤 *yuè bì tāng*)
ephedra (麻黄 *má huáng*, Ephedrae Herba) 6 *liǎng*

gypsum (石膏 *shí gāo*, Gypsum Fibrosum) ½ *jīn*
fresh ginger (生姜 *shēng jiāng*, Zingiberis Rhizoma Recens) 3 *liǎng*
licorice (甘草 *gān cǎo*, Glycyrrhizae Radix) 2 *liǎng*
jujube (大枣 *dà zǎo*, Jujubae Fructus) 15 pieces

Of the above five ingredients, first boil the ephedra (*má huáng*) in six *shēng* of water and remove the scum from the top. Add all [the other] ingredients and boil to get three *shēng*. Divide into three doses and take warm. For aversion to cold, add one piece of aconite (*fù zǐ*) blast-fried. For wind water, add four *liǎng* of [white] atractylodes ([*bái*] *zhú*).

TEXT NOTE, LINE 14.23

[1] Differences of opinion surround the name 越婢汤 *yuè bì tāng*, which consists of 越 *yuè*, meaning to "jump over" or "overstep," and 婢 *bì*, a servant girl. The one most widely accepted explanation and the one on which our translation is based hails from Chén Wú-Jǐ (成无己), who assumes 越 to mean 发越 *fā yuè*, to effuse (move upward and outward) and 婢 to refer to 脾 *pí*, the spleen, which in fact is the character used in the name as it appears in the text *Wài Tái Mì Yào* ("Secrets from the *Wài Tái* Library"). Bó Dé-Xīn (柏德新) interprets 婢 as low, depressed state (卑 *bēi* means "low" or "lowly"), and thus takes *yuè bì* to mean overcoming depression, which, in his opinion, given the pattern and medicinals used, affects lung qì. Qián Huáng (钱潢) believes that the formula is so named because it was effective in curing a servant girl from a place called *Yuè*, hence the commonly used English translation of "Maidservant of Yuè."

SYNOPSIS, LINE 14.23

This line describes the signs and treatment of wind water complicated by depressed heat.

COMMENTARY, LINE 14.23

Wind water is a disease of acute onset that is caused by wind evil assailing the exterior, impairing lung diffusion and regulation, affecting kidney qì transformation, and thereby causing water qì to spill into the fleshy exterior. Since the exterior defense is damaged by wind evil, there is aversion to wind. Water is stirred by the wind and as a result spills in all directions; hence there is generalized swelling. The floating pulse indicates that the disease is located in the exterior, while the absence of thirst indicates that the patient does not yet suffer from an exuberance of interior heat and damage to the fluids.

Alternatively, a number of commentators have followed Yóu Yí 尤怡 who stated that 脉浮不渴 *mài fú bù kě* (floating pulse and absence of thirst) should be read as 脉浮而渴 *mài fú ér kě* (floating pulse and thirst) instead. In his opinion, this combination of symptoms indicates that the present condition is characterized by no great heat in the exterior, but rather exuberant heat in the interior. Because wind is dissipating in nature, there is intermittent spontaneous sweating. Because the sweating is only intermittent, there is no great heat in the exterior. Thus the condition is one dominated by wind and water contending with each other, with the exterior pattern failing to resolve despite sweating, and with the subsistence of depressed heat despite the absence of great heat in the exterior.

For treatment, use Spleen-Effusing Decoction (*yuè bì tāng*), which effuses yáng qì, dissipates water, and clears heat. Ephedra (*má huáng*) combined with fresh ginger (*shēng jiāng*) dissipates water-damp. Gypsum (*shí gāo*) clears depressed heat in the lung and stomach and eliminates thirst. Licorice (*gān cǎo*) and jujube (*dà zǎo*) supplement center qì. For excessively exuberant water-damp, in the text referred to as "wind water," white atractylodes (*bái zhú*) can be added to fortify the spleen and eliminate dampness, so as to enhance the body's capacity to disperse water. The addition of white atractylodes thus makes the formula one that treats both exterior and interior.

Aversion to wind is the key sign of this condition. However, if this symptom is particularly pronounced, signifying severe kidney yáng vacuity and insecurity of defensive qì, you can add aconite (*fù zǐ*) to warm the kidney and assist yáng, thereby fortifying the root and prevening yáng collapse from excessive sweating.

Line 14.24

皮水为病，四肢肿，水气在皮肤中，四肢聂聂动者，防己茯苓汤主之。

防己三两　黄芪三两　桂枝三两　茯苓六两　甘草二两

右五味，以水六升，煮取二升，分温三服。

Pí shuǐ wéi bìng, sì zhī zhǒng, shuǐ qì zài pí fū zhōng, sì zhī zhé zhé dòng zhě, fáng jǐ fú líng tāng zhǔ zhī.

Fáng jǐ sān liǎng; huáng qí sān liǎng; guì zhī sān liǎng; fú líng liù liǎng; gān cǎo èr liǎng

Yòu wǔ wèi, yǐ shuǐ liù shēng, zhǔ qǔ èr shēng, fēn wēn sān fú.

The disease of skin water manifests with swelling of the four limbs, water qì in the skin, and fluttering and twitching of the four limbs.[1] Fangji and Poria Decoction (防己茯苓汤 *fáng jǐ fú líng tāng*) governs.

Fangji and Poria Decoction
(防己茯苓汤 *fáng jǐ fú líng tāng*

- fangji (防己 *fáng jǐ*, Stephaniae Tetrandrae Radix) 3 *liǎng*
- astragalus (黄芪 *huáng qí*, Astragali Radix) 3 *liǎng*
- cinnamon twig (桂枝 *guì zhī*, Cinnamomi Ramulus) 3 *liǎng*
- poria (茯苓 *fú líng*, Poria) 6 *liǎng*
- licorice (甘草 *gān cǎo*, Glycyrrhizae Radix) 2 *liǎng*

Boil the above five ingredients in six *shēng* of water to get two *shēng*. Divide into three doses and take warm.

Text Note, Line 14.24

[1] Fluttering and twitching of the four limbs 四肢聂聂动 *sì zhī zhé zhé dòng*: Fluttering describes the slight movement of tree leaves. In the present context, it describes slight twitching of the flesh, which is mostly a subjective sensation.

SYNOPSIS, LINE 14.24

This line describes the signs and treatment of skin water due to yáng vacuity and qì depression.

COMMENTARY, LINE 14.24

The spleen governs the four limbs. When the spleen is diseased and unable to move and transform water-damp, water accumulates in the flesh and skin of the four limbs. Hence skin water is characterized by swelling of the limbs. This swelling depresses yáng qì and gives rise to a struggle between evil and right, hence the flesh twitches slightly.

The treatment is Fangji and Poria Decoction (*fáng jǐ fú líng tāng*), which penetrates the exterior and dispels dampness on the one hand, and frees yáng and promotes qì transformation on the other. Fangji (*fáng jǐ*) and astragalus (*huáng qí*) penetrate the exterior and dispel dampness, causing the discharge of water with sweat. Cinnamon twig (*guì zhī*) and poria (*fú líng*) free yáng and transform water, causing the discharge of water with urine. Cinnamon twig (*guì zhī*) and astragalus (*huáng qí*) are mutually supportive in freeing yáng and moving impediment, and in rallying defensive yáng. Licorice (*gān cǎo*) harmonizes all the medicinals.

Line 14.25

里水，越婢加朮汤主之，甘草麻黄汤亦主之。

甘草二两　麻黄四两

右二味，以水五升，先煮麻黄，去上沫，内甘草，煮取三升，温服一升，重覆汗出，不汗再服，慎风寒。

Lǐ shuǐ, yuè bì jiā zhú tāng zhǔ zhī, gān cǎo má huáng tāng yì zhǔ zhī.

Gān cǎo èr liǎng; má huáng sì liǎng

Yòu èr wèi, yǐ shuǐ wǔ shēng, xiān zhǔ má huáng, qù shàng mò, nèi gān cǎo, zhǔ qǔ sān shēng, wēn fú yī shēng, zhòng fù hàn chū, bù hàn zài fú, shèn fēng hán.

For interior water, Spleen-Effusing Decoction Plus White Atractylodes[1] (越婢加朮汤 *yuè bì jiā zhú tāng*) governs. Licorice and Ephedra Decoction (甘草麻黄汤 *gān cǎo má huáng tāng*) also governs.

Licorice and Ephedra Decoction (甘草麻黄汤 *gān cǎo má huáng tāng*)
licorice (甘草 *gān cǎo*, Glycyrrhizae Radix) 2 *liǎng* ephedra (麻黄 *má huáng*, Ephedrae Herba) 4 *liǎng*

Of the above two ingredients, first boil the ephedra (*má huáng*) in five *shēng* of water and remove the scum from on top. Add the licorice (*gān cǎo*) and boil to get three *shēng*. Take one *shēng* per dose warm. Heavily cover [the patient] and induce sweating. If there is no sweating, take another dose. Beware of wind-cold.

TEXT NOTE, LINE 14.25

[1] The commentary adds: "For the formula, see above [Appended Formulas, line 5.10). To the formula for Spleen-Effusing Decoction (*yuè bì tāng*), add four liǎng of white atractylodes (*bái zhú*). See also under the chapter for 'Wind-strike.'" The formula is found in line 14.23 above, and also in the "Appended Formulas" section at the end of Chapter 5, "Wind-stroke and Joint Running."

SYNOPSIS, LINE 14.25

This line describes two distinct exterior-dissipating treatments for skin water.

COMMENTARY, LINE 14.25

In the present line, "interior water" actually refers to skin water. In some quotations of this passage, the term 里水 *lǐ shuǐ* is in fact replaced with the term for "skin water," 皮水 *pí shuǐ*. This is a condition of exterior repletion, which in severe cases of swelling is complicated by depressed heat. This pathomechanism becomes clear when we consider the choice of Spleen-Effusing Decoction Plus White Atractylodes (*yuè bì jiā zhú tāng*) as the recommended treatment: It has the effect of dissipating water qì as well as clearing depressed heat, thereby allowing water and heat to be eliminated through exterior resolution.

As an alternative treatment for skin water in its initial stage, when not yet complicated by depressed heat, the present line suggests Licorice and Ephedra Decoction (*gān cǎo má huáng tāng*). This formula contains only licorice (*gān cǎo*), which harmonizes the center and supplements the spleen, thereby promoting lung qì diffusion, and ephedra (*má huáng*), which diffuses the lung and disinhibits water by promoting sweating. As such, it does not contain any medicinal that specifically addresses depressed heat in the interior. Although licorice has a slight heat-clearing action, it is not powerful enough to address the depressed heat on its own. Hence we conclude that Spleen-Effusing Decoction Plus White Atractylodes (*yuè bì jiā zhú tāng*) treats skin water with depressed heat while Licorice and Ephedra Decoction (*gān cǎo má huáng tāng*) treats skin water without depressed heat.

Line 14.26

水之为病，其脉沉小，属少阴。浮者为风；无水，虚胀者为气。水，发其汗即已。脉沉者宜麻黄附子汤，浮者宜杏子汤。

麻黄三两 甘草二两 附子一枚（炮）

右三味，以水七升，先煮麻黄，去上沫，内诸药，煮取二升半，温服八分，日三服。

Shuǐ zhī wéi bìng, qí mài chén xiǎo, shǔ shào yīn. Fú zhě wéi fēng; wú shuǐ, xū zhàng zhě wéi qì. Shuǐ, fā qí hàn jí yǐ. Mài chén zhě yí má huáng fù zǐ tāng, fú zhě yí xìng zǐ tāng.

Má huáng sān liǎng; gān cǎo èr liǎng; fù zǐ yī méi (pào)

Yòu sān wèi, yǐ shuǐ qī shēng, xiān zhǔ má huáng, qù shàng mò, nà zhū yào, zhǔ qǔ èr shēng bàn, wēn fú bā fēn, rì sān fú.

When water causes disease, if the pulse is sunken and small, [the condition] is associated with lesser yīn. If there is no water, vacuity distention is caused by qì. In water [disease], promote sweating to end [the disease]. In [patients with] a sunken pulse, Ephedra and Aconite Decoction (*má huáng fù zǐ tāng*) is appropriate; In [patients with] a floating pulse, Apricot Seed Decoction (杏子汤 *xìng zǐ tāng*) is appropriate.[1]

Ephedra and Aconite Decoction (麻黄附子汤 má huáng fù zǐ tāng)

ephedra (麻黄 *má huáng*, Ephedrae Herba) 3 *liǎng*
licorice (甘草 *gān cǎo*, Glycyrrhizae Radix) 2 *liǎng*
aconite (附子 *fù zǐ*, Aconiti Radix Lateralis Praeparata) 1 piece (blast-fry)

Of the above three ingredients, first boil the ephedra (*má huáng*) in seven *shēng* of water and remove the scum from on top. Add all [the other] ingredients and boil to get two-and-a-half *shēng*. Take eight parts warm, three times a day.

TEXT NOTE, LINE 14.26

[1] The text only gives the formula title. A comment included in the received text reads: "The formula is lost. It could be identical to Ephedra, Apricot Kernel, Licorice, and Gypsum Decoction (*má huáng xìng ren gān cǎo shí gāo tāng*)." This formula is usually referred to in Chinese as 麻杏甘石汤 *má xìng gān shí tāng.*

SYNOPSIS, LINE 14.26

This line describes different treatments for regular water and wind water, and the distinction between water swelling and vacuity distention.

COMMENTARY, LINE 14.26

The terms "regular water" and "wind water" do not appear in this line. Nevertheless, we know that water swelling that manifests in a sunken small pulse is related to the lesser yīn and kidney, because a sunken pulse indicates an interior disease. In this condition, kidney yáng is vacuous and therefore fails to transform qì and move water. It is commonly referred to as regular water. In water swelling with a floating pulse, on the other hand, the pulse indicates that the condition is related to wind, to the exterior, and to the lung. In this type of condition, externally contracted wind impairs lung diffusion and kidney qì transformation. This is referred to as wind water. Both conditions are marked by water in the exterior, and both can be treated by promoting sweating.

The next sentence, "If there is no water, vacuity distention is caused by qì," is an intercalation, indicating that distention and fullness of the abdomen are not necessarily caused by water, but can also be caused by qì. Although such conditions are similar to water disease, they may not be treated by sweating, but must be treated by warming and freeing yáng qì instead.

Regular water is associated with water qì in the exterior and, like wind water, can be treated by sweating, but the fine sunken pulse alerts us that we must also pay attention to kidney yáng and treat the root together with the tip. Hence the text recommends Ephedra and Aconite Decoction (*má huáng fù zǐ tāng*) to warm the channels and promote sweating. In this formula, *má huáng* (Ephedrae Herba) effuses sweat and resolves the exterior, *fù zǐ* (Aconiti Radix Lateralis Praeparata) assists yáng and transforms water, and *gān cǎo* (Glycyrrhizae Radix) regulates the center and supplements the spleen. By contrast, wind water, which is characterized by a floating pulse, is treated by rescuing the lung, using Apricot Seed Decoction (*xìng zǐ tāng*).

Line 14.27

厥而皮水者，蒲灰散主之。

Jué ér pí shuǐ zhě, pú huī sǎn zhǔ zhī.

For reversal[1] and skin water, Charred Dandelion Powder (*pú huī sǎn*) governs.[2]

TEXT NOTES, LINE 14.27

[1] Reversal 厥 *jué*: Counterflow cold of the extremities (手足逆冷 *shǒu zú nì lěng*), i.e., palpable cold up to the elbows and knees.

[2] The formula is missing. A comment included in the received text reads: "For the formula, see the chapter on dispersion-thirst." This formula is found in Chapter 13, "Dispersion-Thirst, Inhibited Urination, and Strangury," line 13.11.

SYNOPSIS, LINE 14.27

This line discusses the signs of skin water, such as a floating pulse, skin swelling, no aversion to wind or thirst, and drum-like distention of the abdomen, and the treatment recommended when it manifests in combination with counterflow cold of the extremities .

COMMENTARY, LINE 14.27

This line describes a condition where the reversal cold is not the regular reversal cold caused by yáng vacuity or qì depression, but is caused by an external exuberance of water evil and internal congestion of damp-heat, which traps yáng qì and prevents it from reaching the limbs. It is thus a sign of exuberant damp-heat, characteristic of skin water. The recommended treatment is Charred Dandelion Powder (*pú huī sǎn*), which clears damp-heat, disinhibits urine, and frees yáng qì.

Line 14.28

问曰：黄汗之为病，身体肿，发热汗出而渴，状如风水，汗沾衣，色正黄如蘗汁，脉自沉，何从得之？师曰：以汗出入水中浴，水从汗孔入得之，宜芪芍桂酒汤主之。

黄芪五两　芍药三两　桂枝三两

右三味，以苦酒一升，水七升，相和煮取三升，温服一升，当心烦，服至六七日乃解。若心烦不止者，以苦酒阻故也。

Wèn yuē: Huáng hàn zhī wéi bìng, shēn tǐ zhǒng, fā rè hàn chū ér kě, zhuàng rú fēng shuǐ, hàn zhān yī, sè zhèng huáng rú bó zhī, mài zì chén, hé cóng dé zhī? Shī yuē: Yǐ hàn chū rù shuǐ zhōng yù, shuǐ cóng hàn kǒng rù dé zhī, yí qí sháo guì jiǔ tāng zhǔ zhī.

Huáng qí wǔ liǎng; sháo yào sān liǎng; guì zhī sān liǎng

Yòu sān wèi, yǐ kǔ jiǔ yī shēng, shuǐ qī shēng, xiāng huó zhǔ qǔ sān shēng, wēn fú yī shēng, dāng xīn fán, fú zhì liù qī rì nǎi jiě. Ruò xīn fán bù zhǐ zhě, yǐ kǔ jiǔ zǔ gù yě.

Question: "The disease of yellow sweat [exhibits] swelling of the body,[1] heat effusion, sweating, and thirst, an appearance like wind water, sweat that dampens the clothing and is true yellow in color like phellodendron juice, and a naturally sunken pulse. How does this arise?" The Master says: "[When a person] enters water for a bath while sweating, the water can enter [the body] through the sweat pores. Thereby, [the person can] contract [this condition]. Astragalus, Peony, Cinnamon Twig, and Vinegar Decoction (黄芪芍桂酒汤主之 *huáng qí sháo guì jiǔ tāng*) governs.

Astragalus, Peony, Cinnamon Twig, and Vinegar Decoction (黄芪芍桂酒汤主之 *huáng qí sháo guì jiǔ tāng*)
astragalus (黄芪 *huáng qí*, Astragali Radix) 5 *liǎng* peony (芍药 *sháo yào*, Paeoniae Radix) 3 *liǎng* cinnamon twig (桂枝 *guì zhī*, Cinnamomi Ramulus) 3 *liǎng*

Boil the above three ingredients in a mixture of one *shēng* of vinegar (*kǔ jiǔ*) and seven *shēng* of water to get three *shēng*. Take one *shēng* [per dose] warm. There should be heart vexation [due to the vinegar]. Take it for six to seven days, and resolution will ensue. If the heart vexation does not stop, it is because the vinegar is causing blockage.[2]

TEXT NOTES, LINE 14.28

[1] Swelling of the body 身体肿 *shēn tǐ zhǒng*: A textual variation has 重 *zhòng* (heaviness) instead.

[2] The commentary adds: "An alternative version of this formula substitutes sacrificial vinegar for [regular] vinegar."

SYNOPSIS, LINE 14.28

This line describes the cause, pathomechanism, signs, and treatment of yellow sweat.

COMMENTARY, LINE 14.28

Yellow sweat is a type of water qì disease that is characterized by effusion of yellow sweat. The symptoms "swelling of the body, heat effusion, sweating, and thirst" also occur in wind water; hence the text mentions that this disease resembles wind water. Nevertheless, we can distinguish these two conditions by the pulse, which in yellow sweat is sunken and in wind water is floating. In addition, wind water is accompanied by aversion to wind, which is absent in yellow sweat, while yellow sweat is characterized by the distinctive yellow coloration of the sweat, which is not seen in wind water.

As the text explains, yellow sweat is caused by sweating that weakens construction and defense qì, coinciding with an invasion of external water-damp. It is thus a combination of internal and external causes. In addition to the cause mentioned in the present line, namely taking a bath while sweating, yellow sweat can occur in any other situation where a person sweats and is exposed to wind, rain, or water; or lives in a damp location, overworks while sweating, or has cold-damp inside the clothing. In these conditions, water can impede construction and defense, transform into heat, and steam in the interstices of the flesh.

The present line recommends Astragalus, Peony, Cinnamon Twig, and Vinegar Decoction (*qí sháo guì jiǔ tāng*) for treating yellow sweat, because this formula has the effect of harmonizing construction and defense, replenishing defense, and dispelling dampness, as well as discharging construction heat. The formula uses cinnamon twig (*guì zhī*) and peony (*sháo yào*) to harmonize construction and defense, and a large amount of astragalus (*huáng qí*) to replenish defense and penetrate the exterior, thereby supporting right and outthrusting evil. Together, these medicinals arouse construction and defense while also moving water-damp. Vinegar, which refers to rice vinegar, can assist peony (*sháo yào*) in containing construction and constraining yīn, as well as discharching the depressed heat in the construction aspect. Altogether, these medicinals replenish defense yáng, boost construction yīn, move qì, and dissipate water-damp. Owing to the acidity in the vinegar, the patient may experience heart vexation after taking this formula. The text informs us that this is a normal effect of the formula and should not stop the patient from continuing to take it for about a week, after which time the medicine will have engendered enough strength to resolve the disease.

Line 14.29

(1)黄汗之病，两胫自冷，假令发热，此属历节；食已汗出，又身常暮卧盗汗出者，此劳气也；若汗出已，反发热者，久久其身必甲错；发热不止者，必生恶疮。

(2)若身重，汗出已，辄轻者，久久必身瞤，瞤即胸中痛，又从腰以上必汗出，下无汗，腰髋弛痛，如有物在皮中状，剧者不能食，身疼重，烦躁，小便不利，此为黄汗，桂枝加黄芪汤主之。

桂枝　芍药各二两　甘草二两　生姜三两　大枣十二枚　黄芪二两

右六味，以水八升，煮取三升，温服一升，须臾，饮热稀粥一升余，以助药力，温覆取微汗，若不汗更服。

(1) Huáng hàn zhī bìng, liǎng jìng zì lěng, jiǎ lìng fā rè, cǐ shǔ lì jié; shí yǐ hàn chū, yòu shēn cháng mù wò dào hàn chū zhě, cǐ láo qì yě; ruò hàn chū yǐ, fǎn fā rè zhě, jiǔ jiǔ qí shēn bì jiǎ cuò; fā rè bù zhǐ zhě, bì shēng wù chuāng.

(2) Ruò shēn zhòng hàn chū yǐ, zhé qīng zhě, jiǔ jiǔ bì shēn shùn shùn, shùn shùn jí xiōng zhōng tòng, yòu cóng yāo yǐ shàng bì hàn chū, xià wú hàn, yāo kuān chí tòng, rú yǒu wù zài pí zhōng zhuàng, jù zhě bù néng shí, shēn téng zhòng, fán

zào, xiǎo biàn bù lì, cǐ wéi huáng hàn, guì zhī jiā huáng qí tāng zhǔ zhī.

Guì zhī, sháo yào gè èr liǎng; gān cǎo èr liǎng; shēng jiāng sān liǎng; dà zǎo shí èr méi; huáng qí èr liǎng

Yòu liù wèi, yǐ shuǐ bā shēng, zhǔ qǔ sān shēng, wēn fú yī shēng, xū yú, yǐn rè xī zhōu yī shēng yú, yǐ zhù yào lì, wēn fù qǔ wēi hàn, ruò bù hàn gèng fú.

(1) In yellow sweat disease, the lower legs are naturally cold. If they effuse heat instead, this is associated with joint running.[1] If the patient sweats after eating or constantly experiences night sweating, this is taxation qì.[2] If [yellow sweat manifests] with heat effusion after sweating, over time the body will inevitably [develop] encrusted skin. If heat effusion is incessant, it will inevitably engender malign sores.

(2) If the body is heavy, after sweating, [this sensation will be] milder. [If yellow sweat persists] over a long time, the body will twitch, and when it twitches, there will be pain in the chest. Furthermore, there will inevitably be sweating above the lumbus and absence of sweating below it, slackness and pain in the lumbus and hip, and a sensation as if there were something in the skin. Severe cases [manifest with] inability to eat, generalized pain and heaviness, vexation and agitation, and inhibited urination. These are [the signs of] yellow sweat. Cinnamon Twig Decoction Plus Astragalus (桂枝加黄芪汤 *guì zhī jiā huáng tāng*) governs.

Cinnamon Twig Decoction Plus Astragalus (桂枝加黄芪汤 guì zhī jiā huáng tāng)

- cinnamon twig (桂枝 *guì zhī*, Cinnamomi Ramulus) 2 *liǎng*
- peony (芍药 *sháo yào*, Paeoniae Radix) 2 *liǎng*
- licorice (甘草 *gān cǎo*, Glycyrrhizae Radix) 2 *liǎng*
- fresh ginger (生姜 *shēng jiāng*, Zingiberis Rhizoma Recens) 3 *liǎng*
- jujube (大枣 *dà zǎo*, Jujubae Fructus) 12 pieces
- astragalus (黄芪 *huáng qí*, Astragali Radix) 2 *liǎng*

Boil the above six ingredients in eight *shēng* of water to get three *shēng*. Take one *shēng* [per dose] heated. After a short while, drink one *shēng* or more of thin gruel to assist the strength of the medicine. Warmly cover up to induce slight sweating. If there is no sweat, take another dose.

TEXT NOTES, LINE 14.29

[1] Joint running 历节 *lì jié*: The name of a disease described in Chapter 5 above. It is characterized by pain and stiffness in multiple joints of the body, and is attributed to contraction of wind, cold, and dampness evil in patients suffering from internal damage to the liver and kidney.

[2] Taxation qì 劳气 *láo qì*: This term does not occur elsewhere in the *Jīn Guì Yào Lüè*. It most likely refers to vacuity taxation. As discussed in Chapter 6 above, this disease category is broad in scope and refers to conditions of chronic debilitation that arise from a variety of causes and manifest in numerous symptoms.

SYNOPSIS, LINE 14.29

This line explains how to distinguish yellow sweat from joint running and taxation qì, and describes the symptoms and treatment of yellow sweat.

COMMENTARY, LINE 14.29

Yellow sweat is characterized by a constant sensation of cold in both lower legs, which is caused by water-damp stagnating in the flesh and skin, leading to depression in the defense level and heat in the construction level. Because dampness is heavy by nature, it pours downward, obstructs yáng qì, and deprives the lower extremities of warmth. By this sign, we can distinguish it from joint running, which manifests in generalized heat effusion, including in the lower legs, and from vacuity taxation, which is mostly caused by dual vacuity of yīn and yáng and manifests in sweating after meals and at night. If yellow sweat persists for a long time, the skin will become dry and scaly, and engender malign sores. This is related to the chronic presence of damp-heat in the skin, depriving it of nourishment, vanquishing qì and blood, and therefore causing rotting in the skin.

The second section describes signs that arise when yellow sweat becomes progressively severe and begins to affect yīn as well as yáng. Yellow sweat is caused by damp-heat depression and can manifest in predominance of heat or dampness. In patients with a constitutional exuberance of yang, and in its initial stages, yellow sweat tends towards repletion heat; in later stages and in patients with constitutional yáng vacuity, it tends toward vacuity cold.

In addition to coldness in the lower legs, yellow sweat manifests with generalized heaviness that is relieved after sweating. This is a manifestation of exuberant dampness, which can be relieved temporarily by eliminating it through the exterior by sweating. However, if yáng vacuity is not also treated, the disease will persist and over time further debilitate yáng qì and exhaust yīn fluids. As a result, the sinews are deprived of nourishment, which results in twitching of the flesh and, owing to insufficiency of yáng qì in the sea of qì, chest pain. Because yáng qì is vacuous in the upper body, sweating occurs above the lumbus. Since water-damp rushes downward and blocks the lower body, there is no sweating, but slackness and lack of strength in the lumbus and hip. In addition, the struggle between evil and right causes a sensation of something crawling under the skin.

The above signs are all manifestations of yáng vacuity and dampness exuberance in the channels and network vessels. In more advanced stages of yellow sweat, we begin to see signs of injury to qì transformation in the bowels and viscera, such as inability to eat, generalized heaviness and pain (due to impaired movement of spleen yáng), vexation and agitation (due to blockage of heart yáng), and inhibited urination (due to nontransformation of kidney qì).

As treatment for yellow sweat, the text recommends Cinnamon Twig Decoction Plus Astragalus (*guì zhī jiā huáng qí tāng*), which regulates and disinhibits construction and defense, diffuses yáng, and expels dampness. In this formula, Cinnamon Twig Decoction (*guì zhī tāng*) can resolve the flesh, harmonize construction and defense, and dissipate external dampness, while at the same time transform qì, regulate yīn and yáng, and restore qì transformation in the bowels and viscera. The addition of astragalus (*huáng qí*) strengthens the formula's effect of supplementing qì, outthrusting the exterior, and expelling dampness, while also disinhibiting the flow of construction and defense qì on the inside and outside, thereby gradually removing dampness evil.

Line 14.30

师曰：寸口脉迟而濇，迟则为寒，濇为血不足；趺阳脉微而迟，微则为气，迟则为寒，寒气不足，则手足逆冷，手足逆冷，则荣卫不利，荣卫不利，则腹满肠鸣相逐；气转膀胱，荣卫俱劳；阳气不通，即身冷，阴气不通即骨疼；阳前通则恶寒，阴前通则痹不仁，阴阳相得，其气乃行，大气一转，其气乃散，实则失气，虚则遗溺，名曰气分。

Shī yuē: Cùn kǒu mài chí ér sè, chí zé wéi hán, sè wéi xuè bù zú; fū yáng mài wēi ér chí, wēi zé wéi qì, chí zé wéi hán, hán qì bù zú, zé shǒu zú nì lěng, shǒu zú nì lěng, zé róng wèi bù lì, róng wèi bù lì, zé fù mǎn cháng míng xiāng zhú; qì zhuǎn páng guāng, róng wèi jù láo; yáng qì bù tōng, jí shēn lěng, yīn qì bù tōng jí gǔ téng; yáng qián tōng zé wù hán, yīn qián tōng zé bì bù rén, yīn yáng xiāng dé, qí qì nǎi xíng, dà qì yī zhuǎn, qí qì nǎi sàn, shí zé shī qì, xū zé yí niào, míng yuē qì fēn.

The Master says: "When the inch opening pulse is slow and rough, slow means cold, and rough means insufficiency of blood. When the instep yáng pulse is faint and slow, faint means qì [vacuity], and slow means cold. Cold with insufficiency of qì[1] means counterflow cold in the extremities. Counterflow cold in the extremities means inhibited flow of construction and defense. Inhibited flow of construction and defense means abdominal fullness, rumbling intestines repelling each other,[2] and if the [cold] qì shifts into the bladder, taxation in both construction and defense.[3] When yáng qì stops, the body is cold; when yīn qì stops, there is bone pain. When yáng flows first, there is aversion to cold; when yīn flows first, there is impediment and insensitivity.[4] [It is only when] yīn and yáng get along that their qì moves, and in one rotation of great qì,[5] [the evil] qì [of water-damp] dissipates. [If the disease develops into a pattern of] repletion, the result is qì loss;[6] [if the disease develops into a pattern of] vacuity, the result is enuresis.[7] [This] is called qì-aspect disease.

TEXT NOTES, LINE 14.30

[1]Cold and insufficiency of qì 寒气不足 *hán qì bù zú*: Presence of cold in conjunction with insufficiency of qì and blood.

[2] Rumbling intestines repelling each other 腹满肠鸣相逐 *fù mǎn chǎng míng xiāng zhú*: Qì and water in the intestines repelling each other.

[3] Taxation in both construction and defense 荣卫俱劳 *róng wèi jù láo*: Debilitation of construction and defense qì.

[4] Impediment and insensitivity 痹不仁 *bì bù rén*: Obstruction of qì and blood causing numbness of the skin and flesh.

[5] Great qì 大气 *dà qì*: Ancestral qì.

[6] Qì loss 失气 *shī qì*: Passing of flatus.

[7] Enuresis 遗尿 *yí niào*: Here, this term denotes the more severe condition of urinary incontinence.

SYNOPSIS, LINE 14.30

This line describes the pulses, signs, and pathomechanisms of qì-aspect disease.

COMMENTARY, LINE 14.30

The inch opening pulse indicates the heart and lung. A slow and rough inch opening pulse indicates a condition of insufficiency of qì and blood that is complicated by the presence of cold evil. The instep yáng pulse indicates the spleen and stomach. A faint and slow instep yáng pulse indicates a condition of spleen qì vacuity with internal generation of cold. Thus we know from the combined pulse manifestations at the inch opening and instep yáng that this line discusses a pathomechanism in which upper and center burner yáng qì is insufficient, qì and blood are both vacuous, and cold evil has overcome the vacuity to distress the inner body. Since the spleen is the source of construction and defense, while the lung is in charge of distributing them, the chief manifestation of this condition is insufficiency of construction and defense qì.

When insufficiency of construction and defense qì and blood is complicated by cold evil, yáng qì is unable to warm the extremities; hence we see counterflow cold in the extremities, which is related to the inhibited movement of construction and defense. In addition, this manifests in distention and fullness in the abdomen, rumbling intestines, and in severe cases, cold qì surging into the bladder. When the movement of qì and blood is inhibited, we see cold and bone pain; when construction and defense are unable to move in harmony, we see aversion to cold and impediment and insensitivity.

The next section of this line discusses the treatment principles of qì-aspect disease. The above-mentioned symptoms are all caused by inhibition, taxation, and disharmony of construction and defense. By making construction and defense qì replete, free-flowing, and harmonious, we are able to restore their normal physiological functions. Construction and defense are the chief constituents of ancestral qì, and when they flow smoothly, ancestral qì is able to move and thereby dissipate the evil qì of water-damp.

The last section differentiates between repletion patterns and vacuity patterns in qì-aspect disease. In this context, "repletion" refers to conditions in which yáng qì is debilitated and ancestral qì fails to move, as a result of which cold qì binds and when discharged into the anus, manifests in flatulence. By contrast, vacuity conditions are related to yáng qì being weakened and losing its ability to contain, which results in the symptom of urinary incontinence.

Line 14.31

气分，心下坚，大如盘，边如旋杯，水饮所作，桂枝去芍加麻辛附子汤主之。

桂枝三两　生姜三两　甘草二两　大枣十二枚　麻黄　细辛各二两　附子（炮）一枚

右七味，以水七升，煮麻黄，去上沫，内诸药，煮取二升，分温三服，当汗出，如虫行皮中即愈。

Qì fēn, xīn xià jiān, dà rú pán, biān rú xuán bēi, shuǐ yǐn suǒ zuò, guì zhī qù sháo jiā má xīn fù zǐ tāng zhǔ zhī.

Guì zhī sān liǎng; shēng jiāng sān liǎng; gān cǎo èr liǎng; dà zǎo shí èr méi; má huáng, xì xīn gè èr liǎng; fù zǐ (pào) yī méi

Yòu qī wèi, yǐ shuǐ qī shēng, zhǔ má huáng, qù shàng mò, nà zhū yào, zhǔ qǔ èr shēng, fēn wēn sān fú, dāng hàn chū, rú chóng xíng pí zhōng jí yù.

Qì-aspect [disease manifests in] hardness below the heart [that is] the size of a plate, with edges like a turned cup.[1] This is created by water-rheum. Cinnamon Twig Decoction Minus Peony Plus Ephedra, Asarum, and Aconite (桂枝去芍药加麻黄细辛附子汤 *guì zhī qù sháo yào jiā má huáng xì xīn fù zǐ tāng*) governs.

Cinnamon Twig Decoction Minus Peony Plus Ephedra, Asarum, and Aconite (桂枝去芍药加麻黄细辛附子汤 *guì zhī qù sháo yào jiā má huáng xì xīn fù zǐ tāng*

cinnamon twig (桂枝 *guì zhī*, Cinnamomi Ramulus) 3 *liǎng*
fresh ginger (生姜 *shēng jiāng*, Zingiberis Rhizoma Recens) 3 *liǎng*
licorice (甘草 *gān cǎo*, Glycyrrhizae Radix) 2 *liǎng*
jujube (大枣 *dà zǎo*, Jujubae Fructus) 12 pieces
ephedra (麻黄 *má huáng*, Ephedrae Herba) 2 *liǎng*
asarum (细辛 *xì xīn*, Asari Radix et Rhizoma) 2 *liǎng*
aconite (附子 *fù zǐ*, Aconiti Radix Lateralis Praeparata) 1 piece (blast-fry)

Of the above seven ingredients, boil the ephedra (*má huáng)* in seven *shēng* of water. Remove the scum from on top, add all [the other ingredients], and boil to get two *shēng*. Divide into three doses and take warm. When sweat issues and there is a sensation like bugs crawling in the skin, recovery will ensue.

TEXT NOTE, LINE 14.31

[1] Hardness below the heart [that is] the size of a plate, with edges like a turned cup 心下坚，大如盘，边如旋杯 *xīn xià jiān, dà rú pán, biān rú xuán bēi*: A lump in the pit of the stomach that feels like the rounded bottom of a cup, elevated in the middle and lower at the edges.

SYNOPSIS, LINE 14.31

This line describes the signs and treatment of qì-aspect disease.

COMMENTARY, LINE 14.31

As described in the previous line, "qì-aspect" disease is a type of water qì disease that is related to yáng qì debilitation and inhibited movement of construction and defense. According to this line, its key sign is "hardness below the heart," which refers to the area of the stomach duct between the center and upper burner. Construction and defense originate in the center burner and diffuse in the upper burner. If they do not move freely and ancestral qì fails to rotate, water-rheum can collect below the heart and cause this symptom. If cold rheum congeals, it takes on a solid shape and can be felt as a large lump with a protruding center that is hard on the outsides and soft on the inside. In addition, qì-aspect disease manifests with the symptoms described in the previous line, such as counterflow cold in the extremities, abdominal fullness and intestinal rumbling, aversion to cold and generalized cold, etc.

Cinnamon Twig Decoction Minus Peony Plus Ephedra, Asarum, and Aconite (*guì zhī qù sháo yào jiā má huáng xì xīn fù zǐ tāng*) has the effect of warming yáng and dissipating cold, freeing the qì dynamic, and moving water-rheum. This formula adds ephedra (*má huáng*), asarum (*xì xīn*), and aconite (*fù zǐ*), to assist yáng, warm the channels, and promote sweating, while cinnamon twig (*guì zhī*) and fresh ginger (*shēng jiāng*) free yáng, transform qì, and dissipate cold rheum, and licorice (*gān cǎo*) and jujube (*dà zǎo*) supplement center qì. As a whole, it arouses yáng qì and moves ancestral qì, purges cold rheum, and dissipates exterior cold. The sensation of something crawling in the skin, mentioned by the text as a sign that the formula is working, indicates that yáng qì has been aroused, is moving throughout the body, and is pushing yīn evil out of the body by outthrusting it through the skin.

Line 14.32

心下坚，大如盘，边如旋盘，水饮所作，枳朮汤主之。

枳实七枚　白朮二两

右二味，以水五升，煮取三升，分温三服，腹中软，即当散也。

Xīn xià jiān, dà rú pán, biān rú xuán pán, shuǐ yǐn suǒ zuò, zhǐ zhú tāng zhǔ zhī.

Zhǐ shí qī méi; bái zhú èr liǎng

Yòu èr wèi, yǐ shuǐ wǔ shēng, zhǔ qǔ sān shēng, fēn wēn sān fú, fù zhōng ruǎn, jí dāng sàn yě.

Hardness below the heart [that is] the size of a plate, with edges like a turned plate, is created by water-rheum. Unripe Bitter Orange and White Atractylodes Decoction (枳朮汤 *zhǐ zhú tāng*) governs.

Unripe Bitter Orange and White Atractylodes Decoction (枳朮汤 *zhǐ zhú tāng*)
unripe bitter orange (枳实 *zhǐ shí*, Aurantii Fructus Immaturus) 7 pieces white atractylodes (白朮 *bái zhú*, Atractylodis Macrocephalae Rhizoma) 2 *liǎng*

Boil the above two ingredients in five *shēng* of water to get three *shēng*. Divide into three doses and take warm. Softness in the center of the abdomen means that [the evil] is dissipating.

SYNOPSIS, LINE 14.32

This line describes another method of treating qì-aspect disease.

COMMENTARY, LINE 14.32

The only difference between the condition described here and the one in the previous line is that the shape of the lump resembles a plate instead of a cup. This could possibly mean that the degree of water accumulation in this line is not as severe as that in the previous one. In any case, the present line discusses a condition of spleen vacuity qì stagnation, as a result of which water-rheum collects internally and binds below the heart. The recommended formula, Unripe Bitter Orange and White Atractylodes Decoction (*zhǐ zhú tāng*) moves qì, dissipates binds, fortifies the spleen, and disinhibits water.

附《外台秘要》方 *Fù «Wài Tài Mì Yào» Fāng*
Formulas from the Wài Tái Mì Yào ("Secrets from the Wài Tái Library")

Fangji and Astragalus Decoction (防己黄芪汤 *fáng jǐ huáng qí tāng*)

治风水，脉浮为在表，其人或头汗出，表无他病，病者但下重，从腰以上为和，腰以下当肿及阴，难以屈身。

Zhì fēng shuǐ, mài fú wéi zài biǎo, qí rén huò tóu hàn chū, biǎo wú tā bìng, bìng zhě dàn xià zhòng, cóng yāo yǐ shàng wéi hé, yāo yǐ xià dāng zhǒng jí yīn, nán yǐ qū shēn.

A treatment for wind water, with a floating pulse, which indicates [an] exterior [pattern]; possibly sweating from the head, [but] no other exterior disease; the patient suffering from heaviness of the lower body only; harmony above the lumbus and swelling below the lumbus that reaches the genitals; and difficulty bending and stretching.[1]

Formula Note, Line 14.32

[1] The commentary adds: "For the formula, see the chapter on Dampness Disease." This refers to line 2.22 of Chapter 2, "Tetany, Dampness, and Thermoplegia".

Formula Synopsis, Line 14.32

This line describes the symptoms and treatment of wind water caused by exterior qì vacuity and exuberance of water-damp.

Formula Commentary, Line 14.32

Fangji and Astragalus Decoction (*fáng jǐ huáng qí tāng*) is the governing formula for treating exterior vacuity-type wind water. The floating pulse indicates the presence of water qì in the exterior. Sweating from the head means that yáng is vacuous and qì is floating. The most important aspect of the present pattern is the exuberance of water-damp, which by nature pours downward and blocks yáng qì; hence we see heaviness in the lower body. This pattern is thus characterized by vacuity of exterior qì in the upper body and exuberance of water-damp in the lower body.

黄疸病脉证治第十五

CHAPTER 15

Jaundice

Pulses, Signs, Treatments

‡ Overview

As the title suggests, this chapter discusses jaundice (疸 *dǎn*), a disease that is characterized by yellowing of the face, skin, eyes, and urine, and whose principal cause is damp-heat. In actuality, however, the scope of this chapter is even more comprehensive, because it also describes conditions of yellowing (发黄 *fā huáng*) which may not be jaundice proper. The translation below has followed Zhāng Jī's example of distinguishing between "jaundice" (疸 *dǎn*) and "yellowing" (发黄 *fā huáng*). Besides yellowing due to damp-heat, the text also discusses the pathomechanisms of yellowing due to cold-damp, yellowing due to fire-forcing (i.e., a treatment method used to force sweating), yellowing due to dryness bind, yellowing due to female taxation, and yellowing due to vacuity.

Zhāng Jī's categorization of jaundice is mostly based on causes. Specifically discussed are grain jaundice, which is related to diet; alcohol jaundice, which is related to excessive consumption of alcohol; female taxation jaundice, which is related to taxation from excessive sexual intercourse; and black jaundice, which results when any of the other forms of jaundice that remain untreated so that over time damp-heat is complicated by stasis. Later physicians have further refined this categorization and added numerous further types to assist in clinical differentiation.

As already mentioned in the *Nèi Jīng*, the pathomechanism of jaundice is related to the internal organs, specifically to the liver, spleen, and kidney. Treatment methods are numerous and include resolving the exterior and effusing sweat, clearing and disinhibiting damp-heat, moistening dryness and expelling stasis, and regulating and supplementing the stomach and spleen. However, the most important treatment method is clearing and disinhibing damp-heat.

‡ Schematic Overview

Jaundice

1. Categorization
   a) Grain jaundice
      Pathomechanism: Food accumulation due to dietary irregularities, impairing splenic movement and transformation and giving rise to damp-heat.
      Signs: Generalized yellowing, dizziness, disquietude in the heart and chest, cold and heat, and abdominal fullness.
   b) Female taxation jaundice
      Pathomechanism: Excessive sexual activity giving rise to kidney depletion with stasis heat brewing internally.
      Signs: Black forehead, lesser abdominal fullness, heat in the hands and feet, spontaneous sweating, and generalized yellowing.
   c) Alcohol jaundice
      Pathomechanism: Excessive alcohol consumption causing damp-heat to brew internally and affect the heart.
      Signs: Anguish in the heart and chest, heat effusion, inability to eat, and periodic vomiting.
2. Pathomechanisms, signs, and treatment
   a) Damp and heat equally prevalent with exuberant lower body heat
      Signs: Cold and heat, inability to eat, disquietude in the heart and chest, persistent yellowness.
      Treatment: Clear heat, disinhibit dampness, and free the bowels, using Virgate Wormwood Decoction (*yīn chén hāo tāng*).
   b) Damp-heat exuberant in the upper body
      Signs: Anguish or hot pain in the heart.
      Treatment: Clear heat and eliminate vexation, using Gardenia and Rhubarb Decoction (*zhī zǐ dà huáng tāng*).
   c) Kidney depletion with stasis heat and dampness
      Signs: Late afternoon aversion to cold, lesser abdominal fullness, generalized yellowing, and black forehead.

Treatment: Dry dampness and dispel stasis with Niter and Alum Powder (*xiāo shí fán shí sǎn*).

d) Dampness more pronounced than heat

Signs: Jaundice with inhibited urination.

Treatment: Fortify the spleen and disinhibit dampness with Virgate Wormwood and Poria Five Powder (*yīn chén wǔ líng sǎn*).

e) Heat more pronounced than dampness with stasis heat binding internally.

Signs: Abdominal fullness, inhibited urination, and spontaneous sweating.

Treatment: Clear heat, break stasis, and free the bowels with Virgate Wormwood and Poria Five Powder (*dà huáng xiāo shí tāng*).

f) Damp-heat in lesser yáng (*shào yáng*)

Signs: Jaundice, abdominal pain, and retching.

Treatment: Harmonize lesser yáng with Minor Bupleurum Decoction (*xiǎo chái hú tāng*).

g) Damp-heat in the exterior with exterior vacuity

Signs: Jaundice with a floating pulse.

Treatment: Promote sweating and resolve the exterior using Cinnamon Twig Decoction Plus Astragalus (*guì zhī jiā huáng qí tāng*).

h) Dryness with stasis

Signs: Withered-yellow complexion and dry bound stool.

Treatment: Moisten the intestines and free the stool using Pork Lard and Hair Brew (*zhū gāo fà jiān*) 猪膏发煎

i) Counterflow ascent of stomach qì

Signs: Jaundice with hiccup.

Treatment: Harmonize the stomach and downbear counterflow using Minor Pinellia Decoction (小半夏汤 *xiǎo bàn xià tāng*).

j) Spleen stomach vacuity cold

Signs: Jaundice in men with uninhibited urination.

Treatment: Supplement the spleen and fortify the stomach with Minor Center-Fortifying Decoction (小建中汤 *xiǎo jiàn zhōng tāng*).

Line 15.1

寸口脉浮而缓，浮则为风，缓则为痹，痹非中风；四肢苦烦，脾色必黄，瘀热以行。

Cùn kǒu mài fú ér huǎn, fú zé wéi fēng, huǎn zé wéi bì, bì fēi zhōng fēng; sì zhī kǔ fán, pí sè bì huáng, yū rè yǐ xíng.

When the inch opening pulse is floating and moderate, floating means wind, and moderate means impediment.[1] [This type of] impediment is not wind-strike.[2] The limbs suffer from vexation, and the spleen's color invariably causes yellowing,[3] which is caused by stasis heat[3] moving [into the exterior].

TEXT NOTES, LINE 15.1

[1] Impediment 痹 *bì*: Obstruction caused by dampness evil.

[2] [This type of] impediment is not wind-strike 痹非中风 *bì fēi zhòng fēng*: The implication of this interpolation is that jaundice is caused by damp-heat stagnating in the spleen and stomach, and not by wind-strike, despite the fact that a floating and moderate pulse also manifests in greater yáng wind-strike patterns.

[3] The spleen's color invariably causes yellowing 脾色必黄 *pí sè bì huáng*: Yellow, the color associated with the spleen, will be in evidence in the skin.

[4] Stasis heat 瘀热 *yū rè*: Blood stasis arising as a result of heat.

SYNOPSIS, LINE 15.1

This line describes the pathomechanism of yellowing.

COMMENTARY, LINE 15.1

This line discusses the pathomechanism of yellowing from the perspective of the pulse. A floating pulse indicates wind evil; a moderate pulse indicates dampness evil. In combination, these two evils obstruct the channels and network vessels, flesh and skin, and joints, and cause yáng to transform into heat. Damp-heat internally encumbers the spleen and follows the channels outward into the limbs where it manifests as vexation. When damp-heat internally invades the blood aspect, it causes blood stasis, and stasis heat consequently spreads all over the body, manifesting in generalized yellowing.

Line 15.2

(1)趺阳脉紧而数，数则为热，热则消谷，紧则为寒，食即为满。尺脉浮为伤肾，趺阳脉紧为伤脾。风寒相搏，食谷即眩，谷气不消，胃中苦浊，浊气下流，小便不通，阴被其寒，热流膀胱，身体尽黄，名曰谷疸。

(2)额上黑，微汗出，手足中热，薄暮即发，膀胱急，小便自利，名曰女劳疸，腹如水状，不治。

(3)心中懊憹而热，不能食，时欲吐，名曰酒疸。

(1) Fū yáng mài jǐn ér shuò, shuò zé wéi rè, rè zé xiāo gǔ , jǐn zé wéi hán, shí jí wéi mǎn. Chǐ mài fú wéi shāng shèn, fū yáng mài jǐn wéi shāng pí. Fēng hán xiāng bó, shí gǔ jí xuàn, gǔ qì bù xiāo, wèi zhōng kǔ zhuó, zhuó qì xià liú, xiǎo biàn bù tōng, yīn bèi qí hán, rè liú páng guāng, shēn tǐ jìn huáng, míng yuē gǔ dǎn.

(2) É shàng hēi, wēi hàn chū, shǒu zú zhōng rè, bó mù jí fā, páng guāng jí, xiǎo biàn zì lì, míng yuē nǚ láo dǎn, fù rú shuǐ zhuàng, bù zhì.

(3) Xīn zhōng ào nóng ér rè, bù néng shí, shí yù tù, míng yuē jiǔ dǎn.

(1) When the instep yáng pulse is tight and rapid, rapid means heat, which results in dispersion of grain,[1] while tight means cold, which results in fullness upon eating. A floating cubit pulse means damage to the kidney; a tight instep yáng pulse means damage to the spleen. [When] wind and cold contend with each other, there will be dizziness upon eating, non-dispersion of grain qì, and suffering from turbidity in the stomach,[2] which flows downward [and causes] urinary stoppage. Yīn contracts cold, heat flows into the bladder, and the body turns yellow throughout. [This] is called grain jaundice.

(2) Blackness on the forehead, slight sweating, heat in the center of the hands and feet, symptoms manifesting at dusk, tension in the bladder, and spontaneous uninhibited urination is called female taxation jaundice. If the abdomen appears as if there was water, it is untreatable.

(3) Anguish and heat in the heart, inability to eat, and periodic desire to vomit is called alcohol jaundice.

TEXT NOTES, LINE 15.2

[1] Dispersion of grain 消谷 *xiāo gǔ*: Swift digestion and rapid hungering.

[2] Suffering from turbidity in the stomach 胃中苦浊 *wèi zhōng kǔ zhuó*: Turbidity refers here specifically to damp-heat.

SYNOPSIS, LINE 15.2

This line describes the pathomechanisms, classification, and main signs of jaundice.

COMMENTARY, LINE 15.2

The first section discusses the pathomechanism of grain jaundice from the perspective of the pulse manifestation. The instep yáng pulse reflects the spleen and stomach. When it is rapid, this indicates heat in the stomach, which causes swift digestion and rapid hungering. When it is tight, this indicates cold in the spleen, which causes dampness to arise, encumber the spleen, and inhibit the movement and transformation of food; hence we see "fullness upon eating." Thus we know from the pulse that grain jaundice is caused by a combination of cold-damp in the spleen and heat in the stomach.

The following sentence explains how we can differentiate between the pulse of grain jaundice (as described above) and the pulse of female taxation jaundice, which is related to vacuity heat in the kidney and therefore manifests in a floating cubit pulse.

The rest of the section further describes the symptoms of grain jaundice: Wind is a yáng evil and here refers to the above-mentioned heat in the stomach, while cold is a yīn evil and refers to dampness in the spleen. Thus, contention between wind and cold describes the pathomechanism of grain jaundice, namely stomach heat and spleen dampness, which bind together into damp-heat. Dizziness in the head after eating is caused by grain entering the stomach and reinforcing heat evil there, so that stomach heat surges upward and interferes with clear yáng. Because cold-damp encumbers the spleen, it is unable to perform movement and transformation; hence we see non-dispersion of grain qì. When cold in the spleen engenders dampness and this transforms into heat, it can combine with damp-heat in the stomach and pour into the bladder, inhibiting qì transformation there and thereby stopping urination. As a result, damp-heat is not discharged but lies depressed, steams, and spills outward. This causes generalized yellowing and thus grain jaundice.

The second section discusses the cause, symptoms, and prognosis of female taxation jaundice, a disease that is caused by taxation from sexual intercourse. Black is the external manifestation of the kidney, which stands in an exterior-interior relationship with the bladder. Sexual taxation damages the kidney, as a result of which vacuity fire follows the bladder channel to flame upward, contend with blood, and cause blackness on the forehead. Kidney vacuity engenders heat; hence we see heat in the center of the hands and feet and slight sweating, which erupt mostly at dusk. Because this disease is caused by kidney vacuity, not by damp-heat, it does not manifest in inhibited urination. If this disease progresses to the point where it spreads from the kidney to the spleen, which manifests in distention of the abdominal region, it becomes increasingly difficult to treat.

The last section describes the symptoms of alcohol jaundice, which is caused by excessive consumption of alcohol damaging the center, so that damp-heat brews internally. When damp-heat steams upward into the heart, the result is oppression, discomfort, and vexing heat in the heart. When it obstructs the center, it inhibits the upbearing and downbearing of the qì dynamic, so that turbid qì is unable to move downward and stomach qì ascends counterflow. Hence the patient is unable to eat and is bothered frequently by nausea.

Line 15.3

阳明病脉迟者，食难用饱，饱则发烦，头眩，小便必难，此欲作谷疸；虽下之，腹满如故，所以然者，脉迟故也。

Yáng míng bìng mài chí zhě, shí nán yòng bǎo, bǎo zé fā fán, tóu xuàn, xiǎo biàn bì nán, cǐ yù zuò gǔ dǎn; suī xià zhī, fù mǎn rú fù, suǒ yǐ rán zhě, mài chí fù yě.

If yáng brightness disease manifests with a slow pulse, difficulty in eating to satiety,[1] vexation after eating to satiety, dizzy head, and inevitably difficult urination, this means that grain jaundice is imminent. Even if you precipitate it, the abdominal fullness remains. The reason for this is that the pulse is slow.

TEXT NOTE, LINE 15.3

[1] Difficulty in eating to satiety 食难用饱 *shí nán yòng bǎo*: The patient likes to stop eating before reaching satiety—in other words, poor appetite.

SYNOPSIS, LINE 15.3

This line describes the pathomechanism of cold transforming into grain jaundice.

COMMENTARY, LINE 15.3

Most cases of grain jaundice are related to damp-heat in yáng brightness and therefore manifest with a rapid pulse. In the present line, however, the pulse is slow, which indicates vacuity cold of greater yīn spleen qì. Because the spleen is vacuous, movement and transformation are impaired, and because it is cold, it is unable to decompose grain and water. Thus we see difficulty in eating to satiety. After eating, the spleen's movement and tranformation is insufficient, so that food is not transformed into essence, but instead into damp turbidity. This obstructs the center burner; hence we see distention and fullness in the stomach duct and abdomen. When damp turbidity interferes with clear yáng in the upper body, we see dizziness in the head. When damp turbidity flows downward and impedes qì transformation, the result is difficult urination and, because damp-heat is not discharged but spills throughout the body, imminent grain jaundice.

This disease is related to cold-damp in greater yīn and should therefore be treated by warming, not by offensive precipitation. If you wrongly diagnose the abdominal distention as a repletion pattern and treat it by precipitating, this will further damage spleen yáng and not relieve the abdominal fullness.

Line 15.4

夫病酒黄疸，必小便不利，其候心中热，足下热，是其证也。

Fū bìng jiǔ huáng dǎn, bì xiǎo biàn bù lì, qí hòu xīn zhōng rè, zú xià rè, shì qí zhèng yě.

The disease of alcohol jaundice invariably manifests with inhibited urination. It is [also] indicated by heat in the heart and under the feet. These are its signs.

SYNOPSIS, LINE 15.4

This line describes the signs of alcohol jaundice.

COMMENTARY, LINE 15.4

The disease of alcohol jaundice is related to excessive consumption of alcohol. Alcohol is by its nature damp and hot and can therefore cause damp-heat to brew internally. If the damp-heat steams upward, it causes vexing heat in the heart; if it pours downward, it causes heat on the underside of the feet. Impeded qì transformation causes inhibited urination, which in turn results in damp-heat spreading throughout the body because it is not discharged through urine. Thus, inhibited urination is the main cause of yellowing and is therefore a key symptom in the diagnosis of this disease.

Line 15.5

酒黄疸者，或无热，靖言了了，腹满，欲吐，鼻燥，其脉浮者先吐之，沉弦者先下之。

Jiǔ huáng dǎn zhě, huò wú rè, jìng yán liǎo liǎo, fù mǎn, yù tù, bí zào, qí mài fú zhě xiān tù zhī, chén xián zhě xiān xià zhī.

Alcohol jaundice can also manifest without heat, and with calm spirit and clear speech, abdominal fullness, desire to vomit, and a dry nose. If the pulse is floating, [treat with] ejection first. If the pulse is sunken and stringlike, [treat with] precipitation first.

SYNOPSIS, LINE 15.5

This line describes further signs and the treatment of alcohol jaundice.

COMMENTARY, LINE 15.5

Alcohol jaundice is generally caused by damp-heat, but can be differentiated by the location of the disease in the upper, middle, or lower part of the body. It needs to be treated accordingly. When dampness is more prevalent than heat, you may not see any heat-related symptoms, and the patient may be calm and speaking clearly. When damp turbidity obstructs the center, you will see abdominal distention and fullness. When it hampers the harmonious downbearing of stomach qì, the result is upflow nausea and desire to vomit. When it impedes the formation and upbearing of the fluids, the nose will be dry. Treat according to these symptoms: A floating pulse means that damp turbidity is congesting the upper body; hence you treat it first by ejection. A sunken stringlike pulse means that the disease evil is lodged in the lower body; hence you treat it first by precipitation.

Line 15.6

酒疸，心中热欲吐者，吐之愈。

Jiǔ dǎn, xīn zhōng rè yù tù zhě, tù zhī yù.

If alcohol jaundice [manifests with] heat in the heart and desire to vomit, [treat it with] ejection to bring about recovery.

Synopsis, Line 15.6

This line discusses the treatment of alcohol jaundice with damp-heat congesting the upper body.

Commentary, Line 15.6

In the condition described in the present line, damp-heat steaming internally results in vexing heat in the heart and desire to vomit. This latter sign is caused specifically by damp turbidity obstructing the center, impairing the stomach's function of harmonious downbearing, and rushing into the upper body. In accordance with this sign, you should treat this type of alcohol jaundice with ejection therapy to eliminate the disease evil through the upper body.

Line 15.7

酒疸下之，久久为黑疸，目青面黑，心中如噉蒜虀状，大便正黑，皮肤爪之不仁，其脉浮弱，虽黑微黄，故知之。

Jiǔ dǎn xià zhī, jiǔ jiǔ wéi hēi dǎn, mù qīng miàn hēi, xīn zhōng rú dàn suàn jī zhuàng, dà biàn zhèng hēi, pí fū zhǎo zhī bù rén, qí mài fú ruò, suī hēi wēi huáng, fù zhī zhī.

When alcohol jaundice [is treated with] precipitation, over time it can turn into black jaundice. [This manifests in] blue-green eyes and a black face, a sensation in the heart as from eating garlic pulp,[1] pure black stool, numbness of the skin when scratched, a weak floating pulse, and blackness [of the skin] that is tinged with yellow. Thereby you know it [has developed out of inappropriate ejection treatment of alcohol jaundice].

Text Note, Line 15.7

[1] Sensation in the heart as from eating garlic pulp 心中如噉蒜虀状 *xīn zhōng rú dàn suàn jí zhuàng*: "Heart" here refers to the stomach. "Pulp" translates 虀 *jí* as pulped garlic, long-stamen onion, and ginger. These condiments are warm-hot in nature and can cause a burning sensation and discomfort in the stomach.

SYNOPSIS, LINE 15.7

This line describes the signs and pulse of black jaundice that is a result of inappropriate precipitation in alcohol jaundice.

COMMENTARY, LINE 15.7

Inappropriate use of ejection in the treatment of alcohol jaundice can over time aggravate the condition and cause it to transform into black jaundice. This is due to the fact that ejection can damage right qì, while at the same time allow damp-heat evil to take advantage of the vacuity, enter the blood aspect, and stagnate yīn-blood. In this case, the green-blue eye-whites indicate that an internal static blood obstruction is depriving the liver orifices of nourishment. The black facial complexion is due to static blood obstruction, preventing blood from nourishing the outside, while the yellow tinge indicates the presence of damp-heat steaming upward.

Because static blood is causing impediment in the network vessels of the skin and flesh, the patient does not feel pain in the skin when scratched. The sensation of burning heat and discomfort in the stomach is caused by damp-heat obstructing the center, while the black stool is due to static blood binding internally and draining into the intestines. The pulse is floating because damp-heat is attacking upward, and weak because qì and blood have already been damaged.

Line 15.8

师曰：病黄疸, 发热烦喘, 胸满口燥者, 以病发时, 火劫其汗, 两热所得。然黄家所得, 从湿得之。一身尽发热, 面黄, 肚热, 热在里, 当下之。

Shī yuē: Bìng huáng dǎn, fā rè fán chuǎn, xiōng mǎn kǒu zào zhě, yǐ bìng fā shí, huǒ jié qí hàn, liǎng rè suǒ de. Rán huáng jiā suǒ dé, cóng shī dé zhī. Yī shēn jìn fā rè, miàn huáng, dǔ rè, rè zài lǐ, dāng xià zhī.

The Master says: "When a jaundice patient presents with heat effusion, vexation, panting, fullness in the chest, and dry mouth, this is due to the fact that sweating was fire-forced[1] at the onset of the disease and the two heats [reinforced each other].[2] However, the yellowing of the patient is caused by contraction of dampness. [This condition manifests with] thorough heat effusion all over the body, yellowing of the face, and heat in the belly.[3] Because the heat is in the interior, you should [treat it with] precipitation.

TEXT NOTES, LINE 15.8

[1] Sweating was fire-forced 火劫其汗 *huǒ jié*: A physician attempted to force sweating by moxibustion, warm needling, or fuming.

[2] Two heats [reinforced each other] 两热 *liǎng rè*: The already present internal heat and the fire added by the treatment combined to create a more severe heat condition.

[3] Heat in the belly 肚热 *dù rè*: Heat in the stomach and abdomen.

SYNOPSIS, LINE 15.8

This line describes the causes, signs, and treatment of jaundice in which heat is more exuberant than dampness.

COMMENTARY, LINE 15.8

In the initial stage of jaundice, a patient can experience heat effusion before the yellow coloration appears. If a physician mis-diagnoses this as externally contracted heat and treats the patient offensively with heat to force sweating and outthrust heat, the internally present heat evil can combine with the externally introduced fire to cause a type of jaundice in which heat evil is particularly exuberant. In such patients, heat signs are more prevalent than dampness signs, and the condition therefore manifests with heat effusion all over the body but particularly in the abdomen, as well as with vexation and agitation, panting, fullness in the chest, and dry mouth. Since the heat repletion is in the interior, the treatment of choice is offensive precipitation.

Interpolating that "Nevertheless, the yellowing of the patient is caused by contraction of dampness," merely reiterates the fact that jaundice is not only caused by heat but also by dampness. Although the present pattern is characterized mostly by heat signs, it would not be a jaundice pattern without dampness.

Line 15.9

脉沉, 渴欲饮水, 小便不利者, 皆发黄。

Mài chén, kě yù yǐn shuǐ, xiǎo biàn bù lì zhě, jiē fā huáng.

A sunken pulse with thirst, desire to drink water, and inhibited urination is always [accompanied by] yellowing.

SYNOPSIS, LINE 15.9

This line describes the pulse and signs of damp-heat yellowing.

COMMENTARY, LINE 15.9

On the basis of the pulse, this line explains the pathomechanism of yellowing due to damp-heat. A sunken pulse indicates that the disease is located in the interior, and that it is related to stagnating dampness. Most cases of damp evil that stagnates and prevents liquid from bearing upward present with thirst, but no increase in drinking fluids. In the present pattern, however, dampness is depressed and transforms into fire, which damages the fluids. Thus we see thirst with desire to drink. Because damp-heat stagnates in the lower body and hampers qì transformation in the bladder, urination is inhibited. Consequently neither damp-heat nor ingested fluids are discharged through the urine; instead they steam and spill inside, causing yellowing.

Line 15.10

腹满，舌痿黄，燥不得眠，属黄家。

Fù mǎn, shé wěi huáng, zào bù dé mián, shǔ huáng jiā.

Abdominal fullness, a withered-yellow tongue,[1] agitation,[2] and inability to sleep [are signs] associated with jaundice patients.

Text Notes, Line 15.10

[1] Withered-yellow tongue 舌痿黄 *shé wěi huǎng*: The commentary notes that this is most likely a mistake and should be read as "withered-yellow body" (身痿黄 *shēn wěi huáng*) instead. This refers to generalized yellowing with lack of sheen.

[2] Agitation 燥 *zào*: While the text literally says "dryness," commentators generally agree that this character should here be interpreted as 躁 *zào* (agitation).

Synopsis, Line 15.10

This line describes the signs of spleen-vacuity yellowing.

Commentary, Line 15.10

The present line focuses on the role of the spleen in the cause of yellowing. The abdomen indicates the spleen. Abdominal fullness is the result of spleen vacuity engendering dampness, which stagnates and causes fullness. Because the spleen is vacuous and therefore unable to move and transform the essence of grain and water to nourish the body, we see a withered-yellow and lusterless complexion all over the body. Yellowing is the external manifestation of the spleen's color. Because spleen dampness is depressed, transforms into heat, and steams upward, the patient suffers from agitation and insomnia. These signs manifest in patients with a constitutional pattern of yellowing due to spleen vacuity.

Line 15.11

黄疸之病，当以十八日为期，治之十日以上瘥，反剧为难治。

Huáng dǎn zhī bìng, dāng yǐ shí bā rì wéi qī, zhì zhī shí rì yǐ shàng chài, fǎn jù wéi nán zhì.

Jaundice disease should last for a period of eighteen days. If treatment [shows an effect] within ten days or so, recovery will ensue. If instead [the condition] becomes more severe, it is hard to treat.

SYNOPSIS, LINE 15.11

This line describes the prognosis for jaundice disease.

COMMENTARY, LINE 15.11

In the majority of cases, jaundice disease should run its course in a period of about eighteen days. If it is treated promptly and appropriately, symptoms should be alleviated in about ten days, which indicates that the condition is easily treated. However, if the condition worsens after ten days, this suggests that evil is exuberant and right is vacuous, which makes treatment increasingly difficult. This line thus emphasizes the need for prompt treatment of jaundice conditions.

Line 15.12

疸而渴者，其疸难治；疸而不渴者，其疸可治。发于阴部，其人必呕；阳部，其人振寒而发热也。

Dǎn ér kě zhě, qí dǎn nán zhì; dǎn ér bù kě zhě, qí dǎn kě zhì. Fā yú yīn bù, qí rén bì ǒu; yáng bù, qí rén zhèn hán ér fā rè yě.

Jaundice that manifests with thirst is difficult to treat. Jaundice that manifests without thirst can be treated. If it begins from the yīn section,[1] the person invariably [suffers from] vomiting. If it begins from the yáng section, the person [suffers from] quivering with cold, and heat effusion.

TEXT NOTE, LINE 15.12

[1] Yīn section 陰部 *yīn bù*: The interior of the body. This contrasts with "yáng section" (阳部 *yáng bù*) mentioned in the next sentence, which refers to the exterior.

SYNOPSIS, LINE 15.12

This line further describes the prognosis of jaundice disease.

Commentary, Line 15.12

Thirst in jaundice patients can have several causes, namely dampness stagnating and preventing liquid from bearing upward; exuberant heat damaging liquid; and qì being so vacuous that it is unable to spread out the fluids. Regardless of the cause, thirst invariably indicates that the disease evil has penetrated into the interior and that evil qì is replete while right qì is vacuous. Because thirst causes the patient to drink, and drinking further aggravates the dampness, this type of jaundice is difficult to treat. By contrast, absence of thirst suggests that the disease evil is still shallow, that heat is not exuberant, that liquid is not damaged, and that right is not vacuous. Thus it can be treated more easily.

Vomiting is generally a sign that occurs in diseases of the interior, while shivering with cold and heat effusion are symptoms of exterior disease. As such, they allow us to differentiate between interior and exterior, deep and shallow, and severe and mild conditions.

Line 15.13

谷疸之为病，寒热不食，食即头眩，心胸不安，久久发黄，为谷疸，茵陈蒿汤主之。

茵陈蒿六两　栀子十四枚　大黄二两

右三味，以水一斗，先煮茵陈，减六升，内二味煮取三升，去滓，分温三服，小便当利，尿如皂角汁状，色正赤，一宿腹减，黄从小便去也。

Gǔ dǎn zhī wéi bìng, hán rè bù shí, shí jí tóu xuàn, xīn xiōng bù ān, jiǔ jiǔ fā huáng, wéi gǔ dǎn, yīn chén hāo tāng zhǔ zhī.

Yīn chén hāo liù liǎng; zhī zǐ shí sì méi dà huáng èr liǎng

Yòu sān wèi, yǐ shuǐ yī dǒu, xiān zhǔ yīn chén, jiǎn liù shēng, nèi èr wèi zhǔ qǔ sān shēng, qù zǐ, fēn wēn sān fú, xiǎo biàn dāng lì, niào rú zào jiǎo zhī zhuàng, sè zhèng chì, yī xiǔ fù jiǎn, huáng cóng xiǎo biàn qù yě.

In the disease of grain jaundice, [we see aversion to] cold and heat [effusion], inability to eat, dizzy head upon eating, disquietude in the heart and chest, and over a long period, the development of yellowing, which constitutes grain jaundice. Virgate Wormwood Decoction (茵陈蒿汤 *yīn chén hāo tāng*) governs.

Virgate Wormwood Decoction (茵陈蒿汤 *yīn chén hāo tāng*)
virgate wormwood (茵陈蒿 *yīn chén hāo*, Artemisiae Scopariae Herba) 6 *liǎng*
gardenia (栀子 *zhī zǐ*, Gardeniae Fructus) 14 pieces
rhubarb (大黄 *dà huáng*, Rhei Radix et Rhizoma) 2 *liǎng*

Of the above three ingredients, first boil the virgate wormwood (*yīn chén*) in one *dǒu* of water until [the liquid] is reduced to six *shēng*. Add the [other] two ingredients and boil to get three *shēng*. Remove the dregs, divide into three doses and take warm. Urination will become uninhibited, with urine that looks like gleditsia (*zào jiá*) juice, of a pure red color. Overnight, the abdomen will be relieved, and the yellowness will be removed through the urine.

Synopsis, Line 15.13

This line describes the signs and treatment of grain jaundice due to damp-heat.

Commentary, Line 15.13

Grain jaundice can arise from food and drink damaging the spleen and stomach and from dampness brewing and transforming into heat. It can furthermore be complicated by externally contracted disease evil. In grain jaundice, aversion to cold and heat effusion are caused by damp-heat steaming outward and by disharmony in construction and defense. When damp-heat obstructs the center, it inhibits the stomach's function of food intake; hence we see inability to eat. Furthermore, water and grain are not transformed into essence but instead assist the dampness in engendering heat. Steaming damp-heat causes vexation, oppression, and discomfort in the heart and chest, and when surging upward, dizziness in the head. Because grain jaundice does not immediately turn the whole body yellow but passes through a stage where damp-heat lies depressed, the text emphasizes that the yellow coloration develops gradually over a long period.

In the treatment of grain jaundice, we concentrate on discharging damp-heat. For this purpose, the text recommends Virgate Wormwood Decoction (*yīn chén hāo tāng*), which is the basic formula for treating damp-heat jaundice. In this formula, virgate wormwood (*yīn chén*) and gardenia (*zhī zǐ*) clear damp-heat, disinhibit jaundice, and abate yellowing, while rhubarb (*dà huáng*) flushes out accumulations, discharges heat, and also abates yellowing. In combination, these medicinals cause stagnant heat to be eliminated through the urine and stool.

Line 15.14

黄家，日晡所发热，而反恶寒，此为女劳得之。膀胱急，少腹满，身尽黄，额上黑，足下热，因作黑疸。其腹胀如水状，大便必黑，时溏，此女劳之病，非水也。腹满者难治，硝石矾石散主之。

硝石　矾石（烧）等分

右二味，为散，以大麦粥汁和服方寸匕，日三服。病随大小便去，小便正黄，大便正黑，是候也。

Huáng jiā, rì bū suǒ fā rè, ér fǎn wù hán, cǐ wéi nǚ láo dé zhī. Páng guāng jí, shào fù mǎn, shēn jìn huáng, é shàng hēi, zú xià rè, yīn zuò hēi dǎn. Qí fù zhàng rú shuǐ zhuàng, dà biàn bì hēi, shí táng, cǐ nǚ láo zhī bìng, fēi shuǐ yě. Fù mǎn zhě nán zhì, xiāo shí fán shí sǎn zhǔ zhī.

Xiāo shí; fán shí (shāo) děng fèn

Yòu èr wèi, wéi sǎn, yǐ dà mài zhōu zhī huó fú fāng cùn bǐ, rì sān fú. Bìng suí dà xiǎo biàn qù, xiǎo biàn zhèng huáng, dà biàn zhèng hēi, shì hòu yě.

People who suffer from yellowing [usually experience] heat effusion in the late afternoon.[1] However, [if they experience] aversion to cold instead, this is caused by female taxation. [Accompanying symptoms are] tension in the bladder, lesser abdominal fullness,[2] thorough yellowing of the body, blackness on the forehead, and heat under the feet. This condition [over time] turns into black jaundice. In such a patient, the abdomen is distended as if [full of] water, and the stool is invariably black and sometimes sloppy. This is female taxation disease, not water [qì disease]. Cases with abdominal fullness are difficult to treat. Niter and Alum Powder (硝石矾石散 *xiāo shí fán shí sǎn*) governs.

Niter and Alum Powder (硝石矾石散 *xiāo shí fán shí sǎn*)
niter (硝石 *xiāo shí*, Nitrum) (burned)[3] alum (矾石 *fán shí*, Alumen) (burned)

Grind equal amounts of the above two ingredients into a powder. Mix a square-inch-spoonful into barley gruel juice and take three doses a day. [As a result] the disease will be removed through the urine and stool, which is indicated by pure yellow urine and pure black stool.

Text Notes, Line 15.14

[1] Late afternoon 日晡 *rì bū*: This refers to the afternoon watch, specifically the time between three and five in the afternoon.

[2] Lesser abdominal fullness 少腹满 *shào fù mǎn*: In the *Qiān Jīn Fāng* ("Thousand Gold Pieces Prescriptions") and *Wài Tái Mì Yào* ("Secrets from the *Wài Tái* Library"), this is written as 小腹满 *xiǎo fù mǎn*, smaller abdominal fullness. The smaller abdomen corresponds to the lower abdomen of modern medicine. The lesser abdomen refers to the lateral region of this area.

[3] Burned 燒 *shāo*: Calcined (煅 *duàn*).

Synopsis, Line 15.14

This line describes the signs and treatment of female taxation jaundice transforming into black jaundice, with static blood and damp-heat.

Commentary, Line 15.14

In patients with habitual yellowing, damp-heat brewing and lying depressed in yáng brightness causes no aversion to cold, and heat effusion from three to five in the afternoon, which is the time when the yáng brightness channel qì exuberates.

As the present line points out, if a patient with yellowing suffers from aversion to cold instead of generalized heat effusion, this indicates a pattern of female taxation jaundice related to vacuity in the kidney and internal heat, not a pattern of yellowing due to damp-heat lying depressed in yáng brightness. In contrast to the generalized heat effusion that occurs in patients with habitual yellowing, the specific sign of female taxation jaundice is localized heat under the feet that arises at dusk, and concurrent aversion to cold. This is related to the fact that yellowing patients suffer from a repletion pattern of exterior heat, while female taxation jaundice is a vacuity pattern of interior heat from kidney vacuity.

Female taxation jaundice is the result of excessive sexual intercourse, which taxes and depletes kidney essence. When detriment to yīn affects yáng, the bladder is deprived of warmth and nourishment; hence we see tension in the bladder. As yáng becomes vacuous on the outside, the fleshy exterior is deprived of warmth, and we see aversion to cold. Because the kidney is vacuous and fails to assist the bladder qì transformation, damp turbidity collects, resulting in abdominal distention and fullness. Because damp turbidity is not discharged to the outside but spills all over the body, we see generalized yellowing, and because female taxation jaundice is a vacuity pattern, the color is invariably dark instead of bright.

Over time, female taxation jaundice can transform into black jaundice, when kidney vacuity engenders heat, vacuity heat scorches the channels and network vessels, and static blood seeps into the intestines. The sign of this is pure black stool. Female taxation jaundice is a disease of the kidney, which will eventually affect the spleen, preventing it from carrying out movement and transformation; hence we see sloppy stool. Spleen vacuity furthermore engenders dampness, and when dampness and static blood combine and stagnate, the abdomen becomes full and distended, as if full of water. As the last sentence emphasizes, abdominal fullness is a sign that the condition has progressed to a critical stage, because both the kidney and spleen fail to perform their functions.

The recommended treatment for this condition is Niter and Alum Powder (*xiāo shí fán shí sǎn*), because it dissipates stasis and transforms dampness. Calcined niter, which is bitter and salty in flavor and cold by nature, enters the blood aspect to dissipate stasis and eliminate heat, while calcined alum, which is cold in nature and sour in flavor, enters the qì aspect to transform dampness and disinhibit water. These two medicinals are taken in barley gruel, which nourishes the stomach and mediates the harshness of the other ingredients.

Line 15.15

酒黄疸，心中懊憹，或热痛，栀子大黄汤主之。

栀子十四枚　大黄一两　枳实五枚　豉一升

右四味，以水六升，煮取二升，分温三服。

Jiǔ huáng dǎn, xīn zhōng ào nóng, huò rè tòng, zhī zǐ dà huáng tāng zhǔ zhī.

Zhī zǐ shí sì méi; dà huáng yī liǎng; zhǐ shí wǔ méi; chǐ yī shēng

Yòu sì wèi, yǐ shuǐ liù shēng, zhǔ qǔ èr shēng, fēn wēn sān fú.

For alcohol jaundice with anguish in the heart and possibly hot pain, Gardenia and Rhubarb Decoction (栀子大黄汤 *zhī zǐ dà huáng tāng*) governs.

Gardenia and Rhubarb Decoction (栀子大黄汤 *zhī zǐ dà huáng tāng*)

- gardenia (栀子 *zhī zǐ*, Gardeniae Fructus) 14 pieces
- rhubarb (大黄 *dà huáng*, Rhei Radix et Rhizoma) 1 *liǎng*
- unripe bitter orange (枳实 *zhǐ shí*, Aurantii Fructus Immaturus) five pieces
- fermented soybean (豉 *chǐ*, Sojae Semen Fermentatum) 1 *shēng*

Boil the above four ingredients in six *sheng* of water to get two *shēng*. Divide into three doses and take warm.

Synopsis, Line 15.15

This line describes the signs and treatment of alcohol jaundice.

COMMENTARY, LINE 15.15

Excessive consumption of alcohol causes damp-heat to brew internally and thereby causes alcohol jaundice. When this damp-heat steams upward into the heart, it causes anguish in the heart, oppression, and discomfort. Damp-heat stagnation inhibits and in severe cases stops the qì dynamic, as a result of which the patient feels hot pain in the heart.

Gardenia and Rhubarb Decoction (*zhī zǐ dà huáng tāng*) is the recommended treatment for this condition, as it clears the heart and eliminates vexation. In the formula, gardenia (*zhī zǐ*) and fermented soybean (*dòu chǐ*) diffuse depressed heat and eliminate vexation. Gardenia (*zhī zǐ*) moves qì and opens binds, while rhubarb (*dà huáng*) discharges damp-heat; hence these two in combination disperse obstruction in the center. As a whole, the formula thus addresses both the heat in the upper body, as well as the repletion in the center.

Line 15.16

诸病黄家，但利其小便，假令脉浮，当以汗解之，宜桂枝加黄芪汤主之。

Zhū bìng huáng jiā, dàn lì qí xiǎo biàn, jiǎ lìng mài fú, dāng yǐ hàn jiě zhī, yí guì zhī jiā huáng qí tāng zhǔ zhī.

In all patients who suffer from yellowing, merely disinhibit urine. If the pulse is floating, use sweating to resolve it. Cinnamon Twig Decoction (桂枝加黄芪汤 *guì zhī jiā huáng qí tāng*) governs.[1]

TEXT NOTE, LINE 15.16

[1] A comment included in the received text reads: "For the formula, see the chapter on Water Qì." This is found in line 14.29 above.

SYNOPSIS, LINE 15.16

This line describes the main principle for treating yellowing, as well as the signs and treatment for evil in the exterior.

COMMENTARY, LINE 15.16

In the majority of patients with yellowing, the disease arises because damp-heat brews internally and causes a breakdown of qì transformation and consequently inhibited urination. As a result, damp-heat is not discharged outward, but instead spills all over the body and thereby causes yellowing. Such conditions are best treated by disinhibiting urine and thereby clearing heat and transforming dampness.

Nevertheless, if a patient presents with a floating pulse, this indicates that the disease evil is still in the exterior, in which case you can resolve the exterior by promoting sweating. The recommended formula for this course of treatment is Cinnamon Twig Decoction Plus Astragalus (*guì zhī jiā huáng qí tāng*), which harmonizes construction and defense, and by effusing sweat, expels the exterior evil.

Line 15.17

诸黄，猪膏发煎主之。
猪膏半斤　乱发（如鸡子大）三枚
右二味，和膏中煎之，发消药成，分再服，病从小便出。

Zhū huáng, zhū gāo fǎ jiān zhǔ zhī.

Zhū gāo bàn jīn; luàn fǎ (rú jī zǐ dà) sān méi

Yòu èr wèi, huó gāo zhōng jiān zhī, fǎ xiāo yào chéng, fēn zài fú, bìng cóng xiǎo biàn chū.

For all yellowing, Pork Lard and Hair Brew (猪膏发煎 *zhū gāo fà jiān*) governs.

Pork Lard and Hair Brew (猪膏发煎 *zhū gāo fà jiān*)
pork lard (猪膏 *zhū gāo*, Suis Adeps) ½ *jīn* hair (乱发 *luàn fǎ*, Crinis) 3 lumps (the size of chicken eggs)

Blend the above two ingredients into a paste and fry. When the hair has dispersed, the medicine is ready. Divide into two doses and take. The disease will come out through the urine.

Synopsis, Line 15.17

This line describes the treatment of yellowing with withered-yellow complexion due to gastrointestinal dryness bind.

Commentary, Line 15.17

While the present line recommends Pork Lard and Hair Brew as treatment for all types of yellowing, the composition of the formula indicates that it specifically addresses yellowing which has progressed to the point where damp-heat has transformed into dryness and has over time desiccated liquid and blood. The symptoms associated with such conditions are dry stool, because the internal organs are deprived of moistening, and dry withered-yellow skin, becasue the skin is not moistened sufficiently. In this formula, pork lard (*zhū gāo*) disinhibits blood in the vessels, resolves wind heat, and moistens dryness bind, while hair (*luàn fǎ*) enters the blood to disperse stasis and free the stool. The formula as a whole frees the stool by moistening the intestines, quickening the blood, and moistening dryness.

Line 15.18

黄疸病，茵陈五苓散主之。
茵陈蒿末十分　五苓散五分
右二味和，先食饮方寸匕，日三服。

Huáng dǎn bìng, yīn chén wǔ líng sǎn zhǔ zhī.

Yīn chén hāo mò shí fēn; wǔ líng sǎn wǔ fēn

Yòu èr wèi huó, xiān shí yǐn fāng cùn bǐ, rì sān fú.

For jaundice disease, Virgate Wormwood and Poria Five Powder (茵陈五苓散 *yīn chén wǔ líng sǎn*) governs.[1]

Virgate Wormwood and Poria Five Powder (茵陈五苓散 *yīn chén wǔ líng sǎn*)
pulverized virgate wormwood (茵陈蒿 *yīn chén hāo*, Artemisiae Scopariae Herba) 10 parts
Poria Five Powder (五苓散 *wǔ líng sǎn*) 5 parts[2]

Mix the above two ingredients. Before meals, take a square-inch-spoonful in fluid, three times a day.

TEXT NOTES, LINE 15.18

[1] A comment included in the received text reads: "An alternative version of the text has: 'Virgate Wormwood Decoction (*yīn chén tāng*) in combination with Poria Five Powder (*wǔ líng sǎn*) governs.' "

[2] A comment included in the received text reads: "For the formula, see the chapter on Phlegm-Rheum." The formula is found in line 12.31 above, in Chapter 12, "Phlegm-Rheum and Cough."

SYNOPSIS, LINE 15.18

This line describes the treatment of jaundice in patterns with dampness more prevalent than heat.

COMMENTARY, LINE 15.18

Again, this line does not specify the type of jaundice for which this formula is recommended. Nevertheless, we can know from the composition and proportion of ingredients that it addresses jaundice conditions in which dampness is more pronounced than heat, because the formula has a strong water-disinhibiting effect. It is therefore recommended for jaundice cases that manifest with prevalent symptoms of dampness, such as nausea and fatigue, generalized heaviness, reduced appetite, scant inhibited urination, light abdominal fullness, a white slimy tongue fur, and a soggy slow pulse.

Virgate Wormwood and Poria Five Powder (*yīn chén wǔ líng sǎn*) has the effect of abating yellowing by both clearing heat and disinhibiting dampness, with virgate wormwood (*yīn chén*) clearing heat and disinhibiting dampness, and Poria Five Powder (*wǔ líng sǎn*) disinhibiting water and eliminating dampness by bland percolation. As such, it is an important and frequently used formula in the treatment of jaundice.

Line 15.19

黄疸，腹满，小便不利而赤，自汗出，此为表和里实，当下之，宜大黄硝石汤。

大黄 黄柏　硝石各四两　栀子十五枚

右四味，以水六升，煮取二升，去滓，内硝更煮取一升，顿服。

Huáng dǎn, fù mǎn, xiǎo biàn bù lì ér chì, zì hàn chū, cǐ wéi biǎo hé lǐ shí, dāng xià zhī, yí dà huáng xiāo shí tāng.

Dà huáng huáng bǎi; xiāo shí gè sì liǎng zhī zǐ shí wǔ méi

Yòu sì wèi, yǐ shuǐ liù shēng, zhǔ qǔ èr shēng, qù zǐ, nà xiāo gèng zhǔ qǔ yī shēng, dùn fú.

If jaundice manifests with abdominal fullness, inhibited voidings of red urine, and spontaneous sweating, this indicates harmony of the exterior, and repletion of the interior. [Treat such conditions with] precipitation. Rhubarb and Niter Decoction (大黄硝石汤 *dà huáng xiāo shí tāng*) is appropriate.

Rhubarb and Niter Decoction (大黄硝石汤 *dà huáng xiāo shí tāng*)

rhubarb (大黄 *dà huáng*, Rhei Radix et Rhizoma) 4 *liǎng*
phellodendron (黄柏 *huáng bǎi*, Phellodendri Cortex) 4 *liǎng*
niter (硝石 *xiāo shí*, Nitrum) 4 *liǎng*
gardenia (栀子 *zhī zǐ*, Gardeniae Fructus) 15 pieces

Of the above four ingredients, boil [everything except the niter] in 6 *shēng* of water to get two *shēng*. Remove the dregs, add the niter (*xiāo*) and boil again to get one *shēng*. Quaff.

Synopsis, Line 15.19

This line describes the signs and treatment of jaundice due to exuberant heat and interior repletion.

Commentary, Line 15.19

In jaundice, damp-heat congests, binds in the interior, and forms interior heat repletion, which results in distention and fullness in the abdominal region. By inhibiting qì transformation in the bladder, it also causes inhibited voidings of red urine. Spontaneous sweating in this context means that repletion heat in the interior is forcing liquid to the outside; it is not a sign of insecurity of the fleshy exterior. Thus the present line states that the exterior is harmonious, and that it is only the interior that is affected by repletion. Accordingly, such conditions are treated by offensive precipitation to free the bowels, discharge heat, and eliminate dampness, thereby abating yellowing.

The recommended formula is Rhubarb and Niter Decoction (*dà huáng xiāo shí tāng*). Among its ingredients, rhubarb (*dà huáng*) drains heat, frees the bowels, cools blood, and moves stasis, while niter (*xiāo shí*) disperses stasis and discharges heat. Together, these two are able to flush out stasis heat. Gardenia (*zhī zǐ*) and phellodendron (*huáng bǎi*) are bitter and cold and drain heat; together they can disinhibit dampness and eliminate yellowing. The formula as a whole has the effect of clearing heat, freeing the stool, disinhibiting dampness, and eliminating yellowing.

This formula is rather strong and therefore should be used only in cases with pronounced signs of repletion heat, like distention and fullness below the rib-side, pain that resists pressure, bound stool, inhibited urination, and a rapid, forceful, and slippery pulse.

Line 15.20

黄疸病，小便色不变，欲自利，腹满而喘，不可除热，热除必哕；哕者，小半夏汤主之。

Huáng dǎn bìng, xiǎo biàn sè bù biàn, yù zì lì, fù mǎn ér chuǎn, bù kě chú rè, rè chú bì yuē; yuē zhě, xiǎo bàn xià tāng zhǔ zhī.

If jaundice [manifests with] no change in the color of urine, [stool] on the verge of spontaneous diarrhea, and abdominal fullness and panting, you must not eliminate heat. If you eliminate heat, [there] will inevitably be hiccup. For hiccup, Minor Pinellia Decoction (小半夏汤 *xiǎo bàn xià tāng*)[1] governs.

TEXT NOTE, LINE 15.20

[1] A comment included in the received text reads: "For the formula, see the chapter on Phlegm-Rheum." The formula is found in Chapter 12, "Phlegm-Rheum and Cough," line 12.28.

SYNOPSIS, LINE 15.20

This line describes the signs and treatment of a transmuted pattern of jaundice due to inappropriate treatment.

COMMENTARY, LINE 15.20

Jaundice normally manifests in red or yellow scant or inhibited urine, which is the result of damp-heat steaming internally. If a jaundice patient presents without a change in the color of urine and stool on the verge of spontaneous diarrhea, this means that the condition is not related to the presence of heat in the interior, but to cold-damp encumbering the spleen and impairing its movement and transformation function. This cold-damp stagnates in the center burner instead of being transformed; hence we see abdominal fullness. This type of abdominal fullness due to vacuity cold is characterized by periodic relief and a liking for warmth and pressure. Because dampness evil stagnates and inhibits the qì dynamic, we also see panting. Being related to an internal exuberance of cold-damp and to spleen vacuity, we treat such a condition with formulas like Center-Rectifying Decoction (*lǐ zhōng tāng*) or Counterflow Cold Decoction (*sì nì tāng*), to warm and move spleen yáng, and to disperse cold and eliminate dampness.

If such a condition is misdiagnosed as an interior heat repletion pattern and treated with bitter cold medicinals to eliminiate heat, this is bound to further damage spleen-stomach yáng qì, which results in counterflow ascent of stomach qì and manifests in hiccup. In that case, use Minor Pinellia Decoction (*xiǎo bàn xià tāng*) to warm the stomach, harmonize the center, downbear counterflow, and suppress hiccup.

Line 15.21

诸黄，腹满而呕者，宜柴胡汤。

Zhū huáng, fù mǎn ér ǒu zhě, yí chái hú tāng.

In all types of yellowing, for abdominal fullness and retching, Bupleum Decoction (*chái hú tāng*) is appropriate.[1]

Text Note, Line 15.21

[1] A comment included in the received text reads: "This must refer to Minor Bupleurum Decoction (*xiǎo chái hú tāng*). For the formula, see the chapter on Vomiting and Retching." This formula is found in Chapter 17, "Retching, Vomiting, Hiccup, and Diarrhea," line 17.15.

Synopsis, Line 15.21

This line describes the signs and treatment of jaundice with lesser yáng symptoms.

Commentary, Line 15.21

In the course of jaundice in the initial stage, abdominal fullness and retching may occur, together with intermittent aversion to cold and heat effusion. By these symptoms, you know that the evil is located in lesser yáng, and that you therefore have to treat by harmonizing and resolving lesser yáng. In such cases, Minor Bupleurum Decoction (*xiǎo chái hú tāng*) is the recommended formula.

Note that Minor Bupleurum Decoction (*xiǎo chái hú tāng*) is not a formula for treating jaundice, but for treating lesser yáng disease. In this formula, ginseng (*rén shēn*) is sweet and warm and can possibly assist dampness in engendering heat. In conditions with pronounced damp-heat, one should therefore replace ginseng (*rén shēn*) with virgate wormwood (*yīn chén*). While this formula does not directly treat jaundice, it can disinhibit and outthrust the qì dynamic by harmonizing and resolving lesser yáng and thereby assist in abating yellowing.

Line 15.22

男子黄,小便自利,当与虚劳小建中汤。

Nán zǐ huáng, xiǎo biàn zì lì, dāng yǔ xū láo xiǎo jiàn zhōng tāng.

If men suffer from yellowing with uninhibited urination, you should give Minor Center-Fortifying Decoction (小建中汤 *xiǎo jiàn zhōng tāng*)[1] for vacuity taxation.

TEXT NOTE, LINE 15.22

[1] A comment included in the received text reads: "For the formula, see the chapter on Vacuity Taxation." This formula is found in Chapter 6, "Blood Impediment and Vacuity Taxation," line 6.13.

SYNOPSIS, LINE 15.22

This line describes the signs and treatment of vacuity taxation with a withered-yellow complexion.

COMMENTARY, LINE 15.22

In patients with yellowing, if urination is not inhibited, this indicates that the yellow coloration is not caused by damp-heat brewing internally, but by spleen-stomach vacuity, insufficiency of qì and blood, and lack of nourishment to the flesh and skin. The resulting withered-yellow complexion is not limited to male patients, but can also arise in women after childbirth or severe bloodloss. In either gender, the yellowing is characterized by a lack of luster, as in dried plants. Because the disease is caused by insufficiency of the spleen and stomach and vacuity of qì and blood, the recommended treatment is Minor Center-Fortifying Decoction (*xiǎo jiàn zhōng tāng*), which fortifies center qì, opens the source of engendering transformation, and makes qì and blood abundant, so that the withered-yellow color disappears by itself.

附方 Appended Formulas, Line 15.22

SINGLE-AGENT MELON STALK DECOCTION (一物瓜蒂汤 *yī wù guā dì tāng*)

瓜蒂汤：治诸黄。

Guā dì tāng: Zhì zhū huáng.

Single-Agent Melon Stalk Decoction (一物瓜蒂汤 *yī wù guā dì tāng*): A treatment for all types of yellowing.[1]

FORMULA NOTE, LINE 15.22

[1] A comment included in the received text reads: "For the formula, see the chapter, "Tetany, Dampness, and Thermoplegia," line 2.27.

EPHEDRA AND PURE WINE DECOCTION (麻黄醇酒汤 *má huáng chún jiǔ tāng*) from the *Qiān Jīn Yào Fāng* ("A Thousand Gold Pieces Prescriptions")

《千金》麻黄醇酒汤：治黄胆。

麻黄三两

右一味, 以美清酒五升, 煮取二升半, 顿服尽。冬月用酒, 春月用水煮之。

«Qiān Jīn» má huáng chún jiǔ tāng: Zhì huáng dǎn.

Má huáng sān liǎng

Yòu yī wèi, yǐ měi qīng jiǔ wǔ shēng, zhǔ qǔ èr shēng bàn, dùn fú jìn. Dōng yuè yòng jiǔ, chūn yuè yòng shuǐ zhǔ zhī.

A treatment for jaundice.

ephedra (麻黄 *má huáng*, Ephedrae Herba) 3 *liǎng*

Boil the above single ingredient in five *shēng* of good clear wine[1] to get two-and-a-half *shēng*. Quaff the entire preparation. In the winter months, use wine; in the spring months, use water to boil it.

FORMULA NOTE, LINE 15.22

[1] Good clear wine 美清酒 *měi qīng jiǔ*: Good quality clear rice wine (non-distilled). This explains 醇酒 *chún jiǔ* in the formula title.

FORMULA COMMENTARY, LINE 15.22

The first of these appended formulas, Single-Agent Melon Stalk Decoction (*yī wù guā dì tāng*), represents an ancient treatment strategy for jaundice that is no longer commonly used. Melon stalk (*guā dì*) is a strong agent for inducing violent ejection. In the early texts, it is used to treat jaundice either by grinding it into a fine powder and blowing it into the patient's nose, or by having the patient ingest it in powder form, in either case inducing violent ejection, which was believed to treat yellowing by elimination.

The second formula for Ephedra and Pure Wine Decoction (*má huáng chún jiǔ tāng*) is a treatment for jaundice that acts by effusing sweat and resolving the exterior. It is appropriate for conditions of exterior repletion that manifest with a floating tight pulse and no sweating.

惊悸吐衄下血胸满瘀血病脉证治第十六

CHAPTER 16

Fright and Palpitation, Blood Ejection, Nosebleed, Lower Body Bleeding, Fullness in the Chest, and Static Blood

Pulses, Signs, Treatments

‡ Overview

This chapter deals with conditions characterized by fright and palpitation, blood ejection, nosebleed, lower body bleeding, fullness in the chest, and static blood. Although fullness in the chest is included in the title, within this chapter it is merely treated as an indicator of static blood, not as a separate disease. The conditions discussed in this chapter can be divided into the two general categories of fright and palpitation on the one hand, and diseases of bleeding on the other hand. They are discussed together here because they are all related to disorders in the heart and blood vessels.

Both "fright" and "palpitation" arise as a result of being frightened and are characterized by a subjective feeling of stirring and disquietude in the heart. Nevertheless, they are differentiated by their causation: Stirring that is due to a stimulus is fright; stirring that is not due to a stimulus is palpitation. In other words, fright is caused by a sudden stimulation from the external environment, which disquiets the spirit. It is generally shallow and therefore less severe, and mostly associated with repletion patterns. Palpitation is a subjective feeling of stirring and disquietude in the heart, which is associated with more severe conditions and mostly occurs in vacuity patterns. However, the two are often interrelated because sudden fright is bound to cause heart palpitation, while ceaseless heart palpitations cause a tendency to fright. The present chapter discusses fright caused by fire evil, and palpitation due to water-rheum, but does not focus on fright palpitation due to other causes.

Blood ejection, nosebleed, lower body bleeding, and static blood are all diseases of the blood and vessels. These three types of bleeding are generally caused either by fire heat forcing blood to move frenetically or by vacuity cold preventing qì from containing blood. Treatment is therefore based on the two major principles of either clearing heat and cooling blood or warming the center and containing blood. Lastly, static blood is only discussed in two lines in this chapter. Nevertheless, these lines contain profound and significant information that provided a basis for the formation and development of theories about static blood in the following centuries.

‡ Schematic Overview

Fright and Palpitation

1. Pulse: A stirred pulse means fright; a weak pulse means palpitation.
2. Treatment
   a) Fright arising when fire evil causes heart yáng to become insufficient and the spirit to float astray: Settle fright and quiet the spirit using Cinnamon Twig Counterflow-Stemming Decoction Minus Peony Plus Dichroa Leaf, Oyster Shell and Dragon Bone (*guì zhī qù sháo yào jiā shǔ qī mǔ lì lóng gǔ jiù nì tāng*).
   b) Palpitation arising when water-rheum intimidates the heart: Eliminate rheum, free yáng, downbear counterflow, and calm palpitation using Pinellia and Ephedra Pill (*bàn xià má huáng wán*).

Bleeding

1. Fire-heat causing frenetic movement of hot blood
   a) *Signs*: Blood ejection or nosebleed.
   b) *Treatment*: Discharging heat with bitterness and cold, downbearing fire, and stanching bleeding.
2. Large intestinal damp-heat
   a) *Signs*: Proximal bleeding (blood followed by stool).
   b) *Treatment*: Clear heat, disinhibit dampness, quicken the blood, and transform stasis using Rice Bean and Chinese Angelica Powder (*chì xiǎo dòu dāng guī sǎn*).
3. Spleen qì vacuity cold
   a) *Signs*: Distal bleeding (stool followed by blood).
   b) *Treatment*: Warm the spleen and contain blood using Yellow Earth Decoction (*huáng tǔ tāng*).

Static Blood

1. This section does not offer any detailed treatments. The main points are:
   a) Static blood is characterized by withered lips and green-blue tongue with dry mouth and a desire to wash the mouth with water rather than swallowing, as well as a subjective sensation of fullness in the chest or abdomen.
   b) Static blood is treated by precipitation.

Line 16.1

寸口脉动而弱，动即为惊，弱即为悸。

Cùn kǒu mài dòng ér ruò, dòng jí wéi jīng, ruò jí wéi jì.

When the inch opening pulse is stirred[1] and weak,[2] stirred means fright, and weakness means palpitation.

TEXT NOTES, LINE 16.1

[1] Pulse is stirred 脉动 *mài dòng*: Short and hasty, running like a bean.

[2] Weak 弱 *ruò*: Fine, soft, and forceless, felt when pressure is applied.

SYNOPSIS, LINE 16.1

This line explains the disease cause and pathomechanism of fright and palpitation in terms of the pulse.

COMMENTARY, LINE 16.1

The heart holds the office of monarch, whence the bright spirit emanates. If it is damaged, qì becomes vacuous and the pulse becomes stirred; this is often seen in fright and timidity. When essence becomes vacuous, the pulse becomes weak; this is often seen in fearful throbbing and heart palpitation. A stirring pulse and fright are generally caused by external stimulation and are therefore related to yáng, while a weak pulse and palpitation are related mostly to depletion of construction and blood, loss of nourishment in the heart vessel, and forceless beating of heart qì. When you diagnose a pulse as weak and stirring at the same time, this indicates the presence of both an internal vacuity of qì and blood, and harassment by external fright.

Line 16.2

师曰：尺脉浮，目睛晕黄，衄未止，晕黄去目睛慧了，知衄今止。

Shī yuē: Chǐ mài fú, mù jīng yùn huáng, nǜ wèi zhǐ, yùn huáng qù mù jīng huì liǎo, zhī nǜ jīn zhǐ.

The Master says: "A floating cubit pulse and eyes with yellow haze [around the pupils][1] means that nosebleed is not yet checked. When the yellow haze is gone and the eyes have cleared,[2] you know that the nosebleed is now checked.

TEXT NOTES, LINE 16.2

[1] Eyes with yellow haze [around the pupils] 目睛晕黄 *mù jīng yùn huáng*: This phrase has two possible meanings: (a) a yellowish circle around the pupils; (b)

clouded yellow vision. Both may be aptly implied.

[2] The eyes have cleared up 目睛慧了 *mù jīng huì liǎo*: Depending on the interpretation of the previous phrase, this can either mean that the yellow ring around the pupils has disappeared, or that the yellow clouded vision has cleared up.

SYNOPSIS, LINE 16.2

This line explains the prognosis of nosebleed on the basis of the pulse.

COMMENTARY, LINE 16.2

The cubit pulse indicates the kidney, and the eyes are the orifice of the liver, which governs the storage of blood and shares a common source with the kidney. The floating cubit pulse described here indicates liver-kidney yīn depletion, which causes ministerial fire to stir internally and vacuity heat to harass the upper body. When vacuity heat from the liver ascends to harass the eyes, the result is a yellow haze around the pupils and clouded vision. The heat also forces blood to move frenetically and damages the yáng network vessels; hence we see nosebleed. When the yellow ring disappears and the vision becomes clear, this indicates that the heat has been eliminated from both the liver and the kidney, and the bleeding is therefore stopped.

Line 16.3

又曰：从春至夏衄者太阳，从秋至冬衄者阳明。

Yòu yuē: cóng chūn zhì xià nǜ zhě tài yáng, cóng qiū zhì dōng nǜ zhě yáng míng.

[The Master] also says: "Nosebleed from spring to summer is [a disease of] greater yáng; nosebleed from autumn to winter is [a disease of] yáng brightness.

SYNOPSIS, LINE 16.3

This line explains the differentiation of nosebleed in terms of exterior heat and interior heat in relation to seasonal weather.

COMMENTARY, LINE 16.3

During the spring and summer, yáng qì is in ascendance, and yáng heat inside the body floats astray to the outside. Nosebleed at this time is therefore mostly caused by an exuberance of heat in the exterior that is damaging the yáng network vessels. This type of condition is related to greater yáng.

In the fall and winter, yáng qì contracts, and yáng heat inside the body consequently hides inside. Nosebleed at this time is mostly caused by an exuberance of heat in the interior that is harassing the blood vessels. This type of condition is related to yáng brightness.

Line 16.4

衄家不可汗，汗出必额上陷，脉紧急，直视不能眴，不得眠。

Nǜ jiā bù kě hàn, hàn chū bì é shàng xiàn, mài jǐn jí, zhí shì bù néng shùn, bù dé mián.

In patients with habitual nosebleed, you must not promote sweating. [In such patients,] sweating is bound to cause a sunken forehead, tight and urgent pulse, straight-staring [eyes] that are unable to roll, and inability to sleep.

SYNOPSIS, LINE 16.4

This line describes a transmuted pattern in patients with nosebleed after inappropriate treatment by promoting sweating.

COMMENTARY, LINE 16.4

As the *Líng Shū* ("Magic Pivot") indicates, "When blood is despoliated, do not effuse sweat; when sweat is despoliated, do not bleed." In patients who have lost blood, yīn-blood is invariably depleted. Since sweat and blood are of the same source, effusing sweat will only further aggravate the damage to yīn-blood. As a result, the channels and network vessels are vacuous; hence the network vessels on the forehead become sunken, and the pulse is tight and urgent. The eyes require blood to be able to see; hence blood depletion deprives the eyes of nourishment and prevents them from turning freely. Because yīn is vacuous and therefore unable to subdue yáng, the patient has difficulty falling asleep.

Line 16.5

病人面无血色，无寒热。脉沉弦者，衄；浮弱，手按之绝者，下血；烦咳者，必吐血。

Bìng rén miàn wú xuè sè, wú hán rè. Mài chén xián zhě nǜ; fú ruò, shǒu àn zhī jué zhě, xià xuè; fán ké zhě, bì tù xuè.

In a patient with a bloodless facial complexion and no aversion to cold or heat effusion, a sunken and stringlike pulse means nosebleed; a floating and weak pulse that expires when pressed means lower body bleeding[1]; and vexation and cough invariably mean blood ejection.[2]

TEXT NOTES, LINE 16.5

[1] Lower body bleeding 下血 *xià xuè*: Precipitation of blood, passing of blood via the anus.

[2] Blood ejection 吐血 *tù xuè*: Expulsion of blood from either the lung or stomach via the mouth. Note that 吐 in Chinese

means simply "to spew." It can mean to spew up the contents of the stomach. When used with 痰 *tán* it means "to spit out phlegm" (in this meaning it is pronounced as *tǔ* in modern Chinese). When blood is expelled via the mouth, the locus of bleeding is not always clearly known. The term 吐血 *tù xuè* can mean expulsion of blood from the lung or stomach. It is translated as "blood ejection" to avoid specifically suggesting bleeding in the lung or digestive tract. In the present line, however, commentators generally agree that bleeding from the lung is the intended meaning.

SYNOPSIS, LINE 16.5

This line describes the differentiation of nosebleed, lower body bleeding, and blood ejection in terms of pulses and signs.

COMMENTARY, LINE 16.5

When a patient presents with a lusterless white facial complexion, this indicates blood desertion. Absence of aversion to cold and heat effusion means that the condition is not an exterior pattern caused by external contraction, but a pattern of internal damage bleeding.

This can manifest in blood ejection, nosebleed, or lower body bleeding, which we can differentiate by pulse and symptoms. A sunken and stringlike pulse indicates that the condition is related to the kidney and liver. In this case, kidney water is vacuous and unable to irrigate liver wood, as a result of which liver fire ascends counterflow, damages the yáng network vessels, and thereby causes nosebleed. By contrast, a floating and weak pulse that disappears when pressed hard indicates that yīn is unable to constrain yáng, as a result of which vacuous yáng floats outward, and that blood is vacuous and the vessels are not filled. As a whole, such a pulse suggests yīn-blood desertion in the lower body and vacuous yáng floating upward. This manifests in lower body bleeding. Lastly, blood ejection manifests in a bloodless facial complexion with vacuity vexation and cough, because it is caused by vacuity heat scorching the lung network vessels.

Line 16.6

夫吐血，咳逆上气，其脉数而有热，不得卧者死。

Fū tù xuè, ké nì shàng qì, qí mài shuò ér yǒu rè, bù dé wò zhě sǐ.

If blood ejection is accompanied by cough and counterflow qì ascent, a rapid pulse, heat [effusion], and inability to sleep, this means death.

SYNOPSIS, LINE 16.6

This line describes the prognosis of critical patterns of blood ejection.

COMMENTARY, LINE 16.6

From the previous line, we know that vexation and cough is a key sign of blood ejection. The present line describes the signs that develop in advanced critical cases of this disease. The combination of blood ejection and cough indicates that the blood is coming from the lung, because coughing has damaged the lung network vessels. Blood ejection inevitably causes depletion of yīn-blood, as a result of which fire becomes exuberant and scorches the lung. This impairs depurative downbearing, which further aggravates the cough and counterflow qì ascent. This is a vicious cycle that in turn prevents yīn from constraining yáng, as a result of which yáng floats outward. This development manifests in generalized heat effusion and a rapid pulse. When vacuity fire floats upward and harasses the heart spirit, it causes vacuity vexation and inability to sleep. At this stage, the depletion of yīn and exuberance of yáng exacerbate each other to the point where yīn and yáng are about to separate. Thus, the prognosis for this pattern is negative, and it becomes difficult to treat.

Line 16.7

夫酒客咳者，必致吐血，此因极饮过度所致也。

Fū jiǔ kè ké zhě, bì zhì tù xuè, cǐ yīn jí yǐn guò dù suǒ zhì yě.

When a drinker[1] suffers from cough, this invariably leads to blood ejection. This is because [the cough] is caused by excessive consumption of alcohol.

TEXT NOTE, LINE 16.7

[1] Drinker 酒客 *jiǔ kè*: A person who habitually drinks alcohol.

SYNOPSIS, LINE 16.7

This line describes the pathomechanism of cough and blood ejection in alcoholics.

COMMENTARY, LINE 16.7

Because alcohol is by nature damp and hot, excessive consumption of alcohol causes damp-heat to brew internally. Collecting in the stomach and damaging the stomach network vessels, it causes blood ejection. Steaming upward and scorching the lung, thereby impairing the lung's ability to depurate the clear and damaging its network vessels, it causes bloody cough. Thus we see how damp-heat can cause coughing and blood ejection by affecting the lung and the stomach. Because both these symptoms manifest in blood being discharged from the mouth, we summarily refer to this symptom as blood ejection.

Line 16.8

寸口脉弦而大，弦则为减，大则为芤，减则为寒，芤则为虚，寒虚相击，此名曰革，妇人则半产漏下，男子则亡血。

Cùn kǒu mài xián ér dà, xián zé wéi jiǎn, dà zé wéi kōu, jiǎn zé wéi hán, kōu zé wéi xū, hán xū xiāng jí, cǐ míng yuē gé, fù rén zé bàn chǎn lòu xià, nán zǐ zé wáng xuè.

When the inch opening pulse is stringlike and large, stringlike means reduced, and large means scallion-stalk; reduced means cold, and scallion-stalk means vacuity. When cold and vacuity contend with each other, this is called drumskin. In women, this means miscarriage or vaginal spotting; in men, it means blood collapse.

Synopsis, Line 16.8

This line describes the pulse of vacuity cold blood collapse.

Commentary, Line 16.8

The text in this line is almost literally the same as line 6.12 in Chapter 6, "Blood Impediment and Vacuity Taxation," the only exception being that line 6.12 includes the symptom of seminal loss at the very end, as one of the manifestations of blood collapse in men. That symptom is most likely left out here because the present chapter discusses diseases related to bleeding. As the commentary to line 6.12 explains, the stringlike and large characteristics of a drumskin pulse are quite specific, referring to a pulse that is large on the outside but hollow inside (hence the reference to scallion-stalk), and reduced when heavy pressure is applied. This indicates vacuity of yīn-blood on the one hand, and stagnation and contraction from congealing cold on the other.

In contrast to a true scallion-stalk pulse, which is the manifestation of rapid blood loss in urgent conditions, a drumskin pulse may be seen resulting from a slowly-developing chronic loss of essence or blood. In clinic, a drumskin pulse is not as common as a scallion-stalk pulse. When observing a drumskin pulse, consider whether the patient could be suffering from chronic loss of blood or essence.

Line 16.9

亡血不可发其表，汗出则寒栗而振。

Wáng xuè bù kě fā qí biǎo, hàn chū zé hán lì ér zhèn.

In blood collapse, you must not effuse the exterior. Sweating will result in shivering with cold.

SYNOPSIS, LINE 16.9

This line describes the transmuted pattern of damage to yáng due to inappropriate sweating in blood collapse.

COMMENTARY, LINE 16.9

Patients who have lost considerable amounts of blood suffer from yīn depletion. Since sweat is also a yīn liquid, effusing sweat will only aggravate the damage to yīn-blood. In addition, sweating forces yáng qì to be discharged outward together with liquid, as a result of which yáng qì is consumed, and defense yáng becomes insufficient for defending the outside. Hence we see shivering and aversion to cold. This pattern is thus one in which depletion of blood and depletion of liquid has transformed into depletion of yáng. Because sweating can not only damage yīn but also yáng, it is contraindicated in any patient with blood loss.

Line 16.10

病人胸满，唇痿，舌青，口燥，但欲漱水不欲咽，无寒热，脉微大来迟，腹不满，其人言我满，为有瘀血。

Bìng rén xiōng mǎn, chún wěi, shé qīng, kǒu zào, dàn yù shù shuǐ bù yù yàn, wú hán rè, mài wēi dà lái chí, fù bù mǎn, qí rén yán wǒ mǎn, wéi yǒu yū xuè.

When a patient presents with fullness in the chest, withered lips,[1] green-blue tongue, dry mouth with desire only to gargle with water but not to swallow, no [aversion to] cold and heat [effusion], a faint, large, and slowly arriving pulse, and no abdominal fullness even though the patient states, "I have fullness,"[2] this means that static blood is present.

TEXT NOTES, LINE 16.10

[1] Withered lips 唇痿 *chún wěi*: Lusterless lips. 痿 *wěi* is here used interchangeably with 萎 *wěi*.

[2] No abdominal fullness even though the person states "I have fullness" 腹不满，其人言我满 *fù bù mǎn, qí rén yán wǒ mǎn*: Fullness that is based only on the patient's subjective feeling but cannot be verified by palpation.

SYNOPSIS, LINE 16.10

This line describes the main pulse and signs of static blood.

COMMENTARY, LINE 16.10

By analyzing the signs of static blood that are mentioned in this line, we can understand the pathomechanism of this disease. Fullness in the chest suggests that static blood is present in the chest, obstructing the qì dynamic and thereby causing qì stagnation. Because static blood is internally obstructed, blood is unable to nourish the upper body; hence we see lusterless lips. The heart governs blood, and the tongue is the sprout of the heart. When static blood stagnates and does not flow freely, the tongue turns purplish green-blue, possibly with purplish green-blue macules or speckles. Dry mouth with desire to only to gargle with water, but not to swallow is caused by a static blood preventing liquid from bearing upward. Because the disease does not involve damage to liquid, the patient only wants to gargle to moisten the mouth, but feels no need to swallow water to supplement liquid.

Line 16.11

病者如热状，烦满，口干燥而渴，其脉反无热，此为阴伏，是瘀血也，当下之。

Bìng zhě rú rè zhuàng, fán mǎn, kǒu gān zào ér kě, qí mài fǎn wú rè, cǐ wéi yīn fú, shì yū xuè yě, dāng xià zhī.

When a patient presents with apparent heat, with vexation and fullness, dry mouth and thirst, but a pulse that [evidences] no heat, this constitutes hidden yīn[1] and means precisely static blood. [Treat this condition by] precipitation.

TEXT NOTE, LINE 16.11

[1] Hidden yīn 陰伏 *yīn fú*: Static blood with depressed heat lying deep in the blood aspect.

SYNOPSIS, LINE 16.11

This line describes the signs and treatment of static blood and depressed heat.

COMMENTARY, LINE 16.11

When static blood lies hidden in the body and becomes depressed, over time it can turn into heat. This causes a subjective feeling of heat effusion and vexation and fullness in the patient. Such a patient will also suffer from thirst and dry mouth because the obstruction by static blood prevents liquid from bearing upward. Yet the pulse will not be slippery, rapid, and surging, as would be the case in true heat conditions, because the heat is lying deeply hidden in the yīn aspect.

We treat such conditions by offensive precipitation, to rid the static blood and thereby resolve depressed heat. Consequently, the various symptoms will disappear unaided.

Line 16.12

火邪者，桂枝去芍药加蜀漆牡蛎龙骨救逆汤主之。

桂枝三两（去皮） 甘草二两（炙）
生姜三两 牡蛎五两（熬） 龙骨四两
大枣十二枚 蜀漆三两（洗去腥）

右为末，以水一斗二升，先煮蜀漆，减二升，内诸药，煮取三升，去滓，温服一升。

Huǒ xié zhě, guì zhī qù sháo yào jiā shǔ qī mǔ lì lóng gǔ jiù nì tāng zhǔ zhī.

Guì zhī sān liǎng (qù pí); gān cǎo èr liǎng (zhì); shēng jiāng sān liǎng; mǔ lì wǔ liǎng (áo) lóng gǔ sì liǎng dà zǎo shí èr méi; shǔ qī sān liǎng (xǐ qù xīng)

Yòu wéi mò, yǐ shuǐ yī dǒu èr shēng, xiān zhǔ shǔ qī, jiǎn èr shēng, nà zhū yào, zhǔ qǔ sān shēng, qù zǐ, wēn fú yī shēng.

For fire evil, Cinnamon Twig Counterflow-Stemming Decoction Minus Peony Plus Dichroa Leaf, Oyster Shell, and Dragon Bone (桂枝救逆汤 *guì zhī qù sháo yào jiā shǔ qī mǔ lì lóng gǔ jiù nì tāng*) governs.

Cinnamon Twig Counterflow-Stemming Decoction Minus Peony Plus Dichroa Leaf, Oyster Shell, and Dragon Bone (桂枝救逆汤 *guì zhī qù sháo yào jiā shǔ qī mǔ lì lóng gǔ jiù nì tāng*)

- cinnamon twig (桂枝 *guì zhī*, Cinnamomi Ramulus) 3 *liǎng* (remove bark)
- licorice (甘草 *gān cǎo*, Glycyrrhizae Radix) 2 *liǎng* (mix-fry)
- fresh ginger (生姜 *shēng jiāng*, Zingiberis Rhizoma Recens) 3 *liǎng*
- oyster shell (牡蛎 *mǔ lì*, Ostreae Concha) 5 *liǎng* (simmer)
- dragon bone (龙骨 *lóng gǔ*, Mastodi Ossis Fossilia) 4 *liǎng*
- jujube (大枣 *dà zǎo*, Jujubae Fructus) 12 pieces
- dichroa leaf (蜀漆 *shǔ qī*, Dichroae Folium) 3 *liǎng* (wash to remove fishy smell)

Of the above seven ingredients, first boil the dichroa leaf (*shǔ qī*) in one *dǒu* and two *shēng* of water and reduce by two *shēng*. Add all [the other] medicinals and boil to get three *shēng*. Remove the dregs and take one *shēng* [per dose] warm.

Synopsis, Line 16.12

This line describes the treatment of fright due to fire-forcing.

Commentary, Line 16.12

The text here merely mentions "fire evil," but does not give any symptoms or pulses to specify the condition to be treated by the formula. Fire evil, which refers here to various heat-related therapies like warm needling, moxibustion, or fumigation, can have a number of negative effects. It can force liquid outward and by sweating damage heart yáng. Strong fire can "eat qì," meaning that heart qì sustains injury. Lastly, it can scorch liquid into phlegm, which then obstructs the orifices of the heart. As a result, spirit qì floats astray, which manifests in fright. Associated signs are heart palpitation, vexation, agitation, fright, and mania, and fidgetiness whether lying down or being up.

This condition is treated with Cinnamon Twig Counterflow-Stemming Decoction Minus Peony Plus Dichroa Leaf, Oyster Shell, and Dragon Bone (*qù sháo yào jiā shǔ qī mǔ lì lóng gǔ jiù nì tāng*) to perfuse heart qì and settle the heart spirit. Because peony (*sháo yào*) supplements yīn it therefore does not serve the purpose of supplementing heart yáng, and is removed from the formula here. Dichroa leaf (*shǔ qī*) flushes out phlegm and expels evil, thereby opening the orifices of the heart, while oyster shell (*mǔ lì*) and dragon bone (*lóng gǔ*) settle fright and quiet the spirit. Altogether, this is a preparation that boosts heart qì and quiets the heart spirit.

Line 16.13

心下悸者，半夏麻黄丸主之。

半夏 麻黄等分

右二味，末之，炼蜜和丸小豆大，饮服三丸，日三服。

Xīn xià jì zhě, bàn xià má huáng wán zhǔ zhī.

Bàn xià, má huáng děng fēn

Yòu èr wèi, mò zhī, liàn mì huò wán xiǎo dòu dà, yǐn fú sān wán, rì sān fú.

For palpitation below the heart, Pinellia and Ephedra Pill (半夏麻黄丸 *bàn xià má huáng wán*) governs.

Pinellia and Ephedra Pill (半夏麻黄丸 *bàn xià má huáng wán*)
pinellia (半夏 *bàn xià*, Pinelliae Rhizoma) ephedra (麻黄 *má huáng*, Ephedrae Herba) in equal proportions

Pulverize the above two ingredients and blend with processed honey (*liàn mì*) to form into pills the size of small beans.[1] Take three pills with fluid, three times a day.

Formula Note, Line 16.13

[1] Small beans 小豆 *xiǎo dòu*: Beans such as adzuki beans or mung beans.

Synopsis, Line 16.13

This line describes the treatment of palpitation due to water-rheum.

Commentary, Line 16.13

"Palpitation" refers to apprehensive stirring, fearful throbbing, and disquietude in the heart. "Below the heart" refers to the area of the stomach duct. When water-rheum collects below the heart and then surges into the heart, heart yáng becomes trapped, causing the patient to experience subjective palpitation and disquietude. Thus you must not effuse the obstructed yáng too strongly or remove the water that is encroaching on the heart too quickly. Therefore, the dosage of this pill preparation is relatively small, and the medicinals are mixed with honey to boost right qì, to remove the evil without damaging right.

Line 16.14

吐血不止者，柏叶汤主之。

柏叶 干姜各　三两　艾三把

右三味，以水五升，取马通汁一升，合煮取一升，分温再服

Tù xuè bù zhǐ zhě, bǎi yè tāng zhǔ zhī.

Bǎi yè, gān jiāng gè sān liǎng; ài yè sān bǎ

Yòu sān wèi, yǐ shuǐ wǔ shēng, qǔ mǎ tōng zhī yī shēng, gě zhǔ qǔ yī shēng, fēn wēn zài fú.

For incessant blood ejection, Arborvitae Leaf Decoction (柏叶汤 *bǎi yè tāng*) governs.

Arborvitae Leaf Decoction
(柏叶汤 *bǎi yè tāng*)

arborvitae leaf (柏叶 *bǎi yè*, Platycladi Cacumen) 3 *liǎng*
dried ginger (干姜 *gān jiāng*, Zingiberis Rhizoma) 3 *liǎng*
mugwort (艾叶 *ài yè*, Artemisiae Argyi Folium) 3 handfuls

Boil the above three ingredients in a mix of five *shēng* of water and 1 *shēng* of horse dung juice (*mǎ tōng zhī*),[1] to get one *shēng*. Divide into two doses and take warm.

TEXT NOTE, LINE 16.14

[1] Horse dung juice 馬通汁 *mǎ tōng zhī*: The strained liquid that is extracted from horse dung after soaking it in water.

SYNOPSIS, LINE 16.14

This line describes the treatment of blood ejection in vacuity cold patterns.

COMMENTARY, LINE 16.14

As in the previous two lines, the text does not give accompanying symptoms or explain the particular cause that is addressed in the formula. Nevertheless, we can deduce the specific condition to which this line refers from the intended effect of the medicinals.

Arborvitae leaf (*bǎi yè*) is bitter, astringent, and slightly cold. By its clearing and downbearing action, it is able to break the force of the counterflow ascent and thus control and stanch bleeding. Dried ginger (*gān jiāng*) and mugwort (*ài yè*) warm yáng and guard the center. Together, they arouse yáng qì to contain blood. Lastly, horse dung juice is slightly warm and conducts blood downward, thereby also stanching bleeding. Because the formula aims at warming the center to stanch bleeding, we know that it addresses a bleeding pattern that is related to vacuity cold.

The causes for this condition are numerous. Over time incessant blood ejection can consume both blood and qì. As a result yáng qì becomes increasingly vacuous. Alternatively, center qì vacuity cold can prevent blood from returning to the channels. Or, excessive consumption of cold fluids can damage yáng qì and impair its ability to warm and contain. Any of these can cause vacuity cold-related blood ejection. This condition manifests with accompanying symptoms of vacuity cold, like withered yellow or somber white facial complexion, pale or dark red blood, fatigued body and spirit, pale tongue with white fur, and a vacuous forceless pulse.

In clinical practice, one can substitute boys' urine for horse dung juice, and charred mugwort (*jiāo ài*) and blast-fried ginger (*pào jiāng*) for mugwort (*ài yè*) and dried ginger (*gān jiāng*) respectively.

Line 16.15

下血，先便后血，此远血也，黄土汤主之。

甘草　干地黄　白朮　附子（炮）
阿胶　黄芩各三两　灶中黄土半斤

右七味，以水八升，煮取三升，分温二服。

Xià xuè, xiān biàn hòu xuè, cǐ yuǎn xuè yě, huáng tǔ tāng zhǔ zhī.

Gān cǎo, gān dì huáng, bái zhú fù zǐ (pào), ē jiāo, huáng qín gè sān liǎng; zào zhōng huáng tǔ bàn jīn

Yòu qī wèi, yǐ shuǐ bā shēng, zhǔ qǔ sān shēng, fēn wēn èr fú.

When lower body bleeding manifests in bleeding after defecating, this is distal bleeding.[1] Yellow Earth Decoction (黄土汤 *huáng tǔ tāng*)[2] governs.

Yellow Earth Decoction
(黄土汤 *huáng tǔ tāng*)

licorice (甘草 *gān cǎo*, Glycyrrhizae Radix) 3 *liǎng*
dried rehmannia (干地黄 *gān dì huáng*, Rehmanniae Radix) 3 *liǎng*
white atractylodes (白朮 *bái zhú*, Atractylodis Macrocephalae Rhizoma) 3 *liǎng*
aconite (附子 *fù zǐ*, Aconiti Radix Lateralis Praeparata) (blast-fry) 3 *liǎng*
ass hide glue (阿胶 *ē jiāo*, Asini Corii Colla) 3 *liǎng*
scutellaria (黄芩 *huáng qín*, Scutellariae Radix) 3 *liǎng*
oven earth (灶中黄土 *zào zhōng huáng tǔ*, Terra Flava Usta) 3 ½ *jīn*

[Take] the above seven ingredients. Using eight *shēng* of water, boil to get three *shēng*. Divide into two and take warm.

TEXT NOTES, LINE 16.15

[1] Distal bleeding 远血 *yuǎn xuè*: Bleeding in the intestinal tract far from the anus.

[2] A comment included in the received text reads: "This [formula] also treats blood ejection and nosebleed."

[3] Oven earth (灶中黄土 *zào zhōng huáng tǔ*, Terra Flava Usta): More commonly called 伏龙肝 *fú lóng gān* in Chinese. The Chinese name literally means "yellow earth in oven," and is sometimes abbreviated to 黄土 *huáng tǔ*, "yellow earth," as in the name of the decoction.

SYNOPSIS, LINE 16.15

This line describes the signs and treatment of bloody stool due to vacuity cold.

COMMENTARY, LINE 16.15

When blood in the stool manifests as bleeding after defecating, this indicates that the blood is coming from above the intestinal tract; hence it is called distal bleeding. This condition is most commonly caused by vacuity cold of spleen qì in the center burner, as a result of which containment is impaired, and blood seeps downward.

The recommended treatment for this condition is Yellow Earth Decoction (*huáng tǔ tāng*), which warms the spleen and nourishes and contains blood. In this formula, oven earth (*huáng tǔ*) has the effect of warming the center, astringing the intestines, and stanching bleeding; aconite (*fù zǐ*) and white atractylodes (*bái zhú*) contain the blood by warming yáng and fortifying the spleen; dried rehmannia (*gān dì huáng*) and ass hide glue (*ē jiāo*) stanch bleeding by enriching yīn and nourishing blood. The above ingredients are assisted by scutellaria (*huáng qín*), which mitigates their warming and drying effect and thereby prevents stirring blood. Lastly, licorice (*gān cǎo*) harmonizes the other medicinals by warming and harmonizing the center.

Line 16.16

下血，先血后便，此近血也，赤小豆当归散主之。

Xià xuè, xiān xuè hòu biàn, cǐ jìn xuè yě, chì xiǎo dòu dāng guī sǎn zhǔ zhī.

When lower body bleeding manifests in bleeding before defecating, this is proximal bleeding.[1] Rice Bean and Chinese Angelica Powder (赤小豆当归散 *chì xiǎo dòu dāng guī sǎn*)[2] governs.

Text Notes, Line 16.16

[1] Proximal bleeding 近血 *jì xuè*: Bleeding in the intestinal tract close to the anus.

[2] The commentary adds: "For the formula, see in the chapter on Fox-Creeper." The formula is found Chapter 3, "Hundred Union Disease, Fox-Creeper, and Yīn-Yáng Toxin," line 3.13.

Synopsis, Line 16.16

This line describes the signs and treatment of bloody stool due to damp-heat.

Commentary, Line 16.16

In contrast to the previous line, the condition discussed in this line is characterized by bleeding occurring before defecation. This indicates that the blood is coming from the intestinal tract. In most cases, this condition is caused by damp-heat brewing and binding in the large intestine, which is forcing the blood to move downward. Because the damp-heat is rotting flesh and forming pus, we can see pus in the stool.

In accord with the disease cause, we treat this condition with Rice Bean and Chinese Angelica Powder (*chì xiǎo dòu dāng guī sǎn*) because this formula stanches bleeding by clearing and disinhibiting damp-heat and invigorating blood. In the formula, rice bean (*chì xiǎo dòu*) clears heat and disinhibits dampness, and expels pus and resolves toxin; Chinese angelica (*dāng guī*) moves blood and dissipates stasis; and sour rice milk clears, cools, and resolves toxin, as well as harmonizes the viscera and bowels. In combination, these ingredients have the effect of dispersing stasis, eliminating pus, clearing heat, and disinhibiting dampness.

Line 16.17

心气不足, 吐血, 衄血, 泻心汤主之。
大黄二两 黄连 黄芩各一两
右三味, 以水三升, 煮取一升, 顿服之。

Xīn qì bù zú, tù xuè, nǜ xuè, xiè xīn tāng zhǔ zhī.
Dà huáng èr liǎng; huáng lián, huáng qín gè yī liǎng
Yòu sān wèi, yǐ shuǐ sān shēng, zhǔ qǔ yī shēng, dùn fú zhī.

For insufficiency of heart qì, with blood ejection and nosebleed, Heart-Draining Decoction (泻心汤 *xiè xīn tāng*)[1] governs.

Heart-Draining Decoction
(泻心汤 *xiè xīn tāng*)

rhubarb (大黄 *dà huáng*, Rhei Radix et Rhizoma) 2 *liǎng*
coptis (黄连 *huáng lián*, Coptidis Rhizoma) 1 *liǎng*
scutellaria (黄芩 *huáng qín*, Scutellariae Radix) 1 *liǎng*

Boil the above three ingredients in three *shēng* of water to get one *shēng*. Quaff.

Text Note, Line 16.17

[1] A comment included in the received text reads: "[This formula] also treats sudden turmoil."

Synopsis, Line 16.17

This line discusses the signs and treatment of blood ejection and nosebleed that is due to exuberant heat.

Commentary, Line 16.17

The heart belongs to fire and governs blood. When heart qì is insufficient, this does not mean that heart fire is insufficient, but that true yīn is insufficient. As a result fire heat becomes exuberant. When heart fire is exuberant, the heart is unable to nourish blood, and blood is forced by the heat to move frenetically into the upper body. Hence we see blood ejection and nosebleed.

This condition is treated by draining the excessive force of fire, for which purpose the text recommends Heart-Draining Decoction (*xiè xīn tāng*). In this formula, coptis (*huáng lián*) excels at draining heart fire; scutellaria (*huáng qín*) drains upper burner fire; and rhubarb (*dà huáng*) conducts fire evil downward by its downbearing and discharging effect. Altogether, these ingredients break the heat by downbearing fire and thereby causing bleeding to stop on its own.

呕吐哕下利病脉证治第十七

CHAPTER 17

Retching and Vomiting, Hiccup, and Diarrhea

Pulses, Signs, Treatments

‡ Overview

This chapter describes the causes, pathomechanisms, signs, pulses, and treatment of retching and vomiting, hiccup, and diarrhea. Retching and vomiting are symptoms of loss of harmonious downbearing in the stomach and are normally used in clinic as a compound term because they tend to appear together. Strictly speaking, though, retching (呕 *ǒu*) refers to the motions of vomiting that produces sound but not matter, while vomiting (吐 *tù*) refers the ejction of matter without any sound. Hiccup (哕 *yuè*) is explained in Chinese medicine as caused by counterflow ascent of qì in the stomach and diaphragm. Diarrhea (下利 *xià lì*) includes not only regular diarrhea but also dysentery. These diseases are discussed together in this chapter because they are all diseases of the stomach and intestines, are mutually conducive, and frequently appear simultaneously.

The conditions described in this chapter all share the same basic pathomechanism of disturbed upbearing and downbearing of the spleen and stomach, but a few are also related to kidney yáng insufficiency or to liver-gallbladder failing to course freely. Spleen qì normally bears upward and stomach qì normally bears downward. Retching, vomiting, and hiccup are all manifestations of counterflow ascent of stomach qì, while diarrhea is the manifestation of a breakdown of spleen qì upbearing.

In all these diseases, treatment generally can be determined on the basis of "repletion indicates yáng brightness; vacuity indicates greater yīn," and "yáng disease belongs to the bowels; yīn disease belongs to the viscera." Repletion and heat patterns are treated by harmonizing the stomach and downbearing counterflow, as well as freeing the bowels and eliminating evil; vacuity and cold patterns are treated by fortifying the spleen and warming the kidney.

To understand the pathomechanisms and treatment of spleen and stomach disease systematically, we will make frequent reference to relevant lines and theories from the *Shāng Hán Lùn* as well as from Chapter 12, "Phlegm-Rheum and Cough," in this text.

‡ Schematic Overview

Vomiting

1. Lesser yáng (*shào yáng*) depressed heat causing liver-stomach disharmony.

   Signs: Vomiting with heat effusion.

   Treatment: Minor Bupleurum Decoction (*xiǎo chái hú tāng*).

2. Gastrointestinal repletion heat.

   Signs: Vomiting after eating.

   Treatment: Rhubarb and Licorice Decoction (*dà huáng gān cǎo tāng*).

3. Stomach cold complicated by liver qì counterflow.

   Signs: Dry retching, ejection of drool and foam, with headache.

   Treatment: Evodia Decoction (*zhū yú tāng*).

4. Spleen-kidney vacuity cold with exuberant yīn repelling yang.

   Signs: Vomiting, weak pulse, uninhibited urination, slight generalized heat effusion, and reversal.

   Treatment: Counterflow Cold Decoction (*sì nì tāng*).

5. Vacuity cold.

   Signs: Vomiting, weak pulse, uninhibited urination, slight generalized heat effusion, and reversal.

   Treatment: Major Pinellia Decoction (*dà bàn xià tāng*).

6. Binding of cold and heat.

   Signs: Vomiting with rumbling intestines and glomus below the heart.

   Treatment: Pinellia Heart-Draining Decoction (*bàn xià xiè xīn tāng*).

7. Water-rheum collecting internally: rheum with qì counterflow.

   Signs: Stomach reflux with thirst and desire to drink water after vomiting.

   Treatment: Poria and Alisma Decoction (*fú líng zé xiè tāng*).

8. Water-rheum collecting internally: insufficiency of center yáng with exuberant internal cold rheum.

   Signs: Dry retching, vomiting counterflow, and vomiting of drool and foam.

Treatment: Pinellia and Dried Ginger Powder (*bàn xià gān jiāng sǎn*).

9. Water-rheum collecting internally: Cold and rheum contending with each other, obstructing chest yáng.

   Signs: [A sensation] in the chest that resembles panting but is not real panting, with [a sensation] that resembles retching but is not real retching, with [a sensation] that resembles hiccup but is not real hiccup, and with unbearable vexation and oppression piercing the heart.

   Treatment: Fresh Ginger and Pinellia Decoction (*shēng jiāng bàn xià tāng*).

Hiccup

1. Evil repletion.

   Signs: Hiccup and abdominal fullness.

   Treatment: For water evil (inhibited anterior section), disinhibit urine; for heat (inhibited posterior section), disinhibit stool.

2. Stomach cold.

   Signs: Dry retching; reversal of the extremities.

   Treatment: Tangerine Peel Decoction (*jú pí tāng*).

3. Stomach vacuity with heat.

   Hiccup.

   Treatment: Tangerine Peel and Bamboo Shavings Decoction (*jú pí zhú rú tāng*).

Diarrhea

1. Method of treatment.

   a) Basic method: Diarrhea and qì (flatus) means exuberant dampness, and is treated by disinhibiting urine.

   b) Contraindication: Vacuity cold diarrhea cannot be treated by attacking the exterior, because this will cause abdominal fullness.

2. Diarrhea.

   a) Vacuity cold diarrhea.

      Signs: Diarrhea, abdominal distention and fullness, generalized pain.

      Treatment: Counterflow Cold Decoction (*sì nì tāng*); Cinnamon Twig Decoction (*guì zhī tāng*).

   b) Cold reversal diarrhea with exuberant yīn repelling yang.

      Signs: Clear-grain diarrhea, sweating, reversal.

      Treatment: Vessel-Freeing Counterflow Cold Decoction (*tōng mài sì nì tāng*).

   c) Vacuity cold intestinal efflux diarrhea.

      Signs: Qì diarrhea.

Treatment: Chebule Powder (*hé lí lè sǎn*).

d) Repletion accumulation diarrhea.

Signs: Hardness below the heart when pressure is applied.

Treatment: Major Qì-Coordinating Decoction (*dà chéng qì tāng*).

e) Qì stagnation and abiding food.

Signs: Diarrhea with a pulse that is slippery, diarrhea not about to stop.

Treatment: Major Qì-Coordinating Decoction (*dà chéng qì tāng*).

f) Dryness binding in the stomach and intestines.

Signs: Diarrhea and delirious speech.

Treatment: Major Qì-Coordinating Decoction (*dà chéng qì tāng*).

3. Dysentery.

a) Vacuity cold.

Signs: Diarrhea with pus and blood in the stool.

Treatment: Peach Blossom Decoction (*táo huā tāng*).

b) Damp-heat.

Signs: Heat diarrhea with tenesmus.

Treatment: Pulsatilla Decoction (*bái tóu wēng tāng*).

4. Aftermath.

a) Vacuity heat.

Signs: Even greater vexation after diarrhea; sogginess below the heart.

Treatment: Gardenia and Fermented Soybean Decoction (*zhī zǐ chǐ tāng*).

b) Residual heat.

Signs: Diarrhea that has stopped, but recurs at set times.

Treatment: Major Qì-Coordinating Decoction (*dà chéng qì tāng*).

Line 17.1

夫呕家有痈脓，不可治呕，脓尽自愈。

Fū ǒu jiā yǒu yōng nóng, bù kě zhì ǒu, nóng nìn zì yù.

If patients with habitual retching have welling-abscess with pus, you must not treat the retching; when the pus has disappeared completely, [the patient] will spontaneously recover.

SYNOPSIS, LINE 17.1

This line describes the treatment of retching due to a purulent welling-abscess of the stomach.

COMMENTARY, LINE 17.1

The causes of retching and vomiting are manifold and include both external evils invading the stomach, and impaired functions of the viscera and bowels themselves. As the *Sù Wèn* ("Plain Questions") states, "When heat gathers in the entrance to the stomach and does not move, it causes welling-abscess in the stomach duct." If a purulent welling-abscess in the stomach is expelled through retching and vomiting, this is the manifestation of right qì expelling evil. In treatment, you must search for the underlying cause and treat the root, instead of simply addressing the vomiting and retching, which is the tip of the condition. The treatment principle is therefore to disperse the welling-abscess and expel pus. When this is achieved, the retching and vomiting will stop on its own. If a physician disregards this advice and focuses on stopping retching and vomiting instead of on expelling pus, the pus toxin will be retained inside, as a result of which the condition is only aggravated further, hence forming a transmuted pattern.

Line 17.2

先呕却渴者，此为欲解；先渴却呕者，为水停心下，此属饮家。呕家本渴，今反不渴者，以心下有支饮故也，此属支饮。

Xiān ǒu què kě zhě, cǐ wéi yù jiě; xiān kě què ǒu zhě, wéi shuǐ tíng xīn xià, cǐ shǔ yǐn jiā.Ǒu jiā běn kě, jīn fǎn bù kě zhě, yǐ xīn xià yǒu zhī yǐn gù yě, cǐ shǔ zhī yǐn.

When retching occurs first and is followed by thirst, this means that [the condition] is about to resolve. When thirst occurs first and is followed by retching, this means that water is collecting below the heart. This is [a symptom] associated with patients with habitual rheum. Patients with habitual retching should generally be thirsty. However, if they are not thirsty, this indicates an association with propping rheum below the heart.

SYNOPSIS, LINE 17.2

This line discusses the pattern differentiation of retching due to water-rheum.

COMMENTARY, LINE 17.2

This line describes three different conditions, on the basis of which we can determine the presence and status of rheum evil: retching first followed by thirst, thirst first followed by retching, and retching that occurs without thirst. In all these, thirst is the key sign for identifying the pattern of rheum collecting in the stomach causing retching and vomiting.

In the first case, retching that is followed by thirst indicates that the patient is about to recover. When we see the symptoms in this order, it means that the water-rheum that was the cause of retching and vomiting has been expelled in the process, that stomach yáng has recovered, that the spleen's function of movement and transformation has been restored, and that we therefore see thirst.

In the second scenario, thirst is followed by retching. The thirst is a sign that rheum is collecting in the stomach, thereby obstructing qì transformation and preventing the fluids from bearing upward. The resulting thirst causes the patient to drink water. Because the rheum impairs the spleen's movement and transformation function and the stomach's harmonious downbearing function, fluid gathers instead of being transformed, ascends counterflow, and causes retching and vomiting. Hence this indicates conditions with habitual rheum.

The last situation is characterized by retching without thirst. As the text stresses, retching generally causes thirst because it consumes the fluids. The absence of thirst in patients with retching is therefore a key sign, indicating that water-rheum is still collecting internally and has not been removed through retching.

Line 17.3

(1) 问曰：病人脉数，数为热，当消谷引食，而反吐者何也？师曰：以发其汗，令阳微膈气虚，脉乃数，数为客热，不能消谷，胃中虚冷故也。

(2) 脉弦者虚也，胃气无余，朝食暮吐，变为胃反；寒在于上，医反下之，今脉反弦，故名曰虚。

(1) Wèn yuē: Bìng rén mài shuò, shuò wéi rè, dāng xiāo gǔ yǐn shí, ér fǎn tù zhě hé yě? Shī yuē: Yǐ fā qí hàn, lìng yáng wēi gé qì xū, mài nǎi shuò, shuò wéi kè rè, bù néng xiāo gǔ wèi zhōng xū lěng gù yě.

(2) Mài xián zhě xū yě, wèi qì wú yú, zhāo? Shí mù tù, biàn wéi wèi fǎn; hán zài yú shàng, yī fǎn xià zhī, jīn mài fǎn xián, gù míng yuē xū.

(1) Question: "In a patient with a rapid pulse, rapid means heat. Hence we should see dispersion of grain with intake of food.[1] If there is vomiting instead, what does this mean?" The Master says:

"[In such patients, inappropriate] promotion of sweating has made yáng faint and diaphragm qì vacuous; hence the pulse is rapid. Rapid [here] means visiting heat,[2] and inability to disperse grain because of vacuity cold in the stomach.

(2) [In such conditions], a stringlike pulse means vacuity. Because stomach qì had no superabundance,[3] what was eaten in the morning was vomited in the evening, transmuting into stomach reflux.[4] There was cold in the upper body, but the physician [wrongly treated with] precipitation. Hence, the pulse has now become stringlike. We call this [a sign of] vacuity.

TEXT NOTES, LINE 17.3

[1] Dispersion of grain with intake of food 消谷引食 *xiāo gǔ yǐn shí*: Swift digestion with rapid hungering.

[2] Visiting heat 客热 *kè rè*: Vacuity heat or false heat.

[3] Stomach qì had no superabundance 胃气无余 *wèi qì wú yú*: Stomach qì had become insufficient, due to inappropriate sweating treatment causing vacuity cold in the stomach.

[4] Stomach reflux 胃反 *wèi fán*: Now usually referred to as 反胃 *fǎn wèi* or 翻胃 *fān wèi*: A stomach disease characterized by vomiting in the morning of food ingested in the evening, and vomiting in the evening of food ingested in the morning.

SYNOPSIS, LINE 17.3

This line describes the pulses, patterns, and pathomechanism of vacuity cold stomach reflux.

COMMENTARY, LINE 17.3

The first part of this line explains the typical pulse in stomach reflux retching and vomiting. Ordinarily, yáng exuberance manifests in a rapid pulse, while yīn exuberance manifests in a slow pulse. Thus a rapid pulse generally should indicate heat, as a result of which a patient should experience swift digestion with rapid hungering. However, in the present case, the patient instead experiences retching and vomiting. This symptom was caused by a physician wrongly treating the patient to achieve promotion of sweating, as a result of which yīn and yáng were debilitated, stomach qì was injured, and vacuity cold in the stomach arose. The rapid pulse is here a reflection of false, temporary heat, which is rooted in a vacuity of stomach yáng; hence the heat is called "visiting heat."

The second part describes a further development of the pathomechanism of vacuity cold stomach reflux, which now manifests in a stringlike pulse. Under normal circumstances, such a pulse indicates cold and pain, but is here explained as indicating vacuity instead. This type of pulse is again caused by incorrect pattern identification and improper treatment: A physician wrongly diagnosed the rapid pulse mentioned in the earlier section as repletion heat in the stomach and intestines, and treated it accordingly with offensive precipitation. However, this only increased the damage to stomach yáng, as a result of which the pulse transmuted from a rapid pulse, indicating visiting heat, to a stringlike pulse, indicating vacuity. In this condition, a stringlike pulse does not indicate water-rheum or yīn cold, but stomach vacuity engendering cold. This cold in the stomach results in a vacuity of ancestral qì, and furthermore causes the spleen and stomach to lose their ability to digest water and grain, so that ingested food is not transformed but lodges in the stomach and is vomited up. In this way, intractable conditions of stomach reflux arise.

Line 17.4

寸口脉微而数，微则无气，无气则营虚，营虚则血不足，血不足则胸中冷。

Cùn kǒu mài wēi ér shuò, wēi zé wú qì, wú qì zé yíng xū, yíng xū zé xuè bù zú, xuè bù zú zé xiōng zhōng lěng.

When the inch opening pulse is faint and rapid, faint means absence of qì; absence of qì means vacuity of construction [qì]; vacuity of construction [qì] means insufficiency of the blood; and insufficiency of the blood means cold in the chest.

Synopsis, Line 17.4

This line describes the pathomechanism of stomach reflux due to dual vacuity of qì and blood, on the basis of the pulse.

Commentary, Line 17.4

In this line, inch opening pulse refers to the pulse at the inch, bar, and cubit positions at both hands. Similar to the previous line, where "[inappropriate] promotion of sweating has made yáng faint and diaphragm qì vacuous; hence the pulse is rapid," the rapid characteristic of the pulse here does not indicate heat, but yáng vacuity, which is due to dual vacuity of qì and blood. The "absence of qì" mentioned here refers to a shortage of yáng qì, which includes defense qì, center qì, and the functional qì in all the viscera and bowels. Since qì and blood, and hence construction-blood and yáng qì, rely on each other for mutual engenderment and nourishment, a debilitation of yáng qì, vacuity of spleen-stomach yáng, and vacuity cold of center qì result in insufficient formation of construction qì, and consequently in vacuity of construction-blood. When construction-blood is insufficient, qì is deprived of nourishment, and yáng qì is unable to upbear and effuse; hence we see yáng vacuity. When qì and blood are both vacuous, there is cold in the chest and vacuity cold in the spleen and stomach, as a result of which the digestion of water and grain is impaired, food collects in the stomach, and is vomited up. This results in stomach reflux retching and vomiting.

Line 17.5

趺阳脉浮而濇，浮则为虚，濇则伤脾，脾伤则不磨，朝食暮吐，暮食朝吐，宿谷不化，名曰胃反。脉紧而濇，其病难治。

Fū yáng mài fú ér sè, fú zé wéi xū, sè zé shāng pí, pí shāng zé bù mó, zhāo shí mù tù, mù shí zhāo tù, sù gǔ bù huà, míng yuē wèi fǎn. Mài jǐn ér sè, qí bìng nán zhì.

When the instep yáng pulse is floating and rough, floating means vacuity, while rough means damage to the spleen. When the spleen is damaged, it [can]not grind;[1] [hence we see] vomiting in the evening of food eaten in the morning, vomiting in the morning of food eaten in the evening, and abiding grain failing to transform. [This] is called stomach reflux. The pulse is tight and rough, and the disease is difficult to treat.

Text Note, Line 17.5

[1] [Can]not grind 不磨 *bù mó*: Cannot digest food.

Synopsis, Line 17.5

This line discusses the pulse, signs, and prognosis of stomach reflux due to dual vacuity of the spleen and stomach.

Commentary, Line 17.5

This line continues the discussion of stomach reflux due to spleen-stomach vacuity and impaired movement and transformation from the preceding two lines. In a healthy person, the instep yáng pulse, which indicates stomach qì, should be not too floating and not too sunken, not too large and not too small, and naturally harmonious and moderate. This indicates that movement and transformation of the spleen and stomach are healthy. The stomach is yáng earth and functions by downbearing harmoniously; hence its pulse should not be floating. A floating instep yáng pulse indicates a lack of downbearing, and hence vacuity of the stomach. The spleen is yīn earth and moves by upbearing; hence its pulse should not be rough. A rough pulse indicates damage to the spleen. When spleen yáng is insufficient, qì fails to transform liquid, liquid and qì are both damaged, and spleen liquid is insufficient. An instep yáng pulse that is both floating and rough thus reflects dual vacuity of the spleen and stomach, as a result of which their functions break down, abiding grain is not transformed, and we see stomach reflux, which manifests in vomiting in the evening of food eaten in the morning, and vomiting in the morning of food eaten in the evening.

Because the root of this condition is dual vacuity of spleen and stomach, and insufficiency of yáng qì, the pulse is not only floating and rough, but also tight, which indicates cold exuberance. This means that the insufficiency of yáng qì has caused vacuity cold. During treatment, assisting yáng will damage yīn, enriching yīn will damage yáng, expelling evil will damage the stomach, and assisting right will entrap evil. Thereby you will cause vomiting above and constipation below, vacuity of right, and repletion of evil, to the point of dual expiry of the spleen and stomach. Thus the text emphasizes the difficulty of treating this condition.

Line 17.6

病人欲吐者，不可下之。

Bìng rén yù tù zhě, bù kě xià zhī.

When the patient is about to vomit, you must not [use] precipitation.

Synopsis, Line 17.6

This line describes the principle that precipitation cannot be used when the patient is about to vomit.

Commentary, Line 17.6

When a patient is about to vomit, it generally means that evil qì is interfering in the stomach and disturbing harmonious downbearing. Vomiting is the force of right qì in expelling the evil outward. Thus, treatment should be based on the principle of helping this process along its course and assisting right qì in overcoming evil, so that the body expel the evil and right qì can become calm on its own. As a result, vomiting will stop.

If you wrongly treat with precipitation when a patient is about to vomit, you act counter to the dynamic of the disease, making right vacuous and trapping evil, thereby aggravating the disease.

Line 17.7

哕而腹满，视其前后，知何部不利，利之即愈。

Yuē ér fù mǎn, shì qí qián hòu, zhī hé bù bù lì, lì zhī jí yù.

In patients with hiccup and abdominal fullness, consider the patient's anterior and posterior [yīn][1] [so as to] know which section is inhibited. [When you] disinhibit that, recovery will ensue.

Text Note, Line 17.7

[1] Anterior and posterior [yīn] 前后 *qián hòu*: Urination and stool.

Synopsis, Line 17.7

This line discusses pattern identification and treatment of repletion hiccup.

Commentary, Line 17.7

When observing the symptoms of hiccup and abdominal fullness occurring together, carefully investigate the cause of the abdominal fullness and differentiate between vacuity and repletion patterns. Because the present line recommends disinhibition as treatment, we know that it discusses repletion hiccup. In most cases, abdominal distention that occurs in conjunction with hiccup is caused by stopped urination and defecation, and qì counterflow distressing the stomach. Stopped urination and stopped defecation can both lead to counterflow ascent of the qì dynamic, which manifests in hiccup.

If hiccup and abdominal fullness are associated with stopped defecation, this is due to internal obstruction by repletion evil, and to stoppage of bowel qì. By contrast, if hiccup and abdominal fullness are associated with stopped urination, the cause is stagnating water-damp and inhibited qì transformation. Both these diseases must be treated in accordance with each pattern. For stopped defecation, this means freeing the bowels and clearing the intestines; for stopped urination, this means freeing and disinhibiting urine.

Line 17.8

呕而胸满者，茱萸汤主之。

吴茱萸一升　人参三两　生姜六两　大枣十二枚

右四味，以水五升，煮取三升，温服七合，日三服。

Ǒu ér xiōng mǎn zhě, zhū yú tāng zhǔ zhī.

Wú zhū yú yī shēng; rén shēn sān liǎng; shēng jiāng liù liǎng; dà zǎo shí èr méi

Yòu sì wèi, yǐ shuǐ wǔ shēng, zhǔ qǔ sān shēng, wēn fú qī gě, rì sān fú.

For retching with fullness in the chest, Evodia Decoction (茱萸汤 *zhū yú tāng*) governs.

Evodia Decoction (茱萸汤 *zhū yú tāng*)

- evodia (吴茱萸 *wú zhū yú*, Evodiae Fructus) 1 *shēng*
- ginseng (人参 *rén shēn*, Ginseng Radix) 3 *liǎng*
- fresh ginger (生姜 *shēng jiāng*, Zingiberis Rhizoma Recens) 6 *liǎng*
- jujube (大枣 *dà zǎo*, Jujubae Fructus) 12 pieces

Boil the above four ingredients in five *shēng* of water to get three *shēng*. Take 7 *gě* [per dose] warm, three times a day.

Synopsis, Line 17.8

This line describes the signs and treatment of retching and vomiting due to stomach vacuity cold.

COMMENTARY, LINE 17.8

Retching and vomiting can occur in both repletion heat patterns and vacuity cold patterns. From the choice of medicinals in the recommended formula, we know that the condition in this line is caused by vacuity cold in the stomach, water-rheum collecting internally, turbid yīn failing to bear downward, and yīn occupying the position of yáng. As a result, yáng in the chest fails to spread out, the qì dynamic is inhibited, and qì counterflow distresses the stomach so that harmonious downbearing breaks down.

The text recommends Evodia Decoction (*zhū yú tāng*) as the formula of choice because it has the effect of warming the center and supplementing vacuity, while also dissipating cold and downbearing counterflow. In this formula, evodia (*wú zhū yú*) and fresh ginger (*shēng jiāng*) warm the stomach and dissipate cold, harmonize the stomach and downbear counterflow, and transform rheum and stop retching. Ginseng (*rén shēn*) and jujube (*dà zǎo*) boost the spleen and calm the stomach, while also warming the center and supplementing vacuity.

Line 17.9

干呕，吐涎沫，头痛者，茱萸汤主之。

Gān ǒu, tù xián mò, tóu tòng zhě, zhū yú tāng zhǔ zhī.

For dry retching, ejection of drool and foam, and headache, Evodia Decoction (*zhū yú tāng*) governs.[1]

TEXT NOTE, LINE 17.9

[1] A comment included in the received text reads: "For the formula, see above." This refers to the preceding line 17.8.

SYNOPSIS, LINE 17.9

This line describes the signs and treatment of vomiting and dry retching with stomach vacuity, collecting rheum, and counterflow ascent of liver qì.

COMMENTARY, LINE 17.9

Dry retching means that the patient makes the sound of vomiting without expelling any matter. It is a symptom of stomach qì counterflow ascent due to liver qì invading the stomach. Ejection of foam and drool is a sign of cold rheum collecting in the stomach. The liver channel rises into the vertex, and when liver qì carries yīn cold evil along its channel to surge upward, the result is headache. As with the previous line, this pathomechanism is also related to stomach qì vacuity cold and to rheum evil flooding upward. Thus, the text again recommends treatment with Evodia Decoction (*zhū yú tāng*), so as to warm yáng and dissipate cold, as well as to downbear counterflow and check retching.

Line 17.10

呕而肠鸣，心下痞者，半夏泻心汤主之。

半夏（洗） 半升 黄芩 干姜 人参各三两 黄连一两 大枣十二枚 甘草三两（炙）

右七味，以水一斗，煮取六升，去滓，再煮取三升，温服一升，日三服。

Ǒu ér cháng míng, xīn xià pǐ zhě, bàn xià xiè xīn tāng zhǔ zhī.

Bàn xià bàn shēng (xǐ); huáng qín, gān jiāng, rén shēn gè sān liǎng; huáng lián yī liǎng; dà zǎo shí èr méi; gān cǎo sān liǎng (zhì)

Yòu qī wèi, yǐ shuǐ yī dǒu, zhǔ qǔ liù shēng, qù zǐ, zài zhǔ qǔ sān shēng, wēn fú yī shēng, rì sān fú.

For retching with rumbling intestines and glomus below the heart, Pinellia Heart-Draining Decoction (半夏泻心汤 *bàn xià xiè xīn tāng*) governs.

Pinellia Heart-Draining Decoction (半夏泻心汤 *bàn xià xiè xīn tāng*)

- pinellia (半夏 *bàn xià*, Pinelliae Rhizoma) ½ *shēng* (wash)
- scutellaria (黄芩 *huáng qín*, Scutellariae Radix) 3 *liǎng*
- dried ginger (干姜 *gān jiāng*, Zingiberis Rhizoma) 3 *liǎng*
- ginseng (人参 *rén shēn*, Ginseng Radix) 3 *liǎng*
- coptis (黄连 *huáng lián*, Coptidis Rhizoma) 1 *liǎng*
- jujube (大枣 *dà zǎo*, Jujubae Fructus) 12 pieces
- licorice (甘草 *gān cǎo*, Glycyrrhizae Radix) 3 *liǎng* (mix-fry)

Boil the above seven ingredients in one *dǒu* of water to get six *shēng*. Remove the dregs and boil again to get three *shēng*. Take one *shēng* [per dose] warm, three times a day.

Synopsis, Line 17.10

This line describes the signs and treatment of retching and vomiting in combined cold and heat patterns.

Commentary, Line 17.10

The signs described in this line include retching and vomiting in the upper body, glomus obstruction in the center, and rumbling intestines in the lower body. Retching and vomiting are caused by stomach qì vacuity cold, turbid evil invading the stomach, and breakdown of harmonious downbearing. Rumbling intestines suggest that vacuity cold in the center burner has caused turbid evil to invade the clear and caused spleen qì to fall downward. Lastly, glomus below the heart means glomus blockage, fullness, and oppression in the stomach duct. This is caused by yáng vacuity in the center burner and by cold and heat binding with each other, as a result of which the stomach fails to downbear the turbid, and the spleen fails to move and transform. This is thus a combined cold and heat pattern with glomus blockage in the center burner causing a breakdown of downbearing and upbearing.

The recommended treatment is Pinellia Heart-Draining Decoction *(xiè xīn tāng*), which is intended to open binds, eliminate glomus, harmonize the stomach, and downbear counterflow. In the formula, dried ginger (*gān jiāng*) and pinellia (*bàn xià*) dissipate cold and downbear counterflow; scutellaria (*huáng qín*) and coptis (*huáng lián*) downbear and clear heat; ginseng (*rén shēn*), licorice (*gān cǎo*), and jujube (*dà zǎo*) supplement and boost center qì. Altogether, these ingredients downbear with bitterness and open with acridity, thereby harmonizing the intestines and stomach.

Line 17.11

干呕而利者，黄芩加半夏生姜汤主之。

黄芩三两 甘草二两（炙） 芍药一两 半夏半升 生姜三两 大枣十二个

右六味，以水一斗，煮取三升，去滓，温服一升，日再、夜一服。

Gān ǒu ér lì zhě, huáng qín jiā bàn xià shēng jiāng tāng zhǔ zhī.

Huáng qín sān liǎng; gān cǎo èr liǎng (zhì); sháo yào yī liǎng; bàn xià bàn shēng; shēng jiāng sān liǎng; dà zǎo shí èr ge

Yòu liù wèi, yǐ shuǐ yī dǒu, zhǔ qǔ sān shēng, qù zǐ, wēn fú yī shēng, rì zài, yè yī fú.

For dry retching with diarrhea, Scutellaria Decoction Plus Pinellia and Fresh Ginger (黄芩加半夏生姜汤 *huáng qín jiā bàn xià shēng jiāng tāng*) governs.

Scutellaria Decoction Plus Pinellia and Fresh Ginger (黄芩加半夏生姜汤 *huáng qín jiā bàn xià shēng jiāng tāng*)

- scutellaria (黄芩 *huáng qín*, Scutellariae Radix) 3 *liǎng*
- licorice (甘草 *gān cǎo*, Glycyrrhizae Radix) 2 *liǎng* (mix-fry)
- peony (芍药 *sháo yào*, Paeoniae Radix) 1 *liǎng*
- pinellia (半夏 *bàn xià*, Pinelliae Rhizoma) ½ *shēng*
- fresh ginger (生姜 *shēng jiāng*, Zingiberis Rhizoma Recens) 3 *liǎng*
- jujube (大枣 *dà zǎo*, Jujubae Fructus) 12 pieces

Boil the above six ingredients in one *dǒu* of water to get three *shēng*. Remove the dregs. Take one *shēng* [per dose] warm, twice a day and once at night.

Synopsis, Line 17.11

This line describes the signs and treatment of dry retching with diarrhea.

Commentary, Line 17.11

Both dry retching and diarrhea are diseases of the stomach and intestines that are caused by invasion of evil heat. Diarrhea results from heat distressing the intestines and preventing the spleen from moving and transforming, so that the turbid is not separated from the clear. Dry retching results from damp-heat evil invading the stomach and causing counterflow ascent of stomach qì. Symptoms should include bitterness in the mouth, a slightly yellow and slimy tongue fur, abdominal pain and rumbling intestines, and distention in the stomach duct.

The focus of this disease is the intestinal tract, and thus in clinic we should concentrate on treatment of the diarrhea. In the recommended formula, Scutellaria Decoction Plus Pinellia and Fresh Ginger (*huáng qín jiā bàn xià shēng jiāng tāng*), Scutellaria Decoction (*huáng qín tāng*) clears heat and checks diarrhea, while the pinellia (*bàn xià*) and fresh ginger (*shēng jiāng*) assist by harmonizing the stomach and downbearing counterflow. Overall, the formula cures both retching and diarrhea by treating damp-heat with acridity for opening and bitterness for downbearing.

Line 17.12

诸呕吐，谷不得下者，小半夏汤主之。

Zhū ǒu tù, gǔ bù dé xià zhě, xiǎo bàn xià tāng zhǔ zhī.

For all [types of] retching and vomiting with inability to get grain down,[1] Minor Pinellia Decoction (小半夏汤 *xiǎo bàn xià tāng*) governs.

Text Notes, Line 17.12

[1] Inability to get grain down 谷不得下 *gǔ bù dé xià*: Inability to eat. "Grain" represents food.

[2] A comment included in the received text reads: "For the formula, see in the chapter on Phlegm-Rheum." (方见痰饮中。) This refers to line 12.28 in Chapter 12, "Phlegm-Rheum and Cough."

Synopsis, Line 17.12

This line describes the signs and treatment of vomiting due to collected rheum in the stomach.

Commentary, Line 17.12

While the presenting signs of retching and vomiting can be rather complex, the pathomechanism is always caused by impaired harmonious downbearing and counterflow ascent of stomach qì. We can differentiate patterns by the presence of cold, heat, vacuity, repletion, and phlegm-rheum. Retching and vomiting most commonly arise as a result of cold and collected rheum in the stomach. Therefore the present line addresses "all [types of] retching and vomiting," and recommends as a general treatment Minor Pinellia Decoction (*xiǎo bàn xià tāng*), which has the effect of dissipating cold, transforming rheum, harmonizing the stomach, and downbearing counterflow. In this formula, pinellia (*bàn xià*) opens rheum bind and downbears counterflow qì, while fresh ginger (*shēng jiāng*) dissipates cold and harmonizes the stomach.

Line 17.13

呕吐而病在膈上，后思水者解，急与之。思水者，猪苓散主之。

猪苓　茯苓　白朮各等分

右三味，杵为散，饮服方寸匕，日三服。

Ǒu tù ér bìng zài gé shàng, hòu sī shuǐ zhě jiě, jí yǔ zhī. Sī shuǐ zhě, zhū líng sǎn zhǔ zhī.

Zhū líng, fú líng, bái zhú, gè děng fèn

Yòu sān wèi, chǔ wéi sǎn, yǐn fú fāng cùn bǐ, rì sān fú.

In cases of retching and vomiting when the disease is above the diaphragm, if the patient after [retching or vomiting] desires [to drink] water, [this means that the condition] is resolving. Urgently give [the patient water to drink]. When [the patient] desires [to drink] water, Polyporus Powder (猪苓散 *zhū líng sǎn*) governs.

Polyporus Powder (猪苓散 *zhū líng sǎn*)
polyporus (猪苓 *zhū líng*, Polyporus) poria (茯苓 *fú líng*, Poria) white atractylodes (白朮 *bái zhú*, Atractylodis Macrocephalae Rhizoma)

Pestle the above three ingredients into a powder and take a square-inch-spoonful in liquid, three times a day.

Synopsis, Line 17.13

This line describes the signs and treatment of retching and vomiting due to water-rheum.

Commentary, Line 17.13

The first phrase, "retching and vomiting when the disease above the diaphragm," means that disease above the diaphragm is manifesting in retching and vomiting. This indicates that the condition is caused by heat in the diaphragm, which is contending with water-rheum collecting in the stomach. The result of this is counterflow ascent of stomach qì and hence retching and vomiting. If such a patient feels thirst after retching and vomiting, this is a positive sign, because it means that the heat and water-rheum in the diaphragm have been removed and that yáng has recovered. Because the water-rheum evil is gone, it is now permissible to gradually give the patient fluid to slowly moisten the dryness and harmonize stomach qì. The signs in the present line were originally caused by heat in the diaphragm and vacuity in the spleen. The heat had caused thirst, but excessive drinking had caused retching when the stomach was unable to disperse water. The retching and vomiting had eliminated the old rheum. Nevertheless, at this stage, if you allow the patient to drink indiscriminately, new rheum can accumulate if the stomach is still weak and therefore unable to disperse water. Thus you must continue medical treatment, for which the text recommends Polyporus Powder (*zhū líng sǎn*) to fortify the spleen and disinhibit water. In the formula, polyporus (*zhū líng*) and poria (*fú líng*) disinhibit water by bland percolation, and white atractylodes (*bái zhú*) fortifies the spleen to move dampness. Because the condition is related to the presence of water-rheum, we prepare the formula in powder form instead of decocting it, to assist stomach qì in dispersing water-rheum.

Line 17.14

呕而脉弱，小便复利，身有微热，见厥者，难治，四逆汤主之。

附子（一枚生用） 干姜一两半 甘草二两（炙）

右三味，以水三升，煮取一升二合，去滓，分温再服。强人可大附子一枚，干姜三两。

Ǒu ér mài ruò, xiǎo biàn fù lì, shēn yǒu wēi rè, jiàn jué zhě, nán zhì, sì nì tāng zhǔ zhī.

Fù zǐ yī méi (shēng yòng); gān jiāng yī liǎng bàn; gān cǎo èr liǎng (zhì)

Yòu sān wèi, yǐ shuǐ sān shēng, zhǔ qǔ yī shēng èr gě, qù zǐ, fēn wēn zài fú. Qiáng rén kě dà fù zǐ yī méi, gān jiāng sān liǎng.

If retching [is followed by] a weak pulse, urination that is again uninhibited, slight heat [effusion] in the body, and there is manifestation of reversal,[1] [the condition] is difficult to treat. Counterflow Cold Decoction (四逆汤 *sì nì tāng*) governs.

Counterflow Cold Decoction (四逆汤 *sì nì tāng*)

- aconite (附子 *fù zǐ*, Aconiti Radix Lateralis Praeparata) 1 piece (use raw)
- dried ginger (干姜 *gān jiāng*, Zingiberis Rhizoma) 1 ½ *liǎng*
- licorice (甘草 *gān cǎo*, Glycyrrhizae Radix) 2 *liǎng* (mix-fry)

Boil the above three ingredients in three *shēng* of water to get one *shēng* and two *gě*. Remove the dregs. Divide into two doses and take warm. For a strong patient, you can use a large piece of aconite (*fù zǐ*) and three *liǎng* of dried ginger (*gān jiāng*).

Text Note, Line 17.14

[1] Reversal 厥 *jué*: Reversal (counterflow) cold of the limbs.

Synopsis, Line 17.14

This line describes the signs and treatment of vacuity cold retching and vomiting with exuberant yīn repelling yáng.

Commentary, Line 17.14

When retching and vomiting manifests with the accompanying symptoms of weak pulse, uninhibited urination, slight generalized heat effusion, and cold in the four limbs, the disease is related to exuberant yīn repelling yáng. In such patients, counterflow ascent of yīn cold and vacuity of yang qì causes retching with a weak pulse. Yīn exuberance in the lower body causes kidney qì to become insecure, thereby increasing urination. When yīn is exuberant inside the body, it repels yáng to the outside; hence we see slight heat effusion in the body, but counterflow cold in the limbs. When you see this constellation of symptoms, yáng qì is critically close to desertion. The text therefore emphasizes that the condition is difficult to treat.

Consequently, you must urgently rescue and restore yáng, for which the text recommends Counterflow Cold Decoction (*sì nì tāng*). In this formula, aconite (*fù zi*) restores yáng and rescues counterflow; dried ginger (*gān jiāng*) warms the center and dissipates cold; and licorice (*gān cǎo*) boosts qì and harmonizes the center. In combination, the formula has the effect of warming the center, dissipating cold, restoring yáng, and rescuing counterflow.

Line 17.15

呕而发热者，小柴胡汤主之。

柴胡半斤　黄芩三两　人参三两　甘草三两　半夏半升　生姜三两　大枣十二枚

右七味，以水一斗二升，煮取六升，去滓，再煎取三升，温服一升，日三服。

Ǒu ér fā rè zhě, xiǎo chái hú tāng zhǔ zhī.

Chái hú bàn jīn; huáng qín sān liǎng; rén shēn sān liǎng; gān cǎo sān liǎng; bàn xià bàn shēng; shēng jiāng sān liǎng; dà zǎo shí èr méi

Yòu qī wèi, yǐ shuǐ yī dǒu èr shēng, zhǔ qǔ liù shēng, qù zǐ, zài jiān qǔ sān shēng, wēn fú yī shēng, rì sān fú.

For retching with heat effusion, Minor Bupleurum Decoction (小柴胡汤 *xiǎo chái hú tāng*) governs.

Minor Bupleurum Decoction (小柴胡汤 *xiǎo chái hú tāng*)

- bupleurum (柴胡 *chái hú*, Bupleuri Radix) ½ *jīn*[1]
- scutellaria (黄芩 *huáng qín*, Scutellariae Radix) 3 *liǎng*
- ginseng (人参 *rén shēn*, Ginseng Radix) 3 *liǎng*
- licorice (甘草 *gān cǎo*, Glycyrrhizae Radix) 3 *liǎng*
- pinellia (半夏 *bàn xià*, Pinelliae Rhizoma) ½ *shēng*
- fresh ginger (生姜 *shēng jiāng*, Zingiberis Rhizoma Recens) 3 *liǎng*
- jujube (大枣 *dà zǎo*, Jujubae Fructus) 12 pieces

Boil the above seven ingredients in one *dǒu* and two *shēng* of water to get six *shēng*. Remove the dregs and boil again to get three *shēng*. Take one *shēng* [per dose] warm, three times a day.

TEXT NOTES, LINE 17.15

[1] One-half jīn 半斤 *bàn jīn*: Several other versions of this formula have "one-half shēng" instead.

SYNOPSIS, LINE 17.15

This line describes the signs and treatment of retching due to lesser yáng evil heat distressing the stomach.

COMMENTARY, LINE 17.15

Retching with heat effusion is a sign of evil heat in lesser yáng distressing the stomach and causing retching and vomiting due to counterflow ascent of stomach qì. In clinical practice, it is accompanied by signs such as bitterness in the mouth, dry throat, and fullness in the chest and rib-side. We treat it with Minor Bupleurum Decoction (*xiǎo chái hú tāng*), so as to course, resolve, and clear heat, and to harmonize the stomach and downbear counterflow. In this formula, bupleurum (*chái hú*) and scutellaria (*huáng qín*) resolve the exterior and clear heat; pinellia (*bàn xià*) and fresh ginger (*shēng jiāng*) downbear counterflow and check retching; and ginseng (*rén shēn*), licorice (*gān cǎo*), and jujube (*dà zǎo*) supplement vacuity and calm the center.

Line 17.16

胃反呕吐者，大半夏汤主之。

半夏二升（洗完用） 人参三两 白蜜一升

右三味，以水一斗二升，和蜜扬之二百四十遍，煮药取二升半，温服一升，余分再服。

Wèi fǎn ǒu tù zhě, dà bàn xià tāng zhǔ zhī.

Bàn xià èr shēng (xǐ wán yòng); rén shēn sān liǎn; bái mì yī shēng

Yòu sān wèi, yǐ shuǐ yī dǒu èr shēng, huó mì yáng zhī èr bǎi sì shí biàn, zhǔ yào qǔ èr shēng bàn, wēn fú yī shēng, yú fēn zài fú.

For stomach reflux retching and vomiting, Major Pinellia Decoction (大半夏汤 *dà bàn xià tāng*) governs.[1]

Major Pinellia Decoction (大半夏汤 *dà bàn xià tāng*)
pinellia (半夏 *bàn xià*, Pinelliae Rhizoma) 2 *shēng* (use after washing)
ginseng (人参 *rén shēn*, Ginseng Radix) 3 *liǎng*
white honey (白蜜 *bái mì*, Mel) 1 *shēng*

Of the above three ingredients, blend the honey into one *dou* and two *shēng* of water, whipping it 240 times. [Add the other] ingredients and boil to get-two and-a-half *shēng*. Take one *shéng* [per dose] warm. Divide the rest into two doses.

TEXT NOTE, LINE 17.16

[1] The commentary adds: "The *Qiān Jīn Fāng* states: 'treats refluxing stomach, inability to receive food, and vomiting after ingesting food.' The *Wài Tái Mì Yào* ("Secrets from the *Wài Tái* Library") states: 'treats retching and glomus and hardness below the heart.'"

SYNOPSIS, LINE 17.16

This line describes treatment of stomach reflux due to vacuity cold.

COMMENTARY, LINE 17.16

When a patient manifests with vomiting in the evening of food eaten in the morning, vomiting in the morning of food eaten in the evening, and vomiting of lodged grain and of clear and cold untransformed substances, this is called stomach reflux retching and vomiting. It is caused by vacuity cold of stomach qì impairing the ripening and rotting of water and grain. When spleen yáng is vacuous, it is unable to transform qì and engender liquid. As a result, the intestinal tract is deprived of moisture, which manifests in dry stool like goat's droppings. It can also cause dryness bind in the stomach and intestines, which impairs the stomach's harmonious downbearing, causing counterflow ascent and resultant vomiting and retching.

This condition is treated with Major Pinellia Decoction (*dà bàn xià tāng*), which opens binds, downbears counterflow, supplements vacuity, and moistens dryness. This formula uses large amounts of pinellia (*bàn xià*) to open binds and downbear counterflow, as well as large amounts of ginseng (*rén shēn*) and white honey (*bái mì*) to supplement vacuity and moisten dryness.

Line 17.17

食已即吐者，大黄甘草汤主之。

大黄四两　甘草一两

右二味，以水三升，煮取一升，分温再服。

Shí yǐ jí tù zhě, dà huáng gān cǎo tāng zhǔ zhī.

Dà huáng sì liǎng; gān cǎo yī liǎng

Yòu èr wèi, yǐ shuǐ sān shēng, zhǔ qǔ yī shēng, fēn wēn zài fú.

For vomiting [occuring] immediately after eating, Rhubarb and Licorice Decoction (大黄甘草汤 *dà huáng gān cǎo tāng*) governs.[1]

Rhubarb and Licorice Decoction (大黄甘草汤 *dà huáng gān cǎo tāng*)
rhubarb (大黄 *dà huáng*, Rhei Radix et Rhizoma) 4 *liǎng* licorice (甘草 *gān cǎo*, Glycyrrhizae Radix) 1 *liǎng*

Boil the above two ingredients in three *shēng* of water to get one *shēng*. Divide into two [doses] and take warm.

TEXT NOTE, LINE 17.17

[1] The commentary adds: "The formula in the *Wài Tái Mì Yào* ("Secrets from the *Wài Tái* Library") further [states that it] treats vomiting of water."

SYNOPSIS, LINE 17.17

This line describes the signs and treatment of vomiting due to gastrointestinal repletion heat.

COMMENTARY, LINE 17.17

When food is immediately vomited up after being ingested, this indicates that repletion heat is congesting the gastrointestinal tract so that bowel qì is stopped. Below, this results in breakdown of conveyance by the intestines and constipation; above, it results in the stomach failing to absorb grain by downbearing and instead forcing it upward in strong urgent surges.

For treatment, the text recommends Rhubarb and Licorice Decoction (*dà huáng gān cǎo tāng*), because of its effect of draining heat and removing repletion, thereby getting rid of repletion heat, freeing stool, and harmonizing stomach qì, so that retching and vomiting stops on its own. In the formula, rhubarb (*dà huáng*) flushes repletion heat out of the stomach and intestines, while licorice (*gān cǎo*) relaxes tension and harmonizes the stomach. Together, these medicinals act by offensive precipitation, but without damaging right.

Line 17.18

胃反，吐而渴，欲饮水者，茯苓泽泻汤主之。

茯苓半斤　泽泻四两　甘草二两　桂枝二两　白朮三两　生姜四两

右六味，以水一斗，煮取三升，纳泽泻再煮取二升半，温服八合，日三服。

Wèi fǎn, tù ér kě, yù yǐn shuǐ zhě, fú líng zé xiè tāng zhǔ zhī.

Fú líng bàn jīn; zé xiè sì liǎng; gān cǎo èr liǎng; guì zhī èr liǎng; bái zhú sān liǎng; shēng jiāng sì liǎng

Yòu liù wèi, yǐ shuǐ yī dǒu, zhǔ qǔ sān shēng, nà zé xiè zài zhǔ qǔ èr shēng bàn, wēn fú bā gě, rì sān fú.

For stomach reflux with thirst and desire to drink water after vomiting, Poria and Alisma Decoction (茯苓泽泻汤 *fú líng zé xiè tāng*)[1] governs.

Poria and Alisma Decoction (茯苓泽泻汤 *fú líng zé xiè tāng*)

poria (茯苓 *fú líng*, Poria) ½ *jīn*
alisma (泽泻 *zé xiè*, Alismatis Rhizoma) 4 *liǎng*
licorice (甘草 *gān cǎo*, Glycyrrhizae Radix) 2 *liǎng*
cinnamon twig (桂枝 *guì zhī*, Cinnamomi Ramulus) 2 *liǎng*
white atractylodes (白朮 *bái zhú*, Atractylodis Macrocephalae Rhizoma) 3 *liǎng*
fresh ginger (生姜 *shēng jiāng*, Zingiberis Rhizoma Recens) 3 *liǎng*

[Take] the above six ingredients. Using one *dǒu* of water, boil to get three *shēng*. Remove the alisma (*zé xiè*), and boil again to get two-and-a-half *shēng*. Take eight *gě* warm, three times a day.

TEXT NOTE, LINE 17.18

[1] The commentary adds : "The *Wài Tái Mì Yào* ("Secrets from the *Wài Tái* Library") [states:] 'To treat dispersion-thirst, expiring pulse, stomach reflux, and vomiting of ingested food, add one *shēng* of wheat (*xiǎo mài*).' "

SYNOPSIS, LINE 17.18

This line describes the signs and treatment of retching and thirst due to rheum obstruction and qì counterflow.

COMMENTARY, LINE 17.18

In the present line, "stomach reflux" does not refer to vacuity cold stomach reflux, but to the pathomechanism of rheum collecting in the stomach, impairing harmonious downbearing, and thereby causing counterflow ascent and retching. Because rheum collects instead of being transformed, and the spleen fails to transport liquid upward, we see thirst and desire to drink liquid. Water-rheum flooding upward causes further retching and vomiting, which again results in thirst and drinking of liquid, which again assists the rheum evil. Hence, vomiting and drinking and thirst exacerbate each other in a vicious cycle.

This condition is treated with Poria and Alisma Decoction (*fú líng zé xiè tāng*) because of its ability to disinhibit water and transform rheum. In this formula, poria (*fú líng*) and alisma (*zé xiè*) act as sovereigns to disinhibit water by bland percolation, with the cooperation of cinnamon twig (*guì zhī*), which frees yáng, and of fresh ginger (*shēng jiāng*), which harmonizes the stomach. These are assisted by white atractylodis (*bái zhú*) and licorice (*gān cǎo*), which fortify the spleen and supplement the center. Together, these ingredients have the effect of transforming qì and moving water, thereby checking retching and thirst.

Line 17.19

吐后渴欲得水而贪饮者，文蛤汤主之。兼主微风脉紧、头痛。

文蛤五两　麻黄　甘草　生姜各三两
石膏五两　杏仁五十个　大枣十二枚

右七味，以水六升，煮取二升，温服一升，汗出即愈。

Tù hòu kě yù dé shuǐ ér tān yǐn zhě, wén gé tāng zhǔ zhī. Jiān zhǔ wēi fēng mài jǐn, tóu tòng.

Wén gé wǔ liǎng; má huáng,, gān cǎo, shēng jiāng gè sān liǎng; shí gāo wǔ liǎng; xìng rén wǔ shí ge; dà zǎo shí èr méi

Yòu qī wèi, yǐ shuǐ liù shēng, zhǔ qǔ èr shēng, wēn fú yī shēng, hàn chū jí yù.

For thirst with desire for water and rapacious drinking after vomiting, Meretrix Clam Shell Decoction (文蛤汤 *wén gé tāng*) governs. It also governs slight wind with a tight pulse and headache.

Meretrix Clam Shell Decoction (文蛤汤 *wén gé tāng*)

meretrix clam shell (文蛤 *wén gé*, Meretricis Concha) 5 *liǎng*
ephedra (麻黄 *má huáng*, Ephedrae Herba) 3 *liǎng*
licorice (甘草 *gān cǎo*, Glycyrrhizae Radix) 3 *liǎng*
fresh ginger (生姜 *shēng jiāng*, Zingiberis Rhizoma Recens) 3 *liǎng*
gypsum (石膏 *shí gāo*, Gypsum Fibrosum) 5 *liǎng*
apricot kernel (杏仁 *xìng rén*, Armeniacae Semen) 50 pieces
jujube (大枣 *dà zǎo*, Jujubae Fructus) 12 pieces

Boil the above seven ingredients in six *shēng* of water to get two *shēng*. Take one *sheng* [per dose] warm. When the patient sweats, recovery will follow.

SYNOPSIS, LINE 17.19

This line describes the signs and treatment of rapacious drinking after vomiting.

COMMENTARY, LINE 17.19

Thirst after vomiting is a normal reaction because vomiting damages liquid and the patient therefore wants to drink liquid to alleviate the dryness. However, "rapacious drinking" after vomiting is a pathological change that occurs when heat and rheum bind in the patient's stomach, and after vomiting, the water is expelled but the heat remains, which then depletes liquid and thereby deprives the body of moisture. This condition possibly manifests also with a tight pulse, headache, and aversion to wind and cold, which indicates that it is caused by a contraction of external evil, which has not resolved.

The recommended treatment is Meretrix Clam Shell Decoction (*wén gé tāng*), because this formula has the effect of clearing heat, engendering liquid, resolving the exterior, and dissipating evil. Among its ingredients, meretrix clam shell (*wén gé*) and gypsum (*shí gāo*) clear heat, engender liquid, moisten dryness, and check thirst; ephedra (*má huáng*) and apricot kernel (*xìng rén*) diffuse the lung and effuse the exterior; and fresh ginger (*shēng jiāng*), jujube (*dà zǎo*), and licorice (*gān cǎo*) calm the center and harmonize construction and defense. In this way, you will resolve the exterior and clear heat, thereby curing the thirst naturally.

Line 17.20

干呕吐逆，吐涎沫，半夏干姜散主之。

半夏　干姜各等分

右二味，杵为散，取方寸匕，浆水一升半，煎取七合，顿服之。

Gān ǒu tù nì, tù xián mò, bàn xià gān jiāng sǎn zhǔ zhī.

Bàn xià, gān jiāng gè děng fèn

Yòu èr wèi, chǔ wéi sǎn, qǔ fāng cùn bǐ, jiāng shuǐ yī shēng bàn, jiān qǔ qī gě, dùn fú zhī.

For dry retching, vomiting counterflow, and vomiting of drool and foam, Pinellia and Dried Ginger Powder (半夏干姜散 *bàn xià gān jiāng sǎn*) governs.

Pinellia and Dried Ginger Powder (半夏干姜散 *bàn xià gān jiāng sǎn*)
pinellia (半夏 *bàn xià*, Pinelliae Rhizoma) dried ginger (干姜 *gān jiāng*, Zingiberis Rhizoma) in equal proportions.

Pestle the above two ingredients into a powder. Mix a square-inch-spoonful with one-and-one-half *shēng* of sour rice milk (*jiāng shuǐ*) and simmer to get seven *gě*. Quaff.

SYNOPSIS, LINE 17.20

This line describes the signs and treatment of vomiting counterflow due to spleen-stomach yáng vacuity and exuberance of cold rheum.

COMMENTARY, LINE 17.20

Symptoms of dry retching, vomiting counterflow, and vomiting of drool and foam that occur together indicate that the patient suffers from insufficiency of center yáng. Vacuity cold in the stomach impairs downbearing of the turbid, and vacuity of spleen yáng impairs dissipation of liquid. Consequently, cold rheum is not transformed and engenders phlegm-drool, which follows stomach qì to ascend counterflow and is ejected as drool and foam. Because the spleen is cold, drool is not contained; because the stomach is cold, its qì ascends counterflow, causing dry retching and vomiting counterflow, and possibly vomiting of drool and foam.

Pinellia and Dried Ginger Powder (*bàn xià gān jiāng sǎn*) is recommended, so as to warm the center and dissipate cold, while at the same time to downbear counterflow and check retching. In this formula, pinellia (*bàn xià*) downbears counterflow, checks retching, and warms and transforms water-rheum, while dried ginger (*gān jiāng*) warms the center and dissipates cold. These ingredients are simmered in sour rice milk (*jiāng shuǐ*), which increases the effect of regulating the center and checking retching. The formula is meant to be quaffed to concentrate the strength of the medicinals and ensure efficacy.

Line 17.21

病人胸中似喘不喘，似呕不呕，似哕不哕，彻心中愦愦然无奈者，生姜半夏汤主之。

半夏半升　生姜汁一升

右二味，以水三升，煮半夏取二升，内生姜汁，煮取一升半，小冷分四服，日三、夜一服，止，停后服。

Bìng rén xiōng zhōng sì chuǎn bù chuǎn, sì ǒu bù ǒu, sì yuē bù yuē, chè xīn zhōng kuì kuì rán wú nài zhě, shēng jiāng bàn xià tāng zhǔ zhī.

Bàn xià bàn shēng; shēng jiāng zhī yī shēng

Yòu èr wèi, yǐ shuǐ sān shēng, zhǔ bàn xià qǔ èr shēng, nà shēng jiāng zhī, zhǔ qǔ yī shēng bàn, xiǎo lěng fēn sì fú, rì sān, yè yī fú, zhǐ, tíng hòu fú.

When a patient presents with [a sensation] in the chest that resembles panting but is not real panting, with [a sensation] that resembles retching but is not real retching, with [a sensation] that resembles hiccup but is not real hiccup, and with unbearable vexation and oppression piercing the heart, Fresh Ginger and Pinellia Decoction (生姜半夏汤 *shēng jiāng bàn xià tāng*) governs.

Fresh Ginger and Pinellia Decoction (生姜半夏汤 *shēng jiāng bàn xià tāng*)

pinellia (半夏 *bàn xià*, Pinelliae Rhizoma) ½ *shēng*

fresh ginger juice (生姜汁 *shēng jiāng zhī*, Zingiberis Rhizoma Recens) 1 *shēng*

Of the above two ingredients, boil the pinellia (*bàn xià*) in three *shēng* of water to get two *shēng*. Add the fresh ginger (*shēng jiāng*) juice and boil to get one-and-one-half *sheng*. When it has cooled slightly, divide into four doses, and take three times a day and once at night. [As soon as the symptoms] are checked, stop taking further doses.

SYNOPSIS, LINE 17.21

This line describes the signs and treatment of cold rheum contending and binding in the chest.

COMMENTARY, LINE 17.21

The chest is the sea of qì, the place where clear qì exits and enters, downbears and upbears. It is also the place where the heart and lung reside and it borders the spleen and stomach below. If cold rheum binds in the chest, it blocks and depresses chest yáng and impedes the upbearing and downbearing and exiting and entering of qì. Thus we see the symptoms of apparent panting, retching, and hiccup, as well as extreme vexation, oppression, and discomfort in the chest. In spite of the fact that the text emphasizes the subjectivity of these sensations, the condition should also objectively manifest in pathological changes that reflect cold rheum binding in the chest, obstructing the qì dynamic, affecting the lung and stomach, and distressing the heart.

Because the condition is caused by cold rheum contending and binding, the recommended treatment is to transform rheum with acridity and warmth, and to open depression and dissipate binds. For this purpose, the text recommends Fresh Ginger and Pinellia Decoction (*shēng jiāng bàn xià tāng*), which contains the same ingredients as Minor Pinellia Decoction (*xiǎo bàn xià tāng*), but in different proportions and for different purposes. While Minor Pinellia Decoction (*xiǎo bàn xià tāng*) uses twice as much pinellia (*bàn xià*) to downbear counterflow and transform rheum, the formula here doubles the amount of fresh ginger (*shēng jiāng*) and uses the juice, to focus on dissipating rheum, removing binds, warming the stomach, and checking vomiting. To avoid an overly stimulating effect, the text recommends letting the preparation cool off a little then to divide it into four doses and take it gradually with attention to the effect.

Line 17.22

干呕，哕，若手足厥者，橘皮汤主之。

橘皮四两　生姜半斤

右二味，以水七升，煮取三升，温服一升，下咽则愈。

Gān ǒu, yuē, ruò shǒu zú jué zhě, jú pí tāng zhǔ zhī.

Jú pí sì liǎng; shēng jiāng bàn jīn

Yòu èr wèi, yǐ shuǐ qī shēng, zhǔ qǔ sān shēng, wēn fú yī shēng, xià yān zé yù.

For dry retching and hiccup, if there is reversal of the extremities, Tangerine Peel Decoction (橘皮汤 *jú pí tāng*) governs.

Tangerine Peel Decoction (橘皮汤 *jú pí tāng*)
tangerine peel (橘皮 *jú pí*, Citri Reticulatae Pericarpium) 4 *liǎng* fresh ginger (生姜 *shēng jiāng*, Zingiberis Rhizoma Recens) ½ *jīn*

Boil the above two ingredients in seven *shēng* of water to get three *shēng*. Take one *shēng* [per dose] warm. When it goes down the throat, recovery ensues.

SYNOPSIS, LINE 17.22

This line describes the signs and treatment of dry retching and hiccup due to stomach cold with qì counterflow.

COMMENTARY, LINE 17.22

Like vomiting and stomach reflux, dry retching and hiccup are also the result of stomach qì ascending counterflow, but in clinic, these symptoms are not as urgent and compelling. If they appear in conjunction with reversal cold in the extremities, this means that the condition is related to stomach cold qì counterflow. In these cases, cold evil has assailed the stomach and trapped stomach yáng, so that it is unable to reach the four tips. Hence we see reversal cold in the extremities. Dry retching and hiccup are the result of stomach qì being obstructed by cold evil, thereby failing to downbear harmoniously, and instead ascending counterflow.

The difference between the present condition and patterns of exuberant yīn and faint yáng, for which Counterflow Cold Decoction (*sì nì tāng*) is the governing formula, is merely a matter of degree, because the cold sensation in the present case is only slight. Therefore the recommended treatment is Tangerine Peel Decoction (*jú pí tāng*), which frees yáng and harmonizes the stomach. In the formula, tangerine peel (*jú pí*) rectifies qì and harmonizes the stomach, and fresh ginger (*shēng jiāng*) dissipates cold and checks retching. Together, they free yáng and get rid of cold, cause stomach qì to downbear harmoniously, and thereby treat dry retching, hiccup, and reversal cold.

Line 17.23

哕逆者，橘皮竹茹汤主之。

橘皮二斤　竹菇二升　大枣三十枚 生姜半斤　甘草五两　人参一两

右六味，以水一斗，煮取三升，温服一升，日三服。

Yuē nì zhě, jú pí zhú rú tāng zhǔ zhī.

Jú pí èr jīn; zhú rú èr shēng; dà zǎo sān shí méi; shēng jiāng bàn jīn; gān cǎo wǔ liǎng; rén shēn yī liǎng

Yòu liù wèi, yǐ shuǐ yī dǒu, zhǔ qǔ sān shēng, wēn fú yī shēng, rì sān fú.

For hiccup, Tangerine Peel and Bamboo Shavings Decoction (橘皮竹茹汤 *jú pí zhú rú tāng*) governs.

Tangerine Peel and Bamboo Shavings Decoction (橘皮竹茹汤 *jú pí zhú rú tāng*)

- tangerine peel (橘皮 *jú pí*, Citri Reticulatae Pericarpium) 2 *jīn*
- bamboo shavings (竹茹 *zhú rú*, Bambusae Caulis in Taenia) 2 *shēng*
- jujube (大枣 *dà zǎo*, Jujubae Fructus) 30 pieces
- fresh ginger (生姜 *shēng jiāng*, Zingiberis Rhizoma Recens) ½ *jīn*
- licorice (甘草 *gān cǎo*, Glycyrrhizae Radix) 5 *liǎng*
- ginseng (人参 *rén shēn*, Ginseng Radix) 1 *liǎng*

Boil the above six ingredients in one *dǒu* of water to get three *shēng*. Take one *shēng* [per dose] warm, three times a day.

Synopsis, Line 17.24

This line describes the treatment of hiccup due to stomach vacuity with heat.

Commentary, Line 17.24

The description of symptoms in this line only mentions hiccup, but we can infer the pattern from the formula recommended. Tangerine Peel and Bamboo Shavings Decoction (*jú pí zhú rú tāng*) has the intended effect of supplementing vacuity, clearing heat, harmonizing the stomach, and downbearing counterflow. Among its ingredients, tangerine peel (*jú pí*) and fresh ginger (*shēng jiāng*) rectify qì, harmonize the stomach, and downbear counterflow; bamboo shavings (*zhú rú*) clears heat and calms the center; ginseng (*rén shēn*), licorice (*gān cǎo*), and jujube (*dà zǎo*) supplement vacuity. Thus we know that the present line addresses a condition of hiccup caused by vacuity heat in the stomach and qì surging up counterflow. Accompanying symptoms should include vacuity vexation and disquietude, shortage of qì, dry mouth, heat in the heart of the palms and soles, and a vacuous rapid pulse. In treatment, hiccup is cured by eliminating vacuity heat, and as a result stomach qì is able to downbear.

Line 17.24

夫六府气绝于外者，手足寒，上气，脚缩；五藏气绝于内者，利不禁；下甚者，手足不仁。

Fū liù fŭ qì jué yú wài zhě, shǒu zú hán, shàng qì jiăo suō, wŭ zàng qì jué yú nèi zhě, lì bù jìn; xià shèn zhě, shǒu zú bù rén.

Expiry of the qì of the six bowels in the outer body[1] [manifests in] coldness of the extremities, qì ascent, and contracted feet. Expiry of the qì of the five viscera in the inner body [manifests in] diarrhea and incontinence. When the diarrhea is severe, the extremities become numb.

Text Note, Line 17.24

[1] Expiry of the qì of the six bowels in the outer body 六府气绝于外 *liù fŭ qì jué yú wài*: Expiry means vacuity. The outer body refers to the external status of the bowels by comparison with the viscera.

Synopsis, Line 17.24

This line describes the pathomechanism and prognosis of retching and vomiting, hiccup, and diarrhea.

Commentary, Line 17.24

In the human body, each bowel and viscera has their assigned functions. The six bowels belong to yáng, which governs defense and the outside; hence their qì flows in the exterior. The five viscera belong to yīn, which governs guarding and the inside; hence their qì flows in the interior. When the present line mentions "expiry of the qì of the six bowels in the outer body" and "expiry of the qì of the five viscera in the inner body," this refers to the pathomechanism of weakness of bowel and visceral qì, as a result of which qì is insufficient to move in the outer body, and to guard and secure and store in the inner body.

Because the stomach is the root of the six bowels and they all receive qì from the stomach, the key to vacuity of bowel qì is found in debilitation of stomach yáng. Similarly, the kidney is the root of earlier heaven in the five viscera, and the qì of all the viscera originates in the kidney. At the same time, the viscera are nourished by later heaven spleen qì, and vacuity of spleen-stomach yáng is bound to affect the kidney. The key to vacuity of visceral qì therefore lies in debilitation of spleen and kidney qì.

If stomach yáng is vacuous, the qì of all the bowels is unable to reach the exterior; hence we see cold of the extremities. Due to the breakdown of the stomach's functions of intake and harmonious downbearing, we see vomiting and hiccup. Because the upper burner is unable to receive qì from the center burner, ancestral qì also becomes vacuous; hence we see qì ascent and hasty panting. Because the sinews are deprived of the warming effected by yáng qì, we see sleeping in a curled position and contracted feet.

If both spleen and kidney qì are debilitated, visceral qì cannot be securely stored, which results in diarrhea. In the initial stage of the disease, spleen disease is more prevalent, which manifests in diarrhea and incontinence because splenic movement breaks down and clear qì falls downward. Over time, disease also affects the kidney by debilitating kidney yáng. Since the lower burner is not united, the diarrhea becomes critically severe. Yīn humor follows the diarrhea and is discharged through the lower body, as a result of which the four limbs and sinews are deprived of moistening and nourishment; hence we see numbness and insensitivity in the extremities.

Line 17.25

下利脉沉弦者，下重；脉大者，为未止；脉微弱数者，为欲自止，虽发热不死。

Xià lì mài chén xián zhě, xià zhòng; mài dà zhě, wéi wèi zhǐ; mài wēi ruò shuò zhě, wéi yù zì zhǐ, suī fā rè bù sǐ.

Diarrhea[1] with a sunken and stringlike pulse means lower-body heaviness.[2] If the pulse is large, it means it has not stopped. If the pulse is faint, weak, and rapid, it means it is about to stop spontaneously. Although there is heat effusion, [the person will] not die.

Text Notes, Line 17.25

[1] Diarrhea 下利 *xià lì*: Here referring to dysentery.

[2] Lower-body heaviness 下重 *xià zhòng*: Abdominal urgency and rectal heaviness.

Synopsis, Line 17.25

This line describes how to infer the signs and prognosis of dysentery from the pulse manifestation.

Commentary, Line 17.25

A sunken pulse indicates the interior, and a stringlike pulse indicates pain and tension. Diarrhea with a sunken stringlike pulse thus suggests that the disease evil has entered the interior and obstructed the qì dynamic so that bowel qì fails to flow freely. Manifestations of this condition are abdominal urgency, rectal heaviness, and abdominal pain.

A large pulse in patients with diarrhea indicates an internal exuberance of heat evil and advancement of the disease; hence the diarrhea is not about to stop. A faint, weak, and rapid pulse, on the other hand, indicates that evil qì is weakening and that yáng qì is gradually recovering; hence the diarrhea is about to stop. Diarrhea with heat effusion is normally a critical sign, indicating that yáng is collapsing on the outside and yīn is collapsing on the inside, while evil qì has not been removed yet. In the present line, however, even though the patient suffers from heat effusion, it will not be severe and will furthermore abate on its own. It is thus a sign that recovery will follow.

Line 17.26

下利，手足厥冷，无脉者，灸之不温，若脉不还，反微喘者死。少阴负趺阳者，为顺也。

Xià lì, shǒu zú jué lěng, wú mài zhě, jiǔ zhī bù wēn, ruò mài bù huán, fǎn wēi chuǎn zhě sǐ. Shào yīn fù fū yáng zhě, wéi shùn yě.

In patients with diarrhea, reversal cold of the extremities, and no [detectable] pulse, moxibustion will not warm [the extremities]. If the pulse does not return but there is slight panting, this means death. If the lesser yīn [pulse] is smaller than the instep yáng [pulse], this means a favorable [prognosis].

Synopsis, Line 17.26

This line explains how to differentiate between a positive and negative prognosis in cases with critical diarrhea.

Commentary, Line 17.26

If a patient presents with diarrhea and concurrent reversal cold of the extremities and no detectable pulse, this indicates an extremely serious situation where yīn and yáng are lost and the patient suffers from dual vacuity of spleen and kidney yáng. Because of the extent to which yáng is debilitated, you will not be able to treat the reversal cold with moxibustion. If the pulse does not return after moxibustion treatment, and you furthermore observe slight panting, this means that yīn qì is exhausted below and yáng qì is deserting above. This is a sign of death due to yīn and yáng separating. If the pulse returns, this is a good sign. The lesser yīn pulse indicates the kidney, and the instep yáng pulse indicates the spleen and stomach. If the lesser yīn pulse is weaker than the instep yáng pulse, this indicates that kidney yáng is being engendered by the spleen and stomach. Because yáng qì of the spleen and stomach has recovered, the patient is about to recover.

Line 17.27

下利, 有微热而渴, 脉弱者, 今自愈。

Xià lì, yǒu wēi rè ér kě, mài ruò zhě, jīn zì yù.

Diarrhea with slight heat [effusion], thirst, and a weak pulse means [the patient] is presently recovering spontaneously.

Synopsis, Line 17.27

This line describes the pulse and signs of yīn-cold diarrhea in the pre-recovery stage.

COMMENTARY, LINE 17.27

When a patient with diarrhea presents with a replete pulse and severe generalized heat effusion, this indicates that right is exuberant and evil replete, and that the dynamic of the disease has not weakened yet. By contrast, if diarrhea is followed by only mild heat effusion, as well as thirst and a desire to drink, and a pulse that may be slightly weak but is otherwise normal and not agitated, this means that the disease is about to be cured. In such cases, the slight heat effusion and thirst indicate that stomach yáng is recovering, and the weak pulse means that evil qì is debilitated and right qì is calm.

Line 17.28

下利脉数，有微热汗出，今自愈；设脉紧为未解。

Xià lì mài shù, yǒu wēi rè hàn chū, jīn zì yù; shè mài jǐn wéi wèi jiě.

In diarrhea, a rapid pulse with slight heat [effusion] and sweating means [the patient is] presently recovering spontaneously. But if the pulse is tight, it means that [the disease] is not yet resolving.

SYNOPSIS, LINE 17.28

This line explains how to determine from the pulse and signs whether spontaneous recovery of vacuity cold diarrhea is imminent or not.

COMMENTARY, LINE 17.28

In damp-heat diarrhea, a rapid pulse indicates that evil heat has not yet resolved and the patient is therefore not yet recovering. Nevertheless, the diarrhea discussed in the present line is related to dual vacuity of the spleen and kidney. In diarrhea from vacuity cold, a rapid pulse after diarrhea does not signify the continued presence of evil qì, but means that yáng qì has recovered, because this type of pulse indicates yáng. In addition, we see slight heat effusion and sweating, which suggest that the evil is removed and right is calm, and that the exterior is harmonious and the interior is resolved, so that yáng qì is moving freely. By contrast, if a patient presents with a tight pulse after diarrhea, this indicates that the exterior evil is not yet resolved, that yáng qì is not yet flowing freely, and that cold evil is still exuberant.

Line 17.29

下利脉数而渴者，今自愈；设不差，必圊脓血，以有热故也。

Xià lì mài shuò ér kě zhě, jīn zì yù; shè bù chài, bì qīng nóng xuè, yǐ yǒu rè gù yě.

In diarrhea, a rapid pulse with thirst means [the patient] is presently recovering spontaneously. If the patient does not recover, there will inevitably be latrine pus and blood.[1] This is caused by the presence of heat.

TEXT NOTE, LINE 17.29

[1] Latrine pus and blood 圊脓血 *qīng nóng xuè*: Pus and blood that the patient discovers in the latrine, i.e., pus and blood in the stool.

SYNOPSIS, LINE 17.29

This line describes the pathomechanism of excessive restoration of yáng in vacuity cold diarrhea.

Line 17.30

下利，脉反弦，发热身汗者，自愈。

Xià lì, mài fǎn xián, fā rè shēn hàn zhě, zì yù.

In diarrhea, a paradoxically stringlike pulse with heat effusion and generalized sweating means spontaneous recovery.

SYNOPSIS, LINE 17.30

This line further describes the pathomechanism, pulses, and signs of spontaneous recovery in vacuity cold diarrhea.

COMMENTARY, LINE 17.30

The above six lines discuss the advance and retreat of the pathomechanism of vacuity cold diarrhea, taking the growth and decline of yáng qì and the exuberance and debilitation of disease evil as the key to determine the prognosis of this disease. Vacuity cold diarrhea is a disease of the interior, and the pulse should therefore be sunken. In the present line, the pulse is not sunken but is stringlike instead. In addition, we see heat effusion and sweating. This combination of signs indicates that yáng qì is restored and that construction and defense are harmonious. Thus the patient is about to recover spontaneously.

Line 17.31

下利气者，当利其小便。

Xià lì qì zhě, dāng lì qí xiǎo biàn.

In patients with diarrhea and qì,[1] disinhibit the urine.

TEXT NOTES, LINE 17.31

[1] Qì 气 *qì*: In this context, the term refers to flatus.

SYNOPSIS, LINE 17.31

This line describes the treatment of diarrhea with flatus.

COMMENTARY, LINE 17.31

"Diarrhea with qì" refers to diarrhea accompanied by flatus. In this case, qì is discharged along with the diarrhea, resulting in constant flatus. This is also known as "qì diarrhea" (气利 *qì lì*). It is mainly caused by spleen vacuity and movement failure, resulting in stagnating dampness and obstructed qì brewing in the intestinal tract. In addition to flatus concurring with diarrhea, it is characterized by rumbling intestines, abdominal distention, and inhibited urination.

While this condition is associated with spleen vacuity, the more important aspect is excessive exuberance of dampness. Therefore, the text recommends treating it by disinhibiting urine. This will disinhibit dampness evil in the intestines and thereby get rid of dampness, move qì, and free the qì dynamic. As a result, the diarrhea will stop on its own.

Line 17.32

下利，寸脉反浮数，尺中自濇者，必圊脓血。

Xià lì, cùn mài fǎn fú shuò, chǐ zhōng zì sè zhě, bì qīng nóng xuè.

In diarrhea, a paradoxically floating and rapid inch pulse and a naturally rough cubit pulse means that inevitably there will be latrine pus and blood.

SYNOPSIS, LINE 17.32

This line describes the pathomechanism of heat diarrhea with pus and blood on the basis of the pulse.

COMMENTARY, LINE 17.32

Diarrhea is a disease of the interior and should therefore manifest with a sunken rather than a floating pulse. Furthermore, the pulse should be slow, and not rapid, because of the presence of cold. The condition in the present line, however, is characterized by an atypical floating and rapid pulse; hence we know that the diarrhea is not caused by yīn cold, but by heat. The inch pulse belongs to yáng and indicates qì. If it is floating and rapid, this is a manifestation of yáng heat exuberance. The cubit pulse belongs to yīn and indicates blood; a rough cubit pulse is a manifestation of yīn-blood insufficiency and of stagnation in the vessels. If yáng heat is hyperactive, yīn-blood is insufficient, and evil toxin stagnates internally, heat will scorch construction and putrefy it. The result of this is diarrhea with pus and blood.

Line 17.33

下利清谷，不可攻其表，汗出必胀满。

Xià lì qīng gǔ, bù kě gōng qí biǎo, hàn chū bì zhàng mǎn.

In clear-grain diarrhea,[1] you must not attack the exterior; sweating will inevitably lead to distention and fullness.

Text Note, Line 17.33

[1] Clear-grain diarrhea 下利清谷 *xià lì qīng gǔ*: Diarrhea characterized by watery, light brown stool containing partially digested food and having no malodor.

Synopsis, Line 17.33

This line describes contraindicated treatment for vacuity cold diarrhea.

Commentary, Line 17.33

Clear-grain diarrhea is caused by vacuity of spleen and kidney yáng and by internal exuberance of yīn cold, which impairs the warming, movement, and transformation of water and grain. In addition to manifesting in diarrhea with interior vacuity cold signs, the debilitation of center yáng impairs external defense, as a result of which we may see signs of external contraction such as aversion to wind or cold. In this situation, interior vacuity cold is the root and is urgent, while externally contracted wind or cold is the tip and not urgent.

In treatment, you must urgently use formulas like Counterflow Cold Decoction (*sì nì tāng*) to warm the center and rescue counterflow, which constitutes treating the root. As a result, center yáng is restored, and exterior cold will then be eliminated on its own. If you treat the tip instead by effusing sweat offensively with acrid dissipating medicinals, sweating will only cause further damage to interior yáng, which will result in congealing cold qì stagnation and hence in the additional symptom of distention and fullness in the center.

Line 17.34

下利脉沉而迟，其人面少赤，身有微热，下利清谷者，必郁冒，汗出而解，病人必微热。所以然者，其面戴阳，下虚故也。

Xià lì mài chén ér chí, qí rén miàn shǎo chì, shēn yǒu wēi rè, xià lì qīng gǔ zhě, bì yù mào hàn chū ér jiě, bìng rén bì wēi rè, suǒ yǐ rán zhě, qí miàn dài yáng, xià xū gù yě.

In diarrhea [with] a sunken and slow pulse, a reddish face, slight generalized heat [effusion], and clear-grain diarrhea, there must be depressed veiling.[1] Sweating will bring about resolution, and the patient inevitably experiences slight heat [effusion].[2] The reason for this is that there is upcast yáng[3] in the face and vacuity in the lower body.

TEXT NOTES, LINE 17.34

[1] Depressed veiling 郁冒汗出 *yù mào hàn chū*: "Veiling" means clouded head as if the head were covered. "Depressed" is generally interpreted as referring to the depressed heat that has caused the veiling.

[2] The patient inevitably experiences slight heat effusion 病人必微热 *bìng rén bì wēi rè*: Alternative editions of this line have 厥 *jué* (reversal) instead of 热 *rè* (heat). The commentaries explain this sign as indicating either that yáng qì is recovering, but still being repelled to the outside by exuberant yīn (in the case of heat effusion), or that yáng qì has not recovered sufficiently to warm and nourish the four limbs (in the case of reversal).

[2] Upcast yáng 戴阳 *dài yáng*: Upfloating of vacuous yáng giving rise to a complexion that is red as if dabbled with rouge.

SYNOPSIS, LINE 17.34

This line describes the pulse, signs, and pathomechanism of vacuity cold diarrhea with vacuous yáng floating upward.

COMMENTARY, LINE 17.34

In diarrhea, a sunken and slow pulse is considered the standard manifestation of yīn cold diarrhea. Three signs—a reddish face, slight generalized heat [effusion], and clear-grain diarrhea—indicate the pathomechanism of exuberant yīn repelling yáng and forcing it to float astray. Exuberant cold in the lower body and upcast yáng in the upper body results in a reddish complexion; yīn exuberance in the inner body repelling yáng to the outside results in slight generalized heat effusion; and yáng debilitation from interior vacuity results in clear-grain diarrhea.

While such a patient suffers from vacuity yáng floating upward and being repelled to the outside, here the diarrhea is also a sign that right qì can yet be aroused and is overcoming evil on the outside. Because yīn and yáng, and right and evil, are repelling and struggling with each other, vacuous yáng is floating in the upper body while yīn cold is located in the lower body. The two do not connect; hence we see slight heat in the extremities, oppression in the heart and chest, and dizziness and veiling in the head. In this case, sweating means that right is prevailing over evil, and that the condition is resolving. This result is achieved by treating with large amounts of yáng-warming, cold-dissipating medicinals, as in Vessel-Freeing Counterflow Cold Decoction (*tōng mài sì nì tāng*), to bring yīn and yáng into harmony and free the upper and lower body.

Line 17.35

下利后脉绝，手足厥冷，晬时脉还，手足温者生，脉不还者死。

Xià lì hòu mài jué, shǒu zú jué lěng, zuì shí mài huán, shǒu zú wēn zhě shēng, mài bù huán zhě sǐ.

In cases of diarrhea followed by an expired pulse and reversal cold of the extremities, return of the pulse within one day[1] and warmth in the extremities means life, and failure of the pulse to return means death.

TEXT NOTE, LINE 17.35

[1] Within one day 晬时 *zuì shí*: A period of twelve watches, i.e., one day. Also called 周时 *zhōu shí*, daily cycle.

SYNOPSIS, LINE 17.35

This line describes the prognosis of vacuity cold diarrhea and yáng debilitation to the point of expiry, on the basis of the pulse and signs.

COMMENTARY, LINE 17.35

An expired pulse and reversal cold of the extremities after diarrhea is a critical sign of yīn exhaustion with yáng debilitation. In such cases, the prognosis hinges on the survival or perishing of yáng qì, which we can determine on the basis of the timely return of the pulse and the presence of warmth in the extremities. If the pulse does not return overnight and the extremities do not warm up, this means that true yáng is expired and that chances for survival are slim.

Line 17.36

下利腹胀满，身体疼痛者，先温其里，乃攻其表。温里宜四逆汤，攻表宜桂枝汤。

桂枝三两（去皮）芍药三两　甘草二两（炙）生姜三两　大枣十二枚

右五味，㕮咀，以水七升，微火煮取三升，去滓，适寒温服一升，服已，须臾啜稀粥一升，以助药力，温覆令一时许，遍身漐漐微似有汗者，益佳，不可令如水淋漓，若一服汗出病差，停后服。

Xià lì fù zhàng mǎn, shēn tǐ téng tòng zhě, xiān wēn qí lǐ, nǎi gōng qí biǎo. Wēn lǐ yí sì nì tāng, gōng biǎo yí guì zhī tāng.

Guì zhī sān liǎng (qù pí); sháo yào sān liǎng; gān cǎo èr liǎng (zhì); shēng jiāng sān liǎng; dà zǎo shí èr méi

Yòu wǔ wèi, fǔ jǔ, yǐ shuǐ qī shēng, wēi huǒ zhǔ qǔ sān shēng, qù zǐ, shì hán wēn fú yī shēng, fú yǐ, xū yú chuò xī zhōu yī shēng, yǐ zhù yào lì, wēn fù lìng yī shí xǔ, biàn shēn zhé zhé wēi sì yǒu hàn zhě, yì jiā, bù kě lìng rú shuǐ lín lí, ruò yī fú hàn chū bìng chài, tíng hòu fú.

In diarrhea with abdominal distention and fullness, and generalized pain, first warm the interior and then attack the exterior. To warm the interior, counterflow Cold Decoction (四逆汤 *sì nì tāng*)[1] is appropriate. To attack the exterior, Cinnamon Twig Decoction (桂枝汤 *guì zhī tāng*) is appropriate.

Cinnamon Twig Decoction (桂枝汤 *guì zhī tāng*)

cinnamon twig (桂枝 *guì zhī*, Cinnamomi Ramulus) 3 *liǎng* (remove the bark)
peony (芍药 *sháo yào*, Paeoniae Radix) 3 *liǎng*
licorice (*gān cǎo*) 2 *liǎng* (mix-fry)
fresh ginger (生姜 *shēng jiāng*, Zingiberis Rhizoma Recens) 3 *liǎng*
jujube (大枣 *dà zǎo*, Jujubae Fructus) 12 pieces

Chew the above five ingredients and boil in seven *shēng* of water over a low flame to get three *shēng*. Remove the dregs. Take one *shēng* [per dose] at a suitable temperature. After taking [the medicine], instantly drink one *shēng* of hot thin gruel to reinforce the strength of the medicine. Cover [up to keep] warm for at least the length of one watch.[2] [If you induce] a light drizzle of sweat all over the body, this is ideal; Do not make [the person sweat] like dripping water. If sweating occurs after a single dose, recovery will ensue, and you should stop taking further [doses].

Text Notes, Line 17.36

[1] A comment included in the received text reads: "For the formula, see above." See line 17.14 of this chapter.

[2] The length of one watch 一時 *yì shí*: A period of two hours.

Synopsis, Line 17.36

This line describes the treatment of vacuity cold diarrhea with concurrent exterior signs.

Commentary, Line 17.36

When treating complex disease of both the interior and exterior, you must carefully decide on the basis of their urgency which pattern to treat initially. If right qì is not vacuous, you can first resolve the exterior and then attack the interior, but if right qì is vacuous, you must first warm the interior before resolving the exterior. In the present line, diarrhea with abdominal distention and fullness means the presence of vacuity cold in the interior. Generalized pain means the presence of exterior evil on the outside. Hence, this is a condition of combined interior and exterior patterns. In this case, the treatment of vacuity cold in the interior is more critical. The text therefore recommends to first warm the interior with Counterflow Cold Decoction (*sì nì tāng*) to make interior qì abundant. If the exterior signs are still present, you may then use Cinnamon Twig Decoction (*guì zhī tāng*) to resolve the exterior evil.

Line 17.37

下利三部脉皆平，按之心下坚者，急下之，宜大承气汤。

Xià lì sān bù mài jiē píng, àn zhī xīn xià jiān zhě, jí xià zhī, yí dà chéng qì tāng.

In diarrhea, if the pulse at all three sections is normal and [you detect] hardness below the heart when pressing, urgently [treat it with] precipitation. Major Qì-Coordinating Decoction (*dà chéng qì tāng*) is appropriate.

SYNOPSIS, LINE 17.37

This line describes the pulse, signs, and treatment of diarrhea in repletion patterns.

COMMENTARY, LINE 17.37

The disease of diarrhea needs to be differentiated into vacuity, repletion, cold, and heat patterns, and treatment needs to be determined accordingly on the basis of supplementing or attacking. In the present line, the healthy pulse in all three sections indicates that this is a case of heat binding in the stomach and intestines, which has not yet affected the regular flow of blood in the vessels. From the fact that there is hardness below the heart, that is, in the area of the stomach duct and abdomen, we know repletion evil is binding internally. Nevertheless, right qì is not vacuous and is trying to expel evil outward, which manifests in the diarrhea. In treatment, we should help this along its course by quickly precipitating the evil repletion, which is called "treating the unstopped by unstopping" (通因通用 *tōng yīn tōng yòng*).

Line 17.38

下利脉迟而滑者，实也，利未欲止，急下之，宜大承气汤。

Xià lì mài chí ér huá zhě, shí yě, lì wèi yù zhǐ, jí xià zhī, yí dà chéng qì tāng.

In diarrhea, a slow and slippery pulse means repletion. If the diarrhea is not about to stop, urgently precipitate. Major Qì-Coordinating Decoction (*dà chéng qì tāng*) is appropriate.

SYNOPSIS, LINE 17.38

This line describes the pulse and signs of diarrhea where precipitation is appropriate.

COMMENTARY, LINE 17.38

A slow pulse in diarrhea means qì stagnation, while a slippery pulse means food accumulation. The condition in the present line is thus one of qì stagnation and food accumulation in the center burner. Consequently splenic movement and transformation is impaired, bowel qì is disharmonious, and diarrhea arises. If the repletion stagnates internally and the evil fails to weaken, the diarrhea will not stop. Hence we should treat in accordance with precedence of pulse over signs and use Major Qì-Coordinating Decoction (*dà chéng qì tāng*) to urgently precipitate it and thereby free the bowels and discharge heat. When the repletion evil is removed, the diarrhea will stop.

Line 17.39

下利脉反滑者，当有所去，下乃愈，宜大承气汤。

Xià lì mài fǎn huá zhě, dāng yǒu suǒ qù, xià nǎi yù, yí dà chéng qì tāng.

In diarrhea, a paradoxically slippery pulse indicates that there may be something to get rid of. Precipitate and recovery will ensue. Major Qì-Coordinating Decoction (*dà chéng qì tāng*) is appropriate.

Synopsis, Line 17.39

This line describes the signs and treatment of diarrhea with a slippery pulse.

Commentary, Line 17.39

If diarrhea is related to repletion heat, the patient's pulse should be rapid; if it is a cold-damp pattern, the pulse should be slow; if it is a case of chronic diarrhea with generalized vacuity, the pulse should be weak. In the present line, however, the pulse is slippery. This is caused by abiding food and should therefore be treated by offensive precipitation. Major Qì-Coordinating Decoction (*dà chéng qì tāng*) is recommended because it frees the bowels, drains repletion, and checks diarrhea by removing repletion evil.

Line 17.40

下利已差，至其年月日时复发者，以病不尽故也，当下之，宜大承气汤。

Xià lì yǐ chài, zhì qí nián yuè rì shí fù fā zhě, yǐ bìng bù jìn gù yě, dāng xià zhī, yí dà chéng qì tāng.

If [a patient] recovers from diarrhea but then suffers recurring attacks at set times,[1] this is because the disease is not eliminated completely. You must precipitate. Major Qì-Coordinating Decoction (大承气汤 *dà chéng qì tāng*)[2] is appropriate.

TEXT NOTES, LINE 17.40

[1] At set times 至其年月日時 *zhì qí nián yuè rì shí*: Literally, "come the year, month, and day."

[2] A comment included in the received text reads: "For the formula, see the chapter on Tetany." This refers to line 2.13 in Chapter 2, "Tetany, Dampness, and Thermoplegia."

SYNOPSIS, LINE 17.40

This line describes the treatment of regularly recurring diarrhea.

COMMENTARY, LINE 17.40

Diarrhea is generally not a condition that recurs in regular cycles. If it does, this indicates that the root of the disease has not been eliminated completely. This can be caused either by inappropriate treatment with astringing and supplementing medicinals too early in the process, or because treatment has not gotten to the bottom of the condition and has allowed the evil to become hidden in the interior of the body. The residual evil stagnates in the stomach and intestines and causes a recurrence of diarrhea under the influence of such factors as seasonal change in weather, imbalanced diet, or internal damage from taxation fatigue. This condition is most common in dysentery and is now also called "intermittent diarrhea" (休息痢 *xiū xī lì*). One should treat this condition based on the root, which means to eliminate the evil completely by unstopping the bowels and draining repletion.

Line 17.41

下利谵语者，有燥屎也，小承气汤主之。

大黄四两　厚朴二两（炙）枳实大者三枚（炙）

右三味，以水四升，煮取一升二合，去滓，分温二服，得利则止。

Xià lì zhān yǔ zhě, yǒu zào shǐ yě, xiǎo chéng qì tāng zhǔ zhī.

Dà huáng sì liǎng; hòu pò èr liǎng (zhì); zhǐ shí dà zhě sān méi (zhì)

Yòu sān wèi, yǐ shuǐ sì shēng, zhǔ qǔ yī shēng èr gě, qù zǐ, fēn wēn èr fú, dé lì zé zhǐ.

Diarrhea with delirious speech indicates the presence of dry stool. Minor Qì-Coordinating Decoction (小承气汤 *xiǎo chéng qì tāng*) governs.

Minor Qì-Coordinating Decoction (小承气汤 *xiǎo chéng qì tāng*)

- rhubarb (大黄 *dà huáng*, Rhei Radix et Rhizoma) 4 *liǎng*
- officinal magnolia bark (厚朴 *hòu pò*, Magnoliae Officinalis Cortex) 2 *liǎng* (mix-fry)
- unripe bitter orange (枳实 *zhǐ shí*, Aurantii Fructus Immaturus) 3 large pieces (mix-fry)

Boil the above three ingredients in four *shēng* of water to get one *shēng* and two *gě*. Remove the dregs, divide into three [doses], and take warm. Stop when you have achieved disinhibition.

SYNOPSIS, LINE 17.41

This line describes the signs and treatment of diarrhea due to gastrointestinal repletion heat.

COMMENTARY, LINE 17.41

Diarrhea with delirious speech can occur in both repletion and vacuity patterns. According to the *Shāng Hán Lùn* ("On Cold Damage"), "In repletion, there is delirious speech, and in vacuity, there is muttering." The difference between these two types of speech disorders is that delirious speech is characterized by a strident voice and deranged speech, while muttering is characterized by a low voice and repetition. The present line is related to repletion heat in the stomach and intestines. Because of internal binding of dry stool and circumfluence of bound heat, this type of diarrhea with delirious speech manifests also with tidal heat, sweating, abdominal fullness with resistance to pressure, foul-smelling sticky stool, yellow dry tongue fur, and slippery pulse. The recommended treatment is to precipitate offensively with Minor Qì-Coordinating Decoction (*xiǎo chéng qì tāng*).

Line 17.42

下利便脓血者，桃花汤主之。

赤石脂一斤（一半剉，一半筛末）
干姜一两　粳米一升

右三味，以水七升，煮米令熟，去滓，温服七合，内赤石脂末方寸匕，日三服，若一服愈，余勿服。

Xià lì biàn nóng xuè zhě, táo huā tāng zhǔ zhī.

Chì shí zhī (yī bàn cuò, yī bàn shāi mò) yī jīn; gān jiāng yī liǎng; jīng mǐ yī shēng

Yòu sān wèi, yǐ shuǐ qī shēng, zhǔ mǐ lìng shóu, qù zǐ, wēn fú qī gě, nà chì shí zhī mò fāng cùn bǐ, rì sān fú, ruò yī fú yù, yú wù fú.

For diarrhea with blood and pus in the stool, Peach Blossom Decoction (桃花汤 *táo huā tāng*) governs.

Peach Blossom Decoction (桃花汤 *táo huā tāng*)
halloysite (赤石脂 *chì shí zhī*, Halloysitum Rubrum) 1 *jīn* (grate half and sift half) dried ginger (干姜 *gān jiāng*, Zingiberis Rhizoma) 1 *liǎng* non-glutinous rice (粳米 *jīng mǐ*, Oryzae Semen) 1 *shēng*

Boil the above three ingredients[1] in seven *shēng* of water until the rice is done. Remove the dregs and take seven *gě* [per dose] warm, adding a square-inch-spoonful of the powdered halloysite (*chì shí zhī*) [to each dose]. Take three times a day. If recovery occurs after the first dose, do not take what remains.

TEXT NOTE, LINE 17.42

[1] The text is somewhat terse here, but the context makes it obvious that you only boil the grated portion of the halloysite (*chì shí zhī*) and reserve the powder to be added as the last stage in the preparation of the medicine.

SYNOPSIS, LINE 17.42

This line describes the signs and treatment of vacuity cold diarrhea with pus and blood in the stool.

COMMENTARY, LINE 17.42

Diarrhea with pus and blood in the stool is most commonly seen in the initial stage of diarrhea, in which case it is related to repletion heat patterns, where exuberant heat has damaged the blood network vessels and putrefied construction. If it arises in chronic incessant diarrhea, on the other hand, it is caused by vacuity cold of visceral qì, insecurity of qì and blood, and efflux desertion and incontinence. Based on the medicinals recommended in this line, we know that in the present case diarrhea with pus and blood clearly falls into the latter category of vacuity cold patterns. In this case, vacuity fall of qì and blood and major damage to center yáng have caused the diarrhea. The precipitated blood will inevitably be dark purple in color, the diarrhea will be red and white mixed together, and the patient will suffer from fatigue and lack of strength. Other symptoms include dull abdominal pain, liking for warmth and pressure, absence of thirst, pale tongue with a white fur, and a faint, fine, and weak pulse.

We treat this condition by warming the center and astringing the intestines to stem desertion. The recommended formula is Peach Blossom Decoction (*táo huā tāng*), the name of which is derived from the fact that the key ingredient, halloysite (*chì shí zhī*), has a color similar to peach blossoms. This medicinal is warm by nature and sweet in flavor, and astringent and heavy. Thus it has the effect of astringing the intestines and securing desertion. Additional ingredients are dried ginger (*gān jiāng*), which warms yáng and dissipates cold, and non-glutinous rice (*jīng mǐ*), which supplements vacuity and calms the center.

Line 17.43

热利下重者，白头翁汤主之。

白头翁二两　黄连　黄柏　秦皮各三两

右四味，以水七升，煮取二升，去滓，温服一升，不愈更服。

Rè lì xià zhòng zhě, bái tóu wēng zhǔ zhī.

Bái tóu wēng èr liǎng; huáng lián, huáng bǎi, qín pí gè sān liǎng

Yòu sì wèi, yǐ shuǐ qī shēng, zhǔ qǔ èr shēng, qù zǐ, wēn fú yī shēng, bù yù gèng fú.

For heat diarrhea with lower-body heaviness, Pulsatilla Decoction (白头翁汤 *bái tóu wēng tāng*) governs.

Pulsatilla Decoction
(白头翁汤 *bái tóu wēng tāng*)

pulsatilla (白头翁 *bái tóu wēng*, Pulsatillae Radix) 2 liǎng
coptis (黄连 *huáng lián*, Coptidis Rhizoma) 3 *liǎng*
phellodendron (黄柏 *huáng bǎi*, Phellodendri Cortex) 3 *liǎng*
ash (秦皮 *qín pí*, Fraxini Cortex) 3 *liǎng*

Boil the above four ingredients in seven *shēng* of water to get two *shēng*. Remove the dregs and take one *shēng* [per dose] warm. If recovery does not ensue, take the second dose.

SYNOPSIS, LINE 17.43

This line describes the signs and treatment of heat diarrhea.

COMMENTARY, LINE 17.43

Heat diarrhea refers to a pathomechanism of heat causing diarrhea and therefore naturally also includes other heat-type symptoms like heat effusion, thirst, red tongue, yellow fur, and rapid pulse. The present line addresses specifically the pathomechanism of damp-heat adhering and binding in the intestines and putrefying and scorching the network vessels in the intestinal tract. As a result, there is malign foul matter, which cannot be expelled, and we see the symptoms of stagnant and ungratifying defecation, diarrhea containing foul-smelling malign pus and blood, and abdominal urgency with rectal heaviness.

The recommended treatment is Pulsatilla Decoction (*bái tóu wēng tāng*) because it clears heat, dries dampness, and cools the blood to check diarrhea. In the formula, pulsatilla Decoction (*bái tóu wēng*) acts as chief ingredient by clearing heat and cooling blood. It is assisted by ash (*qín pí*), which drains heat and astringes the large intestine, and by coptis (*huáng lián*) and phellodendron (*huáng bǎi*), which clear heat, dry dampness, consolidate yīn, and thicken the intestines. These ingredients are well-matched, and thus lend the formula excellent efficacy.

This formula can be modified in accord with symptoms. If heat diarrhea has affected construction-blood, which manifests in strong fever with thirst, vexation and agitation, and a crimson tongue, add medicinals such as lonicera (*jīn yín huā*), rehmannia (*shēng dì huáng*), moutan (*mǔ dān pí*), and red peony (*chì sháo*), to clear heat and resolve toxin, clear construction, and cool the blood. In cases of blood vacuity, you may add ass hide glue (*ē jiāo*) to nourish the blood, while for abdominal pain, add costusroot (*mù xiāng*) and corydalis (*yán hú suǒ*) to disinhibit qì and relieve pain.

Line 17.44

下利后，更烦，按之心下濡者，为虚烦也，栀子豉汤主之。

栀子十四枚　香豉四合（绵裹）
右二味，以水四升，先煮栀子，得二

升半，内豉煮取一升半，去滓，分二服，温进一服，得吐则止。

Xià lì hòu, gèng fán, àn zhī xīn xià rú zhě, wéi xū fán yě, zhī zǐ chǐ tāng zhǔ zhī.

Zhī zǐ shí sì méi; xiāng chǐ sì gě (mián guǒ)

Yòu èr wèi, yǐ shuǐ sì shēng, xiān zhǔ zhī zǐ, dé èr shēng bàn, nà chǐ zhǔ qǔ yī shēng bàn, qù zǐ, fēn èr fú, wēn jìn yī fú, dé tù zé zhǐ.

When diarrhea is followed by even greater vexation and sogginess below the heart[1] when pressed, [this] is vacuity vexation. Gardenia and Fermented Soybean Decoction (栀子豉汤 *zhī zǐ chǐ tāng*) governs.

Gardenia and Fermented Soybean Decoction (栀子豉汤 *zhī zǐ chǐ tāng*)
gardenia (栀子 *zhī zǐ*, Gardeniae Fructus) 14 pieces fermented soybean (香豉 *xiāng chǐ*, Sojae Semen Fermentatum) 4 *gě* (wrap in cotton gauze)

Of the above two ingredients, first boil the gardenia (*zhī zǐ*) in four *shēng* of water to get two-and-a-half *shēng*. Add the fermented soybean (*xiāng chǐ*) and boil to get one-and-a-half *shēng*. Remove the dregs, divide into two [doses], and ingest one dose warm. Stop when you have managed to induce vomiting.

TEXT NOTE, LINE 17.44

[1] Sogginess below the heart 心下濡 *xīn xià rú*: Softness in the pit of the stomach.

SYNOPSIS, LINE 17.44

This line describes the signs and treatments of diarrhea with vacuity vexation.

COMMENTARY, LINE 17.44

If diarrhea is caused by repletion heat, it manifests with heart vexation that is alleviated as soon as the repletion evil is removed through diarrhea. In the present line, however, the heart vexation is not alleviated by the diarrhea, but in fact is even further aggravated. This indicates the continued presence of residual evil that is lying depressed in the chest and diaphragm and harassing the heart spirit. Because the disease-causing repletion evil has been removed, you feel softness rather than hardness when pressing below the heart. This is related to the fact that the condition is due to intangible evil heat harassing the inner body, not to tangible repletion evil binding internally.

This condition is treated with Gardenia and Fermented Soybean Decoction (*zhī zǐ chǐ tāng*), which outthrusts evil and discharges heat, resolves depression, and eliminates vexation. Gardenia (*zhī zǐ*) clears the heart and eliminates vexation, while fermented soybean (*dòu chǐ*) diffuses and discharges depressed heat from inside the chest. In combination, these two ingredients have the effect of eliminating the residual heat and thereby resolving vacuity vexation.

Line 17.45

下利清谷，里寒外热，汗出而厥者，通脉四逆汤主之。

附子大者一枚（生用）干姜三两（强人可四两）甘草二两（炙）

右三味，以水三升，煮取一升二合，去滓，分温再服。

Xià lì qīng gǔ, lǐ hán wài rè, hàn chū ér jué zhě, tōng mài sì nì tāng zhǔ zhī.

Fù zǐ (shēng yòng) dà zhě yī méi; gān jiāng sān liǎng; (qiáng rén kě sì liǎng); gān cǎo èr liǎng (zhì)

Yòu sān wèi, yǐ shuǐ sān shēng, zhǔ qǔ yī shēng èr gě, qù zǐ, fēn wēn zài fú.

For clear-grain diarrhea with interior cold and exterior heat, and sweating and reversal, Vessel-Freeing Counterflow Cold Decoction (通脉四逆汤 *tōng mài sì nì tāng*) governs.

Vessel-Freeing Counterflow Cold Decoction (通脉四逆汤 *tōng mài sì nì tāng*)
aconite (附子 *fù zǐ*, Aconiti Radix Lateralis Praeparata) 1 large piece (use raw) dried ginger (干姜 *gān jiāng*, Zingiberis Rhizoma) 3 *liǎng* (strong patients can take 4 *liǎng*) licorice (甘草 *gān cǎo*, Glycyrrhizae Radix) 2 *liǎng* (mix-fry)

Boil the above three ingredients in three *shēng* of water to get one *shēng* and two *gě*. Remove the dregs, divide into two [doses] and take warm.

SYNOPSIS, LINE 17.45

This line describes the signs and treatment of diarrhea with cold reversal due to yīn exuberance repelling yáng.

COMMENTARY, LINE 17.45

The present pattern of clear-grain diarrhea is related to interior cold and to dual vacuity of spleen and kidney yáng. Because exuberant yīn repels yáng to the outside, we see signs of external heat like generalized heat effusion, red face, and spontaneous sweating. Because exterior heat is related to interior cold, the interior cold is true and is the root of the disease, while the exterior heat is false and is the tip of the disease. "Sweating and reversal" means that sweating occurs simultaneously with reverse flow in the limbs. It is caused by the fact that yīn is exhausted in the lower body as a result of diarrhea, and that yáng has deserted to the outside as a result of sweating; hence yīn and yáng are not connected. Sweating with concurrent reversal therefore indicates the critical nature of this condition.

Treat this condition urgently with Vessel-Freeing Counterflow Cold Decoction (*tōng mài sì nì tāng*), to rescue yáng and contain dissipated qì. In this formula, aconite (*fù zǐ*) is greatly acrid and hot and has the effect of breaking yīn and invigorating yáng, and restoring the flow in the vessels. Dried ginger (*gān jiāng*) is acrid and warm; it warms the center, dissipates cold, and checks diarrhea. Lastly, prepared licorice (*zhì gān cǎo*) fortifies the center and boosts the spleen with sweetness and warmth. In combination, these medicinals increase one another's efficacy and obtain the results of returning yáng and rescuing counterflow.

Line 17.46

下利肺痛，紫参汤主之。

紫参半斤　甘草三两

右二味，以水五升，先煮紫参取二升，内甘草煮取一升半，分温三服。

Xià lì fèi tòng, zǐ shēn tāng zhǔ zhī.

Zǐ shēn bàn jīn; gān cǎo sān liǎng

Yòu èr wèi, yǐ shuǐ wǔ shēng, xiān zhǔ zǐ shēn qǔ èr shēng, nà gān cǎo zhǔ qǔ yī shēng bàn, fēn wēn sān fú.

For diarrhea with lung pain, Bistort Decoction (紫参汤 ***zǐ shēn tāng***) governs.

Bistort Decoction (紫参汤 *zǐ shēn tāng*)
bistort rhizome (紫参 *zǐ shēn*, Bistortae Rhizoma) 5 *liǎng*[2] licorice (甘草 *gān cǎo*, Glycyrrhizae Radix) 3 *liǎng*

Of the above two ingredients, first boil the bistort rhizome (*zǐ shēn*) in five *shēng* of water to get two *shēng*. Add the licorice (*gān cǎo*) and boil to get one-and-one-half *shēng*. Divide into three doses and take warm.[3]

Text Notes, Line 17.46

[1]Lung pain 肺痛 *fèi tòng*: Different opinions have been advanced to explain this phrase. According to one opinion, "lung pain" should be taken at face value. Because the lung and large intestine stand in interior-exterior relationship, disease of the two is mutually conducive. According to a similar opinion, it is possible that diarrhea is associated with disease of the lung, but it should be understood as "chest pain" rather than "lung pain." According to a third opinion, "lung pain" is simply a mistake for "abdominal pain." While it is perhaps easiest to interpret "lung pain" as a textual error for "abdominal pain," a literal reading is also possible. We therefore leave this question open for the discerning reader to consider on their own.

[2] Bistort rhizome (紫参 *zǐ shēn*, Bistortae Rhizoma): The identity of 紫参 *zǐ shēn* has been the subject of some debate. The *Shén Nóng Běn Cǎo Jīng* ("Divine Husbandman's Herbal Foundation Canon") describes it as follows: "It is bitter, acrid, and cold, governs accumulations and gatherings in the heart and abdomen, and evil qì of cold and heat, frees the nine orifices, and disinhibits urine and stool." Because its precise identity is unclear, some commentators have suggested that it is an alternative name for *dān shēn* (Salviae Miltiorrhizae Radix). In modern times, the *Zhōng Yào Dà Cí Diǎn* ("Great Encyclopedia of Chinese Medicinals") suggests that it is a variety of bistort (拳参 *quán shēn*, Bistortae Rhizoma).

[3] A comment included in the received text reads: "It is suspected that this might not be Zhāng Zhòng-Jǐng's formula."

Synopsis, Line 17.46

This line describes the treatment of diarrhea with lung pain.

COMMENTARY, LINE 17.46

As is evident from the text notes above, the interpretation of this line has caused considerable debate among commentators over the centuries, to the point where some question the authenticity of the entire line. If we read the line literally, however, the following meaning can be discerned: Lung pain can be equated with chest pain because the lung resides within the chest. It stands in interior-exterior relationship with the large intestine; hence inhibition in the large intestine can certainly result in disharmony of lung qì, which manifests in oppression, pain, and discomfort in the chest.

From the choice of treatment, we can deduce that the condition described here is diarrhea caused by accumulated heat in the stomach and intestines. Because of diarrhea, the clear and turbid are not separated; hence we should also see inhibited urination. This matches the choice of bistort rhizome (*zǐ shēn*) as the key ingredient in the formula, because it is indicated for accumulations and gatherings in the heart and abdomen, for heat accumulation in the intestines and stomach, for stoppage in the nine orifices, and for inhibited urination and defecation. This effect is assisted by licorice (*gān cǎo*), which clears heat, harmonizes the center, and calms the stomach.

Line 17.44

气利，诃梨勒散主之。

诃梨勒十枚（煨）

右一味，为散，粥饮和，顿服。

Qì lì, hē lí lè sǎn zhǔ zhī.

Hē lí lè shí méi (wēi)

Yòu yī wèi, wéi sǎn, zhōu yǐn huó, dùn fú.

For qì diarrhea, Chebule Powder (诃梨勒散 ***hé lí lè sǎn***) governs.

Chebule Powder (诃梨勒散 *hé lí lè sǎn*)
chebule (诃梨勒 *hē lí lè*, Chebulae Fructus) 10 pieces (roast)

Make a powder with the above single ingredient, mix it with gruel liquid,[1] and quaff.[2]

TEXT NOTES, LINE 17.47

[1] Gruel liquid 粥饮 *zhōu yǐn*: Liquid from cooking rice or other grain gruel, which is used as a medium to drink down the medicine.

[2] A comment included in the received text reads: "It is suspected that this might not be Zhāng Zhòng-Jǐng's formula."

SYNOPSIS, LINE 17.47

This line describes treatment of intestinal efflux qì diarrhea in vacuity cold patterns.

COMMENTARY, LINE 17.47

Qì diarrhea refers to lower body disinhibition and efflux desertion where stool is discharged together with flatus. This condition is most commonly caused by center qì fall and qì vacuity and insecurity. It can arise in repletion or vacuity patterns. Despite the terseness of the present line, we can deduce from the recommended treatment that it addresses a pattern of vacuity cold. The treatment involves the single ingredient chebule (*hē lí lè*), which is warm and astringent and has the effect of constraining the lung, astringing the intestines, checking diarrhea, and stemming desertion. It is thus the ideal medicinal for treating chronic diarrhea in vacuity cold patterns.

Chronic diarrhea will eventually damage the spleen and stomach and cause vacuity cold of center qì. As a result, qì falls and becomes vacuous and insecure. This manifests in efflux desertion and incessant diarrhea. In the recommended formula, chebule (*hē lí lè*) is roasted to increase its effect of astringing the intestines and stemming desertion, and is taken in gruel liquid to boost the intestines and stomach and to fortify center qì.

[附方] APPENDED FORMULAS, LINE 17.47

MINOR QÌ-COORDINATING DECOCTION (小承气汤 *xiǎo chéng qì tāng*) from the *Qiān Jīn Yì Fāng* ("Wings of the Thousand Gold Pieces Prescriptions")

治大便不通，哕数谵语。
Zhì dà biàn bù tōng, yuē, shuò zhān yǔ.

Treats fecal stoppage, frequent hiccup, and delirious speech.[1]

FORMULA NOTE, LINE 17.47

[1]A comment included in the received text reads: "For the formula, see above." This refers to line 17.41 above. This formula comes from the *Qiān Jīn Yì Fāng* ("Wings of the Thousand Gold Pieces Prescriptions"), in the section on sudden turmoil (cholera). The formula consists of 2 liǎng of officinal magnolia bark (*hòu pò*) (mix-fried), 4 liǎng of rhubarb (*dà huáng*), and 5 pieces of unripe bitter orange (*zhǐ shí*) (mix-fried).

FORMULA SYNOPSIS, LINE 17.47

This line describes the signs and treatment of hiccup and delirious speech due to yáng brightness repletion heat.

FORMULA COMMENTARY, LINE 17.47

Hiccup can occur in vacuity and repletion and cold and heat patterns. From the fact that the present line recommends Minor Qì-Coordinating Decoction (*xiǎo chéng qì tāng*), which frees the bowels and discharges heat, we know that this pattern is related to repletion heat. Hence, it should manifest with frequent hiccup, high voice, red tongue, rapid replete pulse, tidal heat in the face, and fecal stoppage. All these are caused by repletion heat in yáng brightness, stoppage of bowel qì, and counterflow ascent of the turbid qì of repletion heat, which stirs the diaphragm, clouds the clear orifices, and affects the brain.

SCUTELLARIA DECOCTION (黄芩汤 *huáng qín tāng*)
from the *Wài Tái Mì Yào* ("Secrets from the *Wài Tái* Library")

治干呕下利。
黄芩 人参 干姜各三两 桂枝一两 大枣十二枚 半夏半升
右六味，以水七升，煮取三升，分温三服。

Zhì gān ǒu xià lì.

Huáng qín, rén shēn, gān jiāng gè sān liǎng; guì zhī yī liǎng; dà zǎo shí èr méi; bàn xià bàn shēng

Yòu liù wèi, yǐ shuǐ qī shēng, zhǔ qǔ sān shēng, fēn wēn sān fú.

Treats dry retching and diarrhea.

Scutellaria Decoction (黄芩汤 *huáng qín tāng*)

scutellaria (黄芩 *huáng qín*, Scutellariae Radix) 3 *liǎng*
ginseng (人参 *rén shēn*, Ginseng Radix) 3 *liǎng*
dried ginger (干姜 *gān jiāng*, Zingiberis Rhizoma) 3 *liǎng*
cinnamon twig (桂枝 *guì zhī*, Cinnamomi Ramulus) 1 *liǎng*
jujube (大枣 *dà zǎo*, Jujubae Fructus) 12 pieces
pinellia (半夏 *bàn xià*, Pinelliae Rhizoma) ½ *shēng*

Boil the above six ingredients in seven *shēng* of water to get three *shēng*. Divide into three [doses] and take warm.

FORMULA SYNOPSIS, LINE 17.47

This line describes the signs and treatment of dry retching with diarrhea in combined cold and heat patterns.

FORMULA COMMENTARY, LINE 17.47

The recommended formula addresses conditions of dry retching and diarrhea that are caused by vacuity cold in the stomach with intestinal heat. Because cold and heat bind in the center burner, the spleen loses its ability to move and transform, and the stomach loses its ability to downbear harmoniously. Cold runs downward, which results in diarrhea. Heat distresses the stomach and impairs its harmonious downbearing, which results in dry retching. In the present line, vacuity cold in the center burner is more severe than intestinal heat; hence the text recommends treatment with Scutellaria Decoction (*huáng qín tāng*). In this formula, dried ginger (*gān jiāng*) and pinellia (*bàn xià*) warm the stomach and check retching, ginseng (*rén shēn*) and jujube (*dà zǎo*) supplement the spleen and boost qì, cinnamon twig (*guì zhī*) warms the center, supplements vacuity, and dissipates cold evil, and scutellaria (*huáng qín*) clears heat. In combination, these medicinals have the effect of contracting and regulating the center, dissipating cold, harmonizing stomach downbearing, supplementing vacuity, and clearing heat.

疮痈肠痈浸淫病脉证并治第十八

CHAPTER 18

Sores, Welling-Abscesses, Intestinal Welling-Abscesses, and Wet Spreading Sores

Pulses, Signs, Treatments

Overview

This chapter discusses the differentiation and treatment of welling-abscesses (痈 *yōng*), intestinal welling-abscess (肠痈 *cháng yōng*), incised wounds (金疮 *jīn chuāng*), and wet-spreading sores (浸淫疮 *jìn yín chuāng*). These are all discussed in one chapter because they are all external medical diseases.

The types of welling-abscesses discussed here all refer to what we now call swollen welling-abscess (痈肿 *yōng zhǒng*). Those that arise on the exterior of the trunk and limbs are called external welling-abscess (外痈 *wài yōng*); those that arise in the interior of the chest, abdomen, trunk, and limbs or in the viscera and bowels are called internal welling-abscess (内痈 *nèi yōng*). Usually, welling-abscesses go through a process of reddening, swelling, heat, and pain, and in severe cases putrefaction, ulceration, and formation of pus; after the pus is eliminated, they turn towards recovery. Welling-abscesses can take the form of either yīn or yáng patterns, a distinction that comes from the *Nèi Jīng* ("Inner Canon"). Yīn patterns are caused by qì depression and cold stagnation causing localized obstruction in the channels and network vessels. Yáng patterns are due to heat toxin stagnating and binding locally in construction-blood, where it can putrefy flesh and form pus.

Intestinal welling-abscess (肠痈 *cháng yōng*) is a type of interior welling-abscess. The key symptoms are pain that refuses pressure on the right side of the lower abdomen, bending and reluctance to stretch in the right lower extremity, aggravated abdominal pain upon stretching, and in severe cases one-sided heat effusion and aversion to cold. In yīn patterns, it is caused by qì and blood stagnation, insufficiency of right qì, and non-transformation of yáng qì, which over time becomes depressed, creates toxins, and forms welling-abscess and swelling in a slow and gradual disease process. In yáng patterns, it is caused by heat toxin gathering internally, binding construction-blood, and putrefying blood and flesh. This is a rather fast process that occurs in critical patterns of right being overcome by repletion evil.

Incised wounds (金疮 *jīn chuāng*), which the title refers to as "sores" (疮 *chuāng*) includes all types of damage to the inner body by metal implements like blades, knives, or axes, as well as exterior wounds. After external damage, the body easily contracts evil qì, which can in serious cases engender sores; hence the disease is called "incised wounds." Its key manifestations are redness, swelling, heat, and pain, as a result of metal blades damaging the skin, flesh, sinew, and bone. Excessive damage to yīn from blood collapse can cause vacuity of qì and blood, and if not treated, in severe cases may be complicated by contraction of evil toxin, causing bursting and formation of pus, and thereby engenderment of sores.

Lastly, wet spreading sores (浸淫疮 *jìn yín chuāng*) are a type of skin disease that starts with the appearance of scabies, gradually discharging yellow fluid that seeps and spreads, until finally forming one piece with itching and unbearable pain. The disease is caused by evil toxin of damp-heat seeping and spreading everywhere. In later times, it came to be called yellow-water sore. It roughly corresponds to impetigo in biomedicine.

The discussions on incised wounds and wet spreading sores are limited to formulas and do not describe signs, hence their clinical value is limited. However, the discussions on intestinal abscesses and swollen welling-abscesses are more complete, and have had far-reaching influence since Zhāng Jī's time.

‡ Schematic Overview

Swollen Abscesses

Initial stage: A pulse that is floating and rapid, heat effusion with aversion to cold as after a soaking (aversion to cold more predominant than heat effusion), and pain of fixed location.

Presence or absence of pus:

Palpable heat means pus is present.

Absence of heat means pus is not present.

Intestinal Welling-Abscesses

When pus has formed:

Signs: Encrusted skin on the body, tension of the abdominal skin, sogginess when pressing like a swelling, [but] no accumulation or gathering in the abdomen, no generalized heat [effusion], and a rapid pulse.

Formula: Coix, Aconite, and Patrinia Powder (*yì yĭ fù zĭ bài jiàng săn*) to expel pus and resolve toxin.

When pus has not formed:

Signs: Swelling and glomus in the lesser abdomen, which when pressed result in pain as in strangury, but with naturally regulated urine, as well as frequent heat effusion, spontaneous sweating, and then again aversion to cold. The pulse is slow and tight.

Formula: Rhubarb and Moutan Decoction (*dà huáng mŭ dān tāng*) to drain heat and expel stasis.

Incised Wounds

Signs: Inch opening pulse floating, rapid, and rough; wounds due to damage by a knife or ax.

Formula: Vaccariae Powder (*wáng bù liú xíng săn*) to disperse stasis, stanch bleeding, and settle pain.

Wet Spreading Sores

Prognosis:

Spreading from the mouth toward the limbs—easy to treat.

Spreading from the limbs to mouth—difficult to treat.

Formula: Powdered Coptis (*huáng lián fĕn*) to drain fire and resolve toxin, and to dry dampness and kill worms.

Line 18.1

诸浮数脉，应当发热，而反洒淅恶寒，若有痛处，当发其痈。

Zhū fú shuò mài, yīng dāng fā rè, ér fǎn sǎ xī wù hán, ruò yǒu tòng chù, dāng fā qí yōng.

All patients with a floating rapid pulse should have heat effusion. However, if they have aversion to cold as after a soaking,[1] and if they have a painful spot, this should indicate that a welling-abscess is erupting.

TEXT NOTE, LINE 18.1

[1] Aversion to cold as if after a soaking 洒淅恶寒 *sǎ xī wù hán*: The patient feels cold as if having been soaked in water.

SYNOPSIS, LINE 18.1

This line describes the pulse, signs, and pathomechanism of swollen welling-abscess in the initial stage.

COMMENTARY, LINE 18.1

Because a floating pulse indicates the exterior and a rapid pulse indicates heat, a rapid floating pulse most commonly manifests in patterns of externally contracted exterior heat. Hence it should be accompanied by heat effusion. Nevertheless, such a pulse can also occur in patterns with exuberant interior heat, in which case it can manifest with aversion to cold, when exterior heat is not yet resolving. In the present line, the patient's condition appears similar to externally contracted exterior heat patterns, but there is discomfort predominantly from aversion to cold. In such cases, check whether this is accompanied by localized redness, swelling, heat, and pain, which is the sign of swollen welling-abscess. This disease is caused by localized congestion of heat toxin, stagnation of qì and blood, and obstruction of construction and defense.

Line 18.2

师曰：诸痈肿欲知有脓无脓，以手掩肿上，热者为有脓，不热者为无脓。

Shī yuē: Zhū yōng zhǒng yù zhī yǒu nóng wú nóng, yǐ shǒu yǎn zhǒng shàng, rè zhě wéi yǒu nóng, bù rè zhě wéi wú nóng.

The Master says: "In all cases of swollen welling-abscess, if you want to know whether it is purulent or not, cover the abscess with a hand. If it is hot, there is pus; if it is not hot, there is no pus."

SYNOPSIS, LINE 18.2

This line describes how to use palpation to determine whether a swollen welling-abscess is purulent or not.

COMMENTARY, LINE 18.2

This line offers a method for diagnosing a swollen welling-abscess as purulent or non-purulent. Lightly place your hand on top of the abscess. If you feel heat, this means that toxin is already gathering; hence there is pus. If you feel no heat, this means that toxin is not yet gathering; hence there is no pus. As the *Líng Shū* ("Magic Pivot") states, "When heat is exuberant, flesh putrefies; when flesh putrefies, it means pus." Later physicians fine-tuned the diagnosis of swollen welling-abscess, and also took into consideration softness or hardness, falling or rising, painful or not, and differences in color, to analyze the pathocondition comprehensively.

Line 18.3

肠痈之为病，其身甲错，腹皮急，按之濡如肿状，腹无积聚，身无热，脉数，此为肠内有痈脓，薏苡附子败酱散主之。

薏苡仁十分　附子二分　败酱五分

右三味，杵为末，取方寸匕，以水二升，煎减半，顿服，小便当下。

Qí shēn jiǎ cuò, fù pí jí, àn zhī rú rú zhǒng zhuàng, fù wú jī jù, shēn wú rè, mài shuò, cǐ wéi cháng nèi yǒu yōng nóng, yì yǐ fù zǐ bài jiàng sǎn zhǔ zhī.

Yì yǐ rén shí fēn; fù zǐ èr fēn; bài jiàng wǔ fēn

Yòu sān wèi, chǔ wéi mò, qǔ fāng cùn bǐ, yǐ shuǐ èr shēng, jiān jiǎn bàn, dùn fú, xiǎo biàn dāng xià.

The disease of intestinal welling-abscess [manifests with] encrusted skin on the body, tension of the abdominal skin, sogginess when pressed like a swelling, [but] no accumulation or gathering in the abdomen, no generalized heat [effusion], and a rapid pulse. This means that there is a purulent welling-abscess in the intestines. Coix, Aconite, and Patrinia Powder (薏苡附子败酱散 *yì yǐ fù zǐ bài jiàng sǎn*) governs.

Coix, Aconite, and Patrinia Powder (薏苡附子败酱散 *yì yǐ fù zǐ bài jiàng sǎn*)
coix (薏苡仁 *yì yǐ rén*, Coicis Semen) 10 parts
aconite (附子 *fù zǐ*, Aconiti Radix Lateralis Praeparata) 2 parts
patrinia (败酱 *bài jiàng*) 5 parts

Pestle the above three ingredients into a powder. Add one square-inch-spoonful to two *shēng* of water and boil to reduce by half. Quaff. [As a sign of recovery, the patient] should discharge urine.

SYNOPSIS, LINE 18.3

This line discusses the signs, pulses, and treatment of intestinal welling-abscess that has already formed.

COMMENTARY, LINE 18.3

In patients with intestinal welling-abscess, construction-blood is chronically depressed in the interior, and the skin and flesh throughout the body lacks nourishment by qì and blood. Hence we see dryness and scaly skin. The skin in the abdominal region is tense and bulging as if swollen because the welling-abscess with pus is binding internally in the intestines, and qì and blood stagnate in the interior. However, we can differentiate welling-abscesses from accumulations and gatherings by the fact that the abdomen is soft when pressed, not hard. When the disease has lasted a long time, heat toxin has already putrefied and transformed into pus, and the right qì is vacuous. Hence there is no generalized heat effusion. Even though there is depressed heat in construction-blood, yáng qì is insufficient, and right cannot overcome evil; hence we see a rapid forceless pulse.

The recommended treatment is Coix, Aconite, and Patrinia Powder (*yì yǐ fù zǐ bài jiàng sǎn*), which expels pus, disperses the welling-abscess, and arouses yáng qì. The formula uses a large amount of coix (*yì yǐ rén*) to expel pus, open congestion, and disinhibit the intestines and stomach, and a small amount of aconite (*fù zǐ*) to arouse yáng qì and dissipate binds, assisted by patrinia (*bài jiàng cǎo*) to break stasis and expel pus. The formula is taken by quaffing so as to concentrate its efficacy, quickly attack the disease, and eliminate the purulent welling-abscess as soon as possible.

Concerning the last statement about discharging urine, commentators differ. Some suggest that it might be a textual error and should actually refer to discharging stool, because the medicine is causing pus and static blood to be expelled in the stool. Others suggest that the medicine restores the free movement of construction and defense, qì and blood, and normalizes qì transformation in the bladder, as a result of which urination is restored.

Line 18.4

肠痈者，少腹肿痞，按之即痛如淋，小便自调，时时发热，自汗出，复恶寒。其脉迟紧者，脓未成，可下之，当有血；脉洪数者，脓已成，不可下也。大黄牡丹汤主之。

大黄四两　牡丹一两　桃仁五十个
芒硝三合　瓜子半升

右五味，以水六升，煮取一升，去滓，内芒硝，再煎沸，顿服之，有脓当下，如无脓，当下血。

Cháng yōng zhě, shào fù zhǒng pǐ, àn zhī jí tòng rú lìn, xiǎo biàn zì tiáo, shí shí fā rè, zì hàn chū, fù wù hán. Qí mài chí jǐn zhě, nóng wèi chéng, kě xià zhī, dāng yǒu xuè; mài hóng shuò zhě, nóng yǐ chéng, bù kě xià yě, dà huáng mǔ dān tāng zhǔ zhī.

Dà huáng sì liǎng; mǔ dān yī liǎng; táo rén wǔ shí ge; máng xiāo sān gě; guā zǐ bàn shēng

Yòu wǔ wèi, yǐ shuǐ liù shēng, zhǔ qǔ yī shēng, qù zǐ, nà máng xiāo, zài jiān fèi, dùn fú zhī, yǒu nóng dāng xià, rú wú nóng, dāng xià xuè.

Intestinal welling-abscess [manifests in] swelling and glomus in the lesser abdomen,[1] which when pressed results in pain as in strangury,[2] but with naturally regulated urine,[3] as well as frequent heat effusion, spontaneous sweating, and then again aversion to cold. If the pulse is slow and tight, pus has not formed yet, and you can [treat it] by precipitation. [In this case, there] ought to be blood [in the precipitated stool]. If the pulse is surging and rapid, pus has already formed, and you must not precipitate.[4] Rhubarb and Moutan Decoction (大黄牡丹汤 *dà huáng mǔ dān tāng*) governs.

Rhubarb and Moutan Decoction (大黄牡丹汤 *dà huáng mǔ dān tāng*)
rhubarb (大黄 *dà huáng*, Rhei Radix et Rhizoma) 4 *liǎng*
moutan (牡丹 *mǔ dān*, Moutan Cortex) 1 *liǎng*
peach kernel (桃仁 *táo rén*, Persicae Semen) 50 pieces
mirabilite (芒硝 *máng xiāo*, Natrii Sulfas) 3 *gě*
wax gourd seed (瓜子 *guā zǐ*, Benincasae Semen) ½ *shēng*

Boil the above five ingredients [except the mirabilite (*máng xiāo*)] in six *shēng* of water to get one *shēng*. Remove the dregs, add the mirabilite (*máng xiāo*), and bring it to a boil again. Quaff. If there is pus, [the medicine] should precipitate it [with the stool]; if there is no pus, it should precipitate blood.

TEXT NOTES, LINE 18.4

[1] Swelling and glomus in the lesser abdomen 少腹肿痞 *shào fù zhǒng pǐ*: A swollen lump with a feeling of blockage. When it is pressed, there is rebound tenderness.

[2] When pressed results in pain as in strangury 按之即痛如淋 *àn zhī jí tòng rú lín*: When palpating an intestinal welling-abscess, pressure results in pain radiating into the bladder and anterior yīn that for the patient feels like the stabbing pain of strangury (e.g., when there are urinary stones).

[3] Naturally regulated urine 小便自調 *xiǎo biàn zì tiáo*: Urine flows normally.

[4] You must not precipitate 不可下也 *bù kě xià yě*: Given the precipitating effect of the following formula, this sentence thus warns against applying it in advanced stages of intestinal welling-abscess.

SYNOPSIS, LINE 18.4

This line describes the pulses, signs, and treatment of intestinal welling-abscess in the critical stage.

COMMENTARY, LINE 18.4

The present pattern is caused by heat toxin gathering internally, by construction-blood stagnating and binding in the intestines, and by stoppage in the channels. Hence we see the symptoms of swelling and glomus in the lesser abdomen, tension and resistance to pressure, and strangury-like pain when pressed. The fact that urination is still normal indicates that the disease has not yet affected the bladder and is still limited to the intestines. By this sign, you can distinguish it from strangury disease. The struggle between right and evil and the depression of construction and obstruction of defense cause frequent heat effusion, spontaneous sweating, and aversion to cold.

In patients with this pattern, a slow, tight, and forceful pulse indicates that construction-blood is trapped by evil qì, heat is latent, blood is static and bound, and pus has not yet formed. Thus, one should urgently treat this by offensively flushing away heat, resolving toxin, breaking up blood, and expelling stasis, to cure the intestinal welling-abscess by precipitating static heat and polluted blood through the stool. In the later, purulent stage of this disease, the pulse becomes surging and rapid, because heat toxin accumulates and repletion heat brews and binds to putrefy blood and vanquish flesh. In this case, offensive treatment with precipitation is contraindicated, because blood-breaking and offensively expelling medicinals can then lead to incessant bleeding, which will deplete right qì. Instead, focus on clearing heat, resolving toxin, expelling pus, and engendering flesh with medicinals like coix (*yì yǐ rén*), patrinia (*bài jiàng cǎo*), lonicera (*jīn yín huā*), Chinese angelica (*dāng guī*), bletilla (*bái jí*), and platycodon (*jié gěng*).

The recommended treatment for intestinal welling-abscesses in the critical stage before pus has formed is Rhubarb and Moutan Decoction (*dà huáng mǔ dān tāng*). In this formula, mirabilite (*máng xiāo*) and rhubarb (*dà huáng*) discharge heat and soften hardness; moutan (*mǔ dān pí*) and peach kernel (*táo rén*) break and cool blood; and trichosanthes seed (*guā lóu zǐ*) clears heat, resolves toxin, dissipates swelling, and expels pus. In combination, these ingredients discharge heat and resolve toxin, break blood, and disperse the abscess.

Line 18.5

问曰：寸口脉浮微而濇，法当亡血，若汗出。设不汗者云何？答曰：若身有疮，被刀斧所伤，亡血故也。

Wèn yuē: Cùn kǒu mài fú wēi ér sè, fǎ dāng wáng xuè, ruò hàn chū, shè bù hàn zhě yún hé? Dá yuē: Ruò shēn yǒu chuāng, bèi dāo fǔ suǒ shāng, wáng xuè gù yě.

Question: "An inch opening pulse that is floating, faint, and rough ought to mean blood collapse or[1] sweating. If there is no sweating, what is the cause?" Answer: "The cause is blood collapse, if the body has wounds[2] due to damage by a knife or ax."

Text Notes, Line 18.5

[1] Or 若 *ruò*: The Chinese 若 usually means "if," but occasionally it can also mean "or." The fact that the original meaning of the character was "choose" helps to explain the relationship between these two meanings.

[2] Wound 疮 *chuāng*: 疮 *chuāng*, which literally means "sore," is here taken to mean 创 *chuāng*, "wound," as the two characters were used interchangeably in early literature.

SYNOPSIS, LINE 18.5

This line describes the pulse and signs of bleeding due to incised wounds.

COMMENTARY, LINE 18.5

A faint floating inch opening pulse indicates vacuity of yáng qì, and roughness indicates an insufficiency of yīn-blood. Altogether, this pulse thus suggests that yáng qì has lost its ability to secure and guard, and that yīn liquid is no longer contained. This sign most commonly occurs in loss of blood and sweat, which share the same source. Blood loss can have a variety of causes, such as blood ejection, nosebleed, lower body bleeding, flooding and spotting, or excessive sweating. If none of these events have occurred in the patient's history, but the patient has wounds on the body from damage by blades or axes, this must mean that blood collapse has caused a floating pulse, with an absence of sweating.

Line 18.6

病金疮，王不留行散主之。

Bìng jīn chuāng, wáng bù liú xíng zhǔ zhī.

王不留行十分（八月八日采） 蒴藋细叶十分（七月七日采） 桑东南根（白皮，三月三日采）十分 甘草十八分 川椒三分（除目及闭口，去汗） 黄芩二分 干姜二分 芍药二分 厚朴二分

Wáng bù liú xíng shí fēn (bā yuè bā rì cǎi); shuò diào xì yè shí fēn (qī yuè qī rì cǎi); sāng dōng nán gēn (bái pí, sān yuè sān rì cǎi) shí fēn; gān cǎo shí bā fēn; chuān jiāo (chú mù jí bì kǒu, qù hàn) sān fēn; huáng qín èr fēn; gān jiāng èr fēn; sháo yào èr fēn; hòu pò èr fēn

右九味，桑根皮以上三味烧灰存性，勿令灰过，各别杵筛，合治之为散，服方寸匕，小疮即粉之，大疮但服之，产后亦可服。如风寒，桑根勿取之。前三物皆阴干百日。

Yòu jiǔ wèi, sāng gēn pí yǐ shàng sān wèi shāo huī cún xìng, wù lìng huī guò, gè bié chǔ shāi, hé zhì zhī wéi sǎn, fú fāng cùn bǐ, xiǎo chuāng jí fěn zhī, dà chuāng dàn fú zhī, chǎn hòu yì kě fú. Rú fēng hán, sāng gēn wù qǔ zhī. Qián sān wù jiē yīn gān bǎi rì.

枳实十六枚 芍药六分 桔梗二分

Zhǐ shí shí liù méi; sháo yào liù fēn; jié gēng èr fēn

右三味，杵为散，取鸡子黄一枚，以药散与鸡黄相等，揉和令相得，饮和服之，日一服。

Yòu sān wèi, chǔ wéi sǎn, qǔ jī zǐ huáng yī méi, yǐ yào sǎn yǔ jī huáng xiāng děng, róu huó lìng xiāng dé, yǐn huó fú zhī, rì yī fú.

甘草二两 桔梗三两 生姜一两 大枣十枚

右四味，以水三升，煮取一升，温服五合，日再服。

Gān cǎo èr liǎng; jié gēng sān liǎng; shēng jiāng yī liǎng; dà zǎo shí méi

Yòu sì wèi, yǐ shuǐ sān shēng, zhǔ qǔ yī shēng, wēn fú wǔ gě, rì zài fú.

For patients with incised wounds, Vaccaria Powder (王不留行散 *wáng bù liú xíng sǎn*) governs.

Vaccaria Powder
(王不留行散 *wáng bù liú xíng sǎn*)

- vaccaria (王不留行 *wáng bù liú xíng*, Vaccariae Semen) 10 parts (pick on the eighth day of the eighth month)
- fine elder leaves (蒴藋細葉 *shuò diào xì yè*, Sambuci Folium Tenue) 10 parts (pick on the seventh day of the seventh month)
- mulberry root bark (桑東南根白皮 *sāng dōng nán gēn bái pí*, Mori Cortex) 10 parts (pick on the third day of the third month)[1]
- licorice (甘草 *gān cǎo*, Glycyrrhizae Radix) 18 parts
- zanthoxylum (川椒 *chuān jiāo*, Zanthoxyli Pericarpium) 3 parts (take out the eyes and [ones with] closed mouths, and remove the sweat)[2]
- scutellaria (黄芩 *huáng qín*, Scutellariae Radix) 2 parts
- dried ginger (干姜 *gān jiāng*, Zingiberis Rhizoma) 2 parts
- peony (芍药 *sháo yào*, Paeoniae Radix) 2 parts
- officinal magnolia bark (厚朴 *hòu pò*, Magnoliae Officinalis Cortex) 2 parts

Of the above nine ingredients, burn the first three ingredients up to mulberry root bark (*sāng gēn pí*) without destroying their nature and turning them to ash, and pestle and sift separately. Then blend them together to form a powder. Take one square-inch-spoonful [per dose]. For a small wound, sprinkle it on; for a large wound, take it [orally]. It can also be taken after childbirth. If there is wind or cold, do not use mulberry root. The first three ingredients can also be prepared by shade-drying for a hundred days.

Pus-Expelling Powder
(排膿散 *pái nóng sǎn*)

- unripe bitter orange (枳实 *zhǐ shí*, Aurantii Fructus Immaturus) 16 pieces
- peony (芍药 *sháo yào*, Paeoniae Radix) 6 parts
- platycodon (桔梗 *jié gěng*, Platycodonis Radix) 2 parts

Pestle the above three ingredients into a powder. Blend one egg yolk with an equal amount of the medicinal powder until thoroughly combined. Take this with fluid, once a day.

Pus-Expelling Decoction
(排脓汤 *pái nóng tāng*)

- licorice (甘草 *gān cǎo*, Glycyrrhizae Radix) 2 *liǎng*
- platycodon (桔梗 *jié gěng*, Platycodonis Radix) 3 *liǎng*
- fresh ginger (生姜 *shēng jiāng*, Zingiberis Rhizoma Recens) 1 *liǎng*
- jujube (大枣 *dà zǎo*, Jujubae Fructus) 10 pieces

Boil the above four ingredients in three *shēng* of water to get one *shēng*. Take five gě [per dose] warm, twice a day.

TEXT NOTES, LINE 18.6

[1] Mulberry root bark 桑東南根白皮 *sāng dōng nán gēn bái pí*: Same as 桑白皮 *sāng bái pí*.

[2] Take out the [ones with] eyes and closed mouths, and remove the sweat 除目及闭口，去汗 *chù mù jí bì kóu, qù hàn*: Remove the seeds that have dropped out of their husk, and remove the closed husks, which still contain seeds. The idea is that the husks are desired, not the seeds.

Synopsis, Line 18.6

This line gives three different formulas for bleeding due to incised wounds.

Commentary, Line 18.6

An incised wound would refer to any external injury from blades, knives, axes, or other metal implements. Damage to the channels in the flesh and skin prevents construction and defense blood and qì from moving freely along the channels. Hence treatment must focus on repairing the interruption in the vessels of the skin and flesh, so as to allow construction and defense to flow without obstruction, and as well as on quickening blood, stanching bleeding, dispersing swelling, relieving pain, and joining sinews and connecting bones. As a result the wound will heal naturally.

Vaccaria Powder (*wáng bù liú xíng sǎn*) is the governing formula for this indication. In this formula, vaccaria (*wáng bù liú xíng*) governs incised wounds by quickening blood, dispersing swelling, and relieving pain; fine elder leaf (*shuò diào xì yè*) disinhibits qì, regulates blood, and unstops impediment and stagnation; and mulberry root bark (*sāng bái pí*) controls damage to the center and interrupted vessels, engendering flesh and stanching bleeding.

These three ingredients should be roasted over a small flame until they are deep yellow in color, or alternatively shade-dried, to preserve their nature and stanch bleeding. Scutellaria (*huáng qín*) and peony (*sháo yào*) clear heat, resolve toxin, constrain yīn, and stanch bleeding; zanthoxylum (*huā jiāo*) and dried ginger (*gān jiāng*) dissipate cold, harmonize yáng, and move stasis, assisted slightly by officinal magnolia bark (*hòu pò*), which moves stasis and disinhibits qì. Lastly, licorice (*gān cǎo*) harmonizes the other medicinals, engenders flesh, and resolves the hundred toxins. The total effect of the formula is to disperse stasis, stanch bleeding, and settle pain. For minor injuries, you can apply it externally to stanch bleeding and relieve pain, but for major wounds with excessive blood loss it should be taken orally so as to strengthen its effect.

Pus-Expelling Powder (*pái nóng sǎn*) is here listed after Vaccaria Powder (*wáng bù liú xíng sǎn*) as it is meant to be used as a supplementary formula in treating incised wounds. In the early stages before incised wounds have become purulent, Vaccaria Powder (*wáng bù liú xíng sǎn*) is the governing formula. When a wound has become infected, however, and begun to form pus, Pus-Expelling Powder (*pái nóng sǎn*) is recommended. This formula uses large proportions of unripe bitter orange (*zhǐ shí*), which breaks stagnant qì, and peony (*sháo yào*), which eliminates blood impediment (inhibited movement of blood), in order to break qì, move stagnation, relieve pain, and quicken blood. Platycodon (*jié gěng*) expels pus and resolves toxin, and egg yolk (*jī zǐ huáng*) supplements vacuity and quiets the center. In combination, these ingredients are the governing formula for expelling pus by dispersing swelling, relieving pain, supporting right, quieting the stomach, and resolving toxin. The formula is therefore used to treat sores and swollen welling-abscesses by expelling pus and resolving toxin.

Pus-Expelling Decoction (*pái nóng tāng*) is a second basic formula for expelling pus and resolving toxin, which can be used for all types of internal and external welling-abscesses as well as for incised wounds with formation of pus. It has the effect of breaking blood, expelling pus, dispersing swelling, and relieving pain, and is particularly suitable in cases with welling-abscess and pus in the upper body. In clinic, it can be used in combination with the preceding decoction formula. In the formula, licorice (*gān cǎo*) resolves toxin, platycodon (*jié gěng*) expels pus, and fresh ginger (*shēng jiāng*) and jujube (*dà zǎo*) harmonize construction and defense, thereby assisting in recovery from incised wounds.

Line 18.7

浸淫疮，从口流向四肢者，可治；从四肢流来入口者，不可治。

Jìn yín chuāng, cóng kǒu liú xiàng sì zhī zhě, kě zhì; cóng sì zhī liú lái rù kǒu zhě, bù kě zhì.

Wet spreading sores that flow[1] from the mouth toward the four limbs can be treated. [Those that] flow from the four limbs to the mouth cannot be treated.

TEXT NOTE, LINE 18.7

[1] Flow 流 *liú*: Spread.

SYNOPSIS, LINE 18.7

This line describes the prognosis of wet spreading sores.

COMMENTARY, LINE 18.7

Wet spreading sores are a type of skin disease that manifests in rather stubborn sores the size of millet seeds. At the onset of the disease, these are limited to a small area with first itching and then pain, then they secrete a yellow fluid that soaks into the skin, and then gradually spread all over the body. Hence they are called wet spreading sores. If they erupt first in the mouth and from there spread to the limbs, this means that the sore toxin is moving from the inside to the outside; hence they are easy to treat. If, on the other hand, they erupt first on the limbs and from there spread to the mouth, this means that the toxin is moving from the outside to the inside; hence this is an unfavorable sign, and the condition is difficult to treat.

Line 18.8

浸淫疮，黄连粉主之。

Jìn yín chuāng, huáng lián fěn zhǔ zhī.

For wet-spreading sores, Coptis Powder (*huáng lián fěn*) governs.[1]

TEXT NOTE, LINE 18.8

[1] The commentary notes that the formula has been lost.

SYNOPSIS, LINE 18.8

This line describes the treatment for wet spreading sores.

COMMENTARY, LINE 18.8

Wet spreading sores are most commonly caused by damp-heat fire toxin. As the *Sù Wèn* ("Plain Questions") states, "All painful and itching sores are related to the heart." Treat them by applying Coptis Powder (*huáng lián fěn*) externally or by taking it internally. Coptis (*huáng lián*) is bitter and cold, can drain heart fire, and has the effect of clearing heat, drying dampness, and resolving toxin.

Most physicians consider that Coptis Powder (*huáng lián fěn*) actually refers to a powder made from coptis (*huáng lián*) as the single ingredient. Others suggest that 粉 *fén* (usually translated as "powder") could refer to 胡粉 *hú fěn* (processed galenite). In contemporary practice, coptis (*huáng lián*) is used as a single ingredient to treat red-eye in small children, fire heat toothache, swollen tongue, dysentery, and all patterns of damp-heat fire toxin like sores and boils, swellings and welling-abscesses.

趺蹶手指臂肿转筋阴狐疝蚘虫病

CHAPTER 19

Hobbled Dorsum of the Foot, Swelling of the Fingers and Arms, Cramping, Yīn Fox-Like Mounting, and Roundworm

Pulses, Signs, Treatment

‡ Overview

This chapter covers hobbled dorsum of the foot (趺蹶 *fū jué*), swelling of the fingers and arms (手指臂肿 *shǒu zhǐ bì zhǒng*), cramping (转筋 *zhuǎn jīn*), yīn fox-like mounting (阴狐疝 *yīn hú shàn*), and roundworm (蚘虫 *huí chóng*). Although these are five different conditions with different symptoms and no relationship to each other, they have been placed together in this chapter because they cannot be classified with any of the other diseases and are not substantial enough to form chapters of their own.

Hobbled dorsum of the foot (趺蹶 *fū jué*) refers to stiffness of the foot from the ankle to the toes, that makes it difficult for the patient to walk. 趺 *fū* means the dorsum or back of the foot; 蹶 *jué* means to have difficulty in walking or to stumble. It is a disease of the foot that is related to a loss of function in the tendons and joints. In addition to wounds from external damage, it is mostly caused by damage to the greater yáng channel that results in hypertonicity in the sinews. Therefore Zhāng Jī recommends acupuncture therapy to relax the sinews.

Swelling of the fingers and arms (手指臂肿 *shǒu zhǐ bì zhǒng*) is a condition characterized by swelling, distention, and pain in the fingers and arms as well as spasms and shaking, possibly accompanied by muscle twitching in various other parts of the body. The pathomechanism of this disease is rooted in wind-damp phlegm-drool stagnating in the joints and channels and network vessels. In treatment, we focus on dispelling wind and eliminating phlegm, as well as nourishing blood and freeing the network vessels.

Cramping (转筋入腹 *zhuǎn jīn*) means that the patient suddenly experiences rigidity and spasmodic pain in the four limbs. It is most commonly due to depressed damp turbidity obstructing the inner body, and over time transforming into heat, which damages liquid. Alternatively, it can be caused by severe vomiting and diarrhea damaging liquid, by a constitutional insufficiency of yīn liquid, qì, and blood, or by severe contraction of cold that is stagnating in the sinews and thereby depriving [the individual] of warmth and nourishment. In treatment, one must consider the specific disease cause and accordingly either clear heat, eliminate dampness, nourish yīn, and increase humor, or warm the channels, dissipate cold, quicken blood, and free the network vessels; or soften the sinews and resolving spasms.

Yīn fox-like mounting qì (阴狐疝气 *yīn hú shàn qì*) is a disease that affects only male patients, making the scrotum now smaller, now larger and accordingly causing intermittent pain. The disease discussed here differs from the type of cold mounting that is described in Chapter 10, "Abdominal Fullness, Cold Mounting, and Abiding Food." Yīn fox-like mounting is caused by cold-damp stagnating in the reverting yīn liver channel and by dual vacuity of the liver and kidney, or by internal damp-heat obstruction. It is therefore treated by warming and freeing yáng, coursing the liver, and regulating qì.

Roundworm (蚘虫 *huí chóng*) is a disease of intestinal parasites that is characterized by frequent severe pain in the abdominal and umbilical region, and in severe cases by vomiting of roundworm. Treatment should focus on treating the tip in the urgent stage, when the worms move and cause violent pain; hence one should urgently calm the roundworm and relieve pain. After this has been achieved, treat the root by expelling roundworm and killing the worms.

‡ Schematic Overview

Hobbled Dorsum of the Foot

Signs: Only being able to [move] forward, but not backward.

Treatment: Needling [to a depth of] two inches.

Swelling of Fingers and Arms

Signs: Swelling and stirring of the fingers and arms; twitching of the body.

Formula: Veratrum and Licorice Decoction (*lí lú gān cǎo tāng*) to eject wind-phlegm above the diaphragm.

CRAMPING

Signs: Rigidity in the arms and legs, and a pulse that [rigidly] moves up and down[1] and is slightly stringlike. Enters the abdomen.

Formula: Chicken's White Droppings Powder (鸡屎白散 *jī shǐ bái sǎn*) to precipitate qì and disperse binds and to clear heat and free the stool.

YĪN FOXLIKE MOUNTING

Signs: [The scrotum] is distorted in size and intermittently ascending and descending.

Formula: Spider Powder (*zhī zhū sǎn*) to disperse cold and discharge binds.

ROUNDWORM

Signs: Ejection of drool and heart pain that arises intermittently.

If toxic medicines do not stop [it], Licorice, Processed Galenite, and Honey Decoction (*gān cǎo fěn mì tāng*) governs.

ROUNDWORM REVERSAL

Signs: Reversal cold of the extremities with violent abdominal pain; vomiting of roundworm, which causes the patient to experience [temporary] calmness and then again intermittent vexation.

Formula: Mume Pill (*wū méi wán*) to dispel cold and quiet roundworm.

Line 19.1

师曰：病趺蹶，其人但能前，不能却，刺腨入二寸，此太阳经伤也。

Shī yuē: Bìng fū jué, qí rén dàn néng qián, bù néng què, cì chuǎi rù èr cùn, cǐ tài yáng jīng shāng yě.

The Master says: "The disease of hobbled dorsum of the foot [manifests in the patient] only being able to [move] forward, but not backward. Needle the calf [to a depth of] two inches. This is [a condition caused by] damage to the greater yáng channel.

SYNOPSIS, LINE 19.1

This line describes the causes, signs, and treatment of hobbled dorsum of the foot.

COMMENTARY, LINE 19.1

As the final phrase explains, hobbled dorsum of the foot is a disease related to the greater yáng channel. Yáng brightness moves the front of the body, and harmony of its sinews allows a person to walk forward. Greater yáng moves the back of the body, and smoothness of its sinews allows a person to move backward. When this channel is damaged, the patient is therefore able to move forward but not backward, which is precisely the sign described in the present line. To treat this condition, needle the calf to drain cold-damp in greater yáng. As soon as the sinews are softened, the patient will be able to move backward again.

Line 19.2

病人常以手指臂肿动，此人身体瞤瞤者，藜芦甘草汤主之。

Bìng rén cháng yǐ shǒu zhǐ bèi zhǒng dòng, cǐ rén shēn tǐ shùn shùn zhě, lí lú gān cǎo tāng zhǔ zhī.

When the patient has frequent swelling and stirring of the fingers and arms, this is twitching of the body. Veratrum and Licorice Decoction (藜芦甘草汤 *lí lú gān cǎo tāng*) governs.

TEXT NOTE, LINE 19.2

[1] The commentary notes that the formula has been lost.

SYNOPSIS, LINE 19.2

This line describes the signs and treatment of swelling and stirring of the fingers and arms.

COMMENTARY, LINE 19.2

Swelling and stirring of the fingers and arms is a disease characterized by swelling and distention in the fingers and arms with simultaneous twitching, and stirring of the muscles all over the body. Traditional texts already point out that "when wind prevails, there is stirring," and "when dampness prevails, there is swelling." Hence we know that the symptoms in the present line are caused by wind-phlegm obstructing the channels and network vessels. Wind-phlegm in the diaphragm attacks, moves, and scurries around. When damp phlegm congeals in the joints, we see swelling; when wind evil invades the channels and network vessels, we see stirring.

The formula for Veratrum and Licorice Decoction (*lí lú gān cǎo tāng*) is lost, but from analyzing the effect of the two mentioned ingredients, we know that the formula was an ejection preparation because veratrum (*lí lú*) ejects wind-phlegm, and licorice (*gān cǎo*) harmonizes the center, but can also induce vomiting. As a result of this effect, wind-damp is removed, and the patient will recover spontaneously.

Line 19.3

转筋之为病，其人臂脚直，脉上下行，微弦。转筋入腹者，鸡屎白散主之。

鸡屎白

右一味，为散，取方寸匕，以水六合，和温服。

Zhuǎn jīn zhī wéi bìng, qí rén bèi jiǎo zhí, mài shàng xià xíng, wēi xián, zhuǎn jīn rù fù zhě, jī shǐ bái sǎn zhǔ zhī.

Jī shǐ bái

Yòu yī wèi, wéi sǎn, qǔ fāng cùn bǐ, yǐ shuǐ liù gě, huó wēn fú.

The disease of cramping [manifests in] rigidity in the arms and legs, and a pulse that goes [straight] up and down[1] and is slightly stringlike. If cramping enters the abdomen, Chicken's White Droppings Powder (鸡屎白散 *jī shǐ bái sǎn*) governs.

Chicken's White Droppings Powder (鸡屎白散 *jī shǐ bái sǎn*)
chicken's white droppings (鸡屎白 *jī shǐ bái*, Galli Excrementum Album)

Grind the above single ingredient into a powder. Blend a square-inch-spoonful with six *gě* of water. Take warm.

TEXT NOTE, LINE 19.2

[1] A pulse that goes [straight] up and down 脉上下行 *mài shàng xià xíng*: This refers to a pulse in the inch, bar, and cubit positions that is stringlike, straight, and forceful, and without softness.

SYNOPSIS, LINE 19.3

This line describes the signs and treatment of cramping entering the abdomen.

COMMENTARY, LINE 19.3

Cramping means pulled tendons due to hypertonicity in the sinews, as a result of which we see restricted movement and pain in the four limbs. There may also be tension and rigidity in the neck, and a pulse that lacks any softness at all, identical to the pulse of tetany. Cramping occurs mostly in the lower limbs, with spasms in the gastrocnemius muscle. In severe cases, it extends from the legs up into the lower abdomen and causes pain there. This is what the text refers to as "cramping enters the abdomen."

From the choice of recommended treatment with Chicken's White Droppings Powder (*jī shǐ bái sǎn*), we know that the present line treats cramping that results from damp turbidity transforming into heat and damaging yīn. In this formula, the single ingredient is chicken's white droppings (*jī shǐ bái*), which is cold in nature, precipitates qì, and disinhibits urination and defecation.

This disease arises not only in cases of damp-heat damaging yīn, but is also very common in critical cases of sudden turmoil vomiting and diarrhea, when excessive consumption of yīn humor has deprived the sinews of warmth. In such cases, treat with Counterflow Cold Powder (*sì nì sǎn*) or Vessel-Freeing Counterflow Cold Powder (*tōng mài sì nì sǎn*), with the addition of evodia (*wú zhū yú*) or chaenomeles (*mù guā*) to warm and nourish. If cramping is caused by lack of nourishment in the sinews due to an invasion of cold evil, use Peony, Licorice, and Aconite Decoction (*sháo yào gān cǎo fù zǐ tāng*) to warm yáng qì, relax tension, and relieve pain.

Line 19.4

阴狐疝气者，偏有大小，时时上下，蜘蛛散主之。

蜘蛛十四枚（熬焦）　桂枝半两

右二味，为散，取八分一匕，饮和服，日再服，蜜丸亦可。

Yīn hú shàn qì zhě, piān yǒu dà xiǎo, shí shí shàng xià, zhī zhū sǎn zhǔ zhī.

Zhī zhū shí sì méi (áo jiāo); guì zhī bàn liǎng

Yòu èr wèi, wéi sǎn, qǔ bā fēn yī bǐ, yǐn huó fú, rì zài fú, mì wán yì kě.

Yīn fox-like mounting qì [manifests in the scrotum] being distorted in size and intermittently ascending and descending. Spider Powder (蜘蛛散 *zhī zhū sǎn*) governs.

Spider Powder (蜘蛛散 *zhī zhū sǎn*)
spider (蜘蛛 *zhī zhū*, Aranea) 14 pieces (simmer till scorched)
cinnamon twig (桂枝 *guì zhī*, Cinnamomi Ramulus) ½ *liǎng*

Make a powder with the above two ingredients. Take an eighth of a spoonful[1] [per dose], mixed into liquid. It can also be [prepared as] honey pills.

TEXT NOTE, LINE 19.4

[1]An eighth of a spoonful 八分一匕 *bā fēn yī bǐ:* It is not clear whether this is a qián-spoonful or a square-inch-spoonful.

SYNOPSIS, LINE 19.4

This line describes the signs and treatment of yīn fox-like mounting.

COMMENTARY, LINE 19.4

Yīn fox-like mounting qì, or fox-like mounting (狐疝 *hú shàn*), refers to a condition in which the testicles intermittently ascend and descend, and the scrotum intermittently grows and shrinks. In this condition, the testicles descend from the abdomen into the scrotum when the patient is standing or walking, as a result of which the scrotum feels distended, large, and as if dropping down. In severe cases, it causes pulling into the lower abdomen and severe pain. When the patient lies flat, the testicles retract into the abdomen, and the scrotum shrinks back to its normal size. The *Líng Shū* ("Magic Pivot") points out that fox-like mounting is a disease of the liver. It is mostly caused by ill-being of the affect-mind, or by cold-damp congealing in the reverting yīn liver channel.

The governing treatment for fox-like mounting is Spider Powder (*zhī zhū sǎn*) because it disinhibits with warmth and acridity. In this formula, spider (*zhī zhū*) breaks stasis and dissipates binds, while cinnamon twig (*guì zhī*) warms the channels and dissipates cold. When cold is dissipated and stasis dispersed, the patient recovers. Note that you have to exercise caution in the use of spider (*zhī zhū*) because it is toxic by nature. In more recent times, physicians have added liver-coursing and qì-regulating medicinals like toosendan (*chuān liàn zǐ*), corydalis (*yán hú suǒ*), costusroot (*mù xiāng*), fennel (*xiǎo huí xiāng*), cyperus (*xiāng fù*), or lindera (*wū yào*).

Line 19.5

问曰：病腹痛有虫，其脉何以别之？师曰：腹中痛，其脉当沉苦弦反洪大，故有蚘虫。

Wèn yuē: Bìng fù tòng yǒu chóng, qí mài hé yǐ bié zhī? Shī yuē: Fù zhōng tòng, qí mài dāng chén kǔ xián fǎn hóng dà, gù yǒu huí chóng.

Question: "When a patient has abdominal pain from worms, how do you differentiate the pulse?" The Master says: "In patients with pain in the abdomen, the pulse should be sunken and stringlike. But if it is surging and large instead, you thereby [know that] there is roundworm.

SYNOPSIS, LINE 19.5

This line describes the pulse diagnosis of roundworm with abdominal pain.

COMMENTARY, LINE 19.5

Abdominal pain is the key symptom of roundworm, but also occurs in numerous other diseases. Therefore, you need additional symptoms to differentiate it correctly. In general, abdominal pain due to interior cold manifests with a sunken and stringlike pulse, because sunken indicates interior cold, and stringlike indicates pain. By contrast, the present condition manifests with a surging and large pulse, but with no heat signs; hence we know that this indicates qì counterflow from stirring roundworms.

Nevertheless, you must corroborate this sign with additional evidence, such as continuous heart and abdominal pain, ejection of drool, blue spots in the white of the eyes, red spots on the surface of the tongue, peeling and eroded tongue fur, white macules on the face, itching in the nostrils, grinding teeth during sleep, insatiable appetite with difficult digestion, abnormal cravings, and irregular bowel movements.

Line 19.6

蚘虫之为病，令人吐涎，心痛发作有时，毒药不止，甘草粉蜜汤主之。

甘草二两　粉一两　蜜四两

右三味，以水三升，先煮甘草取二升，去滓，内粉、蜜，搅令和，煎如薄粥，温服一升，差即止。

Huí chóng zhī wéi bìng, lìng rén tù xián, xīn tòng fā zuò yǒu shí, dú yào bù zhǐ, gān cǎo fěn mì tāngzhǔ zhī.

Gān cǎo èr liǎng; fěn yī liǎng; mì sì liǎng

Yòu sān wèi, yǐ shuǐ sān shēng, xiān zhǔ gān cǎo qǔ èr shēng, qù zǐ, nà fěn, mì, jiǎo lìng huó, jiān rú bó zhōu, wēn fú yī shēng, chài jí zhǐ.

The disease of roundworm [manifests in] ejection of drool and in heart pain that arises intermittently. If toxic medicines do not stop [it], Licorice, Processed Galenite, and Honey Decoction (甘草粉蜜汤 *gān cǎo fěn mì tāng*) governs.

Licorice, Processed Galenite, and Honey Decoction (甘草粉蜜汤 *gān cǎo fěn mì tāng*)
licorice (甘草 *gān cǎo*, Glycyrrhizae Radix) 2 *liǎng*
processed galenite (粉 *fěn*, Galenitum Praeparatum) 1 *liǎng*
honey (蜜 *mì*, Mel) 4 *liǎng*

Of the three above ingredients, first boil the licorice (*gān cǎo*) in three *shēng* of water to get two *shēng*. Remove the dregs, add the processed galenite (*fěn*) and honey (*mì*), stir until blended, and decoct [to a consistency] like thin gruel. Take one *shēng* [per dose] warm. When recovery ensues, stop [taking the medicine].

SYNOPSIS, LINE 19.7

This line describes further signs and treatment for roundworm disease.

COMMENTARY, LINE 19.7

In the present line, "heart pain" refers to pain in the upper abdomen. When roundworms move in the intestines, the result is abdominal pain. When they ascend and harass the gallbladder, there is severe pain in the upper abdomen. When they enter the abdomen, the result is vomiting of roundworm. As the worms stir, they cause pain; as they rest, the pain ceases. This is the special characteristic of pain caused by roundworm. Vacuity cold in the spleen and stomach prevents them from containing fluids; hence liquid spills upward from the spleen and is ejected as clear drool.

In cases when treatment with toxic medicines, intended to kill the worms, has proven ineffective, use the recommended formula, Licorice, Processed Galenite, and Honey Decoction (*gān cǎo fěn mì tāng*) to calm the roundworms and relieve pain, because continued treatment with toxic medicines will only aggravate the pain and furthermore cause other symptoms. When the dynamic of the disease has eased up, you can then again use worm-killing medicines for subsequent treatment. In Licorice, Processed Galenite, and Honey Decoction (*gān cǎo fěn mì tāng*), all three ingredients are sweet, stomach-calming medicinals that will calm the roundworms and relieve pain.

Line 19.7

蚘厥者，当吐蚘，令病者静而复时烦，此为脏寒，蚘上入膈，故烦，须臾复止，得食而呕，又烦者，蚘闻食臭出，其人当自吐蚘。

Huí jué zhě, dāng tù huí, lìng bìng zhě jìng ér fù shí fán, cǐ wéi zàng hán, huí shàng rù gé, fù fán, xū yú fù zhǐ, dé shí ér ǒu, yòu fán zhě, huí wén shí chòu chū, qí rén dāng zì tù huí.

In roundworm reversal,[1] there should be vomiting of roundworm, which causes[2] the patient to experience [temporary] calmness and then again intermittent vexation. This means that there is visceral cold, and roundworm ascending into the diaphragm. Because of this, [we see] vexation that in a short while stops again, vomiting upon eating, and then again vexation. This means that the roundworm smells food and emerges; hence the patient spontaneously vomits roundworm.

TEXT NOTES, LINE 19.7

[1] Roundworm reversal 蚘厥 *huí jué*: Severe abdominal pain with reversal cold of the limbs in patients suffering from roundworm.

[2] Causes 令 *lìng*: The *Jīn Guì Yù Hán Jīng* ("Canon of the Golden Cabinet and Jade Sheath") has 今 *jīn*, "now," which could also make sense in this context. Zhāng Jī uses "now" when describing a clinical case in hand that contrasts with the norm. Thus, this would read: "When there is roundworm reversal, [the person] should vomit roundworm. [However,] now [in the present case] the patient is calm…"

SYNOPSIS, LINE 19.7

This line describes the signs and treatment of roundworm reversal.

COMMENTARY, LINE 19.7

"Roundworm reversal" refers to reversal cold in the extremities that is related to roundworm stirring, causing violent abdominal pain. Vacuity cold in the internal organs and roundworm harassing the chest and diaphragm results in vexation, agitation, and vomiting of roundworm. When roundworm stirs and ascends counterflow, there should be vomiting of roundworm; when roundworm quiets temporarily and then stirs again, the result is that the condition is temporarily calmed and then flares up again as vexation. According to the *Jīn Guì Yào Luè Xīn Diǎn* ("Heart-Insights Classic of the Essential Prescriptions of the Golden Cabinet"), the reason why roundworm quiets temporarily and at other times rises up is that worms like warmth. When there is cold in the viscera, the worms are disquieted and ascend into the diaphragm. Worms also like food. When the viscera are empty, the worms also ascend in search of food.

Line 19.8

蚘厥者，乌梅丸主之。

乌梅三百个　细辛六两　干姜十两　黄连一斤　当归四两　附子六两（炮）　川椒四两（去汗）　桂枝六两　人参六两　黄柏六两

右十味，异捣筛，合治之，以苦酒渍乌梅一宿，去核，蒸之五升米下，饭熟捣成泥，和药令相得，内臼中，与蜜杵二千下，丸如梧子大。先食饮服十丸，日三服，稍加至二十丸。禁生、冷、滑、臭等食。

Huí jué zhě, wū méi wán zhǔ zhī.

Wū méi sān bǎi gè; xì xīn liù liǎng; gān jiāng shí liǎng; huáng lián yī jīn; dāng guī sì liǎng; fù zǐ liù liǎng (pào); chuān jiāo sì liǎng (qù hàn); guì zhī liù liǎng; rén shēn liù liǎng; huáng bǎi liù liǎng

Yòu shí wèi, yì dǎo shāi, gě zhì zhī, yǐ kǔ jiǔ zì wū méi yī xiù, qù hé, zhēng zhī wǔ shēng mǐ xià, fàn shú dǎo chéng ní, huó yào lìng xiāng dé, nà jiù zhōng, yǔ mì chǔ èr qiān xià, wán rú wú zǐ dà. Xiān shí yǐn fú shí wán, rì sān fú, shāo jiā zhì èr shí wán. Jìn shēng, lěng, huá, chòu děng shí.

For roundworm reversal, Mume Pill (乌梅丸 *wū méi wán*) governs.

Mume Pill (乌梅丸 *wū méi wán*)
mume (乌梅 *wū méi*, Mume Fructus) 300 pieces asarum (细辛 *xì xīn*, Asari Radix et Rhizoma) 6 *liǎng* dried ginger (干姜 *gān jiāng*, Zingiberis Rhizoma) 10 *liǎng* coptis (黄连 *huáng lián*, Coptidis Rhizoma) 1 *jīn* Chinese angelica (当归 *dāng guī*, Angelicae Sinensis Radix) 4 *liǎng*

aconite (附子 *fù zǐ*, Aconiti Radix Lateralis Praeparata) 6 *liǎng* (blast-fry)
zanthoxylum (川椒 *chuān jiāo*, Zanthoxyli Pericarpium) 4 *liǎng* (remove the sweat)[1]
cinnamon twig (桂枝 *guì zhī*, Cinnamomi Ramulus) 6 *liǎng*
ginseng (人参 *rén shēn*, Ginseng Radix) 6 *liǎng*
phellodendron (黄柏 *huáng bǎi*, Phellodendri Cortex) 6 *liǎng*

Sift the above ten ingredients separately and combine. Soak the mume (*wū méi*) overnight in vinegar (*kǔ jiǔ*), remove the pits, and steam under five *shēng* of rice. When the rice is cooked, crush the mume (*wū méi*) to form a paste and blend thoroughly with the [other] medicinals. Place in a mortar with [some] honey (*mì*) and pestle two thousand times. Form into pills the size of firmiana seeds. Before meals, take ten pills [per dose] with fluid, three times a day, gradually increasing the dosage up to twenty pills. Raw, cold, slippery, and fetid foods are contraindicated.

TEXT NOTE, LINE 19.8

[1] Remove the sweat 去汗 *qù hàn*: Dry stir-fry to remove the water content.

SYNOPSIS, LINE 19.8

This line further describes the treatment of roundworm reversal.

COMMENTARY, LINE 19.8

Rundworm is a disease commonly seen in clinic and is generally marked by abdominal pain, ejection of drool, and vomiting of roundworm as key signs. Treatment should be based on the following principle: At times when the worms are inactive, concentrate on killing roundworm; at times when the worms stir and harass the gallbladder and stomach, focus on calming roundworm and relieving pain.

The previous line described roundworm associated with vacuity cold in the viscera. Yet in clinic roundworm can also occur in heat patterns or in combined heat and cold patterns. Thus we should carefully select treatment on the basis of pattern identification. The formula recommended in the present line addresses a condition of combined heat and cold pattern, because it employs both warming and cooling medicinals, in addition to stomach-quieting and worm-killing ones.

According to early literature, worms are submerged by sourness; hence we use the sourness of mume (*wū méi*) to submerge them. Worms are quieted by bitterness; hence we use the bitterness of coptis (*huáng lián*) and phellodendron (*huáng bǎi*) to quiet them. Worms are stirred by cold; hence we use cinnamon twig (*guì zhī*), aconite (*fù zǐ*), dried ginger (*gān jiāng*) and zanthoxylum (*huā jiāo*) to warm yáng and dispel cold. Together, these medicinals warm the viscera and quiet roundworm, as a result of which reversal is checked naturally. The formula also contains ginseng (*rén shēn*) and Chinese angelica (*dāng guī*) to boost qì and blood, and to nourish the center and quiet the viscera. Because coptis (*huáng lián*) and phellodendron (*huáng bǎi*) clear heat, while aconite (*fù zǐ*), asarum (*xì xīn*), cinnamon twig (*guì zhī*), and dried ginger (*gān jiāng*) warm the channels and dissipate cold, we know that the roundworm in this condition is related to stomach vacuity with a combination of heat and cold.

妇人妊娠病脉证治第二十

CHAPTER 20

Women's Pregnancy

Pulses, Signs, Treatments

‡ Overview

This and the following two chapters discuss women's diseases in terms of pulses, signs, and treatments under the headings of "Pregnancy" (妊娠 *rèn shēn*), "Postpartum" (产后 *chǎn hòu*), and "Miscellaneous Diseases" (杂病 *zá bìng*). This section is rich in content, comprising 45 lines and 40 formulas, which address menstrual disorders, vaginal discharge, pregnancy, delivery, and miscellaneous other diseases. It is of great value in terms of both theory and clinical application, and served as the foundation from which gynecology was developed several centuries later.

The present chapter deals with commonly occurring diseases of pregnancy. It includes information on the early diagnosis of pregnancy, on differentiating pregnancy from pathological concretions, on treating common diseases of pregnancy like retching and vomiting, abdominal pain, vaginal bleeding, difficult urination, and water swelling, and on nourishing and quieting the fetus. Emphasis is placed on diagnosing pregnancy early and on treating pregnancy-related abdominal pain and vaginal bleeding in accordance with the symptoms, because these aspects directly affect the development of the fetus. Reckless treatment with strong medicinals if pregnancy is misdiagnosed as disease, or a lack of treatment in cases of abdominal pain or vaginal bleeding during pregnancy, can all endanger the safety of the fetus and possibly lead to miscarriage or premature delivery. Therefore, the text discusses these aspects in greater detail.

⸸ Schematic Overview

Diagnosis

1. Diagnosis of early-stage pregnancy: No menstrual period for 60 days, a normal pulse, with thirst, inability to eat, and no [aversion to] cold or heat [effusion].
2. Differentiating pregnancy from concretion.
   a) Concretion: pre-existing concretion disease, with interrupted menstruation for less than three months, incessant spotting, and [a sensation like] stirring fetus above the umbilicus.
   b) Pregnancy: menstruation uninhibited in the three months [before pregnancy] and [fetal] stirring in the sixth month of pregnancy.

Malign Obstruction

1. Spleen-stomach disharmony.
   a) *Signs*: A normal pulse, [but] with slight weakness in the yīn pulses, and with thirst, inability to eat, and no [aversion to] cold or heat [effusion]
   b) *Formula*: Cinnamon Twig Decoction (*guì zhī tāng*).
2. Stomach vacuity and cold rheum.
   a) *Signs*: Incessant retching and vomiting in pregnancy.
   b) *Formula*: Dried Ginger, Ginseng, and Pinellia Pill (*gān jiāng rén shēn bàn xià wán*).

Abdominal Pain

1. Yáng vacuity with exuberant cold.
   a) *Signs*: A stringlike pulse and heat [effusion], abdominal pain, and aversion to cold, and the lesser abdomen feeling as if fanned.
   b) *Formula*: Aconite Decoction (*fù zǐ tāng*) to warm yáng and disperse cold.
2. Liver-Spleen disharmony.
   a) *Signs*: Tense pain in the abdomen.
   b) *Formula*: Chinese Angelica and Peony Powder (*dāng guī sháo yào sǎn*) to harmonize the liver and spleen.

Uterine Obstruction

1. Concretion with vaginal bleeding.
   a) *Signs*: Pre-existing concretion disease, and with interrupted menstruation for less than three months, incessant spotting, and [a sensation like] stirring fetus above the umbilicus.

   b) *Formula*: Cinnamon Twig and Poria Pill (*guì zhī fú líng wán*) to dispel stasis and transform concretions.

2. Thoroughfare and Governing Vessel vacuity cold.
   a) *Signs*: Vaginal bleeding and abdominal pain (called uterine obstruction).
   b) *Formula*: Ass Hide Glue and Mugwort Decoction (*jiāo ài tāng*)

DIFFICULT URINATION

1. Blood vacuity and damp-heat with qì depression transforming into dryness.
   a) *Signs*: Difficult urination with normal eating and drinking.
   b) *Formula*: Chinese Angelica, Fritillaria, and Flavescent Sophora Pill (*dāng guī bèi mǔ kǔ shēn wán*) to nourish the blood, disperse binds, and clear heat.

WATER SWELLING

1. Qì transformation obstructed.
   a) *Signs*: Generalized heaviness, inhibited urination, aversion to cold as if after a soaking, and dizzy head.
   b) *Formula*: Mallow Seed and Poria Powder (*kuí zǐ fú líng sǎn*) to free the orifices and disinhibit water.

DIFFICULT URINATION

1. Blood vacuity with damp-heat causing internal obstruction: Chinese Angelica Powder (*dāng guī sǎn*) to nourish the blood and fortify the spleen and to clear and transform damp-heat.
2. Spleen vacuity with cold-damp collecting: White Atractylodes Powder (*bái zhú sǎn*) to fortify the spleen and warm the center, and eliminate dampness and quiet the fetus.

Line 20.1

师曰：妇人得平脉, 阴脉小弱, 其人渴, 不能食, 无寒热，名妊娠, 桂枝汤主之。于法六十日当有此证, 设有医治逆者, 却一月加吐下者, 则绝之。

Shī yuē: Fù rén dé píng mài, yīn mài xiǎo ruò, qí rén kě, bù néng shí, wú hán rè, míng rèn shēn, guì zhī tāng zhǔ zhī. Yú fǎ liù shí rì dāng yǒu cǐ zhèng, shè yǒu yī zhì nì zhě, què yī yuè jiā tù xià zhě, zé jué zhī.

The Master says: "When a woman [presents with] a normal pulse,[1] [but] with a slight weakness in the yīn pulses,[2] and with thirst, inability to eat, and no [aversion to] cold or heat [effusion], it is called pregnancy. Cinnamon Twig Decoction (*guì zhī tāng*) governs.[3] In standard pregnancies, these signs should appear within sixty days [from the onset of pregnancy]. If a physician has treated [this condition] adversely,[4] and [the condition] persists for a month and is furthermore complicated by vomiting and diarrhea, this will sever [the pregnancy]."[5]

Text Notes, Line 20.1

[1] Normal pulse 平脉 *píng mài*: The pulse of a healthy person with no superabundance or deficiency.

[2] Yīn pulses 阴脉 *yīn mài*: The cubit pulses.

[3] A comment included in the received text reads: "The formula is found in the chapter on diarrhea." This refers to line 17.36 in Chapter 17, "Retching and Vomiting, Hiccup, and Diarrhea."

[4] If a physician has treated [this condition] adversely 设有医治逆者 *shè yǒu yī nì zhě*: If inappropriate treatment is given.

[5] This will sever [the pregnancy] 绝之 *jué zhī*: The woman will miscarry as a result of damage to the fetus from severe morning sickness or inappropriate treatment. Commentators differ on the interpretation of these two characters, due to the fact that the character 绝 *jué* (in its most literal sense, perhaps, to "cut off") has a number of possible meanings. 绝产 *jué chǎn* is a standard term for "severed childbearing," i.e., infertility. An alternative reading interprets 绝之 *jué zhī* as an imperative: "Stop [this treatment]!" or as "Sever [the roots of this condition]!" This can be read as advice to stop and alter the current treatment because it is obviously having adverse affects rather than curing the patient's condition. In either case, it is an indication of the severity of the condition and of the need to adjust treatment to this fact.

Synopsis, Line 20.1

This line describes the signs and treatment of malign obstruction in pregnancy.

Commentary, Line 20.1

As this line points out, standard cases of pregnancy present with a normal healthy pulse, except for slight weakness in the cubit pulse. If this is accompanied by a stopped menstrual period, and by retching and vomiting and inability to eat, but with no signs of external contraction of heat or cold, we know that this is the normal response of the body to pregnancy, which is commonly called "malign obstruction in pregnancy" (妊娠恶阻 *rèn shēn è zǔ*). In the early stage of pregnancy, the yīn pulse is weakened because the fetus is just beginning to bind, channel blood is collecting in the uterus to nourish the fetus, and fetal qì is not yet exuberant. As a result, yīn-blood is clearly insufficient, and the yīn pulse is weaker than the yáng pulse. This pulse occurs only in the first two months of pregnancy, and transforms into a slippery pulse as soon as fetal qì is fortified and blood and qì become abundant in the uterus.

In early pregnancy, the pulse is not diseased, but the body is; hence we should treat the patient with Cinnamon Twig Decoction (*guì zhī tāng*) to transform qì and regulate yīn and yáng, thereby harmonizing the spleen and stomach and curing malign obstruction. In clinic, most patients recover on their own from this condition. Nevertheless, in some cases the condition not only persists but worsens to the point where it can endanger the healthy development of the fetus, due to lack of or inappropriate treatment. If the symptoms do not disappear within one month and we furthermore see diarrhea and vomiting, this is a sign that the safety of the fetus is endangered and miscarriage might occur.

Line 20.2

妇人宿有癥病，经断未及三月，而得漏下不止，胎动在脐上者，为癥痼害。妊娠六月动者，前三月经水利时，胎也。下血者，后断三月衃也。所以血不止者，其癥不去故也，当下其癥，桂枝茯苓丸主之。

桂枝 茯苓 牡丹（去心） 桃仁（去皮尖，熬） 芍药各等分

右五味，末之，炼蜜和丸如兔屎大，每日食前服一丸，不知，加至三丸。

Fù rén sù yǒu zhēng bìng, jīng duàn wèi jí sān yuè, ér dé lòu xià bù zhǐ, tāi dòng zài qí shàng zhě, wéi zhēng gù hài. Rèn shēn liù yuè dòng zhě, qián sān yuè jīng shuǐ lì shí, tāi yě. Xià xuè zhě, hòu duàn sān yuè pēi yě. Suǒ yǐ xuè bù zhǐ zhě, qí zhēng bù qù gù yě, dāng xià qí zhēng, guì zhī fú líng wán zhǔ zhī.

Guì zhī, fú líng, mǔ dān (qù xīn), táo rén (qù pí jiān, áo), sháo yào gè děng fèn

Yòu wǔ wèi, mò zhī, liàn mì huò wán rú tù shǐ dà, měi rì shí qián fú yī wán, bù zhī, jiā zhì sān wán.

If a woman presents with a pre-existing concretion disease,[1] and with interrupted menstruation for less than three months, incessant spotting, and [a sensation like] stirring fetus above the umbilicus, this is harm from intractable concretion disease. In [true fetal] stirring in the sixth month of pregnancy, menstruation was uninhibited in the three months [before pregnancy]. This is the fetus. If there is vaginal bleeding [in the first three months],[2] and afterwards interruption of the menses for three months, this is coagulated blood.[3] The reason why bleeding does not stop is that the concretion is not gone. You must precipitate this concretion. Cinnamon Twig and Poria Pill (桂枝茯苓丸 *guì zhī fú líng wán*) governs.

Cinnamon Twig and Poria Pill (桂枝茯苓丸 *guì zhī fú líng wán*)

cinnamon twig (桂枝 *guì zhī*, Cinnamomi Ramulus)
poria (茯苓 *fú líng*, Poria)
moutan (牡丹 *mǔ dān*, Moutan) (remove the heart)
peach kernel (桃仁 *táo rén*, Persicae Semen) (remove the skin and tips, simmer)
peony (芍药 *sháo yào*, Paeoniae Radix) in equal proportions

Pulverize the above five ingredients. Blend them with processed honey (*liàn mì*) and form them into pills the size of rabbit droppings. Take one pill per day before a meal. If no effect is noticed, increase [the dosage] up to 3 pills.

TEXT NOTES, LINE 20.2

[1] Pre-existing concretion disease 宿有癥病 *sù yǒu zhēng bìng*: Abiding static blood in the abdomen, which binds and forms lumps. This disease existed before the woman became pregnant and is now complicating the pregnancy.

[2] Vaginal bleeding 下血 *xià xuè*: Irregular menstruation with bleeding between periods.

[3] Coagulated blood 衃 *pēi*: Dark purple static blood. In the *Shuō Wén Jiě Zì* ("Explanation of Simple Graphs and Complex Characters"), the character is paraphrased as 凝血也 *níng xuè yě* "This is congealed blood." An alternative textual version has 癥 *zhēng* ("concretion") instead of 衃 *pēi*.

SYNOPSIS, LINE 20.2

This line describes how to differentiate between concretion disease and pregnancy, and how to treat concretion disease.

COMMENTARY, LINE 20.2

The first sentence up to "harm from intractable concretion disease" describes the clinical manifestations of concretion disease with vaginal bleeding. This disease is caused by static blood collecting, binding, and forming lumps. Concretions are masses of fixed form and location that arise in the lower body, often as a result of gynecological diseases. Initially, concretion disease does not affect the menstrual period and women therefore menstruate normally. Over time, though, the menstrual flow becomes inhibited, and in severe cases blocked and stopped. In the present line, the menstrual flow has stopped for less than three months, when the woman suddenly experiences incessant vaginal bleeding, as well as a subjective sensation like stirring fetus above the umbilicus. These signs are not caused by a stirring fetus in a true pregnancy, but by static blood flowing downward, and by qì stirring in response to stirring blood.

The second section up to "this is coagulated blood" explains how to differentiate between a normal pregnancy and concretion disease. If menstruation has been normal in terms of timing, free flow, amount, color, and consistency for three months prior to its interruption, and the uterus has been growing every month since cessation of the menses and feels soft but not painful, the sensation of stirring fetus in the sixth month of pregnancy indicates true stirring fetus in pregnancy. However, if the patient experienced irregular periods and occasional vaginal bleeding for three months before the menses stopped, and afterwards again precipitated dark purple static blood in the third month after the menses stopped, these are the symptoms of concretion disease, not pregnancy.

The last section of this line describes the treatment of concretion disease with vaginal bleeding. In patients with concretion disease, continued vaginal bleeding indicates that the concretion is not eliminated yet. Treatment should therefore focus on removing the concretion, because this will make the bleeding stop on its own and allow new blood to form and nourish the fetus. Cinnamon Twig and Poria Pill (*guì zhī fú líng wán*) is the recommended formula because it disperses stasis and transforms concretions. In the formula, cinnamon twig (*guì zhī*) and peony (*sháo yào*) unstop and regulate blood in the vessels; moutan (*mǔ dān pí*) and peach kernel (*táo rén*) transform stasis and disperse concretions; and poria (*fú líng*) boosts spleen qì. The medicinals are combined with honey and initially taken in small dosages, to minimize or avoid damaging the fetus while expelling the evil.

Cessation of Menses and Vaginal Bleeding	
Concretion Disease	Fetal Spotting
Irregular periods and occasional vaginal bleeding for three months prior to stoppage of menses. Menstrual flow becomes inhibited, in severe cases blocked and stopped.	Menstrual flow normal in timing, flow, amount, color, and consistency for three months prior to interruption.
Precipitation of dark purple static blood in the third month after stoppage of menses; sudden incessant vaginal bleeding; subjective sensation like stirring fetus above the umbilicus less than three months after menstruation has ceased; hardness and pain in the abdomen; static blood flowing downward; qì stirring in response to stirring blood.	Uterus feels soft but not painful, and expanding since cessation of the menses. Sensation of stirring fetus in the lower abdomen after the fifth month of pregnancy. No lumbar or abdominal pain. Non-menstrual bleeding, sometimes incessant.

Line 20.3

妇人怀娠六七月，脉弦发热，其胎愈胀，腹痛恶寒者，少腹如扇，所以然者，子脏开故也，当以附子汤温其脏。

Fù rén huái shēn liù qī yuè, mài xián fā rè, qí tāi yù zhàng, fù tòng wù hán zhě, shào fù rú shàn, suǒ yǐ rán zhě, zǐ zàng kāi fù yě, dāng yǐ gù zǐ tāng wēn qí zàng.

When a woman in the sixth or seventh month of pregnancy [suddenly experiences] a stringlike pulse and heat [effusion], [a sensation of] even greater fetal distention, abdominal pain, and aversion to cold, then the lesser abdomen feels as if fanned.[1] The reason for this is that the uterus is open.[2] Use Aconite Decoction (*fù zǐ tāng*) to warm this viscus.[3]

TEXT NOTES, LINE 20.3

[1] The lesser abdomen feels as if fanned 少腹如扇 *shào fù rú shàn*: This describes a sensation of cold in the lesser abdomen as if cold wind were blowing on it.

[2] The infant's viscus is open 子藏开 *zǐ zàng kāi*: The "infant's viscus" refers to the uterus. "Open" means that it is not constrained.

[3] A commentary in the received text notes here that the formula is lost.

SYNOPSIS, LINE 20.3

This line describes the signs and treatment of abdominal pain in pregnancy due to yáng vacuity and exuberant cold.

COMMENTARY, LINE 20.3

The signs described in the present line indicate a pathomechanism of yáng vacuity and yīn exuberance in a patient in advanced pregnancy. A stringlike pulse in pregnancy indicates vacuity cold. In this pattern, heat effusion is not caused by external contraction, but is a sign that vacuous yáng is floating outward. Because yáng is vacuous and unable to warm the womb, while the qì of yīn cold exuberates internally, the patient experiences a subjective sensation that the fetus is even larger than usual at this stage of pregnancy, accompanied by abdominal pain and aversion to cold, and a feeling as if a cold wind were blowing onto the lower abdomen.

This condition is best treated with Aconite Decoction (*fù zǐ tāng*), to warm yáng, dissipate cold, warm the uterus, and quiet the fetus. While the formula is not listed here, some later physicians have suggested to use the formula for Aconite Decoction (*fù zǐ tāng*) from the *Shāng Hán Lùn* [2 pieces of blast-fried aconite (*fù zǐ*), 3 liǎng each of poria (*fú líng*) and peony (*sháo yào*), 4 liǎng of white atractylodes (*bái zhú*), and 2 liǎng of ginseng (*rén shēn*)].

Line 20.4

师曰：妇人有漏下者，有半产后因续下血都不绝者；有妊娠下血者，假令妊娠腹中痛，为胞阻，胶艾汤主之。

芎藭　阿胶　甘草各二两　艾叶　当

归各三两　芍药四两　干地黄四两
右七味，以水五升、清酒三升，合煮取三升，去滓，内胶令消尽，温服一升，日三服，不差更作。

Shī yuē: Fù rén yǒu lòu xià zhě, yǒu bàn chǎn hòu yīn xù xià xuè dōu bù jué zhě; yǒu rèn shēn xià xuè zhě, jiǎ lìng rèn shēn fù zhōng tòng, wéi bāo zǔ, jiāo ài tāng zhǔ zhī.

Xiōng qióng, ē jiāo, gān cǎo gè èr liǎng; ài yè, dāng guī gè sān liǎng; sháo yào sì liǎng; gān dì huáng

Yòu qī wèi, yǐ shuǐ wǔ shēng, qīng jiǔ sān shēng, gě zhǔ qǔ sān shēng, qù zǐ, nà jiāo lìng xiāo jìn, wēn fú yī shēng, rì sān fú, bù chài gèng zuò.

The Master says: "If a woman experiences spotting, in some cases it is caused by continued and incessant vaginal bleeding after late miscarriage;[1] in some cases it is vaginal bleeding in pregnancy. If it causes pain in the abdomen during pregnancy, this means uterine obstruction.[2] Ass Hide Glue and Mugwort Decoction (芎归胶艾汤 *xiōng guī jiāo ài tāng*) governs.[3]

Ass Hide Glue and Mugwort Decoction (芎归胶艾汤 *xiōng guī jiāo ài tāng*)

- chuanxiong (芎藭 *xiōng qióng*, Chuanxiong Rhizoma) 2 *liǎng*
- ass hide glue (阿胶 *ē jiāo*, Asini Corii Colla) 2 *liǎng*
- licorice (甘草 *gān cǎo*, Glycyrrhizae Radix) 2 *liǎng*
- mugwort (艾叶 *ài yè* Artemisiae Argyi Folium) 3 *liǎng*
- Chinese angelica (当归 *dāng guī*, Angelicae Sinensis Radix) 3 *liǎng*
- peony (芍药 *sháo yào*, Paeoniae Radix) 4 *liǎng*
- dried rehmannia (干地黄 *gān dì huáng*, Rehmanniae Radix) 4 *liǎng*

Boil the above seven ingredients in a blend of five *shēng* of water and three *shēng* of clear wine to get three *shēng*. Remove the dregs, add the ass hide glue (*ē jiāo*), and make it disperse completely. Take one *shēng* [per dose] warm, three times a day. If recovery does not ensue, repeat [the treatment].

TEXT NOTES, LINE 20.4

[1] Late miscarriage 半产 *bàn chǎn*: a technical term that refers to miscarriage in advanced pregnancy, after the fetus has formed but before the normal end of pregnancy. By contrast, if the fetus is lost during the first three months of pregnancy, this is called 堕胎 *duò tāi* ("dropped fetus").

[2] Uterine obstruction 胞阻 *bāo zǔ*: Also called uterine spotting (胞漏 *bāo lòu*, 漏胞 *lòu bāo*). This refers to vaginal bleeding in pregnancy that is accompanied by pain in the abdomen and is not caused by concretions or accumulations.

[3] A comment included in the received text reads: "Another version of this formula adds one liǎng of dried ginger (*gān jiāng*). Dr. Hú does not use dried ginger (*gān jiāng*) when treating women with uterine stirring."

SYNOPSIS, LINE 20.4

This line describes the signs and treatment of two types of vaginal bleeding in pregnancy.

COMMENTARY, LINE 20.4

The symptom of vaginal bleeding occurs most commonly in three circumstances, namely uninterrupted dribbling of menstrual fluid, incessant vaginal bleeding after late miscarriage, and vaginal bleeding due to uterine obstruction during pregnancy (also called uterine spotting). Although these conditions have different causes, their pathomechanism is in each case related to vacuity in the thoroughfare and controlling vessels, as a result of which yīn-blood fails to be contained in the inner body. Therefore, vaginal bleeding in all three circumstances is best treated by regulating and supplementing the thoroughfare and controlling vessels, and by securing the channels and nourishing blood, for which Ass Hide Glue and Mugwort Decoction (*jiāo ài tāng*) is the recommended formula.

If vaginal bleeding during pregnancy is accompanied by abdominal pain, this means uterine obstruction. In this disease, disturbance in the thoroughfare and controlling vessels causes yīn-blood to leak downward instead of entering the uterus to nourish the fetus.

The recommended formula for this condition is Ass Hide Glue and Mugwort Decoction (*jiāo ài tāng*). It consists of Four Agents Decoction (*sì wù tāng*) to nourish and harmonize blood, combined with ass hide glue (*ē jiāo*) to nourish yīn and stanch bleeding, mugwort (*ài yè*) to warm the channels and the uterus, licorice (*gān cǎo*) to harmonize the other medicinals, and clear wine to carry out the force of the other medicinals. In combination, these ingredients thus have the effect of harmonizing blood and stanching bleeding, warming the uterus and the channels, and treating abdominal pain and quieting the fetus. In gynecological practice, this formula is an important treatment for any kind of vaginal bleeding in patterns of blood vacuity and cold stagnation, but must be applied cautiously because of the blood-moving, stasis-conducting effect of Chinese angelica (*dāng guī*), chuanxiong (*chuān xiōng*), and clear wine. It is thus contraindicated in patterns with heat in the blood aspect, or in patterns of incessant vaginal bleeding with only vacuity but no stagnation.

Line 20.5

妇人怀娠腹中㽲痛，当归芍药散主之。

当归三两　芍药一斤　茯苓四两　白术四两　泽泻半斤　芎藭半斤

右六味，杵为散，取方寸匕，酒和，日三服。

Fù rén huái shēn fù zhōng jiǎo tòng, dāng guī sháo yào sǎn zhǔ zhī.

Dāng guī sān liǎng; sháo yào yī jīn; fú líng sì liǎng; bái zhú sì liǎng; zé xiè bàn jīn; xiōng qióng bàn jīn

Yòu liù wèi, chǔ wéi sǎn, qǔ fāng cùn bǐ, jiǔ huó, rì sān fú.

For women's tense pain[1] in the abdomen during pregnancy, Chinese Angelica and Peony Powder (当归芍药散 *dāng guī sháo yào sǎn*) governs.

Chinese Angelica and Peony Powder (当归芍药散 *dāng guī sháo yào sǎn*)

Chinese angelica (当归 *dāng guī*, Angelicae Sinensis Radix) 3 *liǎng*
peony (芍药 *sháo yào*, Paeoniae Radix) 1 *jīn*
poria (茯苓 *fú líng*, Poria) 4 *liǎng*
white atractylodes (白朮 *bái zhú*, Atractylodis Macrocephalae Rhizoma) 4 *liǎng*
alisma (泽泻 *zé xiè*, Alismatis Rhizoma) ½ *jīn*
chuanxiong (芎藭 *xiōng qióng*, Chuanxiong Rhizoma) ½ *jīn*[2]

Pestle the above six ingredients into a powder. Mix a square-inch-spoonful [per dose] with wine, and take this three times a day.

TEXT NOTES, LINE 20.5

[1] Tense pain 疞痛 *jiǎo tòng*: Continuous tension and pain in the abdomen. This is also mentioned under line 21.4 below.

[2] A comment included in the received text reads: "Another version of this formula has 3 liǎng."

SYNOPSIS, LINE 20.5

This line describes the signs and treatment of abdominal pain in pregnancy that is due to liver-spleen disharmony.

COMMENTARY, LINE 20.5

After conception, blood gathers to nourish the fetus, hence yīn-blood becomes relatively vacuous. The liver is the unyielding viscus, and if it is not emolliated and moistened, it is not harmonious. Thus liver blood becomes vacuous and orderly reaching is impaired. Furthermore, emotional excitement causes liver qì to run cross-counterflow and invade spleen earth. The result is liver depression spleen vacuity and liver vacuity qì depression. Therefore, blood stagnates and causes tension and continuous dull pain in the abdomen. This is different from the gripping pain of cold mounting or the stabbing pain of static blood, but is instead related to the pain of vacuity in the center with stagnation.

Because this condition is a pattern of liver depression spleen vacuity, we treat it with Chinese Angelica and Peony Powder (*dāng guī sháo yào sǎn*), to nourish blood and regulate the liver, while also fortifying the spleen and disinhibiting dampness. The formula uses a large dose of peony (*sháo yào*) to regulate the liver, relax tension, and relieve pain, in combination with Chinese angelica (*dāng guī*) and chuanxiong (*chuān xiōng*) to nourish blood and emolliate the liver, as well as disinhibit the qì dynamic. In addition, white atractylodis (*bái zhú*), poria (*fú líng*), and alismatis (*zé xiè*) fortify the spleen and percolate dampness.

Line 20.6

妊娠呕吐不止, 干姜人参半夏丸主之。

干姜　人参各一两　半夏二两

右三味，末之，以生姜汁糊为丸加梧子大，饮服十丸，日三服。

Rèn shēn ǒu tù bù zhǐ, gān jiāng; rén shēn bàn xià wán zhǔ zhī.

Gān jiāng, rén shēn gè yī liǎng; bàn xià èr liǎng

Yòu sān wèi, mò zhī, yǐ shēng jiāng zhī hú wéi wán jiā wú zǐ dà, yǐn fú shí wán, rì sān fú.

For incessant retching and vomiting in pregnancy, Dried Ginger, Ginseng, and Pinellia Pill (干姜人参半夏丸 *gān jiāng rén shēn bàn xià wán*) governs.

Dried Ginger, Ginseng, and Pinellia Pill (干姜人参半夏丸 *gān jiāng rén shēn bàn xià wán*)

- dried ginger (干姜 *gān jiāng*, Zingiberis Rhizoma)
- ginseng (人参 *rén shēn*, Ginseng Radix) 1 *liǎng* each
- pinellia (半夏 *bàn xià*, Pinelliae Rhizoma) 2 *liǎng*

Pulverize the above three ingredients and add fresh ginger juice to make a paste. Form into pills the size of firmiana seeds and take ten pills [per dose] with fluid, three times a day.

Synopsis, Line 20.6

This line describes the signs and treatment of malign obstruction due to stomach vacuity and cold-rheum.

Commentary, Line 20.6

Nausea, retching, and vomiting are the normal response of a woman's body to the changes of pregnancy. These symptoms are mostly caused by stomach vacuity and counterflow ascent of fetal qì. In general, this condition does not last long and cures itself without any need for medical treatment. The present line addresses a condition wherein the symptoms are more severe and moreover are sustained over a longer period of time.

From the choice of recommended medicinals, we know that the condition addressed here is characterized by vomiting of clear fluid or foamy drool, absence of thirst or thirst with a liking for hot drinks, dizziness and heart palpitation, fatigue and somnolence, clear urine and sloppy stool, and a stringlike pulse and slippery tongue fur. The cause of this condition is vacuity cold in the spleen and stomach, and counterflow ascent of cold-rheum. Therefore, we treat it by warming the center, dissipating cold, downbearing counterflow, and checking retching.

In the recommended formula, Dried Ginger, Ginseng, and Pinellia Pill (*gān jiāng rén shēn bàn xià wán*), dried ginger (*gān jiāng*) warms the center and dissipates cold, ginseng (*rén shēn*) supplements the spleen and stomach, and pinellia (*bàn xià*) and fresh ginger (*shēng jiāng*) eliminate rheum and downbear counterflow to check retching. In combination, the four ingredients have the effect of warming the center and supplementing vacuity, eliminating rheum and downbearing counterflow, and harmonizing the stomach and checking retching.

Line 20.7

妊娠小便难，饮食如故，当归贝母苦参丸主之。

当归　贝母　苦参各四两

右三味，末之，炼蜜丸如小豆大，饮服三丸，加至十丸。

Rèn shēn xiǎo biàn nán, yǐn shí rú fù, dāng guī bèi mǔ kǔ shēn wán zhǔ zhī.

Dāng guī, bèi mǔ, kǔ shēn gè sì liǎng

Yòu sān wèi, mò zhī, liàn mì wán rú xiǎo dòu dà, yǐn fú sān wán, jiā zhì shí wán.

For difficult urination with normal eating and drinking in pregnancy, Chinese Angelica, Fritillaria, and Flavescent Sophora Pill (当归贝母苦参丸 *dāng guī bèi mǔ kǔ shēn wán*) governs[1].

Chinese Angelica, Fritillaria, and Flavescent Sophora Pill (当归贝母苦参丸 *dāng guī bèi mǔ kǔ shēn wán*)
Chinese angelica (当归 *dāng guī*, Angelicae Sinensis Radix) 4 *liǎng* fritillaria (贝母 *bèi mǔ*, Fritillariae Bulbus) 4 *liǎng* flavescent sophora (苦参 *kǔ shēn*, Sophorae Flavescentis Radix) 4 *liǎng*

Pulverize the above three ingredients and blend with processed honey (*liàn mì*) to form into pills the size of small beans.[2] Take three pills [per dose] with fluid, increasing the dosage up to 10 pills.

Text Notes, Line 20.7

[1] A comment included in the received text reads: "For male patients, add one-half liǎng of talcum (滑石 *huá shí*)."

[2] Small beans 小豆 *xiǎo dòu*: Beans such as adzuki beans or mung beans.

Synopsis, Line 20.7

This line describes the signs and treatment of inhibited urination in pregnancy, due to blood vacuity and depressed heat.

Commentary, Line 20.7

When a pregnant woman presents with difficult urination but normal eating and drinking, this indicates that the disease is located in the lower burner. This condition occurs after conception due to heat arising from blood vacuity, and depressed qì transforming into dryness. As a result, the fluids in the bladder are insufficient, and urination is inhibited.

This condition is treated with Chinese Angelica, Fritillaria, and Flavescent Sophora Pill (*dāng guī bèi mǔ kǔ shēn wán*). In this formula, Chinese angelica (*dāng guī*) quickens blood and moistens dryness; fritillaria (*bèi mǔ*) disinhibits qì, clears the lung, and resolves depression; flavescent sophora (*kǔ shēn*) clears heat and disinhibits urine, thereby eliminating heat binds. By freeing the upper burner, it also frees the lower burner, in the action of "lifting the pot and removing the lid." Altogether, the formula nourishes vacuous blood, resolves and eliminates depressed heat, regulates the bladder, and thereby disinhibits urine.

Line 20.8

妊娠有水气，身重，小便不利，洒淅恶寒，起即头眩，葵子茯苓散主之。

葵子一斤　茯苓三两

右二味，杵为散，饮服方寸匕，日三服，小便利则愈。

Rèn shēn yǒu shuǐ qì, shēn zhòng, xiǎo biàn bù lì, sǎ xī wù hán, qǐ jí tóu xuàn, kuí zǐ fú líng sǎn zhǔ zhī.

Kuí zǐ yī jīn; fú líng sān liǎng

Yòu èr wèi, chǔ wéi sǎn, yǐn fú fāng cùn bǐ, rì sān fú, xiǎo biàn lì zé yù.

For water qì with generalized heaviness,[1] inhibited urination, aversion to cold as if after a soaking, and dizzy head upon rising, Mallow Seed and Poria Powder (葵子茯苓散 *kuí zǐ fú líng sǎn*) governs.

Mallow Seed and Poria Powder (葵子茯苓散 *kuí zǐ fú líng sǎn*)
mallow seed (葵子 *kuǐ zǐ*, Malvae Semen) 1 *jīn* poria (茯苓 *fú líng*, Poria) 3 *liǎng*

Pestle the above two ingredients into a powder. Take a square-inch-spoonful in fluid, three times a day. When urination is disinhibited, recovery will ensue.

Text Notes, Line 20.8

[1] Generalized heaviness 身重 *shēn zhòng*: Commentators have interpreted this phrase either as referring to a generalized feeling of heaviness due to water-damp lodging in the skin of the body, or as generalized swelling (身肿 *shēn zhǒng*) due to water-damp spilling into the skin.

Synopsis, Line 20.8

This line describes the signs and treatment of water swelling in pregnancy.

Commentary, Line 20.8

Water qì in pregnancy, or "pregnancy swelling" (子肿 *zǐ zhǒng*) as it is now more commonly called, refers to the disease of water swelling due to water-damp during pregnancy. It arises most commonly in the sixth and seventh months of pregnancy when the growth of the fetus affects the upbearing and downbearing of the qì dynamic.

Alternatively, it can be caused by damage from emotions during pregnancy, which prevents the liver from coursing freely, obstructs qì transformation, and causes water-damp to collect. Because qì transformation in the bladder is obstructed, urination is inhibited. When urination is inhibited, water-damp has no pathway for discharge and instead collects in the inner body. Spilling into the skin, it causes water swelling and a feeling of generalized heaviness. Water collects and entraps defense yáng, and the result is aversion to cold, as if the body had been soaked with ice-cold water. Because water qì collects internally, clear yáng is unable to bear upward; hence the patient experiences dizziness.

The condition described in the present line hinges on the fact that qì transformation is obstructed and urination is inhibited. Therefore, it is best treated by disinhibiting water and freeing yáng. When urine is freed, water-damp is removed and consequently yáng qì is freed also. As a result, the various symptoms will disappear on their own.

For this purpose, the text recommends Mallow Seed and Poria Powder (*kuí zǐ fú líng sǎn*). In this formula, mallow seed (*dōng kuí zǐ*) disinhibits and frees the orifices, while poria (*fú líng*) percolates and disinhibits dampness and conducts water downward. Together, these two medicinals disinhibit water and free the orifices, and percolate dampness and free yáng. They are therefore the ideal treatment for repletion patterns of water swelling in pregnancy.

Line 20.9

妇人妊娠，宜常服当归散主之。

当归　黄芩　芍药　芎藭各一斤　白术半斤

右五味，杵为散，酒饮服方寸匕，日再服。妊娠常服即易产，胎无苦疾，产后百病悉主之。

Fù rén rèn shēn, yí cháng fú dāng guī sǎn zhǔ zhī.

Dāng guī, huáng qín, sháo yào, xiōng qióng gè yī jīn; bái zhú bàn jīn

Yòu wǔ wèi, chǔ wéi sǎn, jiǔ yǐn fú fāng cùn bǐ, rì zài fú. Rèn shēn cháng fú jí yì chǎn, tāi wú kǔ jí, chǎn hòu bǎi bìng xī zhǔ zhī.

A pregnant woman should continuously take Chinese Angelica Powder (当归散 *dāng guī sǎn*).

Chinese Angelica Powder (当归散 *dāng guī sǎn*)

- Chinese angelica (当归 *dāng guī*, Angelicae Sinensis Radix) 1 *jīn*
- scutellaria (黄芩 *huáng qín*, Scutellariae Radix) 1 *jīn*
- peony (芍药 *sháo yào*, Paeoniae Radix) 1 *jīn*
- chuanxiong (芎藭 *xiōng qióng*, Chuanxiong Rhizoma) 1 *jīn*
- white atractylodes (白术 *bái zhú*, Atractylodis Macrocephalae Rhizoma) ½ *jīn*

Pestle the above five ingredients into a powder. Take a square-inch-spoonful in wine, twice a day. Taking this [formula] consistently throughout the pregnancy will result in an easy delivery and a fetus free from suffering and disease. All hundred postpartum diseases are governed by it.

SYNOPSIS, LINE 20.9

This line describes the treatment and prevention of stirring fetus due to blood vacuity with damp-heat.

COMMENTARY, LINE 20.9

The ancients knew of numerous methods for nourishing the fetus, the majority of which involved preventative treatments aimed at quieting the fetus. A pregnant woman with a healthy and strong constitution does not need to take medicines for nourishing the fetus. However, if a woman suffers from a weak constitution and tends toward miscarriage and spotting, or has experienced complications in childbirth, or is presenting with existing stirring fetus and red spotting, she requires active medical intervention, which we refer to as "nourishing the fetus" (养胎 *yǎng tāi*) or "quieting the fetus" (安胎 *ān tāi*).

During pregnancy, the most important viscera are the liver, which governs the storage of blood and thereby nurturance of the fetus, and the spleen, which governs movement and transformation and is the source of qì and blood formation.

When liver blood is vacuous, internal heat forms; when the spleen fails to move, dampness forms. Damp-heat obstructs the inner body and affects the fetus, causing it to stir. Thus we use Chinese Angelica Powder (*dāng guī sǎn*) to nourish blood, fortify the spleen, and clear and transform damp-heat.

In this formula, Chinese angelica (*dāng guī*) and peony (*sháo yào*) supplement the liver and nourish blood, and work together with chuanxiong (*chuān xiōng*) to relieve qì and blood stagnation. White atractylodis (*bái zhú*) fortifies the spleen and eliminates dampness, and scutellaria (*huáng qín*) consolidates yīn and clears heat. In this formula, all medicinals together have the effect of supplementing blood vacuity, eliminating damp-heat, and nourishing and quieting the fetus.

The recommendation of the text to consistently take Chinese Angelica Powder needs to be qualified as referring only to patients with liver-spleen vacuity. This also applies to the concluding statement that constant consumption of this formula brings about an easy delivery, healthy fetus, and quick recovery from postpartum discomforts.

Line 20.10

妊娠养胎，白朮散主之。

白朮 芎藭 蜀椒（去汗）三分 牡蛎

右四味，杵为散，酒服一钱匕，日三服，夜一服。但苦痛加芍药；心下毒痛倍加芎藭；心烦吐痛不能食饮，加细辛一两，半夏大者二十枚。服之后，更以醋浆水服之。若呕，以醋浆水服之；复不解者，小麦汁服之；已后渴者，大麦粥服之。病虽愈，服之勿置。

Rèn shēn yǎng tāi, bái zhú sǎn zhǔ zhī.

Bái zhú, xiōng qióng, shǔ jiāo sān fēn (qù hàn); mǔ lì

Yòu sì wèi, chǔ wéi sǎn, jiǔ fú yī qián bǐ, rì sān fú, yè yī fú. Dàn kǔ tòng jiā sháo yào; xīn xià dú tòng bèi jiā xiōng qióng;

xīn fán tù tòng bù néng shí yǐn, jiā xì xīn yī liǎng, bàn xià dà zhě èr shí méi, fú zhī hòu, gèng yǐ cù jiāng shuǐ fú zhī; ruò ǒu, yǐ cù jiāng shuǐ fú zhī, fù bù jiě zhě, xiǎo mài zhī fú zhī; yǐ hòu kě zhě, dà mài zhōu fú zhī. Bìng suī yù, fú zhī wù zhì.

For nourishing the fetus in pregnancy, White Atractylodes Powder (白朮散 *bái zhú sǎn*)[1] governs.

White Atractylodes Powder (白朮散 *bái zhú sǎn*)
white atractylodes (白朮 *bái zhú*, Atractylodis Macrocephalae Rhizoma) chuanxiong (芎藭 *xiōng qióng*, Chuanxiong Rhizoma) zanthoxylum (蜀椒 *shǔ jiāo*, Zanthoxyli Pericarpium) (remove sweat) 3 parts oyster shell (牡蛎 *mǔ lì*, Ostreae Concha)

Pestle the above four ingredients into a powder. Take one qián-spoon in wine, three times a day and once at night. For bitter pain, add peony (*sháo yào*). For toxic pain below the heart, double the chuanxiong (*xiōng qióng*). For heart vexation, vomiting, pain, and inability to eat or drink, add one *liǎng* of asarum (*xì xīn*) and 12 large pieces of pinellia (*bàn xià*). After taking [the medicine], take a further [dose] in sour rice milk. If the patient retches, take it with vinegar water. If it still fails to resolve, take it with wheat juice. If there is thirst afterwards, take it with barley gruel. Even if the patient recovers [sooner], do not discontinue taking [the entirety of the formula].

Text Note, Line 20.10

[1] The commentary notes, "See the *Wài Tái Mì Yào* ("Secrets from the *Wài Tái* Library") [for further information on this formula]." Chapter 33 of the *Wài Tái Mì Yào* contains a formula for White Atractylodes Powder (*bái zhú sǎn*) as a treatment for "repeated damage to the fetus and failure to grow." It consists of four parts each of white atractylodes (*bái zhú*) and chuanxiong (*chuān xiōng*), three parts of zanthoxylum (*huā jiāo*), and two parts of oyster shell (*mǔ lì*), and includes advice that peaches, plums, and sparrow meat are contraindicated. Based on this quotation, we can add the missing amounts for the formula in the present line.

Synopsis, Line 20.10

This line describes the treatment of stirring fetus due to spleen vacuity and cold-damp.

Commentary, Line 20.10

If a pregnant woman has a constitutional shortcoming, this will manifest in corresponding pathological changes as either cold transformation or heat transformation. The previous line described the treatment of damp-heat failing to transform; the present line addresses the treatment of spleen vacuity cold-damp. When the spleen is vacuous and cold-damp obstructs the center, you will see intermittent pain in the stomach duct, retching and vomiting of clear drool, no thought of food and drink, white vaginal discharge, and in severe cases stirring fetus.

This condition is treated with White Atractylodes Powder (*bái zhú sǎn*), which has the effect of quieting the fetus by fortifying the spleen, warming the center, and eliminating cold-damp. In this formula, white atractylodes (*bái zhú*) fortifies the spleen and dries dampness; chuanxiong (*chuān xiōng*) harmonizes the liver and soothes qì, zanthoxylum (*huā jiāo*) warms the center and dissipates cold; and oyster shell (*mǔ lì*) eliminates dampness and disinhibits water. In addition, white atractylodes (*bái zhú*) and chuanxiong (*chuān xiōng*) together have the ability to quiet the fetus by fortifying the spleen and warming blood; and zanthoxylum (*huā jiāo*) matched with oyster shell (*mǔ lì*) has a counterflow-settling and fetus-securing effect.

When we compare the application of White Atractylodes Powder (*bái zhú sǎn*) with that of Chinese Angelica Powder (*dāng guī sǎn*), we realize that both are preparations for eliminating disease and quieting the fetus, and both are used to regulate the liver and spleen. However, Chinese Angelica Powder (*dāng guī sǎn*) emphasizes nourishing blood and regulating the liver; hence it is mostly used in patterns of blood vacuity with nontransformation of damp-heat. By contrast, White Atractylodes Powder (*bái zhú sǎn*) emphasizes warming the center and fortifying the spleen, and is therefore used mostly in patterns with abnormal exuberance of cold-damp.

Line 20.11

妇人伤胎，怀身腹满不得小便，从腰以下重，如有水气状，怀身七月，太阴当养不养，此心气实，当刺泻劳宫及关元，小便微利则愈。

Fù rén shāng tāi, huái shēn fù mǎn bù dé xiǎo biàn, cóng yāo yǐ xià zhòng, rú yǒu shuǐ qì zhuàng, huái shēn qī yuè, tài yīn dāng yǎng bù yǎng, cǐ xīn qì shí, dāng cì xiè láo gōng jí guān yuán, xiǎo biàn wēi lì zé yù.

Damage to the fetus during pregnancy [manifests] in abdominal fullness, inability to urinate, heaviness from the lumbus downward, and an appearance as in water qì [disease]. In the seventh month of pregnancy, the greater yīn [channel] should nourish [the fetus]. If it does not nourish [it], this is heart qì repletion. [For this condition] needle to drain Palace of Toil (*láo gōng*, PC-8) and Origin Pass[1] (*guān yuán*, CV-4). When urine is slightly disinhibited, [the patient will] recover.

TEXT NOTE, LINE 20.11

[1] Palace of Toil (*láo gōng*, PC-8) and Origin Pass (*guān yuán*, CV-4): 劳宫及关元 *láo gōng jí guān yuán*: These are two acupuncture points. Palace of Toil (*láo gōng*, PC-8) is located in the center of the palm on the hand reverting yīn pericardium channel. Origin Pass (*guān yuán*, CV-4) is located three cùn below the umbilicus, on the Controlling Vessel.

SYNOPSIS, LINE 20.11

This line describes the signs and treatment of damage to the fetus due to heart fire exuberance.

COMMENTARY, LINE 20.11

According to TCM theory, damage to the fetus is a condition that most commonly arises in the seventh month of pregnancy, when the fetus is supposed to be nourished by the hand greater yīn lung channel. Typical symptoms include expanded uterus, abdominal fullness, inability to urinate, heaviness below the lumbus, and an appearance as in water qì disease. The pathomechanism of this condition is related to heart qì repletion and heart fire hyperactivity. When heart fire overcomes lung metal, the greater yīn channel is unable to nourish the fetus. Because the fetus is deprived of nourishment, fetal qì is disordered; because the lung fails to regulate and free, the waterways are inhibited. As a result, we see the symptoms described above.

The recommended treatment is to drain heart qì by needling Palace of Toil (*láo gōng*, PC-8), and to normalize fetal qì by needling Origin Pass (*guān yuán*, CV-4). When qì moves, water moves, and when water moves, the various symptoms will disappear. Note that both these points are normally contraindicated in pregnant patients since needling them can result in miscarriage or premature labor. They should therefore be used only by experienced and skilled physicians, with careful attention to the depth of needling.

妇人产后病脉证治第二十一

CHAPTER 21

Women's Postpartum Diseases

Pulses, Signs, Treatments

‡ Overview

This chapter is part of the section that specifically addresses women's conditions. It discusses common postpartum diseases, ranging from damage to qì and blood, and detriment to original qì, to insecurity of the interstices, reduced resistance to disease, so-called "postpartum vacuity of the hundred joints," and susceptibility to external invasion and resulting disease. Furthermore, when the residual blood and turbid fluids after childbirth are not eliminated freely, this tends to engender stagnation, as a result of which we see blood collapse damaging liquid, internal obstruction of static blood, and increased vacuity and stasis.

Under the aspect of vacuity, the text first discusses the three major symptoms of postpartum tetany (产后病痉 *chǎn hòu bìng jìng*), depression and veiling (郁冒 *yù mào*), and difficult defecation (大便难 *dà biàn nán*). While they differ in terms of disease cause, severity, and symptoms, they are all related to the pathomechanism of blood collapse damaging liquid, which is a key principle for identifying patterns and determining treatment in postpartum disease.

Next, the text describes the signs and treatment of postpartum diseases like wind-strike, diarrhea, vexation, derangement, and retching counterflow, and in terms of stasis in particular, postpartum abdominal pain.

In terms of treatment, Zhāng Jī emphasizes the special characteristics of postpartum blood collapse damaging liquid and dual vacuity of qì and blood, but otherwise recommends flexible treatment in accordance with a comprehensive analysis of the clinical patterns in any particular condition. Hence, the skilled physician must not cling blindly to the theory of vacuity in postpartum conditions, but must promote sweating where sweating is needed, or precipitate offensively when offensive precipitation is called for. This dual approach to the treatment of postpartum disease has become known in later times under the principle, "Do not restrict [treatment] to the postpartum [aspect of the disease], and do not forget the postpartum [aspect of the disease]" (无拘于产后，无忘于产后 *wú jū yú chǎn hòu, wú wàng yú chǎn hòu*).

‡ Schematic Overview

Three Diseases After Recent Childbirth

1. Tetany: Blood collapse, damage to liquid, and contraction of wind evil.
2. Depression and veiling: Cold evil exploiting vacuity.
3. Difficult defecation: Loss of moisture in the stomach and intestines.

All are treated by nourishing the blood and restoring fluids.

Pattern Identification and Treatment

1. Depression and veiling with hard stool.

   Signs: Pulse that is slightly weak, inability to eat, hard stool, and sweating from the head.

   Formula: Minor Bupleurum Decoction (*xiǎo chái hú tāng*) to harmonize and disinhibit the pivot and to support right and outthrust the evil.

2. Postpartum abdominal pain.

   a) Blood vacuity with center cold.

   Signs: Postpartum tense pain in the abdomen.

   Formula: Chinese Angelica, Fresh Ginger, and Goat Meat Decoction (*dāng guī shēng jiāng yáng ròu tāng*) to nourish the blood and disperse cold.

   b) Qì and blood depression.

   Signs: Abdominal pain with vexation, fullness, and inability to lie down.

   Formula: For postpartum abdominal pain with vexation, fullness, and inability to lie down, Unripe Bitter Orange and Peony Powder (*zhǐ shí sháo yào sǎn*) will diffuse qì and blood.

   c) Blood stasis.

   Signs: Abdominal pain (that refuses pressure).

   Formula: Static Blood-Precipitating Decoction (*xià yū xuè tāng*) to break blood, expel stasis, and discharge heat.

3. Incomplete elimination of lochia with yáng brightness stomach domain repletion.

Signs: Late afternoon tidal heat, vexation and agitation, inability to eat, delirium, and constipation.

Formula: Major Qì-Coordinating Decoction (*dà chéng qì tāng*) to clear heat and move the blood.

4. Postpartum insufficiency of yīn-blood with vacuity heat cauising internal harassment.

Signs: Vexation and vomiting.

Formula: Major Bamboo Shavings Pill (*zhú pí dà wán*) to quiet the center and boost qì.

5. Postpartum diarrhea.

Signs: Vexation and vomiting.

Formula: Pulsatilla Decoction Plus Licorice and Ass Hide Glue (*bái tóu wēng jiā gān cǎo ē jiāo tāng*) to nourish yīn and clear heat.

6. Postpartum external contraction.

a) Postpartum wind-strike.

Signs: Wind-strike that has lasted for several days, with aversion to cold, heat effusion, sweating, and dry retching.

Formula: Yáng Dawn Decoction (*yáng dàn tāng*) to resolve the exterior and dispel wind.

b) Wind-strike with yáng vacuity.

Signs: Heat effusion, full red complexion, panting, and headache.

Formula: Black Bamboo Leaf Decoction (*zhú yè tāng*) to treat both exterior and interior.

Line 21.1

问曰：新产妇人有三病，一者病痉，二者病郁冒，三者大便难，何谓也？师曰：新产血虚，多汗出，喜中风，故令病痉；亡血复汗，寒多，故令郁冒；亡津液胃燥，故大便难。

Wèn yuē: Xīn chǎn fù rén yǒu sān bìng, yī zhě bìng jìng, èr zhě bìng yù mào, sān zhě dà biàn nán, hé wèi yě? Shī yuē: Xīn chǎn xuè xū, duō hàn chū, xǐ zhōng fēng, fù lìng bìng jìng; wáng xuè fù hàn, hán duō, fù lìng yù mào; wáng jīn yè wèi zào, fù dà biàn nán.

Question: "After recent childbirth, women suffer from three diseases. The first is tetany, the second is depression and veiling,[1] and the third is difficult defecation. What does this mean?" The Master says: "Recent childbirth [that] results in blood vacuity, copious sweating, and a tendency to be struck by wind[2] causes tetany.[3] [It also results in] blood collapse followed by sweating, and increased cold; hence it causes depression and veiling. [It lastly results in] collapse of fluids and stomach dryness;[4] hence it causes difficult defecation."

TEXT NOTES, LINE 21.1

[1] Depression and veiling 郁冒 *yù mào*: Depression denotes feelings of oppression and discomfort; veiling denotes dizzy head and clouded vision, as if the head were covered by something.

[2] Tendency to be struck by wind 喜中风 *xǐ zhòng fēng*: A tendency to contract wind evil. Wind-strike in this context does not mean apoplexy.

[3] Tetany 痉 *jìng*: Various forms of spasm. See Chapter 2.

[4] Stomach dryness 胃燥 *wèi zào*: Zhāng Jī often uses "stomach" to refer loosely to the stomach and intestines. Here, the dryness is located in the intestines.

SYNOPSIS, LINE 21.1

This line describes the pathomechanisms of postpartum tetany, depression and veiling, and difficult defecation.

COMMENTARY, LINE 21.1

Excessive blood loss after childbirth results in dual vacuity of construction and defense, and insecurity of the interstices. As a result, women are particularly susceptible to contracting wind evil during this time. Because liquid is damaged due to blood collapse, it is unable to moisten and nourish the sinews. When this is complicated by wind, which is a yáng evil and can transform into dryness to further damage the sinews, we see spasms and convulsions, or in other words, tetany. Blood collapse followed by sweating causes wearing on blood and damage to liquid. This results not only in susceptibility to invasion by external evils and "increased cold," but also to lack of blood, and yīn vacuity, as a result of which we see abnormal exuberance of yáng qì and upper body reversal. This manifests in dizzy head, distorted vision, and oppression and discomfort, the signs of "depression and veiling." Because childbirth causes double damage to the fluids from blood loss and profuse sweating, the large intestine is deprived of moistening. Consequently, defecation becomes difficult.

All three conditions are common in women after childbirth and, while differing in the particular condition, all are rooted in the identical pathomechanism of blood collapse damaging liquid. Because of this, they are all treated by the same principle of caring for the fluids.

Line 21.2

产妇郁冒，其脉微弱，呕不能食，大便反坚，但头汗出，所以然者，血虚而厥，厥而必冒。冒家欲解，必大汗出。以血虚下厥，孤阳上出，故头汗出。所以产妇喜汗出者，亡阴血虚，阳气独盛，故当汗出，阴阳乃复。大便坚，呕不能食，小柴胡汤主之。

Chǎn fù yù mào, qí mài wēi ruò, ǒu bù néng shí, dà biàn fǎn jiān, dàn tóu hàn chū, suǒ yǐ rán zhě, xuè xū ér jué, jué ér bì mào, mào jiā yù jiě, bì dà hàn chū, yǐ xuè xū xià jué, gū yáng shàng chū, fù tóu hàn chū. Suǒ yǐ chǎn fù xǐ hàn chū zhě, wáng yīn xuè xū, yáng qì dú shèng, fù dāng hàn chū, yīn yáng nǎi fù. Dà biàn jiān, ǒu bù néng shí, xiǎo chái hú tāng zhǔ zhī.

Postpartum depression and veiling [manifests in] a slightly weak pulse, retching and inability to eat, unexpectedly hard stool, and sweating from the head only. The reason for this is that blood is vacuous, and this causes reversal,[1] which inevitably results in veiling. If you want to resolve [disease] in a patient with veiling, you must induce great sweating. Blood vacuity and reversal in the lower body cause solitary yáng to exit from the upper body; hence sweat exits [only] from the head. The reason why a woman after childbirth has a tendency to sweat is that yīn has collapsed and blood is vacuous, and thus yáng qì alone is exuberant. Therefore, you should induce sweating, so as to restore yīn and yáng [to balance]. For hard stool and retching with inability to eat, Minor Bupleurum Decoction (小柴胡汤 *xiǎo chái hú tāng*) governs.[2]

Text Notes, Line 21.2

[1] Reversal 厥 *jué*: Counterflow ascent of qì.

[2] A comment included in the received text reads: "For the formula, see under Retching and Vomiting." The formula is found in Chapter 17, "Retching and Vomiting, Hiccup, and Diarrhea," line 17.15.

Synopsis, Line 21.2

This line describes the cause, pathomechanism, signs, and treatment of postpartum depression and veiling with hard stool.

Commentary, Line 21.2

The previous line pointed out that a condition of depression and veiling is related to the internal cause of "blood collapse followed by sweating" and to the external cause of "increased cold." The present line further elucidates this pathomechanism, emphasizing the significance of blood vacuity and reversal. In other words, the basic pathomechanism is yīn vacuity with yáng exuberance, and counterflow ascent of yáng qì.

Regarding the treatment of postpartum depression and veiling, the text states, "you must induce great sweating." In this context, "great sweating" does not refer to severe dripping sweating, but rather to sweating all over the body. This relates to the fact that sweating from the head only is one of the symptoms of depression veiling. By causing the patient to sweat all over, the abnormal exuberance of yáng is reduced, so that the balance of yīn and yáng is restored. While this type of sweating is achieved with the assistance of dissipating medicinals, the text also mentions another kind of sweating, namely the spontaneous sweating that occurs in patients after childbirth naturally as the body's physiological response to childbirth, with the effect of regulating the balance of yīn and yáng.

As stated in the beginning of this line, the disease of postpartum depression and veiling manifests in sweating from the head only, as well as dizziness, clouded vision, oppression and discomfort, a slightly weak pulse, retching and inability to eat, and hard stool. All these symptoms are caused by a root condition of yīn vacuity and yáng exuberance, which is complicated by an external invasion of cold evil. However, the exterior evil is the tip, and interior vacuity is the root; hence the pulse is weak and not floating. Because yáng qì is abnormally exuberant and moves to the upper body, the stomach loses its ability to downbear harmoniously; there is a lack of fluids in the lower body, and the intestinal tract is deprived of moisture. Thus we see retching with inability to eat, and hard stool.

The general treatment principle for depression and veiling is to resolve the condition by effusing sweat all over the body. More specifically, we treat the tip condition of exterior evil repletion by dissipating, and the root condition of interior vacuity by supplementing. The recommended formula is Minor Bupleurum Decoction (*xiǎo chái hú tāng*), to support right and outthrust evil, to disinhibit the qì dynamic, and to harmonize yīn and yáng, so that the symptoms of depression and veiling are resolved on their own.

Line 21.3

病解能食，七八日更发热者，此为胃实，大承气汤主之。

Bìng jiě néng shí, qī bā rì gèng fā rè zhě, cǐ wéi wèi shí, dà chéng qì tāng zhǔ zhī.

If the disease is resolved and [the patient] is able to eat again, but after seven or eight days again experiences heat effusion, this is stomach repletion. Major Qì-Coordinating Decoction (大承气汤 *dà chéng qì tāng*)[1] governs.

TEXT NOTE, LINE 21.3

[1] A comment included in the received text reads: "For the formula, see the chapter on Tetany." This refers to line 2.13 in Chapter 2, "Tetany, Dampness, and Thermoplegia."

SYNOPSIS, LINE 21.3

This line describes the signs and treatment of resolved depression and veiling transforming into yáng brightness bowel repletion.

COMMENTARY, LINE 21.3

Inability to eat and drink is a key symptom of depression and veiling. When this disease is resolved, the upper burner is disinhibited, the fluids run downward, stomach qì is harmonized, there is generalized sweating, and the patient is able to eat and drink again. However, if residual evil is not eliminated completely, it can cause stagnation and bind with food to form a pattern of stomach repletion. As a result, you see heat effusion after seven or eight days. This type of heat effusion is not related to disease of the exterior, but to disease in the interior. In addition to heat effusion, you will see other symptoms of interior repletion, such as abdominal fullness and pain, hard bound stool, a sunken and replete pulse, and a thick yellow tongue fur.

Despite the fact that postpartum patients tend to suffer from blood vacuity, the recommended treatment is offensive precipitation with Major Qì-Coordinating Decoction (*dà chéng qì tāng*), which expels evil and rids repletion.

Line 21.4

产妇腹中㽲痛，当归生姜羊肉汤主之。并治腹中寒疝，虚劳不足。

Chǎn fù fù zhōng jiǎo tòng, dāng guī shēng jiāng yáng ròu tāng zhǔ zhī. Bìng zhì fù zhōng hán shàn, xū láo bù zú.

For tense pain in the abdomen after childbirth, Chinese Angelica, Fresh Ginger, and Goat Meat Decoction (当归生姜羊肉汤 *dāng guī shēng jiāng yáng ròu tāng*) governs.[2] [This formula] also treats cold mounting in the abdomen, vacuity taxation, and insufficiency.

TEXT NOTES, LINE 21.4

[1] Tense pain 㽲痛 *jiǎo tòng*: Continuous tension and pain in the abdomen. This is also mentioned under line 20.5 above.

[2] A comment included in the received text reads: "For the formula, see under Cold Mounting." This refers to line 10.18 in Chapter 10, "Abdominal Fullness, Cold Mounting, and Abiding Food."

SYNOPSIS, LINE 21.4

This line describes the signs and treatment of postpartum abdominal pain from blood vacuity and interior cold.

COMMENTARY, LINE 21.4

When cold evil exploits vacuity and enters the interior, it causes tension and pain in the abdomen. Because the pattern is related to vacuity cold, the pain is continuous and dull, and likes warmth and pressure. In addition, there may be physical cold and fear of cold, a pale tongue with a moist white tongue fur, and a vacuous and moderate, or sunken and fine pulse. This condition arises due to excessive blood loss during delivery and emptiness in the thoroughfare and controlling vessels. Because blood is scant and qì is weak, they move without force. Furthermore, cold evil exploits the vacuity and invades the blood chamber, resulting in blood vacuity with cold stagnation, disharmony in the channels and network vessels, and tension and dull pain in the abdomen.

The recommended formula is Chinese Angelica, Fresh Ginger, and Goat/Lamb Meat Decoction (*dāng guī shēng jiāng yáng ròu tāng*) to supplement vacuity, nourish blood, dissipate cold, and relieve pain. In this formula, Chinese angelica (*dāng guī*) nourishes blood and supplements vacuity; fresh ginger (*shēng jiāng*) warms the center and dissipates cold; and goat/lamb meat (*yáng ròu*), as a medicinal with affinity to flesh and blood, supplements vacuity and engenders blood. This formula can also be used to treat cold mounting due to cold from blood vacuity, as well as vacuity taxation and insufficiency due to yáng vacuity and blood cold.

Line 21.5

产后腹痛，烦满不得卧，枳实芍药散主之。

枳实（烧令黑，勿太过）芍药等分

右二味，杵为散，服方寸匕，日三服，并主痈脓，以麦粥下之。

Chǎn hòu fù tòng, fán mǎn bù dé wò, zhǐ shí sháo yào sǎn zhǔ zhī.

Zhǐ shí (shāo lìng hēi, wù tài guò); sháo yào děng fēn

Yòu èr wèi, chǔ wéi sǎn, fú fāng cùn bǐ, rì sān fú, bìng zhǔ yōng nóng, yǐ mài zhōu xià zhī.

For postpartum abdominal pain with vexation, fullness, and inability to lie down, Unripe Bitter Orange and Peony Powder (枳实芍药散 *zhǐ shí sháo yào sǎn*) governs.

Unripe Bitter Orange and Peony Powder (枳实芍药散 *zhǐ shí sháo yào sǎn*)
unripe bitter orange (枳实 *zhǐ shí*, Aurantii Fructus Immaturus) (burn until black, but not excessively) peony (芍药 *sháo yào*, Paeoniae Radix) in equal proportions

Pestle the two above ingredients into a powder. Take one square-inch-spoonful three times a day. [This formula] also governs welling-abscesses with pus. Down it with barley gruel.

SYNOPSIS, LINE 21.5

This line describes the signs and treatment of postpartum abdominal pain due to repletion from qì depression and blood stasis.

COMMENTARY, LINE 21.5

Abdominal pain after childbirth can arise in both vacuity and repletion patterns. If it is not accompanied by vexation and fullness, but by liking for pressure and warmth, we know that the disease is related to interior vacuity and to cold. In the present line, we know from the accompanying signs that the condition is related to interior repletion. After childbirth, qì and blood can become depressed and stagnant, and consequently form repletion and cause obstruction in the qì dynamic. The fact that the condition here is characterized by "vexation, fullness, and inability to lie down," indicates that the distention is more severe than the pain, and hence that the key factor in this pathomechanism is qì stagnation. Vexation is the result of qì depression transforming into heat, and depressed heat harassing the heart; fullness is the result of stagnation and inhibition of the qì dynamic; and pain is the result of stoppage of both qì and blood.

In accord with the pathomechanism, the condition is best treated by breaking qì, dissipating binds, harmonizing blood, and relieving pain. The recommended treatment is Unripe Bitter Orange and Peony Powder (*zhǐ shí sháo yào sǎn*). In this formula, unripe bitter orange (*zhǐ shí*) breaks qì and dissipates binds. Being burned until blackened, it also has the effect of entering the blood aspect and moving qì within blood; peony (*sháo yào*) harmonizes blood and relieves pain. These two ingredients are taken in relatively small dosage and in equal proportions because this condition is not severe and is therefore treated gradually. It is best taken with barley gruel because barley is sweet, salty, and cool by nature, and enters the spleen and stomach channels to eliminate heat, boost qì, and harmonize the stomach and calm the center.

Line 21.6

师曰：产妇腹痛，法当以枳实芍药散，假令不愈者，此为腹中有干血着脐下，宜下瘀血汤主之。亦主经水不利。

Shī yuē: Chǎn fù fù tòng, fǎ dāng yǐ zhǐ shí sháo yào sǎn, jiǎ lìng bù yù zhě, cǐ wéi fù zhōng yǒu gān xuè zhù qí xià, yí xià yū xuè tāng zhǔ zhī. Yì zhǔ jīng shuǐ bù lì.

大黄三两　桃仁二十枚　䗪虫（熬，去足）二十枚

Dà huáng sān liǎng; táo rén èr shí méi; zhè chóng (áo, qù zú) èr shí méi

右三味，末之，炼蜜和为四丸，以酒一升，煎一丸，取八合，顿服之，新血下如豚肝。

Yòu sān wèi, mò zhī, liàn mì hé wéi sì wán, yǐ jiǔ yī shēng, jiān yī wán, qǔ bā gě, dùn fú zhī, xīn xuè xià rú tún gān.

The Master says: "The standard treatment for women with abdominal pain after childbirth is Unripe Bitter Orange and Peony Powder (*zhǐ shí sháo yào sǎn*). However, if recovery does not occur, this means that there is dry blood fixed in the abdomen below the umbilicus. Static Blood-Precipitating Decoction (下瘀血汤 *xià yū xuè tāng*) governs. [This formula] also governs inhibited menstrual flow.

Static Blood-Precipitating Decoction (下瘀血汤 *xià yū xuè tāng*)

rhubarb (大黄 *dà huáng*, Rhei Radix et Rhizoma) 3 *liǎng*
peach kernel (桃仁 *táo rén*, Persicae Semen) 20 pieces
ground beetle (蟅虫 *zhè chóng*, Eupolyphaga seu Steleophaga) 20 pieces (simmer and remove legs)

Pulverize the above three ingredients and blend with processed honey (*liàn mì*) to form into four pills. Decoct one pill in one *shēng* of wine to get eight *gě*. Quaff. New blood will descend like piglet's liver.

SYNOPSIS, LINE 21.6

This line describes the signs and treatment of postpartum abdominal pain due to stasis heat binding in the uterus.

COMMENTARY, LINE 21.6

If postpartum abdominal pain is related to qì and blood stagnation, we treat it with Unripe Bitter Orange and Peony Powder (*zhǐ shí sháo yào sǎn*) to move qì and harmonize blood. The present line describes a condition where such treatment has been ineffective and the abdominal pain continues. The reason for this is that the medicine was too mild for the condition, because blood stasis is more severe than qì stagnation, and "dry blood is fixed in the abdomen below the umbilicus." Dry blood forms when static blood collects for a time, is trapped and transforms into heat, and heat scorches the blood. Below the umbilicus refers to the location of the uterus. This condition is characterized by stabbing pain in the lower abdomen, resistance to pressure, possibly small lumps, and pain more severe than distention.

In such conditions, we need to switch the formula to Static Blood-Precipitating Decoction (*xià yū xuè tāng*) to break blood, expel stasis, and discharge heat. In this formula, rhubarb (*dà huáng*) enters the blood aspect to flush out heat and expel stasis, removing the old and instituting the new; apricot kernel (*táo rén*) quickens blood, transforms stasis, and moistens dryness; and ground beetle (*zhè chóng*) attacks dry blood by expelling stasis and breaking binds. In combination, these three medicinals have a fierce blood-breaking effect, which is mitigated by blending them with honey to form pills. We can also use this formula to treat other conditions of static heat binding internally, such as inhibited menstrual flow, menstrual pain, and blocked menstruation. Nevertheless, note that this formula should given only to strong patients with repletion patterns.

Line 21.7

产后七八日，无太阳证，少腹坚痛，此恶露不尽。不大便，烦躁发热，切脉微实，再倍发热，日晡时烦躁者，不食，食则谵语，至夜即愈，宜大承气汤主之。热在里，结在膀胱也。

Chǎn hòu qī bā rì, wú tài yáng zhèng, shào fù jiān tòng, cǐ wù lù bù jìn, bù dà biàn, fán zào fā rè, qiē mài wēi shí, zài bèi fā rè, rì bū shí fán zào zhě, bù shí, shí zé zhān yǔ, zhì yè jí yù, yí dà chéng qì tāng zhǔ zhī. Rè zài lǐ, jié zài páng guāng yě.

If on the seventh or eighth day after giving birth a woman has no greater yáng signs, but hardness and pain in the lesser abdomen, this means incomplete elimination of lochia.[1] [This will be accompanied by] inability to defecate, vexation, agitation, and heat effusion, a pulse that feels slightly replete, a further doubling of heat effusion, vexation and agitation in the late afternoon [so severe that] she is unable to eat, delirious speech on eating, and relief in the evening. Major Qì-Coordinating Decoction (*dà chéng qì tāng*) governs.[2] There is heat in the interior, and binding in the bladder.

Text Notes, Line 21.7

[1] Incomplete elimination of the lochia 恶露不尽 *è lù bù jìn*: Lochia is a clotted bloody discharge via the vagina after delivery. The Chinese term 恶露 *è lù* literally means "malign dew." If retained in the uterus after childbirth it is considered one of the major pathogenic agents of women's diseases.

[2] A comment included in the received text reads: "For the formula, see under Tetany." See line 2.13 in Chapter 2, "Tetany, Dampness, and Thermoplegia."

Synopsis, Line 21.7

This line describes the signs and treatment of postpartum stasis obstruction and interior repletion.

Commentary, Line 21.7

When a woman experiences lesser abdominal hardness and pain on the seventh or eighth day after childbirth, with no defecation, heat effusion, vexation, and agitation, inability to eat, delirious speech upon eating, and a slightly replete pulse, these are the symptoms of static blood obstructing the inner body, complicated by interior heat in yáng brightness. The absence of greater yáng signs indicates that the condition is not an exterior pattern. This condition arises when lochia is not eliminated completely and static blood collects in the uterus. When this static blood obstructs the uterine network vessels, the woman feels pain.

The list of symptoms from "inability to defecate" to "relief in the evening" describes the signs of yáng brightness bowel repletion. Late afternoon is the time when yáng brightness qì is hyperactive; hence the symptoms of vexation, agitation, and heat effusion are particularly severe during this time, and abate afterwards. Severe heat effusion in the late afternoon, also called "late afternoon tidal heat," is a special characteristic of yáng brightness bowel repletion. Repletion bind in the stomach and intestines causes inability to eat. If the patient is compelled to eat, the food inevitably increases stomach heat, which exuberates and harasses the spirit light upward because the stomach network vessels are connected to the heart. As a result, we see delirious speech. When night falls, yīn grows and yáng vanishes, the qì of yáng brightness weakens, and evil heat is reduced, thereby relieving the symptoms.

The final sentence states, "There is heat in the interior, and binding in the bladder." In this context, "interior" refers to yáng brightness, and "bladder" to the lesser abdomen. This means that the heat is not located in the exterior, but in yáng brightness, and that static blood is not located in the upper or center burners, but in the lower burner. Thus it describes the location of binding heat evil and of internally obstructing static blood, and emphasizes that both these factors must be taken into consideration in treatment.

The present pattern is a complex and critical condition that combines stasis obstruction with interior heat. Because the interior heat signs are more critical and severe, the text recommends Major Qì-Coordinating Decoction (*dà chéng qì tāng*) to precipitate stomach repletion. If you only were to treat blood bind and neglect the stomach, you may eliminate the blood but not eliminate the yáng brightness heat. This would only worsen the patient's condition. Therefore use Major Qì-Coordinating Decoction (*dà chéng qì tāng*), which not only discharges heat and frees the stool, thereby treating yáng brightness repletion heat, but also precipitates static blood together with the eliminated heat and freed stool. If this treatment fails to completely eliminate static blood and lesser abdominal hardness, and if pain persists, employ blood-breaking stasis-freeing preparations like Static Blood-Precipitating Decoction (*xià yū xuè tāng*) to eliminate the static blood.

Line 21.8

产后风，续之数十日不解，头微痛，恶寒，时时有热，心下闷，干呕汗出，虽久，阳旦证续在耳，可与阳旦汤。

Chăn hòu fēng, xù zhī shù shí rì bù jiě, tóu wēi tòng wù hán, shí shí yŏu rè, xīn xià mèn, gān ŏu hàn chū, suī jiŭ, yáng dàn zhèng xù zài ĕr, kĕ yŭ yáng dàn tāng.

Postpartum wind [strike] that continues for several tens of days without resolution [manifests in] slight headache, aversion to cold, frequent heat effusion, oppression below the heart, dry retching, and sweating. Even though [the condition] is enduring, yáng dawn signs continue to be present. You can give Yáng Dawn Decoction (*yáng dàn tāng*).[1]

TEXT NOTE, LINE 21.8

[1] A comment included in the received text reads: "This is the same as Cinnamon Twig Decoction (*guì zhī tāng*). For the formula, see under Diarrhea." See Chapter 17, "Retching and Vomiting, Hiccup, and Diarrhea," line 17.36.

SYNOPSIS, LINE 21.8

This line describes the signs and treatment of enduring postpartum wind-strike.

COMMENTARY, LINE 21.8

After childbirth, qì and blood are both vacuous. The body's resistance is weakened, and it can easily contract exterior evil. If wind evil assails the outside, it will cause disease in the exterior, which manifests with signs of greater yáng wind-strike, such as slight headache, aversion to cold, frequent heat effusion, and sweating. The fact that the condition in the present line continues without resolution indicates that the exterior pattern of wind-strike in greater yang, though having persisted for some time, is still present. According to Xú Zhōng-Kě 徐忠可, oppression in the chest and dry retching are signs that "greater yáng evil wants to enter the inner body, but the inner body will not receive it." Hence we know that the evil is still in greater yáng in the exterior and can therefore still be treated with Yáng Dawn Decoction (*yáng dàn tāng*) to resolve the exterior and dispel evil.

Commentators have interpreted Yáng Dawn Decoction as follows:

—As an alternate name for Cinnamon Twig Decoction (*guì zhī tāng*). This is the view is held by Wáng Shū-Hé 王叔和, Lín Yì 林亿, Sūn Sī-Miǎo 孙思邈, Chéng Wú-Jǐ 成无已, and many others. Chéng Wú-Jǐ says that *yáng dàn* (阳旦) is an alternate name for cinnamon twig.

—As Cinnamon Twig Decoction (*guì zhī tāng*) with the addition of scutellaria (*huáng qín*). This view is represented by Yù Jiā-Yán 喻嘉言.

—As Cinnamon Twig Decoction (*guì zhī tāng*) with the addition of aconite (*fù zǐ*) because it is aimed at treating wind. This view is represented by Wèi Niàn-Tíng 魏念庭.

—As Cinnamon Twig Decoction (*guì zhī tāng*) with an increased amount of cinnamon twig (*guì zhī*) and the addition of aconite (*fù zǐ*). This view is represented by Chén Xiū-Yuán 陈修园.

—As a yáng-upbearing formula, principally *chái hú* (Bupleuri Radix). This view is represented by Táo Hóng-Jǐng 陶弘景.

In any case, the formula is most likely either identical to or a derivative of Cinnamon Twig Decoction (*guì zhī tāng*).

Line 21.9

产后中风，发热，面正赤，喘而头痛，竹叶汤主之。

竹叶一把　葛根三两　防风一两　桔梗 桂枝　人参　甘草各一两　附子（炮）一枚　大枣十五枚　生姜五两

右十味，以水一斗，煮取二升半，分温三服，温覆使汗出。颈项强，用大附子一枚，破之如豆大，煎药扬去沫，呕者，加半夏半升洗。

Chǎn hòu zhōng fēng, fā rè, miàn zhèng chì, chuǎn ér tóu tòng, zhú yè tāng zhǔ zhī.

Zhú yè yī bǎ; gé gēn sān liǎng; fáng fēng yī liǎng; jié gěng, guì zhī, rén shēn, gān cǎo gè yī liǎng; fù zǐ (pào) yī méi; dà zǎo shí wǔ méi; shēng jiāng wǔ liǎng

Yòu shí wèi, yǐ shuǐ yī dǒu, zhǔ qǔ èr shēng bàn, fēn wēn sān fú, wēn fù shǐ hàn chū. Jǐng xiàng qiáng, yòng dà fù zǐ yī méi, pò zhī rú dòu dà, jiān yào yáng qù mò, ǒu zhě, jiā bàn xià bàn shēng xǐ.

For postpartum wind-strike with heat effusion, a full red face, panting, and headache, Black Bamboo Leaf Decoction (竹叶汤 *zhú yè tāng*) governs.

Black Bamboo Leaf Decoction
(竹叶汤 *zhú yè tāng*)

black bamboo leaf (竹叶 *zhú yè*, Bambusae Folium) 1 handful
pueraria (葛根 *gé gēn*, Puerariae Radix) 3 *liǎng*
saposhnikovia (防风 *fáng fēng*, Saposhnikoviae Radix) 1 *liǎng*
platycodon (桔梗 *jié gěng*, Platycodonis Radix) 1 *liǎng*
cinnamon twig (桂枝 *guì zhī*, Cinnamomi Ramulus) 1 *liǎng*
ginseng (人参 *rén shēn*, Ginseng Radix) 1 *liǎng*
licorice (甘草 *gān cǎo*, Glycyrrhizae Radix) 1 *liǎng*
aconite (附子 *fù zǐ*, Aconiti Radix Lateralis Praeparata) 1 piece (blast-fry)
jujube (大枣 *dà zǎo*, Jujubae Fructus) 15 pieces
fresh ginger (生姜 *shēng jiāng*, Zingiberis Rhizoma Recens) 5 *liǎng*

Boil the above ten ingredients in one *dǒu* of water to get two-and-a-half *shēng*. Divide into three doses and take warm. Warmly cover up [the patient] to induce sweating. For stiffness of the neck and nape, use one large piece of aconite (*fù zǐ*), crushed to bean-sized pieces. Decoct the medicine and remove the scum. For retching, add half a *shēng* of washed pinellia (*bàn xià*).

SYNOPSIS, LINE 21.9

This line describes the signs and treatment of postpartum wind-strike with yáng vacuity.

COMMENTARY, LINE 21.9

In the present line, wind is contracted from the outside, and the disease evil is located in the exterior; hence we see heat effusion and headache. However, in addition we see redness of the face and panting, which are symptoms of vacuous yáng straying upward. This condition is caused by severe vacuity of right qì after childbirth, as a result of which original qì is not guarded securely in the lower body but strays upward, and exterior evil is easily contracted and fails to resolve. Thus the condition is one of right vacuity and evil repletion, of tip heat and root cold.

If you consider only the disease evil in the exterior and consequently treat this condition solely by resolving the exterior and dissipating evil, floating yáng is in danger of desertion. If you consider only the vacuity of right qì and consequently treat by supplementing right, the exterior evil will fail to resolve. Thus you must both support right and expel evil, and treat the exterior and interior condition simultaneously. The formula recommended is Black Bamboo Leaf Decoction (*zhú yè tāng*).

In this formula, black bamboo leaf (*zhú yè*), pueraria (*gé gēn*), saposhnikovia (*fáng fēng*), platycodon (*jié gěng*), and cinnamon twig (*guì zhī*) track down wind and dissipate evil to resolve the outside. Ginseng (*rén shēn*) and aconite (*fù zǐ*) warm yáng and boost qì to secure the vacuity desertion in the interior. Licorice (*gān cǎo*), fresh ginger (*shēng jiāng*), and jujube (*dà zǎo*) regulate construction and defense. Black bamboo leaf (*zhú yè*) is the chief medicinal and hence gives the formula its name. Wind is a yáng evil; if not resolved it can transform into heat, which can scorch the sinews and form tetany.

Line 21.10

妇人乳中虚，烦乱，呕逆，安中益气，竹皮大丸主之。

生竹茹二分　石膏二分　桂枝一分
甘草七分　白薇一分

右五味，末之，枣肉和丸弹子大，以饮服一丸，日三、夜二服。有热者，倍白薇；烦喘者，加柏实一分。

Fù rén rǔ zhōng xū, fán luàn, ǒu nì, ān zhōng yì qì, zhú pí dà wán zhǔ zhī.

Shēng zhú rú èr fēn; shí gāo èr fēn; guì zhī yī fēn; gān cǎo qī fēn; bái wēi yī fēn

Yòu wǔ wèi, mò zhī, zǎo ròu huò wán dǎn zǐ dà, yǐ yǐn fú yī wán, rì sān, yè èr fú. Yǒu rè zhě, bèi bái wēi, fán chuǎn zhě, jiā bǎi shí yī fēn.

Center vacuity in lactating women[1] [manifests in] vexation and retching counterflow. [Treat this by] quieting the center and boosting qì. Major Bamboo Shavings Pill (竹皮大丸 *zhú pí dà wán*) governs.

Major Bamboo Shavings Pill
(竹皮大丸 *zhú pí dà wán*)

- raw bamboo shavings (生竹茹 *shēng zhú rú*, Bambusae Caulis in Taenia) 2 parts
- gypsum (石膏 *shí gāo*, Gypsum Fibrosum) 2 parts
- cinnamon twig (桂枝 *guì zhī*, Cinnamomi Ramulus) 1 part
- licorice (甘草 *gān cǎo*, Glycyrrhizae Radix) 7 parts
- black swallowwort (白薇 *bái wēi*, Cynanchi Atrati Radix) 1 part

Pulverize the above five ingredients. Blend with jujube paste and form into pills the size of slingshot pellets. Take one pill [per dose] with fluid, three times a day and twice at night. For heat [effusion], double the amount of black swallowwort (*bái wēi*). For vexation and panting, add one part of arborvitae seed (*bǎi shí*).

TEXT NOTE, LINE 21.10

[1] Center vacuity in lactating women 妇人乳中虛 *fù rén rǔ zhōng xū*: The interpretation of this phrase varies among commentators, depending on the understanding of 乳 *rǔ* and the grammatical function of 中 *zhōng*. The term 乳 *rǔ* can refer to either lactation, breastfeeding, or breast. Accordingly, the phrase can be read as "For women's vacuity in the breasts" or, as in our translation above, as "center vacuity in lactating women" This refers to the period after childbirth, which is supported by the fact that an alternative version of this line in the *Mài Jīng* ("Pulse Canon") has 产 *chǎn* "in childbed" instead of 乳 *rǔ*.

SYNOPSIS, LINE 21.10

This line describes the signs and treatment of vacuity heat vexation and retching in women during lactation.

COMMENTARY, LINE 21.10

Due to profuse bleeding during childbirth, women in childbed tend to suffer from insufficiency of yīn-blood. This is compounded by the fact that yīn-blood ascends to become breast milk and feed the newborn child. Profuse lactation therefore further consumes blood and compounds the insufficiency of the source of qì and blood that arises from the strain of delivery. Vacuity of yīn-blood engenders internal heat, which ascends to harass the heart. Hence we see vexation. Because vacuity heat harasses and invades the stomach, the stomach fails to downbear harmoniously, as a result of which retching and qì counterflow arise.

The recommended treatment for this condition aims at quieting the center and boosting qì by clearing heat, downbearing counterflow, and supplementing center qì. In the governing formula, Major Bamboo Shavings Pill (*zhú pí dà wán*), bamboo (*zhú rú*) and gypsum (*shí gāo*) are cold and sweet. They clear stomach heat, eliminate vexation, check retching, and thereby quiet the center. Black swallowwort (*bái wēi*) clears vacuity heat. Cinnamon twig (*guì zhī*) is able to calm surging and downbear counterflow with acrid warmth, while its warming and drying effect is reduced by combining it with cold medicinals. Gypsum (*shí gāo*) is very cold, but in combination with acrid warm medicinals is able to clear stomach heat without injuring stomach yáng. The formula uses a large amount of licorice (*gān cǎo*), assisted by jujube paste, to effectively boost center qì and engender fluids.

Line 21.11

产后下利虚极，白头翁加甘草阿胶汤主之。

白头翁　甘草　阿胶各二两　秦皮
黄连　柏皮各三两

右六味，以水七升，煮取二升半，内胶令消尽，分温三服。

Chǎn hòu xià lì xū jí, bái tóu wēng jiā gān cǎo ē jiāo tāng zhǔ zhī.

Bái tóu wēng, gān cǎo, ē jiāo gè èr liǎng; qín pí, huáng lián, bǎi pí gè sān liǎng

Yòu liù wèi, yǐ shuǐ qī shēng, zhǔ qǔ èr shēng bàn, nà jiāo lìng xiāo jìn, fēn wēn sān fú.

For postpartum diarrhea and extreme vacuity, Pulsatilla Decoction Plus Licorice and Ass Hide Glue (白头翁加甘草阿胶汤 *bái tóu wēng jiā gān cǎo ē jiāo tāng*) governs.

Pulsatilla Decoction Plus Licorice and Ass Hide Glue (白头翁加甘草阿胶汤 *bái tóu wēng jiā gān cǎo ē jiāo tāng*)
pulsatilla (白头翁 *bái tóu wēng*, Pulsatillae Radix) 2 *liǎng* licorice (甘草 *gān cǎo*, Glycyrrhizae Radix) 2 *liǎng* ass hide glue (阿胶 *ē jiāo*, Asini Corii Colla) 2 *liǎng* ash (秦皮 *qín pí*, Fraxini Cortex) 3 *liǎng* coptis (黄连 *huáng lián*, Coptidis Rhizoma) 3 *liǎng* arborvitae bark (柏皮 *bǎi pí*, Platycladi Cortex) 3 *liǎng*

Boil the above six ingredients in seven *shēng* of water to get two and half *shēng*. Add the ass hide glue (*ē jiāo*) and let it melt completely. Divide into three doses and take warm.

SYNOPSIS, LINE 21.11

This line describes the signs and treatment of postpartum heat diarrhea with damage to yīn.

COMMENTARY, LINE 21.11

If postpartum vacuity of qì and blood is complicated by damage to yīn from diarrhea, the result is extreme vacuity. According to Táng Róng-Chuān 唐容川 "diarrhea" here refers to dysentery with pus and blood in the stool. It is therefore most likely accompanied by symptoms like heat effusion and abdominal pain, tenesmus, and sticky sloppy stool containing blood and pus.

Treatment should therefore aim at clearing heat and checking diarrhea, as well as nourishing blood and enriching yīn, for which Pulsatilla Decoction Plus Licorice and Ass Hide Glue (*bái tóu wēng jiā gān cǎo ē jiāo tāng*) is recommended. Pulsatilla Decoction (*bái tóu wēng tāng*) is the governing formula for damp-heat dysentery, by attacking and clearing heat, drying dampness, and cooling blood, to check diarrhea. Licorice (*gān cǎo*) is added to supplement the center, nourish stomach yīn, and thereby engender fluids, and ass hide glue (*ē jiāo*) is added to enrich yīn and nourish blood.

[附方] Appended Formulas

THREE AGENTS SCUTELLARIA DECOCTION (三物黄芩汤 *sān wù huáng qín tāng*) from the *Qiān Jīn Fāng* ("Thousand Gold Pieces Prescriptions")

治妇人在草蓐，自发露得风。四肢苦烦热，头痛者，与小柴胡汤；头不痛但烦者，此汤主之。

黄芩一两　苦参二两　干地黄四两

右三味，以水六升，煮取二升，温服一升，多吐下虫。

Zhì fù rén zài cǎo rù zì fā lù dé fēng. Sì zhī kǔ fán rè, tóu tòng zhě, yǔ xiǎo chái hú tāng; tóu bù tòng dàn fán zhě, cǐ tāng zhǔ zhī.

Huáng qín yī liǎng; kǔ shēn èr liǎng; gān dì huáng sì liǎng

Yòu sān wèi, yǐ shuǐ liù shēng, zhǔ qǔ èr shēng, wēn fú yī shēng, duō tù xià chóng.

To treat women's bitter vexing heat in the four limbs from exposure to wind in childbed, if there is headache, give Minor Bupleurum Decoction (*xiǎo chái hú tāng*); if there is no headache and only vexation, [Three Agents Scutellaria Decoction (三物黄芩汤 *sān wù huáng qín tāng*)] governs.

Three Agents Scutellaria Decoction (三物黄芩汤 *sān wù huáng qín tāng*)

scutellaria (黄芩 *huáng qín*, Scutellariae Radix) 1 *liǎng*
flavescent sophora (苦参 *kǔ shēn*, Sophorae Flavescentis Radix) 2 *liǎng*
dried rehmannia (干地黄 *gān dì huáng*, Rehmanniae Radix) 4 *liǎng*

Boil the above three ingredients in six *shēng* of water to get two *shēng*. Take one *shēng* [per dose] warm. [The formula will cause] increased vomiting and precipitation of worms.

FORMULA COMMENTARY, LINE 21.11

This formula treats contraction of wind in childbed. An unclean environment or inattentive care during delivery can cause a parturient woman to contract disease evil. If you see heat effusion and vexation in the extremities in combination with headache, it indicates that the evil is predominantly in the exterior and upper body, that wind has not yet transformed into heat, and that the condition must therefore be treated by harmonizing and clearing heat. For this, Minor Bupleurum Decoction (*xiǎo chái hú tāng*) is the recommended formula. If the patient does not experience headache, we know that the disease evil has already entered the interior and that there is heat in the blood aspect. Treatment should therefore focus on clearing heat by cooling and nurturing blood.

For this purpose, the recommended formula is Three Agents Scutellaria Decoction (*sān wù huáng qín tāng*). Scutellaria (*huáng qín*) and flavescent sophora (*kǔ shēn*) clear heat and eliminate vexation, while dried rehmannia (*gān dì huáng*) cools and nourishes blood. Because the bitter and cold nature of flavescent sophora (*kǔ shēn*) can damage stomach qì, this formula may induce vomiting and, in patients with roundworm, discharge of worms.

INTERNALLY SUPPLEMENTING CHINESE ANGELICA CENTER-FORTIFYING DECOCTION
(内补当归建中汤 *nèi bǔ xiāng guī jiàn zhōng tāng*)
from the *Qiān Jīn Fāng* ("Thousand Gold Pieces Prescriptions")

治妇人产后虚羸不足，腹中刺痛不止，吸吸少气，或苦少腹中急，摩痛引腰背，不能食饮。产后一月，日得服四五剂为善，令人强壮，宜。

当归四两　桂枝三两　芍药六两　生姜三两　甘草二两　大枣十二枚

右六味，以水一斗，煮取三升，分温三服，一日令尽。若大虚，加饴糖六两，汤成内之，于火上暖令饴消。若去血过多，崩伤内衄不止，加地黄六两，阿胶二两，合八味，汤成内阿胶。若无当归，以穹藭代之。若无生姜，以干姜代之。

Zhì fù rén chǎn hòu xū léi zú, fù zhōng cì tòng bù zhǐ, xī xī shǎo qì, huò kǔ shào fù zhōng jí, mó tòng yǐn yāo bèi, bù néng shí yǐn. Chǎn hòu yī yuè, rì dé fú sì wǔ jì wéi shàn, lìng rén qiáng zhuàng yí.

Dāng guī sì liǎng; guì zhī sān liǎng; sháo yào liù liǎng; shēng jiāng sān liǎng; gān cǎo èr liǎng; dà zǎo shí èr méi

Yòu liù wèi, yǐ shuǐ yī dǒu, zhǔ qǔ sān shēng, fēn wēn sān fú, yī rì lìng jìn. Ruò dà xū, jiā yí táng liù liǎng, tāng chéng nà zhī, yú huǒ shàng nuǎn lìng yí xiāo, ruò qù xuè guò duō, bēng shāng nèi nǜ bù zhǐ, jiā dì huáng liù liǎng, ē jiāo èr liǎng, gě bā wèi, tāng chéng nà ē jiāo, ruò wú dāng guī, yǐ xiōng qióng dài zhī, ruò wú shēng jiāng, yǐ gān jiāng dài zhī.

Treats women's postpartum vacuity emaciation and insufficiency with incessant stabbing pain in the abdomen, strong inhalations with shortage of qì, possibly tension, contractions, and pain in the lesser abdomen stretching into the lumbus and back, and inability to eat and drink. In the month after delivery, it is excellent to take four or five doses a day. It will make the patient strong.

Internally Supplementing Chinese Angelica Center-Fortifying Decoction (内补当归建中汤 *nèi bǔ xiāng guī jiàn zhōng tāng*)

Chinese angelica (当归 *dāng guī*, Angelicae Sinensis Radix) 4 *liǎng*
cinnamon twig (桂枝 *guì zhī*, Cinnamomi Ramulus) 3 *liǎng*
peony (芍药 *sháo yào*, Paeoniae Radix) 6 *liǎng*
fresh ginger (生姜 *shēng jiāng*, Zingiberis Rhizoma Recens) 3 *liǎng*
licorice (甘草 *gān cǎo*, Glycyrrhizae Radix) 2 *liǎng*
jujube (大枣 *dà zǎo*, Jujubae Fructus) 12 pieces

Boil the above six ingredients in one *dǒu* of water to get three *shēng*. Divide into three doses and take warm, finishing it in one day. For major vacuity, add six *liǎng* of malt sugar (*yí táng*). Add it after the decoction is done, and keep it warm over the flame until the malt sugar is melted. For excessive blood loss through incessant internal bleeding, add six *liǎng* of rehmannia (*dì huáng*) and two *liǎng* of ass hide glue (*ē jiāo*). Combine the [first] eight ingredients, and after the decoction is done, add the ass hide glue (*ē jiāo*). If Chinese angelica (*dāng guī*) is unavailable, use chuanxiong (*xiōng qióng*) instead. If fresh ginger (*shēng jiāng*) is unavailable, use dried ginger (*gān jiāng*).

Formula Commentary, Line 21.11

Childbirth results in dual vacuity of qì and blood, and inevitably in emptiness in the sea of blood. If movement and transformation in the central region is smooth, qì and blood will recover. However, vacuity cold in the center burner can impair movement and transformation and cause insufficiency in the source of transformation. As a result, the vacuity of qì and blood is increased, and they are insufficient for moistening the bowels and viscera and nurturing the channels and vessels. The result is tension and pain in the abdomen, and possibly contractions and pain in the smaller abdomen stretching to the lumbus and back. Reduced moistening of the skin and flesh and nourishing of the formal body causes vacuity emaciation and insufficiency. Spleen-stomach vacuity causes shortage of qì and reduced eating.

Treating this condition with Internally Supplementing Chinese Angelica Center-Fortifying Decoction (*nèi bǔ xiāng guī jiàn zhōng tāng*) has the effect of fortifying the center region, boosting qì and blood, relaxing tension, and relieving pain.

This formula is identical with Minor Center-Fortifying Decoction (*xiǎo jiàn zhōng tāng*) with the addition of Chinese angelica (*dāng guī*). In this formula, Chinese angelica (*dāng guī*) harmonizes and nourishes blood, while Minor Center-Fortifying Decoction (*xiǎo jiàn zhōng tāng*) regulates yīn and yáng, fortifies center qì, and relaxes tension to relieve pain. It can be used in any condition related to blood vacuity and cold. It can also be used as a supplement for childbearing women, but should not be taken by patients with constitutional yīn vacuity and stomach yīn insufficiency, because it is predominantly warming.

妇人杂病脉证并治第二十二

CHAPTER 22

Women's Miscellaneous Diseases

Pulses, Signs, Treatments

‡ OVERVIEW

This chapter discusses the causes, signs, and treatments of women's miscellaneous diseases (妇人杂病 *fù rén zá bìng*), a term that covers a variety of women's conditions related to menstruation, vaginal discharge, the genitalia, and emotional disturbances. It includes diseases like heat in the blood chamber, visceral agitation, plum-pit qì, "a sensation in the throat like a lump of roasted meat," inhibited menstrual flow, vaginal discharge, spotting, abdominal pain, shifted bladder, and vaginal sores, but focuses particularly on menstrual disorders, vaginal discharge, and abdominal pain.

The three major causes of women's diseases in this chapter are vacuity of qì and blood, accumulated cold, and qì bind, which refers to binding oppression of the qì dynamic. All these can disorder the menses and, in severe cases, cause a range of gynecological conditions related to menstrual block.

The diagnosis of women's diseases is based on a careful analysis of the pulse in terms of yīn and yáng, heat and cold, and vacuity and repletion. Treatment is varied, including both internal and external application, with internal preparations like salves, decoctions, powder, pills, and wines, and external therapies like acupuncture, washes, and suppositories. This chapter thus has served in subsequent centuries as an important foundation for the practice of identifying patterns and determining treatment in women's miscellaneous diseases.

‡ Schematic Overview

Miscellaneous Women's Diseases

1. General Features
   a) Causes and pathomechanisms: Vacuity, accumulated cold, and bound qi.
   b) Principles of treatment: Differentiate yīn and yáng, identify vacuity and repletion, and apply acupuncture or medicinal therapy.
2. Determining treatment on the basis of patterns identified.
   a) Heat entering the blood chamber.
      Signs: On the seventh or eighth day after wind-strike, with extended aversion to cold and heat effusion that break out at [regular] times, the woman happens to experience interrupted menstrual flow.
      Treatment: Minor Bupleurum Decoction (*xiǎo chái hú tāng*) and needling of Cycle Gate (*qī mén*, LV-14).
   b) Lump in the throat (plum-pit qì).
      Signs: [A sensation] in the throat like a lump of roasted meat.
      Treatment: Pinellia and Officinal Magnolia Bark Decoction (*bàn xià hòu pò tāng*).
   c) Visceral agitation.
      Signs: Tendency to sorrow and desire to weep, as if possessed by spirits, and frequent yawning and stretching.
      Treatment: Channel-Warming (Menses-Warming) Decoction (*wēn jīng tāng*) to warm and nourish qì and blood and to disperse stasis.
   d) Spotting.
      Signs: "Channel fall" with black spotting that fails to resolve.
      Treatment: Ass Hide Glue and Ginger Decoction (*jiāo jiāng tāng*) to warm and supplement the thoroughfare and controlling vessels.

Inhibited Menstruation

1. Blood stasis menstrual irregularities.
   Signs: Disease below the girdle with inhibited menstrual flow, lesser abdominal fullness and pain, and periods coming twice in one month.
   Treatment: Cucumber Gourd Root Powder (*tǔ guā gēn sǎn*) to quicken the blood, transform stasis, and stanch bleeding.
2. Blood stasis menstrual block.
   Signs: Inhibited descent of a woman's menses.
   Treatment: Dead-On Decoction (*dǐ dàng tāng*) expels stasis and breaks accumulations.
3. Blood and water binding in the blood chamber.
   Signs: Postpartum lower abdominal fullness that appears like a serving bowl, with slight difficulty in urination and no thirst.

Treatment: Rhubarb and Kansui Decoction (*dà huáng gān suì tāng*) to break stasis and expel water.

Abdominal Pain

1. Wind and blood contending with each other.

   Signs: Blood and qì stabbing pain in the abdomen.

   Treatment: Carthamus Wine (*hóng lán huā jiǔ*) to quicken the blood, dinshibit qì, and relieve pain.

2. Liver-spleen disharmony.

   Signs: All abdominal pain in women.

   Treatment: Chinese Angelica and Peony Powder (*dāng guī sháo yào sǎn*) to harmonize the liver and spleen.

3. Center qì vacuity cold.

   Signs: Women's abdominal pain.

   Treatment: Minor Center-Fortifying Decoction (*xiǎo jiàn zhōng tāng*) to warm the center and nourish blood.

Vaginal Discharge

1. Damp-heat vaginal discharge.

   Signs: Blocked and inhibited menstrual flow with discharge of white matter.

   Treatment: Alum Pill (*fán shí wán*) to transform dampness. Note that this is a topical formula.

2. Cold-damp vaginal discharge.

   Signs: Cold in the vagina.

   Treatment: Cnidium Seed Powder (*shé chuáng zǐ sǎn*) to expel cold-damp from the vagina.

Shifted Bladder

This disease is caused by the bladder tie being twisted.

Signs: Eating and drinking as normal, but vexing heat with inability to sleep, propped breathing, and inability to urinate.

Treatment: Kidney Qì Pill (*shèn qì wán*) to invigorate kidney qì and disinhibit urine.

Disease of the Anterior Yīn

1. Yīn sores.

   Signs: A lesser yīn pulse that is slippery and rapid; putrefying eroding sores in the vagina.

   Treatment: Langya Decoction (*láng yá tāng*) to clear heat and dry dampnesss and to kill worms and relieve itching.

2. Vaginal flatulence (passing gas via the vagina).

   Signs: Downward draining of stomach qì with yīn flatulence in continuous blasts means repletion of grain qì.

   Treatment: Lard and Hair Brew (*gāo fà jiān*) to moisten the intestines and free the stool.

Line 22.1

妇人中风七八日，续来寒热，发作有时，经水适断，此为热入血室。其血必结，故使如疟状，发作有时，小柴胡汤主之。

Fù rén zhòng fēng qī bā rì, xù lái hán rè, fā zuò yǒu shí, jīng shuǐ shì duàn, cǐ wéi rè rù xuè shì. Qí xuè bì jié, gù shǐ rú nüè zhuàng, fā zuò yǒu shí, xiǎo chái hú tāng zhǔ zhī.

If on the seventh or eighth day following [contraction of] wind-strike, a woman experiences extended [aversion to] cold and heat [effusion] occurring at [regular] intervals, and happens to experience interruption of menstrual flow, this is heat entering the blood chamber.[1] [In such patients,] the blood is inevitably bound, and this is causing [the condition] to appear like malaria, with regular outbreaks. Minor Bupleurum Decoction (*xiǎo chái hú tāng*) governs.[2]

Text Notes, Line 22.1

[1] Heat entering the blood chamber 热入血室 *rè rù xuè shì*: Commentators throughout the centuries have disagreed on the meaning of the term "blood chamber." According to one school, it has a narrow meaning, referring to the uterus. Another school suggests that it broadly refers to all entities related to the production, storage, and movement of blood in the lower part of the female body, therefore including the liver and the thoroughfare and controlling vessels as well as the uterus.

[2] A comment included in the received text reads: "For the formula, see under Retching and Vomiting." The formula is found in Chapter 17, "Retching and Vomiting, Hiccup, and Diarrhea," line 17.15.

Synopsis, Line 22.1

This line describes the signs and treatment of heat entering the blood chamber.

Commentary, Line 22.1

When women suffer from greater yáng wind-strike symptoms, they experience signs like aversion to cold, heat effusion, and sweating, but these should have abated by the seventh or eighth day. The condition in the present line is marked by the continued presence of these signs, by their occurrence at regular intervals as in malaria conditions, and lastly by the complication of interrupted menstruation. From this combination of symptoms we know that exterior evil has exploited vacuity in the channels and entered the blood chamber. Heat and blood contend with each other, and as a result channel blood is depressed and binds instead of moving. This is referred to by the phrase "heat entering the blood chamber." Because the blood chamber belongs to the liver, which stands in exterior-interior relationship with the gallbladder, we see the lesser yáng symptom of malaria-like heat effusion and aversion to cold.

This condition is treated with Minor Bupleurum Decoction (*xiǎo chái hú tāng*), which harmonizes and resolves lesser yáng, thereby eliminating the exterior evil, while it also dissipates evil heat bind in the blood chamber. By resolving evil heat, the formula naturally restores the flow of bound blood. To treat this condition, later physicians have tended to aim treatment not only toward resolving evil qì in lesser yáng, but also to cooling blood. In modern clinical practice, we therefore add salvia (*dān shēn*), peony (*sháo yào*), moutan (*mǔ dān pí*), and similar blood-cooling and blood-quickening ingredients to increase the effect.

Line 22.2

妇人伤寒发热，经水适来，昼日明了，暮则谵语，如见鬼状者，此为热入血室。治之无犯胃气及上二焦，必自愈。

Fù rén shāng hán fā rè, jīng shuǐ shì lái, zhòu rì míng liǎo, mù zé zhān yǔ, rú jiàn guǐ zhuàng zhě, cǐ wéi rè rù xuè shì. Zhì zhī wú fàn wèi qì jí shàng èr jiāo, bì zì yù.

If a woman with cold damage related heat effusion incidentally starts menstruating and is clear[-headed] during the day, but speaks deliriously in the evening, as if she were seeing ghosts, this is heat entering the blood chamber. In treatment, do not harm stomach qì and the two upper burners. You must allow the patient to recover naturally.

Synopsis, Line 22.2

This line describes further signs and treatment contraindications of heat entering the blood chamber.

Commentary, Line 22.2

In the condition described in this line, a female patient suffering from heat effusion due to cold damage also experiences mental derangement and delirious speech.

The key characteristic of this symptom is that it coincides with the incidental onset of her menstrual period and that it occurs only in the evening, but not during the day. From this we know that although her menstrual flow is uninhibited, evil qì has exploited vacuity and entered the blood chamber. As a result, heat is again harassing the blood aspect. Because blood is yīn and is therefore particularly vulnerable during the night, her mind is clear during the day, but deranged and confused at night.

This symptom is not caused by yáng brightness bowel repletion, but by heat entering the blood chamber and by exuberant heat in the blood aspect. Thus you may not treat it by offensive precipitation, which would damage stomach qì in the center burner, or with sweat-effusing substances, which would damage clear qì in the upper burner. We know from the healthy flow of menstrual blood that the evil has not yet entered deeply and bound with blood. Therefore you can treat it with outwardly discharging medicinals in accordance with the menstrual cycle; or, according to some commentators' interpretation of the final phrase, wait for a natural recovery without medical treatment, because the evil will discharge on its own with the menstrual blood.

Line 22.3

妇人中风，发热恶寒，经水适来，得之七八日，热除，脉迟，身凉和，胸胁满，如结胸状，谵语者，此为热入血室也，当刺期门，随其实而取之。

Fù rén zhōng fēng, fā rè wù hán, jīng shuǐ shì lái, dé zhī qī bā rì, rè chú, mài chí, shēn liáng hé, xiōng xié mǎn, rú jié xiōng zhuàng, zhān yǔ zhěn zhě, cǐ wéi rè rù xuè shì yě, dāng cì qī mén, suí qí shí ér qǔ zhī.

If a woman with wind-strike-related heat [effusion] and [aversion to] cold incidentally starts menstruating, and if on the seventh or eighth day following [wind] contraction she has eliminated the heat and presents with a slow pulse and cool and harmonious body, but with fullness in the chest and rib-side as in chest bind,[1] and with delirious speech, this is heat entering the blood chamber. You should needle Cycle Gate (*qī mén*, LV-14)[2] to address the condition in accordance with the repletion.

Text Note, Line 22.3

[1] Chest bind 结胸 *jié xiōng*: Pain with hardness and fullness above the diaphragm and below the heart.

Synopsis, Line 22.3

This line describes the signs and treatment of heat entering the blood chamber with exterior heat having disappeared.

Commentary, Line 22.3

The present line describes a condition in which a woman happens to start menstruating while suffering from heat effusion and aversion to cold due to greater yáng wind-strike. The heat abates after seven or eight days and her pulse and body temperature return to normal, but she experiences distention and fullness in the chest and rib-side, as well as delirious speech. These symptoms indicate that the exterior heat has been eliminated but static heat is binding in the blood chamber. The blood chamber belongs to the liver, and the liver channel nets the rib-side. Static heat causes inhibition in the liver channel; hence we see fullness in the chest and rib-side, as in chest bind. The delirious speech is here not a symptom of yáng brightness bowel repletion, but of hot blood heat ascending and harassing the spirit light.

The text recommends treating this condition by needling Cycle Gate (*qī mén*, LV-14), which is a point on the liver channel. By draining repletion heat in the liver channel, you will be able to dissipate static heat in the blood chamber.

Line 22.4

阳明病，下血谵语者，此为热入血室，但头汗出，当刺期门，随其实而泻之，濈然汗出即愈。

Yáng míng bìng, xià xuè zhān yǔ zhě, cǐ wéi rè rù xuè shì, dàn tóu hàn chū, dāng cì qī mén, suí qí shí ér xiè zhī, jí rán hàn chū jí yù.

If yáng brightness disease [manifests] with vaginal bleeding and delirious speech, this is heat entering the blood chamber. [It is marked by] sweating from the head only. You should needle Cycle Gate (*qī mén*, LV-14), draining it in accord with the repletion. Pouring sweat indicates recovery.

Synopsis, Line 22.4

This line describes the signs and treatment of yáng brightness disease with heat entering the blood chamber.

Commentary, Line 22.4

If women who suffer from yáng brightness disease experience vaginal bleeding outside their menstrual cycle, as well as delirious speech and sweating from the head only, these are signs that yáng brightness interior heat is blazing, that heat evil has followed the channels to enter the blood chamber, and that interior heat is sweltering and forcing blood to move frenetically. Delirious speech is the result of heat harassing the blood aspect and disquieting the spirit light, not of interior heat in yáng brightness bowel repletion. Thus it should appear during the day, but calm down in the evening. Sweating from the head only is caused by heat in the blood chamber sweltering and ascending with the liver and the controlling and thoroughfare vessels.

As in the previous line, this condition is treated by needling Cycle Gate (*qī mén*, LV-14) to drain repletion heat in the liver and blood chamber. By removing evil heat, yīn and yáng are harmonized, as a result of which the entire body effuses sweat profusely and the patient recovers.

This line concludes the discussion of patterns of heat entering the blood chamber, which began in line 22.1 of this chapter. Regardless of whether the menstrual flow is incidentally interrupted or started, whether the exterior pattern is already resolved or evil heat has fallen into the inner body, or whether yáng brightness heat exuberates and forces blood to move downward, all these conditions are equally treated by draining heat, whether with medicinals or with acupuncture. However, you must take into consideration whether blood is bound or not. In cases without blood bind, treatment should aim at clearing heat and cooling blood; in cases with blood bind, treatment should aim at clearing heat and moving stasis.

Line 22.5

妇人咽中如有炙脔, 半夏厚朴汤主之。

半夏一升　厚朴三两　茯苓四两　生姜五两　干苏叶二两

右五味, 以水七升, 煮取四升, 分温四服, 日三, 夜一服。

Fù rén yān zhōng rú yǒu zhì luán, bàn xià hòu pò tāng zhǔ zhī.

Bàn xià yī shēng; hòu pò sān liǎng; fú líng sì liǎng; shēng jiāng wǔ liǎng; gān sū yè èr liǎng

Yòu wǔ wèi, yǐ shuǐ qī shēng, zhǔ qǔ sì shēng, fēn wēn sì fú, rì sān, yè yī fú.

When a woman has a [sensation] in the throat like a lump of roasted meat, Pinellia and Officinal Magnolia Bark Decoction (半夏厚朴汤 *bàn xià hòu pò tāng*)[1] governs.

Pinellia and Officinal Magnolia Bark Decoction (半夏厚朴汤 *bàn xià hòu pò tāng*

pinellia (半夏 *bàn xià*, Pinelliae Rhizoma) 1 *shēng*
officinal magnolia bark (厚朴 *hòu pò*, Magnoliae Officinalis Cortex) 3 *liǎng*
poria (茯苓 *fú líng*, Poria) 4 *liǎng*
fresh ginger (生姜 *shēng jiāng*, Zingiberis Rhizoma Recens) 5 *liǎng*
dried perilla leaf (干苏叶 *gān sū yè*, Perillae Folium Exsiccatum) 2 *liǎng*

Boil the above five ingredients in seven *shēng* of water to get four *shēng*. Divide into four doses and take warm, three times a day and once at night.

TEXT NOTE, LINE 22.5

[1] A comment included in the received text reads: "[As indications for this formula] the *Qiān Jīn Fāng* ("Thousand Gold Pieces Prescriptions") has fullness in the chest, hardness below the heart, and a stuck sensation in the throat as if from a lump of roasted meat that can neither be ejected nor swallowed."

SYNOPSIS, LINE 22.5

This line describes the signs and treatment of qì stagnation and congealing phlegm in the throat.

COMMENTARY, LINE 22.5

This condition is mostly caused by seven-affect binding depression, which inhibits the qì dynamic. As a result, qì stagnates and phlegm congeals, ascending counterflow into the throat. The result is a subjective feeling of obstruction in the throat, as if something were stuck that cannot be expelled either by ejection or by swallowing. Nevertheless, it does not obstruct the ingestion of food or drink. This disease has since become known as "plum-pit qì" (梅核气 *méi hé qì*).

The recommended treatment is Pinellia and Officinal Magnolia Bark Decoction (*bàn xià hòu pò tāng*), which opens binds and transforms phlegm, and normalizes qì and downbears counterflow. In this formula, pinellia (*bàn xià*), officinal magnolia bark (*hòu pò*), and fresh ginger (*shēng jiāng*) dissipate binds with their acridity and downbear counterflow with their bitterness. They are assisted by poria (*fú líng*), which disinhibits rheum and transforms phlegm, and by aromatic perilla leaf (*zǐ sū yè*), which diffuses qì and resolves depression. In combination, these medicinals normalize qì and dissipate phlegm, as a result of which the sensation of roasted meat in the throat is cured.

Line 22.6

妇人脏躁，喜悲伤欲哭，像如神灵所作，数欠伸，甘麦大枣汤主之。

甘草三两　小麦一升　大枣十枚

右三味，以水六升，煮取三升，温分三服，亦补脾气。

Fù rén zàng zào, xǐ bēi shāng, yù kū, xiàng rú shén líng suǒ zuò, shuò qiàn shēn, gān mài dà zǎo tāng zhǔ zhī.

Gān cǎo sān liǎng; xiǎo mài yī shēng; dà zǎo shí méi

Yòu sān wèi, yǐ shuǐ liù shēng, zhǔ qǔ sān shēng, wēn fēn sān fú, yì bǔ pí qì.

Women's visceral agitation [manifests in] a tendency to sorrow and desire to weep, as if possessed by spirits, and frequent yawning and stretching. Licorice, Wheat, and Jujube Decoction (甘麦大枣汤 *gān mài dà zǎo tāng*) governs.

Licorice, Wheat, and Jujube Decoction (甘麦大枣汤 *gān mài dà zǎo tāng*)
licorice (甘草 *gān cǎo*, Glycyrrhizae Radix) 3 *liǎng* wheat (小麦 *xiǎo mài*, Tritici Semen) 1 *shēng* jujube (大枣 *dà zǎo*, Jujubae Fructus) 10 pieces

Boil the above three ingredients in six *shēng* of water to get three *shēng*. Divide into three doses and take warm. [This formula] also supplements spleen qì.

Synopsis, Line 22.6

This line describes the signs and treatment of visceral agitation.

Commentary, Line 22.6

Typical manifestations of visceral agitation include disturbed emotions, sorrow and crying without reason, frequent stretching and yawning, and mental fatigue. Physicians now generally agree that this disease is caused by affect-mind ill-being or excessive thought and preoccupation, which causes liver depression transforming into fire, damaging yīn and consuming humor, and resulting in a dual vacuity of the spleen and heart. It is treated with Licorice, Wheat, and Jujube Decoction (*gān mài dà zǎo tāng*), to supplement the spleen, nourish the heart, relax tension, and check agitation, with special emphasis placed on supplementing the spleen.

Commentators disagree regarding the location of visceral agitation. The theory that visceral agitation is associated with the uterus and is caused by blood vacuity in the uterus and contraction of wind transforming into heat is unlikely, given the fact that the disease affects not only women, but occasionally also men. A second theory explains "viscus" in "visceral agitation" as referring to the heart viscus, because the heart stores the spirit and the key symptom is agitation and disquietude of the spirit due to damage from the seven affects. Some scholars have also associated visceral agitation with the lung because sorrow and desire to weep are associated with this viscus. Alternatively, Chén Xiū-Yuán 陈修园 has stated that "the viscera belong to yīn, and when yīn is vacuous, fire exploits it; hence there is agitation, regardless of which viscus is affected." By contrast, Huáng Shù-Zēng 黄树曾 has emphasized that "viscus refers to all five viscera (heart, liver, spleen, lung, and kidney), and visceral agitation refers to insufficiency of fluids, yīn, and blood in all the five viscera, or a part thereof."

A last theory emphasizes the connection of this disease to the liver and heart in particular, on the basis of ingredients in the recommended formula. In conclusion, it appears from the associated symptoms that this disease affects all the viscera comprehensively. Joy, anger, and sorrow are the affects associated with the heart, liver, and lung respectively.

According to the *Nèi Jīng* ("Inner Canon"), kidney disease manifests in a tendency to frequent yawning and stretching. Spleen disease as well manifests in stretching, related to the fact that the spleen governs the four limbs. Thus we can conclude that this disease starts in the liver and from there affects the heart, spleen, lung, and kidney. Treatment focuses particularly on the spleen because it governs movement and transformation and is the source of the fluids and of yīn-blood.

Line 22.7

妇人吐涎沫，医反下之，心下即痞，当先治其吐涎沫，小青龙汤主之。涎沫止，乃治痞，泻心汤主之。

Fù rén tù xián mò, yī fǎn xià zhī, xīn xià jí pǐ, dāng xiān zhì qí tù xián mò, xiǎo qīng lóng tāng zhǔ zhī. Xián mò zhǐ, nǎi zhì pǐ, xiè xīn tāng zhǔ zhī.

If a physician inappropriately treats by precipitation a woman who presents with drool foaming at the mouth, the result will be glomus below the heart. You must first treat the drool foaming at the mouth, for which Minor Black Dragon Decoction (小青龙汤 *xiǎo qīng lóng tāng*) governs.[1] When the drool and foam cease, then treat the glomus, for which Heart-Draining Decoction (泻心汤 *xiè xīn tāng*) governs.[2]

TEXT NOTES, LINE 22.7

[1] A comment included in the received text reads: "For the formula, see under Phlegm-Rheum." This refers to line 12.23 in Chapter 12, "Phlegm-Rheum and Cough."

[2] A comment included in the received text reads: "For the formula, see under Fright and Palpitation." This refers to line 16.17 in Chapter 16, "Fright and Palpitation, Blood Ejection, Nosebleed, Lower Body Bleeding, Fullness in the Chest, and Static Blood."

SYNOPSIS, LINE 22.7

This line describes the prognosis and treatment of glomus resulting from inappropriate precipitation of cold rheum in the upper burner.

COMMENTARY, LINE 22.7

Drool foaming at the mouth is a sign of cold rheum in the upper burner. It should be treated by warming and transforming cold rheum, not by offensive precipitation. If a physician misdiagnoses the cause of drool and inappropriately treats with offensive precipitation, it will damage the patient's center yáng, and cold rheum will bind internally, causing the formation of glomus below the heart. This is similar to the formation of glomus from inappropriate precipitation treatment in cold damage conditions.

In conditions where this type of glomus coexists with cold rheum, we must first rid the cold rheum by warming and dissipating it with Minor Black Dragon Decoction (*xiǎo qīng lóng tāng*) before treating the glomus with Heart-Draining Decoction (*xiè xīn tāng*).

Line 22.8

(1)妇人之病，因虚积冷结气，为诸经水断绝，至有历年，血寒积结胞门，寒伤经络凝坚。

(2)在上呕吐涎唾，久成肺痈，形体损分。在中盘结，绕脐寒疝；或两胁疼痛，与脏相连；或结热中，痛在关元，脉数无疮，肌若鱼鳞，时着男子，非止女身。在下未多，经候不匀，令阴掣痛，少腹恶寒；或引腰脊，下根气街，气冲急痛，膝胫疼烦。奄忽眩冒，状如厥癫；或有忧惨，悲伤多嗔，此皆带下，非有鬼神。

(3)久则羸瘦，脉虚多寒；三十六病，千变万端；审脉阴阳，虚实紧弦；行其针药，治危得安；其虽同病，脉各异源；子当辨记，勿谓不然。

(1) Fù rén zhī bìng, yīn xū jī lěng jié qì, wéi zhū jīng shuǐ duàn jué, zhì yǒu lì nián, xuè hán jī jié bāo men, hán shāng jīng luò níng jiān.

(2) Zài shàng, ǒu tù xián tuò, jiǔ chéng fèi yōng, xíng tǐ sǔn fēn; zài zhōng pán jié, rào qí hán shàn, huò liǎng xié téng tòng, yǔ zàng xiāng lián, huò jié rè zhōng, tòng zài guān yuán, mài shuò wú chuāng, jī ruò yú lín, shí zhuó nán zǐ, fēi zhǐ nǚ shēn; zài xià wèi duō, jīng hòu bù yún, lìng yīn chè tòng, shào fù wù hán, huò yǐn yāo jǐ, xià gēn qì jiē, qì chōng jí tòng, xī jìng téng fán, yǎn hū xuàn mào, zhuàng rú jué diān, huò yǒu yōu cǎn, bēi shāng duō chēn, cǐ jiē dài xià, fēi yǒu guǐ shén.

(3) Jiǔ zé léi shòu, mài xū duō hán, sān shí liù bìng, qiān biàn wàn duān, shěn mài yīn yáng, xū shí jǐn xián, xíng qí zhēn yào, zhì wēi dé ān, qí suī tóng bìng, mài gè yì yuán, zǐ dāng biàn jì, wù wèi bù rán.

(1) Women's diseases are caused by vacuity, accumulated cold, and bound qì, which cause the menstrual fluids to stop flowing. If this continues for a number of years, blood and cold accumulate and bind in the mouth of the uterus, and cold damages the network vessels so that they become congealed and hard.

(2) In the upper [body], [this results in] retching and vomiting of drool and spittle, and over time in the formation of pulmonary welling-abscess and a distinct decrease in the physical body.[1] Coiling and binding[2] in the center [of the body], [it results in] cold mounting around the umbilicus, either with pain in both rib-sides linking the viscera [of the spleen and liver], or with binding heat in the center, pain at Origin Pass (*guān yuán*, CV-4), a rapid pulse but no sores, and scaly skin. [These diseases can] sometimes affect males and are not limited to the female body. In the lower [body], [the result is] copious foam,[3] an uneven menstrual cycle, pulling pain in the genitals, and aversion to cold in the lesser abdomen. It can also reach into the lumbar spine, and descend to the root at the qì street,[4] where surging qì[5] [causes] pain and tension, and pain and vexation in the knees and lower legs, sudden dizzy veiling, as in [clouding] reversal or [mania and] withdrawal, or possibly anxiety, sorrow, and irascibility. [These signs are] all [attributable to] disease below the girdle;[6] they do not indicate the presence of ghosts and spirits.

(3) Over time, the result will be marked emaciation, a vacuous pulse, and increased cold. [Women's diseases are known as] the thirty-six diseases,[7] but there are myriad variations. Determine whether the pulse is marked by yīn or yáng, vacuity or repletion, and a tight or stringlike quality. [Then] apply needles and medicinals to treat critical [conditions] and secure well-being. Although the disease may be the same, each pulse has a different source. Any master will identify and take note [of this]. Do not disregard this fact.

TEXT NOTES, LINE 22.8

[1] A distinct decrease in the formal body 形体损分 *xíng tǐ sǔn fēn*: The traditional explanation for this is dramatic weight loss that makes the patient look so different from before the onset of illness that one would think that it was a different person. 分 *fēn* is understood as "separate" or "different."

[2] Coiling and binding 盘结 *pán jié*: Accumulation and congealing.

[3] Copious foam 未多 *wèi duō*: The literal meaning of these two characters, "not much," is subject to debate. We can either understand it as referring to "not much bleeding," in the sense of scant menstruation, or alternatively follow Sūn Shì-Yáng (孙世扬) who suggests that 未 *wèi* is a mistake for 沫 *mò*, foam, which in this context can be interpreted as vaginal discharge.

[4] Qì street 气街 *qì jiē:* The *Líng Shū* ("Magic Pivot") mentions four qì streets, which are severally located in the head, chest, abdomen, and lower leg. Opinion differs as to which is meant here. Modern texts say that the qì street of the abdomen is meant, and specifically an acupuncture point by the same name: Qì Street (*qì jiē*, ST-30). However, it could refer to the qì street of the lower leg, since the lower leg is mentioned a little further ahead.

[5] Surging qì 气冲 *qì chōng:* This probably refers to a movement of qì. It is unlikely to refer to the acupuncture point Surging Qì (*qì chōng*, ST-30), since this is a synonym for Qì Street (*qì jiē*, ST-30), which has just been mentioned in the text (see note 4 above).

[6] Disease below the girdle 带下 *dài xià*: In a medical context, the Chinese term, which literally means "below the girdle," also carries the technical meaning of "women's disease" in general, or "vaginal discharge" more specifically. From the context, it is clear that it refers to women's diseases in general.

[7] Thirty-six diseases 三十六病 *sān shí liù bìng*: This is a technical term referring to the varieties of women's diseases, which is mentioned in line 1.13. It is explained in the *Zhū Bìng Yuán Hòu Lùn* ("Origin and Indicators of Disease") as follows: "The thirty-six diseases spoken of in the various formularies are the twelve concretions, nine pains, seven injuries, five damages, and three intractable diseases." In the *Qiān Jīn Fāng* ("Thousand Gold Pieces Prescriptions"), line 4:3 has 带下三十六疾 *dài xià sān shí liù jí*, "thirty-six diseases below the girdle," which differs only slightly.

SYNOPSIS, LINE 22.8

This line describes the causes, pathomechanisms, symptoms, and treatment principles of women's diseases.

COMMENTARY, LINE 22.8

This line consists of three sections discussing the causes, symptoms, and treatment of women's diseases. The first section explains the causes of women's miscellaneous diseases under the three aspects of vacuity, accumulated cold, and bound qì. In this context, vacuity refers to shortage of qì and blood; accumulated cold to a chronic accumulation of cold; and bound qì to a binding depression of the qì dynamic. Any of these can cause disharmony between qì and blood, disturb the function of the viscera and bowels, and damage the thoroughfare and controlling vessels. Over time, this leads to inhibited menstruation and in severe cases menstrual block and stoppage. When menstruation is disordered, cold accumulates in the uterus, and the uterine vessels are obstructed by congealing cold, qì stagnation, and blood stasis. By contrast, if qì and blood are abundant, the blood flows freely in the vessels, the qì dynamic is regulated, and the menses descend in a timely manner.

The second section describes the pathological changes that arise in the upper, center, and lower burner as a result of the above-mentioned three causes of women's disease, namely vacuity, accumulated cold, and bound qì. When vacuity, cold, or bound qì affect the upper burner, cold rheum in the lung will result in coughing and vomiting of drool and spittle. Over time, depressed cold can transform into heat and damage the lung network vessels to cause pulmonary welling-abscess and physical emaciation.

In the center burner, vacuity, cold, and bound qì will affect the functions of the spleen and liver, manifesting differently depending on the patient's constitution. In a patient with yáng vacuity and a tendency toward cold, the result will be cold mounting with pain around the umbilicus, and, if vacuity cold ascends counterflow from below, abdominal pain that connects these viscera to each other, or pain in both rib-sides. In a patient with yáng hyperactivity, the disease will result from heat scorching and drying blood, causing static blood. This will manifest in pain in Origin Pass (*guān yuán*, CV-4) below the navel, a rapid pulse, and, due to the presence of static blood internally and the failure to supply new blood to the outside, desiccated scaly skin.

The symptoms described above for the upper and center burner occur not only in women, but can also manifest in men. By contrast, the symptoms of the lower burner are specific to women. They constitute what medical texts refer to as either "below the girdle" (带下 *dài xià*) or the "thirty-six diseases" (三十六病 *sān shí liù bìng*), both of which are generic terms for gynecological conditions in Chinese medicine and center around the three diseases of vaginal discharge, menstrual irregularities, and abdominal masses. The present line mentions specifically increased vaginal discharge (or in an alternative interpretation, scant menses), irregular menstruation, pulling pain in the genitals, aversion to cold in the lesser abdomen, and pain that is rooted in Qì Thoroughfare (*qì jiē*, ST-30), also called Surging Qì (*qì chōng*, ST-30), and that stretches to the lumbar spine. These symptoms result from disease in the liver and kidney, particularly liver depression and kidney vacuity, as a result of which essence and blood are insufficient, the sea of blood is empty or spills without constancy, and the thoroughfare and controlling vessels are damaged. In severe cases, the patient may also suffer from sudden dizziness and veiling, as in diseases like clouding reversal or mania and withdrawal, or emotional abnormalities like increased anxiety, sorrow, and irascibility. Lastly, Zhāng Jī emphasizes that these symptoms are not due to supernatural causes like spirit possession, but by disturbed physiological functions in women's reproductive organs, i.e., "disease below the girdle."

The last section of this line discusses the particulars of treating women's chronic diseases, which are characterized by marked emaciation, a vacuous pulse, and increased cold. In general, it is essential to use careful pulse diagnosis and analysis as the basis for identifying the specific pattern, and then to apply internal and external treatment accordingly. By correctly identifying the roots of each individual's condition, the careful physician will avoid inappropriate treatment.

Line 22.9

问曰：妇人年五十所，病下利数十日不止，暮即发热，少腹里急，腹满，手掌烦热，唇口干燥，何也？师曰：此病属带下。何以故？曾经半产，瘀血在少腹不去。何以知之？其证唇口干燥，故知之。当以温经汤主之。

吴茱萸三两　当归　芎藭　芍药各二两　人参 桂枝　牡丹皮（去心）　阿胶　生姜　甘草各二两　半夏半升　麦门冬（去心）一升

右十二味，以水一斗，煮取三升，分温三服。亦主妇人少腹寒，久不受胎，兼取崩中去血，或月水来过多，及至期不来。

Wèn yuē: Fù rén nián wǔ shí suǒ, bìng xià lì shù shí rì bù zhǐ, mù jí fā rè, shào fù lǐ jí, fù mǎn, shǒu zhǎng fán rè, chún kǒu gān zào, hé yě? Shī yuē: Cǐ bìng shǔ dài xià. Hé yǐ fù? Céng jīng bàn chǎn, yū xuè zài shào fù bù qù. Hé yǐ zhī zhī? Qí zhèng chún kǒu gān zào, gù zhī zhī. Dāng yǐ wēn jīng tāng zhǔ zhī.

Wú zhū yú sān liǎng; dāng guī, xiōng qióng, sháo yào gè èr liǎng; rén shēn, guì zhī, mǔ dān pí (qù xīn) èr liǎng; ē jiāo, shēng jiāng, gān cǎo gè èr liǎng; bàn xià bàn shēng; mài mén dōng (qù xīn) yī shēng

Yòu shí èr wèi, yǐ shuǐ yī dǒu, zhǔ qǔ sān shēng, fēn wēn sān fú. Yì zhǔ fù rén shào fù hán, jiǔ bù shòu tāi, jiān qǔ bēng zhōng qù xuè, huò yuè shuǐ lái guò duō, jí zhì qī bù lái.

Question: "When a woman of about fifty years of age suffers from vaginal bleeding for several tens of days without stopping, with heat effusion at dusk, lesser abdominal urgency, abdominal fullness, vexing heat in the palms of the hands, and dry lips and mouth, what is this?" The Master says: "This disease is ascribed to [disorder] below the girdle. How is it caused? [The woman must have] previously experienced a miscarriage, as a result of which static blood is present in the lesser abdomen instead of having been eliminated. How can you know this? You know this by the sign of dry lips and mouth. Use Channel-Warming (Menses-Warming) Decoction (温经汤 *wēn jīng tāng*) to govern it."

Channel-Warming (Menses-Warming) Decoction (温经汤 *wēn jīng tāng*)

evodia (吴茱萸 *wú zhū yú*, Evodiae Fructus) 3 *liǎng*
Chinese angelica (当归 *dāng guī*, Angelicae Sinensis Radix) 2 *liǎng*
xiongqiong (芎藭 *xiōng qióng*, Chuanxiong Rhizoma) 2 *liǎng*
peony (芍药 *sháo yào*, Paeoniae Radix) 2 *liǎng*
ginseng (人参 *rén shēn*, Ginseng Radix) 2 *liǎng*
cinnamon twig (桂枝 *guì zhī*, Cinnamomi Ramulus) 2 *liǎng*
moutan (牡丹皮 *mǔ dān pí*, Moutan Cortex) (remove core) 2 *liǎng*
ass hide glue (阿胶 *ē jiāo*, Asini Corii Colla) 2 *liǎng*
fresh ginger (生姜 *shēng jiāng*, Zingiberis Rhizoma Recens) 2 *liǎng*
licorice (甘草 *gān cǎo*, Glycyrrhizae Radix) 2 *liǎng*
pinellia (半夏 *bàn xià*, Pinelliae Rhizoma) ½ *shēng*
ophiopogon (麦门冬 *mài mén dōng*, Ophiopogonis Radix) (remove core) 1 *shēng*

Boil the above twelve ingredients in one *dǒu* of water to get three *shēng*. Divide into three doses and take warm. [This formula] also governs women's lesser abdominal cold and chronic failure to conceive; it also helps to eliminate blood from flooding or excessive menstrual bleeding or failure of the menses to arrive [at their proper] time.

TEXT NOTE, LINE 22.9

[1] Vaginal bleeding 下利 *xià lì*: Literally, "disinhibition in the lower body." Commentators generally agree that 利 *lì* is a textual corruption for 血 *xuè* "blood" and thus that this term should be understood as vaginal bleeding.

SYNOPSIS, LINE 22.9

This line describes the signs and symptoms of flooding and spotting due to vacuity cold in the thoroughfare and controlling vessels, together with an internal obstruction by static blood.

COMMENTARY, LINE 22.9

As noted in the *Nèijīng*, women after the age of seven times seven experience vacuity of essence-blood, debilitation of kidney qì, exhaustion of tiānguǐ (reproductive viability), and cessation of menstruation. The present line, however, describes a condition with pathological vaginal bleeding for several tens of days, which is referred to as "flooding and spotting" (崩漏 *bēng lòu*). This condition results from vacuity cold in the thoroughfare and controlling vessels, following a miscarriage where static blood is not eliminated but lodges in the lesser abdomen. This causes abdominal fullness and urgency, possibly with one-sided stabbing pain or resistance to pressure. In addition, continuous bleeding over such a long time wears on yīn-blood. The resulting yīn vacuity engenders internal heat, which manifests in signs like heat effusion in the evening and vexing heat in the palms of the hands. When static blood is not eliminated, new blood is not engendered, and the fluids fail to moisten the upper body. Hence we see dry lips and mouth. All these symptoms relate to deficiency in the lower origin, vacuity cold in the thoroughfare and controlling vessels, and static blood collecting internally.

The recommended treatment is Channel-Warming (Menses-Warming) Decoction (*wēn jīng tāng*) to warm and nourish the blood in the channels. By supplementing vacuity cold and moving static blood, this formula achieves the effect of warming the channels/menses and moving stasis.

In the formula, evodia (*wú zhū yú*), fresh ginger (*shēng jiāng*), and cinnamon twig (*guì zhī*) warm the channels, dissipate cold, and warm blood; ass hide glue (*ē jiāo*), Chinese angelica (*dāng guī*), chuanxiong (*chuān xiōng*), peony (*sháo yào*), and moutan (*mǔ dān pí*) nourish the blood, harmonize construction, and move stasis; ophiopogon (*mài dōng*) and pinellia (*bàn xià*) moisten dryness and downbear counterflow; and licorice (*gān cǎo*) and ginseng (*rén shēn*) supplement and boost center qì. In combination, they warm and supplement the thoroughfare and controlling vessels, nourish blood and move stasis, and support right and dispel evil.

Line 22.10

带下经水不利，少腹满痛，经一月再见者，土瓜根散主之。

土瓜根 芍药 桂枝 蟅虫各三分

右四味，杵为散，酒服方寸匕，日三服。

Dài xià jīng shuǐ bù lì, shào fù mǎn tòng, jīng yī yuè zài jiàn zhě, tǔ guā gēn sǎn zhǔ zhī.

Tǔ guā gēn, sháo yào, guì zhī, zhè chóng gè sān fèn

Yòu sì wèi, chǔ wéi sǎn, jiǔ fú fāng cùn bǐ, rì sān fú.

For disease below the girdle, with inhibited menstrual flow, lesser abdominal fullness and pain, and periods coming twice in one month, Cucumber Gourd Root Powder (土瓜根散 *tǔ guā gēn sǎn*)[1] governs.

Cucumber Gourd Root Powder (土瓜根散 *tǔ guā gēn sǎn*)

cucumber gourd root (土瓜根 *tǔ guā gēn*, Trichosanthis Cucumeroidis Radix) 3 parts
peony (芍药 *sháo yào*, Paeoniae Radix) 3 parts
cinnamon twig (桂枝 *guì zhī*, Cinnamomi Ramulus) 3 parts
ground beetle (蟅虫 *zhè chóng*, Eupolyphaga seu Steleophaga) 3 parts

Pestle the above four ingredients into a powder. Take a square-inch-spoonful in wine, three times a day.

TEXT NOTE, LINE 22.10

[1] A comment included in the received text reads: "Yīn bulging and genital swelling is also governed by this formula."

SYNOPSIS, LINE 22.10

This line describes the signs and treatment of menstrual irregularities owing to blood stasis.

COMMENTARY, LINE 22.10

The gynecologic conditions of inhibited menstruation or shortened menstrual cycles are generally caused by abiding stasis and are therefore accompanied by fullness and pain in the lesser abdomen and possibly hardness or lumps in the lesser abdomen when pressed, scant purple menses with clots, a dark purple tongue, and a rough pulse. Alternatively, inhibited menstruation can also be caused by blood vacuity, in which case you will not see distention and pain in the abdomen, but only symptoms of insufficiency of qì and blood.

Treatment of inhibited menstruation due to blood stasis should center on quickening the blood and freeing stasis. For this purpose, the text recommends Cucumber Gourd Root Powder (*tǔ guā gēn sǎn*). In this formula, cinnamon (*guì zhī*) and peony (*sháo yào*) harmonize construction, while cucumber gourd root (*tǔ guā gēn*) and ground beetle (*zhè chóng*) dispel stasis and break blood. (*Tǔ guā gēn* is also called 王瓜根 *wáng guā gēn.*) With the addition of wine to activate the strength of the medicinals, the formula removes stasis, as a result of which the menstrual flow is naturally regulated.

Line 22.11

寸口脉弦而大，弦则为减，大则为芤，减则为寒，芤则为虚，寒虚相搏，此名曰革。妇人则半产漏下，旋覆花汤主之。

Cùn kǒu mài xián ér dà, xián zé wéi jiǎn, dà zé wéi kōu, jiǎn zé wéi hán, kōu zé wéi xū, hán xū xiāng bó, cǐ míng yuē gé. Fù rén zé bàn chǎn lòu xià, xuán fù huā tāng zhǔ zhī.

When the inch opening pulse is both stringlike and large, stringlike means reduced, and large means scallion-stalk; reduced indicates cold, and scallion-stalk indicates vacuity. Cold and vacuity contend with each other, and this is called a drumskin [pulse]. In women, [this type of pulse] means miscarriage and spotting. Inula Decoction (旋覆花汤 *xuán fù huā tāng*)[1] governs.

TEXT NOTE, LINE 22.11

[1] A comment included in the received text reads: "For the formula, see the chapter, 'Wind and Cold in the Five Viscera and Accumulations and Gatherings'." This refers to Chapter 11, line 11.7.

SYNOPSIS, LINE 22.11

This line describes the pulse and treatment of miscarriage and spotting.

COMMENTARY, LINE 22.11

A variation of this line is found in Chapter 6, "Blood Impediment and Vacuity Taxation," line 6.12. There, the text adds: "In men, it means blood collapse and seminal loss," but no recommended treatment is given. See the commentary to line 6.12 for a discussion of this pulse and the related pathomechanism.

Inula Decoction (*xuán fù huā tāng*) is administered to course the liver, dissipate binds, rectify the blood, and free the network vessels; as such it does not appear to be related to the condition described in this line. Some texts such as the *Yī Zōng Jīn Jiàn* ("Golden Mirror of Medicine") have therefore suggested that the recommended formula is a textual corruption. By contrast, Xū Zhōng-Kě 须忠可, for example, points out that vacuity combined with cold means that evil is present. This must be treated by opening binds to arrest the spotting, and blood will be engendered naturally without any need for supplementation. On the other hand, if you supplement in the presence of evil, you will only make evil exuberant and aggravate the spotting, which will cause detriment before achieving benefit.

Line 22.12

妇人陷经，漏下黑不解，胶姜汤主之。

Fù rén xiàn jīng, lòu xià hēi bù jiě, jiāo jiāng tāng zhǔ zhī.

For women's channel fall, with black spotting that fails to resolve, Ass Hide Glue and Ginger Decoction (*jiāo jiāng tāng*) governs.[1]

TEXT NOTE, LINE 22.12

[1] A comment included in the received text reads: "Chén Yì 臣亿 et al., consulted all the versions without finding any formula for Ass Hide Glue and Ginger Decoction (*jiāo jiāng tāng*). Hence they assume that this refers to the formula for Ass Hide Glue and Mugwort Decoction (*jiāo ài tāng*) in the chapter on Pregnancy."

SYNOPSIS, LINE 22.12

This line describes the signs and treatment of women's channel fall.

COMMENTARY, LINE 22.12

Channel fall refers to downward fall of channel qì, which manifests in incessant vaginal bleeding. The condition described herein is caused by vacuity cold in the thoroughfare and controlling vessels, so that they are unable to contain blood. The recommended treatment is Ass Hide Glue and Ginger Decoction (*jiāo jiāng tāng*), intended to warm and supplement the thoroughfare and controlling vessels, and to nourish blood and check bleeding.

Commentators have stressed the significance of the statement in this line that the condition manifests with spotting of black-colored blood. In most circumstances, profuse vaginal bleeding is characterized by blood that is bright red in color, which is caused by fire in the thoroughfare and controlling vessels. By contrast, if the blood lost is scant or is retained for a longer period, it must be purple or black, which invariably indicates that it is related to vacuity cold. However, this sign can also be caused by static blood and depressed heat, with fire in the thoroughfare and controlling vessels. Thus we must take into account not only the black spotting, but also accompanying symptoms of vacuity cold, before we can safely use the recommended treatment.

Line 22.13

妇人少腹满，如敦状，小便微难而不渴，生后者，此为水与血，俱结在血室也，大黄甘遂汤主之。

大黄四两　甘遂二两　阿胶二两

右三味，以水三升，煮取一升，顿服之，其血当下。

Fù rén shào fù mǎn, rú duì zhuàng, xiǎo biàn wēi nán ér bù kě, shēng hòu zhě, cǐ wéi shuǐ yǔ xuè, jù jié zài xuè shì yě, dà huáng gān suì tāng zhǔ zhī.

Dà huáng sì liǎng; gān suì èr liǎng; ē jiāo èr liǎng

Yòu sān wèi, yǐ shuǐ sān shēng, zhǔ qǔ yī shēng, dùn fú zhī, qí xuè dāng xià.

Women's lower abdominal fullness that appears like a serving bowl,[1] with slight difficulty in urination and no thirst, when arising after giving birth,[2] means both water and blood binding in the blood chamber.[3] Rhubarb and Kansui Decoction (大黄甘遂汤 *dà huáng gān suì tāng*) governs.

Rhubarb and Kansui Decoction (大黄甘遂汤 *dà huáng gān suì tāng*)
rhubarb (大黄 *dà huáng*, Rhei Radix et Rhizoma) 4 *liǎng* kansui (甘遂 *gān suì*, Kansui Radix) 2 *liǎng* ass hide glue (阿胶 *ē jiāo*, Asini Corii Colla) 2 *liǎng*

Boil the above three ingredients in three *shēng* of water to get one *shēng*. Quaff, and the blood should descend.

TEXT NOTES, LINE 22.13

[1] Serving bowl 敦 *duì*: 敦 is an obsolete name for an ancient vessel used for serving food. It is round, flat at the edges, and deep and rounded in the middle.

[2] After giving birth 生后 *shēng hòu*: The Chinese 生 *shēng* in the narrow sense means "to give birth," but the word has many general usages, one of which is in the combination 生病 ("to fall sick"). Thus an alternative interpretation of the phrase 生后 *shēng hòu* in this context is "after falling sick." See the commentary below.

[3] Blood chamber 血室 *xuè shì*: This refers quite literally to the place where blood gathers in the female body. What the "blood chamber" is and where it is located is not specified in early texts. It has been variously explained as referring to the liver, the uterus, and the thoroughfare vessel.

SYNOPSIS, LINE 22.13

This line describes the signs and treatment of water and blood binding in the blood chamber.

COMMENTARY, LINE 22.13

Women's lesser abdominal fullness can be caused by an amassment of either water or blood. If it manifests with uninhibited urination, this indicates amassment of blood; if it manifests with inhibited urination and thirst, it means water amassment. The present case is characterized by abdominal fullness to the point that the abdomen protrudes like an upturned bowl, accompanied by slightly inhibited urination, and no thirst. Thus, we can diagnose this condition as one of both water and blood binding in the blood chamber.

Commentators have suggested three different interpretations of the phrase 生后 *shēng hòu*, which is translated above as "after giving birth." They have either translated it, as we have done, by equating it to 产后 *chǎn hòu*, "after childbirth." Some have deemed it equivalent to 生病后 *shēng bìng hòu*, "after falling sick"; or others have determined its meaning as 曾生育过之妇 *céng shēng yù guò zhī fù*, "in a woman who has given birth in the past."

While the first interpretation is perhaps the most literal, the second reading of "after falling sick" appears to make more sense from a clinical perspective, since this condition can arise in any woman, regardless of her reproductive experience. Moreover, if this line merely addressed women during the postpartum stage, it would be found in the chapter on women's postpartum diseases, not in the present chapter on women's miscellaneous diseases.

Treatment should focus on simultaneously attacking water and blood, for which purpose the text recommends Rhubarb and Kansui Decoction (*dà huáng gān suì tāng*) to break blood and expel water. This formula attacks and expels water and blood bind with rhubarb (*dà huáng*), which attacks stasis, and kansui (*gān suì*), which expels water, assisted by ass hide glue (*ē jiāo*) to nourish blood and support right, so that evil is removed without damaging right.

Line 22.14

妇人经水不利下，抵当汤主之。

水蛭三十个（熬） 虻虫三十枚（熬，去翅足） 桃仁二十个（去皮尖） 大黄三两(酒浸)

右四味，为末，以水五升，煮取三升，去滓，温服一升。

Fù rén jīng shuǐ bù lì xià, dǐ dāng tāng zhǔ zhī.

Shuǐ zhì sān shí ge (áo); méng chóng sān shí méi (áo, qù chì zú); táo rén èr shí gè (qù pí jiān); dà huáng sān liǎng (jiǔ jìn)

Yòu sì wèi, wéi mò, yǐ shuǐ wǔ shēng, zhǔ qǔ sān shēng, qù zǐ, wēn fú yī shēng.

For inhibited descent of a woman's menses,[1] Dead-On Decoction (抵当汤 *dǐ dàng tāng*) governs.[2]

Dead-On Decoction (抵当汤 *dǐ dàng tāng*)

- leech (水蛭 *shuǐ zhì*, Hirudo) 30 pieces (simmer)
- tabanus (虻虫 *méng chóng*, Tabanus) 30 pieces (simmer and remove the wings and legs)
- peach kernel (桃仁 *táo rén*, Persicae Semen) 20 pieces (remove the skin and tips)
- rhubarb (大黄 *dà huáng*, Rhei Radix et Rhizoma) 3 *liǎng* (steep in wine)

Pulverize the above four ingredients and boil in five *shēng* of water to get three *shēng*. Remove the dregs. Take one *shēng* per dose warm.

Text Notes, Line 22.14

[1] Inhibited descent of the menses 经水不利下 *jīng shuǐ bù lì xià*: In early literature, 经水不利 *jīng shuǐ bù lì*, inhibited menstrual flow, is a much more common expression for this condition. The addition of 下 *xià* here may be a textual error, or alternatively could denote that the condition described is more severe or of a slightly different nature than the more general "inhibited menstrual flow," which is mentioned, for example, in line 22.10 above and treated by quickening blood and moving stasis. By contrast, the condition here requires the powerful stasis-attacking blood-breaking action of Dead-On Decoction (*dǐ dàng tāng*).

[2] A comment included in the received text reads: "Also treats men's fullness, urgency, and presence of static blood in the bladder."

Synopsis, Line 22.14

This line describes the signs and treatment of inhibited menstruation in stasis bind repletion patterns.

COMMENTARY, LINE 22.14

The present line describes a condition of menstrual block and stoppage that is caused by static blood binding internally and forming repletion. Therefore, we must first remove the stasis bind before restoring an uninhibited menstrual flow.

The recommended formula is Dead-On Decoction (*dǐ dàng tāng*), in which leech (*shuǐ zhì*) and tabanus (*méng chóng*) attack the stasis, and rhubarb (*dà huáng*) and apricot kernel (*táo rén*) precipitate the blood. When static blood is removed, new blood is engendered, and the menses once again will flow uninhibitedly. On the basis of this treatment, we know that this condition should also manifest with lesser abdominal hardness, fullness, bind, and pain, or with no objective abdominal fullness, but only a subjective sensation of fullness, as well as with black stool, uninhibited urine, and a sunken and rough pulse.

Line 22.15

妇人经水闭不利，脏坚癖不止，中有干血，下白物，矾石丸主之。

矾石三分（烧）　　杏仁一分

右二味，末之，炼蜜和丸枣核大，内脏中，剧者再内之。

Fù rén jīng shuǐ bì bù lì, zàng jiān pǐ bù zhǐ, zhōng yǒu gān xuè, xià bái wù, fán shí wán zhǔ zhī.

Fán shí (shāo) sān fēn; xìng rén yī fēn

Yòu èr wèi, mò zhī, liàn mì huò wán zǎo hé dà, nà zàng zhōng, jù zhě zài nà zhī.

For women's blocked and inhibited menstrual flow, with a hard aggregation in the uterus[1] that does not go away, which means dry blood in the center, and with discharge of white matter,[2] Alum Pill (矾石丸 *fán shí wán*) governs.

Alum Pill (矾石丸 *fán shí wán*)
alum (矾石 *fán shí*, Alumen) 3 parts (calcined) apricot kernel (杏仁 *xìng rén*, Armeniacae Semen) 1 part

Pulverize the above two ingredients and blend with processed honey (*liàn mì*) to form into pills the size of jujube pits. Insert one into the uterus; in severe cases insert a second one.

TEXT NOTES, LINE 22.15

[1] Hard aggregation in the uterus 脏坚癖 *zàng jiān pì*: An aggregation is an morbid accumulation of matter in the abdomen characterized by a lump. Here, 脏 *zàng* (literally, "viscus") is an abbreviation for 子脏 *zǐ zàng*, "uterus."

[2] Discharge of white matter 下白物 *xià bái wù*: White vaginal discharge.

SYNOPSIS, LINE 22.15

This line describes the external treatment of dry blood menstrual block with damp-heat vaginal discharge.

COMMENTARY, LINE 22.15

The present line explains a condition in which white vaginal discharge is caused by blocked or inhibited menstruation, by dry blood fixed internally and depressed, and by damp-heat forming and putrefying over time. Thus, this condition is initially caused by static blood, but is also related to the presence of damp-heat.

The recommended treatment is Alum Pill (*fán shí wán*), to be inserted as a vaginal suppository. This formula consists of alum (*fán shí*), which is sour, astringent, and cold, and hence promotes contraction, dries dampness, resolves toxin, and kills worms; apricot kernel (*xìng rén*), which is bitter and moist, to disinhibit qì and moisten dryness; and honey (*fēng mì*), which enriches and moistens. It is thus intended to eliminate damp-heat and thereby stop vaginal discharge. Nevertheless, this preparation merely treats the tip and usually therefore it would be accompanied by internal preparations to disperse stasis and free the menses as treatment of the root. Note that the above formula is not recommended in cases with vaginal erosion.

Line 22.16

妇人六十二种风，及腹中血气刺痛，红蓝花酒主之。

红蓝花一两

右一味，以酒一大升，煎减半，顿服一半，未止再服。

Fù rén liù shí èr zhǒng fēng, jí fù zhōng xuè qì cì tòng, hóng lán huā jiǔ zhǔ zhī.

Hóng lán huā yī liǎng

Yòu yī wèi, yǐ jiǔ yī dà shēng, jiān jiǎn bàn, dùn fú yī bàn, wèi zhǐ zài fú.

For sixty-two kinds of wind in women, with blood and qì stabbing pain in the abdomen, Carthamus Wine (红蓝花酒 *hóng lán huā jiǔ*)[1] governs.

Carthamus Wine (红蓝花酒 *hóng lán huā jiǔ*)
carthamus (红蓝花 *hóng lán huā*, Carthami Flos)

Boil the above ingredient in one large *shēng* of wine until reduced to half. Quaff half as one dose. [If the pain] does not stop, take a second dose.

TEXT NOTE, LINE 22.16

[1] A comment included in the received text reads: "It is doubtful whether this is Zhāng Jī's formula."

SYNOPSIS, LINE 22.16

This line describes the signs and treatment of abdominal pain from blood stasis and qì stagnation.

COMMENTARY, LINE 22.16

The sixty-two kinds of wind refers comprehensively to the various types of wind evil that cause disease. Commentators disagree on whether this refers only to external wind invading the body from the outside, or also to internally engendered wind. Regarding the former, it is well-known in Chinese medicine that women are particularly susceptible to wind exploiting vacuity and invading the abdomen after childbirth. Alternatively, wind can also be engendered internally as a result of the liver being deprived of nourishment. In either case, wind contends with blood and qì, as a result of which blood congeals and stops; hence we see stabbing abdominal pain.

The recommended treatment is Carthamus Wine (*hóng lán huā jiǔ*), which is intended to quicken blood, move stasis, disinhibit qì, and relieve pain. In this formula, Carthami Flos (*hóng lán huā*) quickens blood, frees the channels/menses, and relieves pain with acridity and warmth, while wine has the ability to move blood. Because wind naturally disappears when blood moves, this formula does not need to use further wind-expelling medicinals.

Line 22.17

妇人腹中诸疾痛，当归芍药散主之。

Fù rén fù zhōng zhū jí tòng, dāng guī sháo yào sǎn zhǔ zhī.

For all abdominal pain in women, Chinese Angelica and Peony Powder (当归芍药散 *dāng guī sháo yào sǎn*)[1] governs.

TEXT NOTE, LINE 22.17

[1] A comment included in the received text reads: "For the formula, see above under Pregnancy." This refers to line 20.5 in Chapter 20, "Pregnancy."

SYNOPSIS, LINE 22.17

This line describes the treatment of women's abdominal pain.

COMMENTARY, LINE 22.17

The causes of women's abdominal pain are numerous, including cold, heat, vacuity, repletion, qì, or food, but are most often related to qì stagnation and congealing blood. From the choice of medicinals in the recommended formula, we can deduce that this line refers to abdominal pain that is caused by liver-spleen disharmony, spleen vacuity with damp obstruction, and qì and blood stasis, a pathomechanism that is most likely caused by affect-mind damage.

The recommended formula, Chinese Angelica and Peony Powder (*dāng guī sháo yào sǎn*) harmonizes the liver and spleen, rectifies qì and blood, and disinhibits water-damp, thereby relieving pain. Deducing the signs on the basis of the ingredients in this formula, the cases treated may also manifest with inhibited urination, abdominal distention and fullness, and slight swelling of the head, face, and limbs.

Line 22.18

妇人腹中痛，小建中汤主之。

Fù rén fù zhōng tòng, xiǎo jiàn zhōng tāng zhǔ zhī.

For women's abdominal pain, Minor Center-Fortifying Decoction (小建中汤 *xiǎo jiàn zhōng tāng*)[1] governs.

TEXT NOTE, LINE 22.18

[1] A comment included in the received text reads: "For the formula, see under Vacuity Taxation above." This refers to line 6.13 in Chapter 6, "Blood Impediment and Vacuity Taxation."

SYNOPSIS, LINE 22.18

This line describes the treatment of women's abdominal urgency and pain due to spleen-stomach vacuity cold.

COMMENTARY, LINE 22.18

In cases where women's abdominal pain is caused by spleen-stomach vacuity cold in the center burner, you will see abdominal pain that likes pressure, heart palpitation and vacuity vexation, a lusterless facial complexion, fatigued spirit and reduced food intake, sloppy thin stool, a pale red tongue, and a fine rough pulse. Because vacuity cold in the spleen and stomach disables engendering transformation and causes insufficiency of qì and blood, the channels in the bowels and viscera are deprived of nourishment, and the movement of qì and blood is inhibited; hence, abdominal pain arises.

We use Minor Center-Fortifying Decoction (*xiǎo jiàn zhōng tāng*), which warms the center and banks up earth, and thereby restores the source of engendering transformation and of spleen-stomach movement and transformation. As a result, qì and blood are made abundant and flow freely, and the abdominal pain is relieved naturally.

Line 22.19

问曰：妇人病，饮食如故，烦热不得卧，而反倚息者，何也？师曰：此名转胞，不得溺也。以胞系了戾，故致此病，但利小便则愈，宜肾气丸主之。

干地黄八两　薯蓣四两　山茱萸四两
泽泻三两　茯苓三两　牡丹皮三两
桂枝 附子（炮）各一两

右八味，末之，炼蜜和丸梧子大，酒下十五丸，加至二十五丸，日再服。

Wèn yuē: fù rén bìng, yǐn shí rú gù, fán rè bù dé wò, ér fǎn yǐ xī zhě, hé yě? Shī yuē: cǐ míng zhuǎn bāo, bù dé niào yě. Yǐ bāo xì liǎo lì, gù zhì cǐ bìng, dàn lì xiǎo biàn zé yù, yí shèn qì wán zhǔ zhī.

Gān dì huáng bā liǎng; shǔ yù sì liǎng; shān zhū yú sì liǎng; zé xiè sān liǎng; fú líng sān liǎng; mǔ dān pí sān liǎng; guì zhī, fù zǐ (pào) gè yī liǎng

Yòu bā wèi, mò zhī, liàn mì hé wán wú zǐ dà, jiǔ xià shí wǔ wán, jiā zhì èr shí wǔ wán, rì zài fú.

Question: "When a woman presents with eating and drinking as normal, but vexing heat with inability to sleep, and propped breathing,[1] what disease is this?" The Master says: "This is called shifted bladder.[2] It [results in] inability to urinate. This disease is caused by the bladder tie being twisted.[3] You need only to disinhibit the urine and recovery will ensue. Kidney Qì Pill (肾气丸 *shèn qì wán*) governs."

Kidney Qì Pill (肾气丸 *shèn qì wán*)
dried rehmannia (干地黄 *gān dì huáng*, Rehmanniae Radix) 8 *liǎng*
dioscorea (薯蓣 *shǔ yù*, Dioscoreae Rhizoma) 4 *liǎng*
cornus (山茱萸 *shān zhū yú*, Corni Fructus) 4 *liang*
alisma (泽泻 *zé xiè*, Alismatis Rhizoma) 3 *liǎng*
poria (茯苓 *fú líng*, Poria) 3 *liǎng*
moutan (牡丹皮 *mǔ dān pí*, Moutan Cortex) 3 *liǎng*
cinnamon twig (桂枝 *guì zhī*, Cinnamomi Ramulus) 1 *liǎng*
aconite (附子 *fù zǐ*, Aconiti Radix Lateralis Praeparata) 1 *liǎng* (blast-fry)

Pulverize the above eight ingredients and blend with processed honey (*liàn mì*) to form into pills the size of firmiana seeds. Down 15 pills [per dose] with wine, increasing [the dosage] up to 25 pills, twice a day.

TEXT NOTES, LINE 22.19

[1] Propped breathing 倚息 *yǐ xī*: A condition in which the patient can only breathe comfortably in reclining posture.

[2] Shifted bladder 转胞 *zhuǎn bāo*: 胞 *bāo* can refer to the uterus or to the bladder, but based on context clearly refers to the bladder in this line. Shifted bladder is a condition that occurs in pregnancy when the enlarged uterus displaces the bladder, causing difficulty in urination.

[3] Twisted bladder tie 胞系了戾 *bāo xì liǎo lì*: This describes a condition where the bladder connector, which appears to refer to the ureter, is twisted and entangled, as a result of which urine is unable to pass smoothly.

SYNOPSIS, LINE 22.19

This line describes the signs and treatment of shifted bladder.

COMMENTARY, LINE 22.19

The key symptoms of women's shifted bladder are tension and pain below the umbilicus and urinary stoppage; its main cause is kidney qì vacuity resulting in stopped bladder qì transformation. Because the disease is not located in the stomach, eating and drinking are normal. Because it is located in the bladder, on the other hand, we see lesser abdominal distention and fullness, and inability to urinate. When water qì does not move, turbid yīn ascends counterflow and vacuous yáng harasses the upper body; hence there is vexing heat with inability to sleep, and propped breathing.

We treat this condition with Kidney Qì Pill (*shèn qì wán*) to warm yáng and transform qì. When kidney yáng is abundant, qì transformation is restored and urine is disinhibited.

Line 22.20

蛇床子散方，温阴中坐药。

蛇床子仁

右一味，末之，以白粉少许，和令相得，如枣大，绵裹内之，自然温。

Shé chuáng zǐ sǎn fāng, wēn yīn zhōng zuò yào.

Shé chuáng zǐ rén

Yòu yī wèi, mò zhī, yǐ bái fěn shǎo xǔ , hé lìng xiāng dé, rú zǎo dà, mián guǒ nà zhī, zì rán wēn.

Cnidium Seed Powder (蛇床子散 *shé chuáng zǐ sǎn*) formula is a suppository[1] that warms the inside of the vagina.

Cnidium Seed Powder (蛇床子散 *shé chuáng zǐ sǎn*)
cnidium seed (蛇床子仁 *shé chuáng zǐ rén*, Cnidii Fructus)

Pulverize the above single ingredient and blend with a little processed galenite (*qiān fěn*) until thoroughly combined. Take an amount the size of a jujube, wrap it in gauze, and insert it [into the vagina]. [The vagina] will spontaneously become warm.

Text Note, Line 22.20

[1] Suppository 坐药 *zuò yào*: Vaginal suppository, i.e., medicine inserted into the vagina. The Chinese means "sitting medicine," and is apparently so named because in ancient times women would sit with their knees on the ground with their buttocks resting on their heels before applying it.

Synopsis, Line 22.20

This line describes the external treatment of vaginal cold with cold-damp vaginal discharge.

Commentary, Line 22.20

From the intended effect of this treatment, namely that it "warms the inside of the vagina," we know that the patient suffers from a subjective sensation of cold in the genitals. On the basis of the single ingredient, we can deduce that this pattern should be accompanied by vaginal discharge, soreness and heaviness in the lumbus, and vaginal itching. This condition is caused by the evil of yīn cold damp turbidity congealing in the lower burner. Cnidium Seed Powder (*shé chuáng zǐ sǎn*) applied as a suppository has the effect of directly warming the location of the evil, warming the uterus, eliminating dampness, killing worms, and stopping itching.

Line 22.21

少阴脉滑而数者，阴中即生疮，阴中蚀疮烂者，狼牙汤洗之。

狼牙三两

右一味，以水四升，煮取半升，以绵缠筯如茧，浸汤沥阴中，日四遍。

Shào yīn mài huá ér shuò zhě, yīn zhōng jí shēng chuāng, yīn zhōng shí chuāng làn zhě, láng yá tāng xǐ zhī.

Láng yá sān liǎng

Yòu yī wèi, yǐ shuǐ sì shēng, zhǔ qǔ bàn shēng, yǐ mián chán jīn rú jiǎn, jìn tāng lì yīn zhōng, rì sì biàn.

A lesser yīn pulse that is slippery and rapid indicates engenderment of sores in the vagina. For putrefying eroding sores in the vagina, wash it with Langya[1] Decoction (狼牙汤 *láng yá tāng*).

Langya Decoction (狼牙汤 *láng yá tāng*)
Langya (狼牙 *láng yá*) 3 *liǎng*

Boil the above single ingredient in four *shēng* of water to get half a *shēng*. Wrap silk fibers around a chopstick like a cocoon, steep it in the decoction, and [use this to] trickle [the decoction] into the inside of the vagina, four times a day.

Text Note, Line 22.21

[1] Langya 狼牙 *láng yá*: This is likely the root of *Agrimonia pilosa* (downy agrimony or cocklebur) or *Potentilla cryptotaenia* (a species of cinquefoil), both of the rose family (Rosaceae). In the *Běn Cǎo Jīng Jí Zhù* ("Variorum of the Herbal Foundation Canon"), Táo Hóng-Jǐng offers 狼牙 as synonym for 牙子 *yǎ zǐ*. He describes it as a highly toxic plant, used mostly as a vermifuge, but also specifically for the treatment of women's genital erosion.

Commentators disagree on the identity of this medicinal, but sometimes suggest substituting 狼毒 Chinese wolfsbane (*láng dú*). This is, however, highly toxic and should therefore not be used for a long time or in patients with open sores.

Synopsis, Line 22.21

This line describes the pulse and treatment of vaginal sores due to lower burner damp-heat.

Commentary, Line 22.21

Lesser yīn belongs to the kidney, which governs the two yīn, that is, the anal and genital orifices. A slippery and rapid lesser yīn pulse thus indicates damp-heat brewing in the lower burner. If damp-heat gathers in the genitals, it will over time invariably cause itching, pain, and erosion inside the vagina, accompanied by turbid dribbling discharge. The recommended treatment consists of washing the vagina with a concentrated decoction of agrimony (*láng yá*). This will have the effect of clearing heat, drying dampness, killing worms, and stopping itching.

Line 22.22

胃气下泄，阴吹而正喧，此谷气之实也，膏发煎导之。

Wèi qì xià xiè, yīn chuī ér zhèng xuān, cǐ gǔ qì zhī shí yě, gāo fǎ jiān dǎo zhī.

Downward draining of stomach qì with yīn flatulence[1] in continuous blasts means repletion of grain qì.[2] Lard and Hair Brew (膏发煎 *gāo fà jiān*)[3] abducts it.

TEXT NOTES, LINE 22.22

[1] Yīn flatulence 阴吹 *yīn chuī*: A condition characterized by the passing of gas via the vagina; vaginal flatulence.

[2] Repletion of grain qì 谷气之实 *gǔ qì zhī shí*: Firmness of the stool, i.e., constipation.

[3] A comment included in the received text reads: "For the formula, see under 'Jaundice' above." This refers to line 15.17, in chapter 15, "Jaundice," where the formula is called 猪膏发煎 *zhū gāo fà jiān*, consisting of the two ingredients pork lard and hair.

SYNOPSIS, LINE 22.22

This line describes the cause, signs, and treatment of yīn flatulence.

COMMENTARY, LINE 22.22

This line discusses yīn flatulence, a condition common in older women, women who have given birth excessively, and women with habitual excessive vaginal discharge. In this pathomechanism, dryness bind in the stomach and intestines and inhibition of bowel qì causes turbid qì to drain downward and reach the genitals, which results in flatulence from qì exiting from the vagina. Given the recommended treatment, we know that the condition addressed here stems from blood vacuity and lack of liquid, which results in constipation. This prevents downward-moving stomach qì from exiting through the anus, so that it is forced into the vagina instead. The recommended treatment, Lard and Hair Brew (*gāo fà jiān*), nourishes blood and moistens dryness, thereby freeing and abducting stool and allowing qì to return to its regular pathway.

Line 22.23

雄黄　葶苈

Xióng huáng; tíng lì

右二味，末之，取腊月猪脂，熔，以槐枝绵裹头四五枚，点药烙之。

Yòu èr wèi, mò zhī, qǔ là yuè zhū zhī, róng, yǐ huái zhī mián guǒ tóu sì wǔ méi, diǎn yào lào zhī.

[Infantile Worm-Eaten Tooth Formula (小儿疳虫蚀齿方 *xiǎo ér gān chóng shí chǐ fāng*)][1]

realgar (雄黄 *xióng huáng*, Realgar)
lepidium/descurainiae (葶苈 *tíng lì*, Lepidii/Descurainiae Semen)

Pulverize the above two ingredients. Melt twelfth-month pork lard.[2] Take four or five pagoda tree twigs with the tips wrapped in silk floss. Dip the medicine in this and ignite it [to apply it to the teeth].

TEXT NOTES, LINE 22.23

[1] A comment included in the received text reads: "It is doubtful whether this is Zhāng Jī's formula."

[2] 12th month pork lard (腊月猪脂 *là yuè zhū zhī*): Pork fat rendered at the end of the lunar year.

SYNOPSIS, LINE 22.23

This line describes the external treatment for gān-worms eroding the teeth.

COMMENTARY, LINE 22.23

It is commonly considered that this line is not part of the original text by Zhāng Jī. Nevertheless, it is worthy of discussion. When children fail to receive appropriate nourishment, and food and drink stagnate, symptoms of spleen-stomach vacuity detriment and malnourishment result, such as eating followed by rapid hungering, sloppy bound irregular stool, disquieted sleep, increased sweating, grinding of the teeth, yellow facial complexion, and emaciation of the flesh. This is gān accumulation. In small children, gān accumulation is caused by stagnation of food and drink in the stomach, which easily transforms into damp-heat. This causes dental disease like erosion of the gums, engenderment of worms due to depressed damp-heat, and cavities.

The recommended formula can be used as an external treatment for this condition. In the formula, realgar (*xióng huáng*), lepidii/descurainiae (*tíng lì zǐ*), lard, and pagoda tree tips all have the effect of moving and quickening blood, dispersing swelling, and killing worms. This is reinforced by igniting the pork lard and heating the affected tooth, thereby killing the "worms" directly.

杂寮疗方第二十三

CHAPTER 23

Miscellaneous Formulas

Pulses, Signs, Treatments

‡ Overview

Most scholars since the Míng and Qīng periods onward assume that the following three chapters are not in fact part of the original text by Zhāng Jī, but were perhaps added during the Sòng period by Lín Yì 林亿 and his collaborators when they reorganized the text for publication. They are therefore most likely formulas that originated from the experience of later physicians or from popular transmission, added to complement the book's content. For this reason, some of these scholars do not even include these chapters in their editions of the *Jīn Guì Yào Lüè* ("Essential Prescriptions of the Golden Cabinet"). Other scholars have argued that these formulas do in fact stem from Zhāng Jī, as can be seen from quotations in the *Zhǒu Hòu Bèi Jí Fāng* ("Emergency Standby Remedies"), *Qiān Jīn Fāng* ("Thousand Gold Pieces Prescriptions"), *Wài Tái Mì Yào* ("Secrets from the *Wài Tái* Library"), *Xiǎo Pǐn Fāng* ("Small Formulary"), and *Gǔ Jīn Lù Yàn* ("Ancient and Modern Records Tested"). As such, they reflect Zhāng Jī's efforts at collecting and editing efficacious formulas among the people on the basis of ancient medical records. We have therefore included them here for their obvious historical value.

The following three chapters are rich in content and have established the foundation for later developments in the areas of emergency treatments, dietary therapy, and preventative medicine, in both theory and clinical application. Some of the methods found here are in common use to this day.

The present chapter on "Miscellaneous Formulas" contains 16 lines with 22 formulas and more than ten disease patterns. Except for lines 1, 2, and 4, which discuss treatment methods for vacuity heat in the five viscera and recuperative care after cold damage, the remaining 13 lines all describe emergency treatments in various critical conditions like sudden death, suicide from hanging, or drowning.

In treating the critical conditions four goals are important: restoring consciousness; restoring respiration; safeguarding yáng qì; eliminating evil qi. Medicinals used to restore consciousness include long-stamen onion juice, garlic chive juice, acorus flakes, cinnamon flakes, horse dung, and cow slop.

Line 23.1

退五藏虚热：
冬三月加柴胡八分　白朮八分　陈皮五分　大腹槟榔（并皮子用）四枚　生姜五分　桔梗七分；春三月加枳实减白朮共六味；夏三月加生姜三分　枳实五分　甘草三分共八味　秋三月加陈皮三分共六味
右各㕮咀，分为三贴，一贴以水三升，煮取二升，分温三服，如人行四五里进一服。如四体壅，添甘草少许，每贴分作三小贴，每小贴以水一升，煮取七合，温服，再合滓为一服，重煮都成四服。

Tuì wŭ zàng xū rè:

Dōng sān yuè jiā chái hú bā fēn; bái zhú bā fēn; chén pí wŭ fēn; dà fù bīng láng (bìng pí zĭ yòng) sì méi; shēng jiāng wŭ fēn; jié gēng qī fēn. Chūn sān yuè jiā zhĭ shí; jiăn bái zhú gòng liù wèi.; Xià sān yuè jiā shēng jiāng sān fēn; zhĭ shí wŭ fēn; gān căo sān fēn, gòng bā wèi. Qiū sān yuè jiā chén pí sān fēn, gòng liù wèi.

Yòu gè fŭ jŭ, fēn wéi sān tiē, yī tiē yĭ shuĭ sān shēng, zhŭ qŭ èr shēng, fēn wēn sān fú, rú rén xíng sì wŭ lĭ jìn yī fú. Rú sì tĭ yōng, tiān gān căo shăo xŭ, mĕi tiē fēn zuò sān xiăo tiē, mĕi xiăo tiē yĭ shuĭ yī shēng, zhŭ qŭ qī gĕ, wēn fú, zài gĕ zĭ wéi yī fú, chóng zhŭ dōu chéng sì fú.

To abate vacuity heat in the five viscera.
In the three winter months, use:

[Seasonally Varied Bupleurum Drink (四时加减柴胡饮子 *sì shí jiā jiăn chái hú yĭn zĭ*)]

bupleurum (柴胡 *chái hú*, Bupleuri Radix) 8 parts
white atractylodes (白朮 *bái zhú*, Atractylodis Macrocephalae Rhizoma) 8 parts
tangerine peel (陈皮 *chén pí*, Citri Reticulatae Pericarpium) 5 parts
areca (槟榔 *bīng láng*, Arecae Semen) 4 pieces (use with skin and seed)
fresh ginger (生姜 *shēng jiāng*, Zingiberis Rhizoma Recens) 5 parts
platycodon (桔梗 *jié gĕng*, Platycodonis Radix) 7 parts

In the three spring months, add:

unripe bitter orange (枳实 *zhĭ shí*, Aurantii Fructus Immaturus)

Remove white atractylodes (白朮 *bái zhú*, Atractylodis Macrocephalae Rhizoma), to make a total of six ingredients.

In the three summer months, add:

fresh ginger (生姜 *shēng jiāng*, Zingiberis Rhizoma Recens) 3 parts
unripe bitter orange (枳实 *zhĭ shí*, Aurantii Fructus Immaturus) 5 parts
licorice (甘草 *gān căo*, Glycyrrhizae Radix) 3 parts

to make a total of eight ingredients.

In the three autumn months, add:

tangerine peel (陈皮 *chén pí*, Citri Reticulatae Pericarpium) 3 parts

to make a total of six ingredients.

Chew the above ingredients and divide into three packets. Boil each packet with three *shēng* of water to get two *shēng*. Divide into three doses and take warm, separating doses by the time it takes to walk four or five lĭ.[1] If there is congestion in the limbs, slightly increase the amount of licorice (*gān căo*), divide each packet into three small packets, and boil each packet with one *shēng* of water to get seven *gĕ*. Take warm. Further, combine the dregs to make another packet and boil this again to create a total of four doses.[2]

TEXT NOTES, LINE 23.1

[1] Separating doses by the time it takes to walk four or five lǐ 如人行四五里进一服 *rú rén xíng sì wǔ lǐ*: About 30 minutes.

[2] A comment included in the received text reads: "It is doubtful whether this is Zhāng Jī's formula."

SYNOPSIS, LINE 23.1

This line describes a seasonally varied treatment for vacuity heat in the viscera.

COMMENTARY, LINE 23.1

Cold or heat contraction in the five viscera can be treated with Seasonally Varied Bupleurum Drink (*sì shí jiā jiǎn chái hú yǐn zǐ*), but this formula must be modified in accordance with the seasons. In this formula, bupleurum (*chái hú*) is the chief medicinal, as it harmonizes the exterior and interior and yīn and yáng. White atractylodis (*bái zhú*) supports and nourishes spleen earth. Platycodon (*jié gěng*) and tangerine peel (*chén pí*) disinhibit qì in the upper and center burners. Areca (*bīng láng*) outthrusts qì from inside the abdomen. Lastly, fresh ginger (*shēng jiāng*) assists in the diffusing and outthrusting action of bupleurum (*chái hú*) and in the dispersing and abducting action of areca (*bīng láng*).

In the winter, increase the amount of bupleurum (*chái hú*) to assist engenderment of qì. In the spring, add unripe bitter orange (*zhǐ shí*) to activate the mechanism of effusing the old, and remove white atractylodis (*bái zhú*) because it might dry the spleen and impede the orderly reaching of liver qì. In the summer, exuberant heat can cause damage to qì, while exuberant dampness can cause qì stagnation. Therefore, we add licorice (*gān cǎo*) to assist white atractylodis (*bái zhú*) in helping qì overcome dampness, and we increase the amount of fresh ginger (*shēng jiāng*) and unripe bitter orange (*zhǐ shí*) to diffuse qì stagnation. Lastly, in the autumn, the climate is even, and we only need to slightly increase tangerine peel (*chén pí*) to warm the center and regulate the spleen.

Line 23.2

诃黎勒　陈皮　厚朴各三两
右三味，末之，炼蜜丸如梧子大，酒饮服二十丸，加至三十丸。

Hē lí lè　chén pí　hòu pò　gè sān liǎng

Yòu sān wèi, mò zhī, liàn mì wán rú wú zǐ dà, jiǔ yǐn fú èr shí wán, jiā zhì sān shí wán.

[Extended-Use Chebule Pill (长服诃黎勒丸 *cháng fú hē lí lè wán*)[1]

chebule (诃黎勒 *hē lí lè*, Chebulae Fructus) 3 *liǎng*
tangerine peel (陈皮 *chén pí*, Citri Reticulatae Pericarpium) 3 *liǎng*
officinal magnolia bark (厚朴 *hòu pò*, Magnoliae Officinalis Cortex) 3 *liǎng*

Pulverize the above three ingredients and [blend with] processed honey (*liàn mì*) to form into pills the size of firmiana seeds. Take twenty pills per dose with wine, increasing [the dosage] up to thirty pills.

TEXT NOTE, LINE 23.2

[1] A comment included in the received text reads: "It is doubtful whether this is Zhāng Jī's formula."

SYNOPSIS, LINE 23.2

This line presents a formula to treat dietary irregularities that can be taken over an extended period.

COMMENTARY, LINE 23.2

Stagnation in the intestines and stomach due to dietary irregularities is a common cause of disease. The ancients therefore extensively used many dispersing and abducting medicinals in their formulas for cultivating health, to prevent congestion in the interstices and blockage in the nine orifices, and to harmonize qì and blood. In modern times, by contrast, people prefer to take enriching medicinals to supplement and nourish, which can cause qì congestion and stagnation of evils. The three ingredients in the present formula all disinhibit qì and move stagnation, and when taken as honey pills in wine, also prevent stagnation of qì in the blood aspect. The main ingredient, chebule (*hē lí lè*), astringes the intestines and precipitates qì, and can therefore treat chronic diarrhea or dysentery, prolapse of the rectum, and bloody stool. Extended-Use Chebule Pill (*cháng fú hē lí lè wán*) is thus a preparation that secures the spleen and disinhibits qì, while attending to right and evil at the same time.

Line 23.3

大黄一两　干姜一两　巴豆（去皮心，熬，外研如脂）一两

右药各须精新，先捣大黄，干姜为末，研巴豆内中，合治一千杵，用为散，蜜和丸亦佳，密器中贮之，莫令歇。主心腹诸卒暴百病。若中恶客忤，心腹胀满，卒痛如锥刺，气急口噤，停尸卒死者，以暖水若酒服大豆许三四丸，或不下，捧头起，灌令下咽，须臾当差，如未差，更与三丸，当腹中鸣，即吐下便差。若口噤，亦须折齿灌之。

Dà huáng yī liǎng　gān jiāng yī liǎng　bā dòu (qù pí xīn, áo, wài yán rú zhī) yī liǎng

Yòu yào gè xū jīng xīn, xiān dǎo dà huáng, gān jiāng wéi mò, yán bā dòu nà zhōng, gě zhì yī qiān chǔ, yòng wéi sǎn, mì huò wán yì jiā, mì qì zhōng zhù zhī, mò lìng xiē. Zhǔ xīn fù zhū cù bào bǎi bìng. Ruò zhòng è kè wǔ, xīn fù zhàng mǎn, cù tòng rú zhuī cì, qì jí kǒu jìn, tíng shī cù sǐ zhě, yǐ nuǎn shuǐ ruò jiǔ fú dà dòu xǔ sān sì wán, huò bù xià, pěng tóu qǐ, guàn lìng xià yàn, xū yú dāng chài, rú wèi chài, gèng yǔ sān wán, dāng fù zhōng míng, jí tù xià biàn chài. Ruò kǒu jìn, yì xū zhé chǐ guàn zhī.

Three Agents Emergency Standby Pill (三物备急丸 *sān wù bèi jí wán*)[1]
rhubarb (大黄 *dà huáng*, Rhei Radix et Rhizoma) 1 *liǎng* dried ginger (干姜 *gān jiāng*, Zingiberis Rhizoma) 1 *liǎng* croton (巴豆 *bā dòu*, Crotonis Fructus) 1 *liǎng* (remove the skin and core, simmer, grind separately until resembling fat)

The above ingredients each need to be of choicest quality and fresh. First crush the rhubarb (*dà huáng*) and dried ginger (*gān jiāng*) into a powder; grind the croton (*bā dòu*) and add to these. Then pestle them all together a thousand times. Using this as a powder, or blended with honey (*mì*) into pills, is good. Store in a tightly [sealed] container, so as not to [let the medicinal strength] leak. [This formula] governs the hundred sudden and fulminant diseases of the heart and abdomen. For malignity striké and visiting hostility,[3] distention and fullness in the heart and abdomen, sudden pain as if being stabbed with an awl, rapid breathing and clenched jaw, stopping corpse,[4] and sudden death[liness],[5] take three or four pills the size of soybeans with warm water or wine. If [the patient] cannot get them down, support the head with two hands and pour [the medicine into the mouth so that it goes] down the throat. Recovery should ensue in a moment. If the patient fails to recover, give a further dose of three pills. There should be rumbling in the abdomen, and soon thereafter vomiting and diarrhea; then recovery will ensue. If the jaw is clenched, you may also have to knock out teeth to pour [the medicine] in.

TEXT NOTES, LINE 23.3

[1] A comment included in the received text reads: "According to the *Qiān Jīn Fāng* ("Thousand Gold Pieces Prescriptions"), you may also use *Sī Kōng Péi Xiù* made into pills. First combine to make a juice, then turn the mouth to make it enter between the teeth. You will achieve excellent results."

[2] Malignity strike 中恶 *zhòng è*: A condition described in the *Zhū Bìng Yuán Hòu Lùn* ("Origin and Indicators of Disease") caused by evil strike and demons exerting evil influences, and manifesting in sudden stabbing pain in the heart and abdomen, oppression and derangement as if [the person] were about to die, enlarged abdomen with fullness, and in severe cases blood ejection.

[3] Visiting hostility 客忤 *kè wǔ*: A condition described in the *Zhū Bìng Yuán Hòu Lùn* ("Origin and Indicators of Disease") caused by the sudden invasion of evil visiting qì, giving rise to clouding collapse and asphyxiation. If not treated immediately, the patient will die.

[4] Stopping corpse 停尸 *tíng shī*: A condition in which morbid qì has stopped in the flesh, causing abdominal fullness, distention, and stabbing pain with rapid panting respiration, attacking the rib-sides, and surging up into the heart and chest. These symptoms recur after the patient recovers.

[5] Sudden death[liness] 卒死 *cù sǐ*: One of the indicators of malignity strike. It arises when a patient suffering from vacuity is

exposed to bandit wind. The body's yīn qì is exhausted internally, while yáng qì is repelled externally. Such sudden expiration of physical strength gives rise to the appearance of death. It is possibly accompanied by pain in the heart and abdomen, generalized heaviness, and inability to eat.

SYNOPSIS, LINE 23.3

This line presents a formula for sudden and fulminant illness.

COMMENTARY, LINE 23.3

The various fulminant diseases of the heart and abdomen, such as malignity stroke, visiting hostility, stopping corpse, and sudden deathliness, are generally caused by cold evil accumulating and stagnating, causing blockage of the qì dynamic. They are extremely critical, and we therefore use croton (*bā dòu*), which is acrid and hot, for drastic precipitation, to open and free the blockage. Dried ginger (*gān jiāng*) warms the center and assists croton (*bā dòu*) in expelling cold, while rhubarb (*dà huáng*) flushes the intestines and stomach, to remove the old and institute the new. In combination, these three ingredients have the effect of offensively expelling accumulated cold. This formula treats suddenly arising fulminant and critical conditions of cold repletion. If not given immediately, you will be unable to obtain results. Therefore it is called "emergency standby" in the title, which means that you should always have this ready to be able to respond to critical situations.

Line 23.4

治伤寒令愈不复：

紫石英　白石英　赤石脂　钟乳（碓炼）　栝蒌根　防风　桔梗　文蛤　鬼臼各十分　太乙余粮（烧）十分　干姜 附子（炮去皮）　桂枝（去皮）各四分

右十三味，杵为散，酒服方寸匕。

Zhì shāng hán lìng yù bù fù:

Zǐ shí yīng, bái shí yīng, chì shí zhī zhōng rǔ shí (duì liàn), guā lóu gēn fáng fēng, jié gēng, wén gé, guǐ jiù gè shí fèn; tài yǐ yú liáng (shāo) shí fèn; gān jiāng, fù zǐ (pào qù pí), guì zhī (qù pí) gè sì fèn

Yòu shí sān wèi, chǔ wéi sǎn, jiǔ fú fāng cùn bǐ.

To treat cold damage, curing it without recurrence [use the formula below][1]:

Fluorite Cold Food Powder (紫石寒食散 *zǐ shí hán shí sǎn*)

- fluorite (紫石英 *zǐ shí yīng*, Fluoritum) 10 parts
- white quartz (白石英 *bái shí yīng*, Quartz Album)[2] 10 parts
- halloysite (赤石脂 *chì shí zhī*, Halloysitum Rubrum) 10 parts
- stalactite (钟乳石 *zhōng rǔ shí*, Stalactitum) 10 parts (refine by pounding)
- trichosanthes root (栝蒌根 *guā lóu gēn*, Trichosanthis Radix) 10 parts
- saposhnikovia (防风 *fáng fēng*, Saposhnikoviae Radix) 10 parts
- platycodon (桔梗 *jié gěng*, Platycodonis Radix) 10 parts
- meretrix clam shell (文蛤 *wén gé*, Meretricis Concha) 10 parts

common dysosma (鬼臼 *guǐ jiù*, Dysosmae Versipellis Rhizoma) 10 parts
limonite (太乙余粮 *tài yǐ yú liáng*, Limonitum) 10 parts (burned)
dried ginger (干姜 *gān jiāng*, Zingiberis Rhizoma) 4 parts
aconite (附子 *fù zǐ*, Aconiti Radix Lateralis Praeparata) (blast-fry and remove skin) 4 parts
cinnamon twig (桂枝 *guì zhī*, Cinnamomi Ramulus) (remove bark) 4 parts

Pestle the above thirteen ingredients to a powder. Take a square-inch-spoonful [per dose] in wine.

TEXT NOTES, LINE 23.4

[1] A comment included in the received text reads: "See the *Qiān Jīn Yì* (Wings of the Thousand Gold Pieces Prescriptions)."

[2] The *Qiān Jīn Yì* as well as some commentaries note that white quartz (*bái shí yīng*) here should be replaced with glauberite (*hán shuǐ shí*). Accordingly, the title of this formula in the *Qiān Jīn Yì* is Fluorite and Glauberite Powder (*zǐ shí hán shí sǎn*).

SYNOPSIS, LINE 23.4

This line presents a formula for treating and preventing recurrence of cold damage.

COMMENTARY, LINE 23.4

After cold damage disease, liver-kidney yáng is vacuous, and the defense yáng exterior is loose, so that external cold can easily penetrate. Thus we must warm the liver and kidney and secure defense yáng, as well as engender liquid and check thirst, as preventative and recuperative treatment. In *Gāo Zhù Jīn Guì Yào Lüè* ("Gāo's Annotated Essential Prescriptions of the Golden Cabinet"), Gāo Xuē-Shān (高学山) explains, "[The present formula] uses warming and moistening fluorite (*zǐ shí yīng*) to supplement liver qì and blood; acrid, salty, and cold glauberite (*hán shuǐ shí*) to supplement kidney essence; acrid, sweet, warm, and astringing halloysite (*chì shí zhī*) to bank up vacuity in the intestines and stomach; acrid, warm, water-removing, and qì-staying stalactite (*zhōng rǔ shí*) to warm the life gate fire; and warm, salty, slightly cold, and water-disinhibiting qì-retaining limonite (*tài yǐ yú liáng*) to warm and transform water in the bladder. Acrid, warm, qì-supplementing dried ginger (*gān jiāng*) and aconite (*fù zǐ*) enter the bowels and viscera to gather and root visceral qì, while evil-expelling and penetrating common dysosma (*guǐ jiù*) seals securely and causes direct [downward] movement. These actions are assisted by platycodon (*jié gěng*), which opens and raises the channels; cinnamon twig (*guì zhī*), which frees and moves defense yáng; and saposhnikovia (*fáng fēng*), which secures tightly. As a result, the bowels and viscera are warmed internally, defense qì is replete on the outside, and further strikes by cold evil are avoided. Since patients recovering from cold damage tend to suffer from vexing thirst, which can cause water-rheum conditions, the formula also contains liquid-engendering trichosanthes root (*guā lóu gēn*), thirst-checking meretrix clam shell (*wén gé*), and water-disinhibiting limonite (*tài yǐ yú liáng*)."

Line 23.5

薤捣汁灌鼻中

Xiè dǎo zhī guàn bí zhōng

[Sudden Death Rescue Formula (救卒死方 *jiù cù sǐ fāng*)] Crush long-stamen onion (薤 *xiè*)[1] and pour the juice into the nose.

TEXT NOTE, LINE 23.5

[1] Long-stamen onion 薤 *xiè*: This presumably refers to 薤白 *xiè bái*, Allii Macrostemonis Bulbus, the white bulb of the plant, although this is not specified.

SYNOPSIS, LINE 23.5

This line and its formulas give emergency treatments for various forms of sudden death, i.e., states resembling death.

COMMENTARY, LINE 23.5

Sudden deathliness is caused by a separation of yīn and yáng, by stoppage between above and below, and by one-sided exhaustion. If yīn evil is blocking the orifices, pouring the juice from crushed long-stamen onion (*xiè bái*) down the nose can have the effect of repelling yīn evil and freeing yáng qì. Since the lung governs qì and opens at the nose, external evil that has entered through the nose can therefore also be discharged through the nose by inducing sneezing to arouse the spirit.

又方 *Yòu fāng* Additional Formulas, Line 23.5

雄鸡冠割取血，管吹内鼻中。

Xióng jī guàn gē qǔ xuè, guǎn chuī nà bí zhōng.

Cut off a rooster's comb and take the blood. Use a tube to blow it into the nose.

猪脂如鸡子大，苦酒一升，煮沸，灌喉中。

Zhū zhī rú jī zǐ dà, kǔ jiǔ yī shēng, zhǔ fèi, guàn hóu zhōng.

Boil [a lump of] lard the size of a chicken's egg in one *shēng* of vinegar (苦酒 *kǔ jiǔ*). Pour into the throat.

鸡肝及血涂面上, 以灰围四旁, 立起。

Jī gān jí xuè tú miàn shàng, yǐ huī wéi sì páng, lì qǐ.

Smear the liver and blood from a chicken on the [patient's] face and surround it with ash on all sides. [The patient] will immediately rise.

大豆二七粒，以鸡子白并酒和，尽以吞之。

Dà dòu èr qī lì, yǐ jī zǐ bái bìng jiǔ hé, jìn yǐ tūn zhī.

Mix two times seven soybeans (*dà dòu*) with egg white and wine. Swallow it all.

FORMULA COMMENTARY, LINE 23.5

This line and its formulas describe emergency measures to save patients from sudden death[liness].

The first additional formula employs the method of overcoming yīn disaster with a yáng substance. A rooster's comb signifies the location where yáng qì gathers, and the blood from there is therefore yáng from the summit. Blowing it into the patient's nose means that a healthy person takes it into their mouth, either pure or mixed with wine, and then blows qì mixed with this blood into the patient's nose. In this way, the medicine can descend down the throat, qì can move, and the clenched jaw can open naturally. Hence, this treatment has the effect of killing evil and rescuing the patient from sudden death[liness].

In the second additional formula, lard is used because it can lubricate the orifices, assist stomach qì, and free yang in the skin. Boiled in vinegar, the aroma can affect the nose, while it is poured into the throat to collect right and expel evil, with the effect of arousing the brain.

The third additional formula recommends applying chicken liver and blood to the patient's face. Wind qì flows to the liver, and the face is the meeting place for all yáng. This treatment is thus intended to summon qì and blood with wind and fire. Furthermore, surrounding it with ashes causes the warmth of fire and earth to warm defensive qì, making it replete on the outside.

In the fourth additional formula, soybean (*dà dòu*) has the effect of resolving the hundred toxins, as well as engendering stomach yáng. Egg white breaks abiding blood and frees kidney yáng. In combination with liquid, which frees and moves yáng qì, this treatment method is able to rescue a patient from malignity strike and sudden death.

Line 23.6

救卒死而壮热者方。

矾石半斤，以水一斗半煮消，以渍脚令没踝。

Jiù cù sǐ ér zhuàng rè zhě fāng.

Fán shí bàn jīn, yǐ shuǐ yī dǒu bàn zhǔ xiāo, yǐ zì jiǎo lìng mò huái.

A formula to rescue [a patient] from sudden death with vigorous heat [effusion]:

Boil half a *jīn* of alum (*fán shí*) in one *dǒu* of water until dispersed. Soak the feet in this, submerging the ankles.

COMMENTARY, LINE 23.6

When blood and qì together run into the upper body, the result is great reversal and fulminant death. In such cases, vigorous heat effusion indicates that sudden death is caused by reversing yáng that is moving alone. Alum (*fán shí*), which promotes astriction, is here prepared in a warm decoction to soak the feet up to above the ankles. This has the effect of astringing counterflow qì and causing heat to move downward.

Line 23.7

救卒死而目闭者方。
骑牛临面，捣薤汁灌耳中，吹皂荚末鼻中，立效。

Jiù cù sǐ ér mù bì zhě fāng.

Qí niú lín miàn, dǎo xiè zhī guàn ěr zhōng, chuī zào jiá mò bí zhōng, lì xiào.

A formula to rescue from sudden death with closed eyes:

Ride an ox right up to [the patient's] face. Pound long-stamen onion and pour the juice into the [patient's] ears. Blow powdered gleditsia (*zào jiá*) into the nose. Immediate efficacy.

COMMENTARY, LINE 23.7

Sudden death with closed eyes is caused by yáng qì fall and evil qì fixed internally. As treatment, this line recommends to hold the patient up and bring an ox right up to them, so that the breath of the ox connects with the breath of the patient and affects it. The breath of the ox may warm the patient, the foul odor may stimulate the patient's yáng qì. Pouring long-stamen onion (*xiè bái*) juice into the patient's ear will free heart and kidney qì, while blowing powdered gleditsia (*zào jiá*) into the nose will induce sneezing and thereby open the orifices and cause qì to connect upward with the chest.

Line 23.8

救卒死而张口反折者方。
灸手足两爪后十四壮了，饮以五毒诸膏散。

Jiù cù sǐ ér zhāng kǒu fǎn zhé zhě fāng.

Jiǔ shǒu zú liǎng zhǎo hòu shí sì zhuàng liǎo, yǐn yǐ wǔ dú zhū gāo sǎn.

A formula to rescue from sudden death with gaping mouth stretched backward.[1]

Burn fourteen cones of moxa on the nails of both hands and feet. Drink the various types of Five Toxin pastes and powders.[2]

TEXT NOTES, LINE 23.8

[1] Gaping mouth stretched backward 张口反折 *zhāng kǒu fǎn zhé*: An alternative interpretation of this phrase reads this as "gaping mouth and arched-back rigidity (角弓反张 *jiǎo gōng fǎn zhāng*)."

[2] A comment included in the received text reads: "Some of these contain croton (*bā dòu*)."

COMMENTARY, LINE 23.8

Gaping mouth with arched-back rigidity indicates that there is evil in the channels. Therefore you must first burn moxa on the hands and feet, which is the location where the twelve channels begin and end, to guide back yáng qì, returning yáng and freeing qì. The formula for Five Toxins Powder (*wǔ dú sǎn*) is unfortunately lost, but if it is related to the formula for Péi Gōng's Eight Toxins Pastes (*péi gōng bā dú gāo*) from the *Qiān Jīn Fāng* ("Thousand Gold Pieces Prescriptions"), it governs sudden strike by wind or toxin, gripping or stabbing abdominal pain, and corpse reversal with sudden failure to recognize people, by warming and freeing yáng qì.

Line 23.9

救卒死而四肢不收失便者方

马屎一升，水三斗，煮取二斗以洗之；又取牛洞(稀粪也)一升，温酒灌口中，灸心下一寸、脐上三寸，脐下四寸各一百壮，差。

Jiù zú sǐ ér sì zhī bù shōu shī biàn zhě fāng

Mǎ shǐ yī shēng, shuǐ sān dǒu, zhǔ qǔ èr dǒu yǐ xǐ zhī; yòu qǔ niú dòng (xī fèn yě) yī shēng, wēn jiǔ guàn kǒu zhōng, jiǔ xīn xià yī cùn, qí shàng sān cùn, qí xià sì cùn gè yī bǎi zhuàng, chài.

A formula to rescue from sudden death[liness] with loss of use of the limbs and incontinence.

Boil one *shēng* of horse dung with three *dǒu* of water to get two *dǒu*. Use this to wash [the patient]. Another: Take one *shēng* of cow slop,[1] [mix it with warm wine] and pour it into the mouth. Burn a hundred cones of moxa each one *cùn* below the heart, three *cùn* above the umbilicus, and four *cùn* below the umbilicus. Recovery [will ensue].

TEXT NOTE, LINE 23.9

[1] Cow slop 牛洞 *niú dòng*: Watery excrement of cattle.

COMMENTARY, LINE 23.9

When sudden death[liness] is accompanied by loss of the use of the limbs, this indicates that yáng qì is not reaching the four tips, but is deserting to the outside.

Fecal and urinary incontinence means that right qì is so debilitated that it is unable to contain, and that yáng is about to desert downward. The stench of animals is able to resolve toxin and kill evil. Horse dung is by nature warm; washing the patient with a boiled mixture of horse dung and water can astringe yáng qì. Cow slop enters the spleen to warm the gastrointestinal downpour. Pouring it into the patient's mouth with warm wine is intended to stem the downward desertion of yáng qì. Burning moxa on the upper, center, and lower burner—that is, on Great Tower Gate (*jù què*, CV-14), Interior Strengthening (*jiàn lǐ*, CV-11), and Central Pole (*zhōng jí*, CV-3)—can restore triple burner yáng and return expiring qì.

Line 23.10

救小儿卒死而吐利不知是何病方

狗屎一丸，绞取汁以灌之。无湿者，水煮干者取汁。

Jiù xiǎo ér cù sǐ ér tù lì bù zhī shì hé bìng fāng

Gǒu shǐ yī wán, jiǎo qǔ zhī yǐ guàn zhī. Wú shī zhě, shuǐ zhǔ gān zhě qǔ zhī.

A formula to rescue from infantile sudden death[liness] with vomiting and diarrhea regardless of what disease it is:

Wring out one piece of dog feces to get the liquid. Pour this [into the patient's mouth]. If you do not have a moist one, you can boil a dry one in water to get the liquid.

Commentary, Line 23.10

According to Lǐ Shí-Zhēn, dog feces are hot by nature, slightly toxic, and can treat cholera and food accumulations, and resolve all toxins. Because vomiting and diarrhea are here caused by cold strike and food accumulation, dog feces can treat this condition by effusing yáng qì, warming the center, and transforming stagnation.

Line 23.11

尸蹶脉动而无气，气闭不通，故静而死也，治方：

菖蒲屑，内鼻两孔中吹之，令人以桂屑着舌下。又方：剔取左角发方寸烧末，酒和，灌令入喉，立起。

Shī jué mài dòng ér wú qì, qì bì bù tōng, gù jìng ér sǐ yě, zhì fāng:

Chāng pú xiè, nà bí liǎng kǒng zhōng chū zhī, lìng rén yǐ guì xiè zhuó shé xià. Yòu fāng: Tī qǔ zuǒ jiǎo fà fāng cùn shāo mò, jiǔ hé, guàn lìng rù hóu, lì qǐ.

A formula to treat corpse reversal[1] with stirring pulse but no breathing, and qì blockage and stoppage causing stillness and then death:[2]

Insert acorus (*shí chāng pú*) flakes into both nostrils and insufflate them. Have the patient hold cinnamon flakes under the tongue. Another formula: Scrape off a square-inch area of hair from the left corner [of the head] and char to a powder. Mix with wine and pour it down the throat. [The patient] will immediately rise.

TEXT NOTES, LINE 23.11

[1] Corpse reversal 尸蹶 *shī jué*: The character 蹶, which in other contexts means "to hobble" or "to stumble," is related to 厥 *jué*, as which it should be read here. Corpse reversal is a condition marked by sudden clouding collapse with comatose loss of consciousness.

[2] A comment included in the received text reads: "For the pulse and signs, see the previous fascicle." 脉证见上卷。)

COMMENTARY, LINE 23.11

In corpse reversal, if the pulse has not stopped yet but still stirs, this indicates that construction qì is not expired yet, even if the patient has stopped breathing. Insufflating acorus (*shí chāng pú*) flakes into the nose is intended to free and harmonize lung qì, arouse the spirit with aroma, and open the orifices and clear up infection. In addition, cinnamon flakes under the tongue have the effect of opening the orifice of the heart and freeing blood in the vessels, thereby speeding up the effect.

The second method is adopted from the *Sù Wèn* ("Plain Questions"). The left corner of the head is where yáng qì is located and where the five network vessels (that is, the network vessels of the hand and foot lesser yīn and greater yīn, and the foot yáng mín channels) revolve. Scraping off the hair (which is the surplus of blood) at this location can supplement the desertion, and when mixed with wine and poured down the patient's throat, assists the strength of the medicine to move qì and blood and effuse yáng qì.

Line 23.12

救卒死，客忤死，还魂汤主之。
麻黄（去节）三两（一方四两） 杏仁（去皮尖）七十个 甘草（炙）一两
右三味，以水八升，煮取三升，去滓，分令咽之。通治诸感忤。
韭根一把 乌梅二七个 吴茱萸(炒)半升
右三味，以水一斗煮之，以病人栉内中，三沸，栉浮者生，沉者死。煮取三升，去滓，分饮之。

Jiù zú sǐ kè wǔ sǐ huán hún tāng zhǔ zhī fāng

Má huáng (qù jié) sān liǎng (yī fāng sì liǎng); xìng rén (qù pí jiān) qī shí gè; gān cǎo (zhì) yī liǎng

Yòu sān wèi, yǐ shuǐ bā shēng, zhǔ qǔ sān shēng, qù zǐ, fēn lìng yàn zhī. Tōng zhì zhū gǎn wǔ.

Jiǔ gēn yī bǎ; wū méi èr qī ge; wú zhū yú (chǎo) bàn shēng

Yòu sān wèi, yǐ shuǐ yī dǒu zhǔ zhī, yǐ bìng rén zhì nà zhōng, sān fèi, zhì fú zhě shēng, chén zhě sǐ. Zhǔ qǔ sān shēng, qù zǐ, fēn yǐn zhī.

To rescue from sudden death[liness] and visiting hostility death[liness], Ethereal Soul-Restoring Decoction (还魂汤 *huán hún tāng*) governs.[1]

Ethereal Soul-Restoring Decoction (还魂汤 *huán hún tāng*)
ephedra (麻黄 *má huáng*, Ephedrae Herba) 3 *liǎng* (remove skin; another version of this formula uses 4 *liǎng*)
apricot kernel (杏仁 *xìng rén*, Armeniacae Semen) 70 pieces (remove skin and tip)
licorice (甘草 *gān cǎo*, Glycyrrhizae Radix) 1 *liǎng* (mix-fry)[1]

Boil the above three ingredients in eight *shēng* of water to get three *shēng*. Remove the dregs, divide [into three doses], and make [the patient] swallow it. This completely treats all [types of] hostility contractions.

[An Additional Formula]
garlic chive root (韭菜根 *jiǔ cài gēn*, Allii Tuberosi Radix) 1 handful
mume (乌梅 *wū méi*, Mume Fructus) 14 pieces
evodia (吴茱萸 *wú zhū yú*, Evodiae Fructus) ½ *shēng* (stir-fry)

Boil the above three ingredients in 1 *dǒu* of water. Take the patient's comb and place it in [the decoction]. Bring it to a boil three times. If the comb floats, [the patient] will live; if it sinks, [the patient] will die. Boil it to get three *shēng*, remove the dregs, and divide into [three doses]. [Have the patient] drink it.

TEXT NOTE, LINE 23.12

[1] The commentary quotes the *Qiān Jīn Fāng* ("Thousand Gold Pieces Prescriptions"): "It governs sudden hostility, attacks by demons, flying corpse, all sudden expiry of qì with failure to regain consciousness, and possibly already death with clenched mouth that cannot be opened. Remove some teeth to pour the decoction in. If the decoction is in the mouth but is not going down the throat, divide the patient's hair, grasp it on the right and left, and pull, guiding the patient's shoulders. When the medicine is down, give another dose of one shēng, and the patient will revive in just a moment." A comment included in the received text reads: "The *Qiān Jīn Fāng* adds shaved cinnamon bark (*guì xīn*), two liǎng."

COMMENTARY, LINE 23.12

The various conditions of sudden deathliness and visiting hostility deathliness are mostly caused by a failure of right to overcome evil, as a result of which yáng qì is blocked and death ensues. Ethereal Soul-Restoring Decoction (*huán hún tāng*) frees the exterior and dissipates evil to restore right. In the formula, ephedra (*má huáng*) upbears yáng and outthrusts evil to the exterior; apricot kernel (*xìng rén*) disinhibits the lung; and mix-fried licorice (*gān cǎo*) regulates the center and supports right.

The second treatment involves a preparation of garlic chive root (*jiǔ gēn*), mume (*wū méi*), and evodia (*wú zhū yú*). In this formula, *jiǔ gēn* acts by freeing yáng with warmth and acridity; *wū méi* is sour and astringent, enters the liver, and has the ability to open gates; and *wú zhū yú* downbears turbid yīn and warms liver yáng with bitterness and warmth. When yīn is borne down, yáng is freed, and the gates are opened, the ethereal soul returns on its own.

Following the formula, the text offers a method for prognosticating the patient's death or survival, depending on whether a comb sinks or floats in this decoction. Xú Bīn 徐彬 suggests that this is related to the fact that floating is associated with yáng, and sinking with yīn, floating meaning that the patient's yáng qì is not yet expired, and sinking meaning death because the patient has only yīn left but no yáng.

Line 23.13

救自缢死，旦至暮虽已冷，必可治；暮至旦，小难也，恐此当言忿气盛故也。然夏时夜短于昼，又热，犹应可治。又云：心下若微温者，一日以上，犹可治之。

徐徐抱解，不得截绳，上下安被卧之。一人以脚踏其两肩，手少挽其发，常弦弦勿纵之；一人以手按据胸上，数动之；一人摩捋臂胫，屈伸之。若已僵，但渐渐强屈之，并按其腹。如此一炊顷，气从口出，呼吸眼开，而犹引按莫置，亦勿苦劳之，须臾，可少桂枝汤及粥清，含与之，令濡喉，渐渐能咽，及稍止。若向令两人以两管吹其两耳，罙好。此法最善，无不活也。

Jiù zì yì sì, dàn zhì mù suī yǐ lěng, bì kě zhì; mù zhì dàn, xiǎo nán yě, kǒng cǐ dāng yán fèn qì shèng gù yě. Rán xià shí yè duǎn yú zhòu, yòu rè, yóu yīng kě zhì. Yòu yún: Xīn xià ruò wēi wēn zhě, yī rì yǐ shàng, yóu kě zhì zhī fāng.

Xú xú bào jiě, bù dé jié shéng, shàng xià ān bèi wò zhī. Yī rén yǐ jiǎo tà qí liǎng jiān, shǒu shǎo wǎn qí fà, cháng xián xián wù zòng zhī; yī rén yǐ shǒu àn jù xiōng shàng, shù dòng zhī; yī rén mó lǚ bì jìng, qū shēn zhī. Ruò yǐ jiāng, dàn jiàn jiàn qiáng qū zhī, bìng àn qí fù. Rú cǐ yī chuī qīng, qì cóng kǒu chū, hū xī yǎn kāi, ér yóu yǐn àn mò zhì, yì wù kǔ láo zhī, xū yú, kě shǎo guì zhī tāng jí zhōu qīng, hán yǔ zhī, lìng rú hóu, jiàn jiàn néng yàn, jí shāo zhǐ. Ruò xiàng lìng liǎng rén yǐ liǎng guǎn chuī qí liǎng ěr, shēn hǎo. Cǐ fǎ zuì shàn, wú bù huó yě.

To rescue from suicide from hanging. If it has been from dawn until dusk [since the person hanged themselves before they were found], even if the body is already cold, you should be able to treat [such a person]. If it has been from dusk until dawn, it is a little difficult. The reason for this may be angry words or exuberant qì. During the summer, nights are shorter than days, and it is furthermore hot. [Therefore,] you should likely be able to treat this. It is also said that if there is slight warmth below the heart, even if it has been more than one day, you should still be able to treat it.

Gently embrace and release the person; do not cut the rope above or below, and lay the body on a blanket. Have one person use their feet to step on both shoulders while using the hands to pull slightly on the hair, keeping it tight and not releasing it. Have another person press on the chest with the hands, moving it rapidly. Have yet another person rub and stroke the arms and shins, bending and stretching them. If the body is already stiff, force it little by little to bend, and at the same time press the abdomen. Continue with this for about as long as it takes to cook a meal, and qì should come out of the mouth, the person should inhale and exhale, and the eyes should open. Continue to stretch and press, and do not desist yet, but do not belabor and tax the person either. In a moment, you can give a little Cinnamon Twig Decoction (*guì zhī tāng*) and clear gruel, having the patient hold it in the mouth, moisten the throat, and gradually swallow it as they are able to, then gradually stop. If you can also have two people blow into both ears with two tubes, this is very good. This method is the best, and survival is ensured.

COMMENTARY, LINE 23.13

This line offers an emergency treatment for people who have attempted suicide by hanging. As the text points out, the chance for survival is better if the person is found in the evening after hanging him/herself in the morning, because during the day there is a surplus of yáng qì, and yáng governs life. Night, on the other hand, is associated with yīn, which governs death; hence, treatment is more difficult if the person is found in the morning after a whole night has passed. Similarly, prognosis is more positive in the summer, because days are longer than nights, and the weather is warm, which both means a surplus of yáng. Lastly, if you can feel a little warmth still below the heart, this means that true qì is still present in the bowels and viscera, and heart yáng has not expired yet, in spite of the fact that yīn and yáng and the channels and network vessels are blocked.

The recommended treatment describes a physical manipulation that involves three people. One person steps on the patient's shoulders and pulls slightly on the hair to lift the head up and straighten and free the neck; while a second person massages and presses on the chest to restore chest breathing, and a third person massages and bends and stretches the arms and legs and rubs the abdominal region to restore abdominal breathing. After a while, give Cinnamon Twig Decoction (*guì zhī tāng*), to diffuse and free yáng qì, and gruel, to moisten and nourish stomach qì. Having two people blow into the patient's ears has the effect of freeing qì and therefore increases the efficacy of this treatment.

Line 23.14

凡中暍死，不可使得冷，得冷便死，疗之方

屈草带，绕暍人脐，使三两人溺其中，令温。亦可用热泥和屈草，亦可扣瓦椀底，按及车缸以着暍人，取令溺，须得流去，此谓道路穷，卒无汤，当令溺其中，欲使多人溺，取令温若汤，便可与之，不可泥及车缸，恐此物冷，暍既在夏月，得热泥土、暖车缸，亦可用也。

Fán zhōng yē sǐ, bù kě shǐ dé lěng, dé lěng biàn sǐ, liáo zhī fāng

Qū cǎo dài, rào yē rén qí, shǐ sān liǎng rén niào qí zhōng, lìng wēn. Yì kě yòng rè ní hé qū cǎo, yì kě kòu wǎ wǎn dǐ àn jí chē wǎ yǐ zhuó yē rén, qǔ lìng niào, xū dé liú qù, cǐ wèi dào lù qióng, cù wú tāng, dāng lìng niào qí zhōng, yù shǐ duō rén niào, qǔ lìng wēn ruò tāng, biàn kě yǔ zhī, bù kě ní jí chē gāng, kǒng cǐ wù lěng, yē jì zài xià yuè, dé rè ní tǔ, nuǎn chē gāng, yì kě yòng yě.

In all cases of death from thermoplegia, do not expose the person to cold, as any exposure to cold will result in death. A formula to treat it:

Make a belt out of grass and bend it to encircle the umbilicus of the person with thermoplegia. Have three or two people urinate in the middle, to warm [this area]. You can also use hot mud together with the bent grass. You can also cover [the umbilicus] with the bottom of a ceramic bowl and press on this with the linchpin from a cart to make it adhere to the patient['s umbilicus]. Make somebody urinate on this until it runs off. This is what is called the roadway poverty [method]. In emergencies, when all of a sudden there is no hot water to use, you can make someone urinate on the center. You want to make a number of people urinate on it until it is warm like hot water. You can give [the patient] this, instead of using mud or a cart's linchpin, for fear that these things might be cold. If the heat strike occurs in the summer months, and you are able to get hot mud and warm the linchpin, you may use them.

COMMENTARY, LINE 23.14

In the summer, thermoplegia can cause clouding, collapse, and death. This is mostly brought on by right vacuity and dietary irregularities, or by excessive taxation from overwork. As a result, summerheat is able to invade, guest evil is depressed, and the orifices are blocked. Do not use cold water or other cold substances to make a cold compress or bathe the patient, because this will entrap the summerheat internally and prevent it from effusing. Cold and heat will only excite each other, and the condition will be aggravated. Encircling the umbilical region with a belt made from grass and urinating on this to warm the area is an emergency treatment to be used as a last resort when hot water is not available, as in remote undeveloped areas. Treating with warmth is indicated by the fact that points like Sea of Qì (*qì hǎi*, CV-6) and Origin Pass (*guān yuán*, CV-4) are located below the umbilicus, and that applying heat to them will free yáng and open the orifices.

Line 23.15

救溺死方

取灶中灰两石余，以埋人，从头至足，水出七孔，即活。

右疗自缢溺暍之法，并出自张仲景为之，其意殊绝，殆非常情所及，本草所能关，实救人之大术矣。伤寒家数有暍病，非此遇热之暍。

Jiù nì sǐ fāng

Qǔ zào zhōng huī liǎng dàn yú, yǐ mái rén, cóng tóu zhì zú, shuǐ chū qī kǒng, jí huó.

Yòu liáo zì yì niào yē zhī fǎ, bìng chū zì zhāng zhòng jǐng wéi zhī, qí yì shū jué, dài fēi cháng qíng suǒ jí, běn cǎo suǒ néng guān, shí jiù rén zhī dà shù yǐ. Shāng hán jiā shù yǒu yē bìng, fēi cǐ yù rè zhī yē.

A formula to rescue from death by drowning:

Take two *dàn* or more of ashes from inside a stove and bury the person in this from head to toes. When water comes out of the seven orifices, this means life.

The treatment methods above for suicide by hanging, and for drowning and thermoplegia, all stem directly from Zhāng Jī's hand. Their significance is exceedingly special; they are neither based on common sense nor related to the herbal foundation.[1] They truly constitute the great art of rescuing people. Cold damage people have many forms of thermoplegia disease, [though not] the thermoplegia of exposure to heat [described] here.[2]

TEXT NOTES, LINE 23.15

[1] The text here appears corrupted with statements that most likely were not from the original *Jīn Guì Yào Lüè*. Zhāng Jī is referred to in the third person. Versions of this part of the text vary considerably. Most scholars simply choose one version and do not bother explaining the other variations.

[2] A comment included in the received text reads: "Lines from the *Wài Tái Mì Yào* ("Secrets from the *Wài Tái* Library") and *Zhǒu Hòu Bèi Jí Fāng* ("Emergency Standby Remedies")." In other words, both works contain this line on death by drowning. Obviously, the text contained in this paragraph was not written by Zhāng Jī himself.

COMMENTARY, LINE 23.15

As a result of drowning, water enters from the orifices to pour into the viscera and bowels, block the qì dynamic, and cause death from asphyxiation. Covering the patient under warm dry ashes from a stove will warm yáng qì on the outside and percolate water-damp on the inside. Hence the flow of qì and blood is restored, and water exits from the orifices.

Line 23.16

治马坠及一切筋骨损方

大黄（切浸，汤成下）一两 绯帛(烧灰)如手大 乱发（烧灰用）如鸡子大 久用炊单布（烧灰）一尺 败蒲（一握三寸）桃仁（去皮尖熬）四十九个 甘草（炙剉）如中指节

右七味，以童子小便量多少煎汤成，内酒一大盏，次下大黄，去滓，分温三服。先剉败蒲席半领，煎汤浴，衣被盖覆，斯须通利数行，痛楚立差。利及浴水赤，勿怪，即瘀血也。

Zhì mǎ zhuì jí yī qiè jīn gǔ sun fāng

Dà huáng (qiē jìn, tāng chéng xià) yī liǎng fēi bó (shāo huī) rú shǒu dà luàn fà (shāo huī yòng) rú jī zǐ dà jiǔ yòng chuī dān bù (shāo huī) yī chǐ bài pú (yī wò sān cùn) táo rén (qù pí jiān áo) sì shí jiǔ gè gān cǎo (zhì cuò) rú zhōng zhǐ jié

Yòu qī wèi, yǐ tóng zǐ xiǎo biàn liàng duō shǎo jiān tāng chéng, nà jiǔ yī dà zhǎn, cì xià dà huáng, qù zǐ, fēn wēn sān fú. Xiān cuò bài pú xí bàn lǐng, jiān tāng yù, yī bèi gài fù, sī xū tōng lì shù xíng, tòng chǔ lì chài. Lì jí yù shuǐ chì, wù guài, jí yū xuè yě.

A formula to treat falling from a horse and all injuries of the sinews and bones:[1]

rhubarb (大黄 *dà huáng*, Rhei Radix et Rhizoma) 1 *liǎng* (cut and soak; add when the decoction is done)
crimson silk (绯帛 *fēi bó*) a hand-sized piece (char into ashes)
hair (乱发 *luàn fà*, Crinis Crinis) an egg-sized piece (char into ashes)
a cloth that has long been used for cooking (久用炊单布 *jiǔ yòng chuī dān bù*) 1 *chǐ* (char into ashes)
rotten typha (败蒲 *bài pú*, Typhae Pollen) 1 handful, 3 *cùn* long
peach kernel (桃仁 *táo rén*, Persicae Semen) 49 pieces (remove the skin and tips, simmer)
licorice (甘草 *gān cǎo*, Glycyrrhizae Radix) a piece the size of the middle finger joint (mix-fry and grate)

Decoct the above seven ingredients [except for the rhubarb (*dà huáng*)] in an appropriate amount of child's urine until the decoction is done. Add 1 large cup of wine, and then the rhubarb (*dà huáng*). Remove the dregs, divide into three doses, and take warm. Alternatively,[2] cut up half of a rotten typha mat, decoct it, and bathe [the patient] in this. Then cover up the patient, wait a while,[3] and after several bouts of diarrhea, the pain will be relieved. Do not worry if the diarrhea and bath water turn red. This is static blood.

TEXT NOTES, LINE 23.16

[1] A comment included in the received text reads: "See the formula in the *Zhǒu Hòu Bèi Jí Fāng* ("Emergency Standby Remedies")."

[2] Alternatively 先 *xiān*: The translation is based on a textual variation that has 别 *bié* instead, since 先 *xiān*, "first," makes little sense in the context.

[3] Wait a while 斯须 *sī xū*: A textual variation has 服药须 *fú yào xū*, "take the medicine, and wait."

COMMENTARY, LINE 23.16

Falling from a horse or another high place not only damages the sinews and bones internally, but also causes static blood and qì bind. Thus we must first quicken blood, move stasis, and settle pain. The recommended formula here contains *táo rén* (Persicae Semen) and *dà huáng* (Rhei Radix et Rhizoma), both of which expel stasis. Crimson silk (*fēi bó*) can treat bleeding from incised wounds, disperse swelling, and relieve pain; hair (*luàn fà*) disperses stasis and checks bleeding; child's urine (*tóng biàn*) conducts stasis downward; cooking cloth (*chuī bù*) dissipates stagnation and disperses swelling; licorice (*gān cǎo*) relaxes tension and harmonizes the various medicinals; and wine strengthens the effect of the medicinals to treat static blood and stagnant qì in the viscera. This action is reinforced by bathing the patient in rotten cattail (*bài pú*), which breaks blood and moves qì, and by warming the patient under covers to hasten the movement of qì and blood in the channels and network vessels throughout the body.

禽兽鱼虫禁忌并治第二十四

CHAPTER 24

Fowl, Beasts, Fish, and Insects

Contraindications and Treatments

‡ Overview

Dietary therapy is a key aspect of Chinese medicine. The present chapter, "Fowl, Beasts, Fish, and Insects," and the following one, "Fruits, Vegetables, and Grains" discuss dietetic hygiene and thereby offer an important contribution to the science of food.

The present chapter focuses on dietary hygiene, prevention of food poisoning, and on medicinal treatment of food poisoning. It discusses the causes and treatment for contraindicated unclean food, disease of the five viscera with contraindications of the five flavors and seasonally appropriate food rules, methods for differentiating the various types of unclean food of animal origin, diseases caused by food poisoning, and the reasoning behind food combinations that are detrimental to health, contraindicated foods in pregnancy. It concludes with treatment methods and formulas for food poisoning.

To modern readers, this chapter appears to contain unsubstiantiable statements and even superstitious elements. For example, "Horses without night eyes on the legs are inedible" apparently reflects a belief that horses have a spot on their legs that enables them to see at night. Interestingly, we find many contraindications about eating animal products, which suggests that the practice was prevalent in Hàn times. Set against this are what moderns regard as sensible admonitions against eating food contaminated by insects and other substances. In general, the contents of this chapter, though interesting from the historical perspective, are not emphasized in modern Chinese medical education in China.

Line 24.1

凡饮食滋味，以养于身，食之有妨，反能为害，自非服药炼液，焉能不饮食乎？切见时人，不闲调摄，疾疢竞起，若不因食而生，苟全其生，须知切忌者矣。所食之味，有与病相宜，有与身为害，若得宜则益体，害则成疾，以此致危，例皆难疗。凡煮药饮汁，以解毒者，虽云救急，不可热饮，诸毒病得热更甚，宜冷饮之。

Fán yǐn shí zī wèi, yǐ yǎng yú shēn, shí zhī yǒu fáng, fǎn néng wéi hài, zì fēi fú yào liàn yè, yān néng bù yǐn shí hū? Qiē jiàn shí rén, bù xián tiáo shè, jí chèn jìng qǐ, ruò bù yīn shí ér shēng, gǒu quán qí shēng, xū zhī qiē jì zhě yǐ. Suǒ shí zhī wèi, yǒu yǔ bìng xiāng yí, yǒu yǔ shēn wéi hài, ruò dé yí zé yì tǐ, hài zé chéng jí, yǐ cǐ zhì wēi, lì jiē nán liáo. Fán zhǔ yào yǐn zhī, yǐ jiě dú zhě, suī yún jiù jí, bù kě rè yǐn, zhū dú bìng dé rè gèng shèn, yí lěng yǐn zhī.

All the flavors of food and drink can be used to nourish the body. But there are foods that hinder it and are able to do harm instead. If you do not have a diet limited to medicinal and refined alchemical foods,[1] how could you not eat and drink? If I look closely at my contemporaries, they do not occupy themselves with regulating and conserving [their health], and the diseases that arise are all engendered by food. Whoever wishes to keep their life whole must know all the contraindications. Among the flavors of food, some are appropriate for [treating] disease, and some are harmful to the body. If you consume what is appropriate, it boosts the body; if you consume what is harmful, it creates disease. Because of this, critical conditions arise which are difficult to cure. Whenever you boil medicines and drink the juice to resolve toxin, even in so-called emergency rescue situations, you may not drink them hot, because the various types of poisoning are aggravated by heat. [Therefore] you should drink them cold.

TEXT NOTE, LINE 24.1

[1] Diet limited to medicinal and refined alchemical foods 服药炼液 *fēi fú yào liàn yè*: This refers to serious practitioners of the Daoist art of immortality, who in the advanced stages of the pursuit of longevity discontinue the consumption of meat, grain, or ordinary food, limiting their diet to such substances as pine cone, mushroom, and alchemical preparations.

SYNOPSIS, LINE 24.1

This line describes the influence of diet on the human body, and the rule that toxin-resolving medicinals should be consumed when cold.

Line 24.2

肝病禁辛，心病禁咸，脾病禁酸，肺病禁苦，肾病禁甘；春不食肝，夏不食心，秋不食肺，冬不食肾，四季不食脾。辨曰：春不食肝者，为肝气王，脾气败，若食肝，则又补肝，脾气败尤甚，不可救。又肝王之时，不可以死气入肝，恐伤魂也。若非王时即虚，以肝补之佳。余脏准此。

Gān bìng jìn xīn, xīn bìng jìn xián, pí bìng jìn suān, fèi bìng jìn kǔ, shèn bìng jìn gān; chūn bù shí gān, xià bù shí xīn, qiū bù shí fèi, dōng bù shí shèn, sì jì bù shí pí. Biàn yuē: Chūn bù shí gān zhě, wéi gān qì wàng, pí qì bài, ruò shí gān, zé yòu bǔ gān, pí qì bài yóu shèn, bù kě jiù. Yòu gān wàng zhī shí, bù kě yǐ sǐ qì rù gān, kǒng shāng hún yě. Ruò fēi wàng shí jí xū, yǐ gān bǔ zhī jiā. Yú zàng zhǔn cǐ.

In liver disease, acridity is contraindicated; in heart disease, saltiness is contraindicated; in spleen disease, sourness is contraindicated; in lung disease, bitterness is contraindicated; and in kidney disease, sweetness is contraindicated. In the spring, do not eat liver; in the summer, do not eat heart; in the fall, do not eat lung; in the winter, do not eat kidney; and in all four seasons, do not eat spleen. This is explained by saying: "The reason why we do not eat liver in the spring is that [at this time] liver qì is effulgent, but spleen qì is vanquished. If you eat liver, you will further supplement the liver and thereby further aggravate the vanquishing of spleen qì [to the point] where it cannot be rescued. Furthermore, at the time when the liver is effulgent, you must not allow dead qì to enter the liver, because it might damage the ethereal soul. At times when [the liver] is not effulgent but vacuous, it is excellent to supplement it by eating liver. [Treat] the other viscera according to the same principle."

Synopsis, Line 24.2

This line describes dietary contraindications in terms of flavor and season in relation to the five viscera.

Commentary, Line 24.2

The liver belongs to wood, and if a patient with liver disease eats acrid foods, the acridity can cause the lung to further damage the liver; hence acrid foods are contraindicated in liver disease. The heart belongs to fire, and if a patient with heart disease eats salty foods, the saltiness can cause the kidney to further damage heart; hence salty foods are contraindicated in heart disease. Similarly, sour foods are contraindicated in spleen disease because sourness assists the liver in damaging the spleen; bitter foods are contraindicated in lung disease because bitterness assists the heart in damaging the lung; and sweet foods are contraindicated in kidney disease because sweetness assists the spleen in damaging the kidney.

Furthermore, seasonal contraindications are related to the fact that in every season one viscus is effulgent and another one vanquished. If you consume foods that are associated with that season, such as liver in the spring, you will supplement the effulgence of the liver further and enable it to overcome the spleen, which is vacuous at this time. In addition, eating liver in the spring will not only weaken the spleen, but will also damage the ethereal soul, since liver wood stores the ethereal soul. By contrast, it is excellent to eat liver at the time when the liver is vacuous, because it will supplement it. All the viscera follow this rule.

Line 24.3

凡肝脏自不可轻噉，自死者弥甚。

Fán gān zàng zì bù kě qīng dàn àn, zì sǐ zhě mí shèn.

In all [animals], the liver may not be eaten lightly. This is especially so if [the animal] has died a natural death.

Synopsis, Line 24.3

Starting with this line, the following section describes various preventive methods to be observed to avoid food poisoning when consuming meat.

Commentary, Line 24.3

It is an ancient belief that if animals were frightened at the time of slaughter and there was anger in the liver, the expiring qì would return to the liver, which would therefore become inappropriate for human consumption. Furthermore, the liver is the viscus that resolves toxin and stores toxic substances. Thus it may not be eaten lightly, particularly when the animal has died on its own, possibly due to poisoning or epidemic pestilence.

Line 24.4

凡心皆为神识所舍，勿食之，使人来生复其报对矣。

Fán xīn jiē wéi shén shì suǒ shè, wù shí zhī, shǐ rén lái shēng fù qí bào duì yǐ.

In all [animals], the heart is the abode of the mind. Do not eat it, because it causes the reincarnated person to return for compensation.

Commentary, Line 24.4

This line expresses the combination of the Buddhist concept of reincarnation, which became popular in China beginning with the late Hàn period, and indigenous Chinese ideas about the ethereal and corporeal souls. According to the doctrine of reincarnation, humans are reborn in a variety of forms after dying, and any animal can therefore in fact constitute a human reincarnation. This prohibition against eating heart does not reflect modern traditional Chinese medical ideas.

Line 24.5

凡肉及肝，落地不着尘土者，不可食之。猪肉落水浮者，不可食。

Fán ròu jí gān, luò dì bù zhuó chén tǔ zhě, bù kě shí zhī. Zhū ròu luò shuǐ fú zhě, bù kě shí.

Any flesh as well as liver that when dropped on the ground does not get stained with dust is inedible. Pork that is dropped in water and floats is inedible.

COMMENTARY, LINE 24.5

When meat is spoiled or contaminated, it putrefies and swells with water. Therefore, dust does not stick to it when it is dropped to the ground. Similarly, when meat begins to putrefy, qì is engendered; hence it floats when dropped into water. Both of these are signs that the meat is spoiled and therefore not fit for human consumption.

Line 24.6

诸肉及鱼，若狗不食，鸟不啄者，不可食之。

Zhū ròu jí yú, ruò gǒu bù shí, niǎo bù zhuó zhě, bù kě shí zhī.

Any flesh and fish that dogs do not eat and birds do not peck at is inedible.

Line 24.7

诸肉不干，火炙不动，见水自动者，不可食之。

Zhū ròu bù gān, huǒ zhì bù dòng, jiàn shuǐ zì dòng zhě, bù kě shí zhī.

Any flesh that is not dried, if it does not move when roasted in the fire or if it moves on its own in water, is inedible.

COMMENTARY, LINE 24.7

Any meat that is not dry should contract when exposed to high heat. If it fails to do so, this is a sign of water swelling and hence spoilage. Similarly, decomposition engenders qì inside the meat. Under water, the emission of gas will make the meat move and hence indicates spoilage.

Line 24.8

肉中有如朱点者，不可食之。

Ròu zhōng yǒu rú zhū diǎn zhě, bù kě shí zhī.

When meat has red spot-like marks, it is inedible.

COMMENTARY, LINE 24.8

Red spots on meat are stasis macules that are caused by malign blood gathering. This invariably indicates that the animal has died from epidemic pestilence or that the meat is contaminated by an infestation with cysticerci. In any case, the meat can not be eaten.

Line 24.9

六畜肉热血不断者，不可食之。父母及本身命肉，食之令人神魂不安。

Liù chù ròu rè xuè bù duàn zhě, bù kě shí zhī. Fù mǔ jí běn shēn mìng ròu, shí zhī lìng rén shén hún bù ān.

The flesh of the six domestic animals[1] must not be eaten when hot blood has not stopped flowing yet. Eating meat associated with one's own and one's parents' fate[2] will make the person's spirit and ethereal soul disquieted.

TEXT NOTES, LINE 24.9

[1] Six domestic animals 六畜 *liù chù*: Pig, ox, goat, horse, fowl, and dog.

[2] Meat associated with one's own and one's parents' fate 父母及本身命肉 *fù mǔ jí běn shēn mìng ròu*: Meat that is associated with one's own or one's parents' time of birth. For example, the time from 1–3 AM belongs to 丑 *chǒu*, which is associated with the ox. Hence, persons born at this time or whose parents were born at this time should avoid this type of meat.

Line 24.10

食肥肉及热羹，不可饮冷水。

Shí féi ròu jí rè gēng, bù kě yǐn lěng shuǐ.

When eating fatty meat and hot meat broth, you must not drink cold water.

Line 24.11

诸五脏及鱼，投地尘土不污者，不可食之。

Zhū wǔ zàng jí yú, tóu dì chén tǔ bù wū zhě, bù kě shí zhī.

If any of the five organ [meats] and fish do not stain when tossed to the ground, [they] are inedible.

COMMENTARY, LINE 24.11

See line 24.5 above.

Line 24.12

秽饭、馁鱼、臭肉，食之皆伤人。

Huì fǎn, něi yú, chòu ròu, shí zhī jiē shāng rén.

Eating dirty rice, spoiled fish, and malodorous meat will all damage a person.

Line 24.13

自死肉，口闭者，不可食之。

Zì sǐ ròu, kǒu bì zhě, bù kě shí zhī.

All flesh [from animals] having died on their own with mouth closed is inedible.

Line 24.14

六畜自死，皆疫死，则有毒，不可食之。

Liù chù zì sǐ, jiē yì sǐ, zé yǒu dú, bù kě shí zhī.

When [any of] the six domestic animals die on their own, it is always death from epidemics. Therefore they contain poison and are inedible.

Line 24.15

兽自死，北首及伏地者，食之杀人。

Shòu zì sǐ, běi shǒu jí fú dì zhě, shí zhī shā rén.

Eating [meat of] beasts that have died a natural death, while facing north and bending to the ground, will kill a person.

COMMENTARY, LINE 24.15

This prohibition apparently relates to the belief that this manner of death indicates that the animal has contracted the qì of yīn cold toxic pestilence from the north, and is therefore unfit for consumption.

Line 24.16

食生肉，饱饮乳，变成白虫。

Shí shēng ròu, bǎo yǐn rǔ, biàn chéng bái chóng.

Eating raw meat or drinking milk to satiety can transform into whiteworm disease.[1]

TEXT NOTE, LINE 24.16

[1] A comment included in the received text reads: "A textual variation has 血蛊 *xuè gǔ*, blood gǔ, instead."

Line 24.17

疫死牛肉，食之令病洞下，亦致坚积，宜利药下之。

Yì sǐ niú ròu, shí zhī lìng bìng dòng xià, yì zhì jiān jī, yí lì yào xià zhī.

Eating beef from oxen that have died from epidemic causes the disease of throughflux diarrhea. It can also result in hard accumulations, in which case you should precipitate with disinhibiting medicinals.

COMMENTARY, LINE 24.17

Beef from oxen that have died from pestilence is poisonous. Throughflux diarrhea is the body's natural response to eliminate the toxin. However, if the toxin becomes congested, causing qì stagnation and static blood, it can also cause hardness, glomus, accumulations, and gatherings. In that case, the patient must be treated with offensive precipitation to disperse accumulation, conduct stagnation, and eliminate pestilential toxin to the outside.

Line 24.18

脯藏米瓮中，有毒，及经夏食之，发肾病。

Fǔ cáng mǐ wèng zhōng, yǒu dú, jí jīng xià shí zhī, fā shèn bìng.

Dried meat that has been stored in a rice jar contains toxin. If you eat [this] as well as [dried meat that has been stored] for a whole summer, kidney disease will arise.

Commentary, Line 24.18

Storing dried meat in an earthenware jar can cause depressed steaming damp-heat. Alternatively, dried meat can also become moldy when stored in the summer. Because putrefied qì enters the kidney, kidney disease arises.

Line 24.19

治自死六畜肉中毒方

黄檗屑

捣服方寸匕。

Zhì zì sǐ liù chù ròu zhòng dú fāng

Huáng bó xiè

Dǎo fú fāng cùn bǐ.

A formula to treat poisoning from [eating] the flesh of the six domestic animals that have died a natural death.

phellodendron (黄柏 *huáng bǎi*, Phellodendri Cortex) (grate)

Pound and take a square-inch-spoonful [per dose].

Synopsis, Line 24.19

This line introduces the next section of this chapter, which discusses treatments for various types of food poisoning.

Commentary, Line 24.19

When domestic animals die on their own, this is caused by toxic epidemic. Eating the flesh of such animals therefore causes "toxin strike" or poisoning, which manifests with nausea, retching and vomiting, fullness in the chest and diaphragm, vexation and oppression, abdominal pain and diarrhea, and in severe cases with heat effusion and tremors. Phellodendron (*huáng bǎi*), which is bitter and cold, is a heat-clearing toxin-resolving medicinal, which disinhibits the lower burner, drains the bladder, and conducts heat toxin outward.

Line 24.20

治食郁肉漏脯中毒方
烧犬屎，酒服方寸匕，每服人乳汁亦良。饮生韭汁三升，亦得。

Zhì shí yù ròu lòu fǔ zhòng dú fāng

Shāo quǎn shǐ, jiǔ fú fāng cùn bǐ, měi fú rén rǔ zhī yì liáng. Yǐn shēng jiǔ zhī sān shēng, yì dé.

A formula to treat poisoning from eating depressed meat and leaked-on dried meat.[1]

Char dog feces and take a square-inch-spoonful per dose in wine. Taking it in human breast milk is also good. Drinking three *shēng* of fresh garlic chive juice is also possible.

TEXT NOTE, LINE 24.20

[1] A comment included in the received text reads: "Depressed meat refers to meat that has been stored overnight in a tightly sealed container. Leaked-on dried meat refers to meat that has been preserved in a leaky thatched hut and has been soaked."

COMMENTARY, LINE 24.20

Both charred dog feces and fresh scallion juice have the effect of warming yáng qì in the stomach to transform putrefaction, while human breast milk moistens dryness and also has a toxin-resolving action.

Line 24.21

治黍米中藏干脯食之中毒方
大豆
浓煮汁饮数升即解。亦治狸肉漏脯等毒。

Zhì shǔ mǐ zhōng cáng gān fǔ shí zhī zhòng dú fāng

Dà dòu

Nóng zhǔ zhī yǐn shù shēng jí jiě. Yì zhì lí ròu lòu fǔ děng dú.

A formula to treat poisoning from eating dried meat that has been stored in broomcorn millet:

yellow soybean (大豆 *dà dòu*, Sojae Semen Flavum)

Boil into a concentrated liquid and drink several *shēng* to resolve [the toxin]. [This formula] also treats toxin from fox meat, leaked-on dried meat, etc.

Line 24.22

治食生肉中毒方

掘地深三尺，取其下土三升，以水五升煮数沸，澄清汁，饮一升，即愈。

Zhì shí shēng ròu zhòng dú fāng

Jué dì shēn sān chǐ, qǔ qí xià tǔ sān shēng, yǐ shuǐ wǔ shēng zhǔ shù fèi, chéng qīng zhī, yǐn yī shēng, jí yù.

A formula to treat poisoning from eating raw meat:

Dig [a hole] into the earth three *chǐ* deep and take out three *shēng* of earth from the bottom. Boil it in five *shēng* of water, bringing it to a boil several times. Let [the dirt] settle and drink one *shēng* per dose of the clear liquid. Recovery will ensue.

COMMENTARY, LINE 24.22

This line constitutes the method of resolving toxin with yellow earth water (地浆 *dì jiāng*), which clears heat, resolves toxin, and harmonizes the center.

Line 24.23

治食六畜鸟兽肝中毒方

水浸豆豉，绞取汁，服数升愈。

Zhì shí liù chù niǎo shòu gān zhòng dú fāng

Shuǐ jìn dòu chǐ, jiǎo qǔ zhī, fú shù shēng yù.

A formula to treat poisoning from eating the liver of the six domestic animals and wild birds and beasts.

Soak fermented soybean (*dòu chǐ*, Sojae Semen Fermentatum) in water. Squeeze it out to get the juice. Take several *shēng* to recover [from the poisoning].

COMMENTARY, LINE 24.23

Fermented soybean (*dòu chǐ*) is produced by fermenting black soybeans. It is able to resolve the various toxins, and also has the effect of inducing ejection. Taking it can therefore treat toxin strike.

Line 24.24

马脚无夜眼者，不可食之。

Mǎ jiǎo wú yè yǎn zhě, bù kě shí zhī.

Horses without night eyes on the legs are inedible.

SYNOPSIS, LINE 24.24

Beginning with this line, the rest of this chapter lists a variety of contraindicated foods and food combinations, as well as a handful of treatments.

COMMENTARY, LINE 24.24

"Night eyes on the legs" refers to spots on the horse's front legs on top of the knee that supposedly allow the horse to see at night. If a horse lacks this feature, it is unable to go about at night and therefore is most likely diseased.

Line 24.25

食酸马肉，不饮酒，则杀人。

Shí suān mǎ ròu, bù yǐn jiǔ, zé shā rén.

Eating galloping horse meat[1] without drinking wine will kill the person.

TEXT NOTE, LINE 24.25

[1] Galloping horse meat 酸酸马肉 *suān mǎ ròu*: 酸 *suān* is most likely a textual corruption for 骏 *jùn*, a character that refers to the qualities of an excellent swift horse. By association, this quality is often used in materia medica literature to refer to the effect of horse meat.

COMMENTARY, LINE 24.25

Horse flesh is acrid, bitter, cold, toxic, and always "galloping." Because of its strength, it is difficult to digest, which can be resolved by drinking wine.

Line 24.26

马肉不可热食，伤人心。

Mǎ ròu bù kě rè shí, shāng rén xīn.

Horse meat must not be eaten hot, or it will damage the person's heart.

COMMENTARY, LINE 24.26

The horse is associated with fire, and the heart is the viscus of fire and is averse to heat. Hence, eating hot horse meat will cause an exuberance of fire qì and thereby damage the heart.

Line 24.27

马鞍下肉，食之杀人。

Mǎ ān xià ròu, shí zhī shā rén.

Eating meat from under a horse's hoof will kill the person.

COMMENTARY, LINE 24.27

According to Lǐ Wén 李彣, meat from under a horse's hoof is not penetrated by wind qì, but is soaked by sweat and dampness. Thus it easily putrefies and forms toxin. Eating it will therefore kill the person.

Line 24.28

白马黑头者，不可食之。

Bái mǎ hēi tóu zhě, bù kě shí zhī.

White horses with black heads are inedible.

Line 24.29

白马青蹄者，不可食之。

Bái mǎ qīng tí zhě, bù kě shí zhī.

White horses with greenish black hooves are inedible.

Line 24.30

马肉、豘肉共食，饱醉卧，大忌。

Mǎ ròu, tún ròu gòng shí, bǎo zuì wò, dà jì.

Eating horse meat with piglet meat, and falling asleep on a full stomach when intoxicated are greatly contraindicated.

COMMENTARY, LINE 24.30

Horse meat is associated with fire while pork is associated with water. Eating these two meats at the same time causes disharmony. Falling asleep intoxicated with a full stomach damages spleen qì.

Line 24.31

驴、马肉合猪肉食之，成霍乱。

Lǘ, mǎ ròu hé zhū ròu shí zhī, chéng huò luàn.

Eating donkey and horse meat in combination with pork causes cholera.

COMMENTARY, LINE 24.31

Donkey meat is effusing, and eating it stirs wind; horse meat is fierce; and pork is slimy. These meats are adverse to each other by nature. Eating them in combination can cause gastrointestinal disease like vomiting and retching or diarrhea.

Line 24.32

马肝及毛，不可妄食，中毒害人。

Mǎ gān jí máo, bù kě wàng shí, zhòng dú hài rén.

Horse liver and hair must not be eaten recklessly. [Such] poisoning will harm the person.

Line 24.33

治马肝毒中人未死方

雄鼠屎二七粒, 末之, 水和服, 日再服。

又方：人垢, 取方寸匕，服之佳。

Zhì mǎ gān dú zhòng rén wèi sǐ fāng

Xióng shǔ shǐ èr qī lì, mò zhī, shuǐ huò fú, rì zài fú.

Yòu fāng: rén gòu, qǔ fāng cùn bǐ, fú zhī jiā.

A formula to treat poisoning from horse liver, when the person has not yet died:

Pulverize 2 × 7 droppings from a male mouse. Take it mixed with water, two doses a day.[1]

Another formula: Take a square-inch-spoonful of human filth.[2] Taking this is highly efficacious.

TEXT NOTES, LINE 24.33

[1] A comment included in the received text reads: "If the droppings are pointy, they are it." (屎尖者是。)

[2] Human filth 人垢 *rén gòu*: More commonly called "head filth" (头垢 *tóu gòu*), this refers to dirt and grease from the head, which has the medicinal effect of inducing vomiting and resolving toxin.

Line 24.34

治食马肉中毒欲死方
香豉二两　杏仁三两
右二味, 蒸一食顷熟, 杵之服, 日再服。
又方：煮芦根汁饮之良。

Zhì shí mǎ ròu zhōng dú yù sǐ fāng
Xiāng chǐ èr liǎng; xìng rén sān liǎng
Yòu èr wèi, zhēng yī shí qīng shú, chǔ zhī fú, rì zài fú.
Yòu fāng: zhǔ lú gēn zhī yǐn zhī liáng.

A formula to treat poisoning from eating horse meat, verging on death:

fermented soybean (香豉 *xiāng chǐ*, Glycines Semen Fermentatum) 2 *liǎng*
apricot kernel (杏仁 *xìng rén*, Armeniacae Semen) 3 *liǎng*

Steam the above 2 ingredients for as long as it takes to eat a meal, and pestle thoroughly. Take this twice a day.

Another formula: Drinking boiled phragmites (*lú gēn*) juice is good.

COMMENTARY, LINE 24.34

Toxin strike and abdominal distention from eating horse meat can be treated with fermented soybean (*xiāng chǐ*), which resolves toxin and downbears qì, and apricot kernel (*xìng rén*), which disinhibits the lung and discharges qì.

Horses have a natural liking for phragmites (*lú gēn*), which is sweet and cold, can resolve all meat toxin, and disinhibits urine. It is thus an excellent medicinal for resolving toxin from diseased horses.

Line 24.35

疫死牛，或目赤，或黄，食之大忌。

Yì sǐ niú, huò mù chì, huò huáng, shí zhī dà jì.

Eating ox that has died from epidemic, whether its eyes are red or yellow, is greatly contraindicated.

Line 24.36

牛肉共猪肉食之，必作寸白虫。

Niú ròu gòng zhū ròu shí zhī, bì zuò cùn bái chóng.

Eating beef together with pork invariably causes inch whiteworm.

COMMENTARY, LINE 24.36

Beef is by nature stagnant while pork stirs wind. When they enter the stomach without dissipating, they ferment and form damp-heat, thereby engendering inch whiteworm.

Line 24.37

青牛肠，不可合犬肉食之。

Qīng niú cháng, bù kě hé quǎn ròu shí zhī.

Intestines from greenish-black ox must not be eaten together with dog meat.

COMMENTARY, LINE 24.37

Water buffalo intestine is by nature warm and difficult to digest, while dog meat is hot. Thus they should not be eaten in combination.

Line 24.38

牛肺从三月至五月，其中有虫如马尾，割去勿食，食则损人。

Niú fèi cóng sān yuè zhì wǔ yuè, qí zhōng yǒu chóng rú mǎ wěi, gē qù wù shí, shí zé sǔn rén.

From the third to the fifth month, ox lung contains worms that resemble hair from a horse's tail. Cut them up and do not eat it. Eating it will injure the person.

COMMENTARY, LINE 24.38

The third to the fifth month describes the transition from spring to summer, which is the season when insects multiply. They enter the oxen's lung directly by being breathed in, or via the stomach through food and water. Eating the lung of oxen diseased by worms is detrimental to health.

Line 24.39

牛，羊，猪肉，皆不得以楮木，桑木蒸炙，食之令人腹内生虫。

Niú, yang, zhū ròu, jiē bù dé yǐ chǔ mù, sāng mù zhēng zhì, shí zhī lìng rén fù nèi shēng chóng.

Beef, goat meat, and pork must all not be steamed or roasted over wood from the paper mulberry or mulberry. Eating it will cause the person to engender worms inside the abdomen.

Line 24.40

啖蛇牛肉杀人。何以知之？啖蛇者，毛发向后顺者是也。

Dàn shé niú ròu shā rén. Hé yǐ zhī zhī? Dàn shé zhě, máo fà xiàng hòu shùn zhě shì yě.

Eating beef from an ox that has been bitten by a snake kills the person. How can you know this? When bitten by a snake, the [ox's] hair will point backwards.

Line 24.41

治啖蛇牛肉食之欲死方

饮人乳汁一升，立愈。

又方: 以泔洗头，饮一升愈。牛肚细切，以水一斗，煮取一升，暖饮之，大汗出者愈。

Zhì dàn shé niú ròu shí zhī yù sǐ fāng

Yǐn rén rǔ zhī yī shēng, lì yù.

Yòu fāng: yǐ gān xǐ tóu, yǐn yī shēng yù. Niú dǔ xì qiē, yǐ shuǐ yī dǒu, zhǔ qǔ yī shēng, nuǎn yǐn zhī, dà hàn chū zhě yù.

A formula to treat [a patient] on the verge on death after eating meat from an ox that has been bitten by a snake:

Drinking one *shēng* of human breast milk will cause immediate recovery.

Another formula: Wash the head with water that rice has been rinsed in, then drink 1 *shēng* [of this]. Recovery [will ensue]. Finely chop an oxen's stomach and boil it in 1 *dǒu* of water to get 1 *shēng*. Drink it warm. Great sweating means recovery.

COMMENTARY, LINE 24.41

Water that rice has been rinsed in is sweet and cool. After it is used to wash the head, it also contains head filth, which has the effect of ejecting toxin. Hence it can be used as a medicinal to resolve toxin here. Ox stomach is sweet and warm, boosts qì, supplements the spleen and stomach, and is also able to resolve toxin. Drinking it warm to cause great sweating induces the toxin to be discharged along with the sweat.

Line 24.42

治食牛肉中毒方
甘草
煮汁饮之，即解。
Zhì shí niú ròu zhòng dú fāng
Gān cǎo
Zhǔ zhī yǐn zhī, jí jiě.

A formula to treat poisoning from eating beef:

licorice (甘草 *gān cǎo*, Glycyrrhizae Radix)

Boil and drink the juice, to resolve [the toxin].

COMMENTARY, LINE 24.42

Licorice (*gān cǎo*) is said to "resolve the hundred toxins." It is still used widely in current clinical practice in formulas to resolve the toxins of various medicinal substances.

Line 24.43

羊肉其有宿热者，不可食之。
Yáng ròu qí yǒu sù rè zhě, bù kě shí zhī.

Goat meat must not be eaten by persons with abiding heat.

COMMENTARY, LINE 24.43

Goat meat is greatly hot by nature. A person with latent heat disease or with constitutional heat should therefore avoid eating goat meat, because it may cause heat effusion.

Line 24.44

羊肉不可共生鱼、酪食之，害人。
Yáng ròu bù kě gòng shēng yú, lào shí zhī, hài rén.

Goat meat must not be eaten together with raw fish or koumiss [fermented milk]. It harms the person.

Line 24.45

羊蹄甲中有珠子白者，名羊悬筋，食之令人癫。

Yáng tí jiǎ zhōng yǒu zhū zǐ bái zhě, míng yáng xuán jīn, shí zhī lìng rén diān.

When there is a white pearl inside a goat's hoof, this is called "goat's suspended sinew." Eating it causes the person [to suffer from] withdrawal.

Line 24.46

白羊黑头，食其脑，作肠痈。

Bái yáng hēi tóu, shí qí nǎo, zuò cháng yōng.

Eating the brain of a white goat with a black head causes intestinal welling-abscess.

Line 24.47

羊肝共生椒食之，破人五脏。

Yáng gān gòng shēng jiāo shí zhī, pò rén wǔ zàng.

Eating goat liver together with raw pepper will break the person's five viscera.

COMMENTARY, LINE 24.47

Goat meat and pepper are both acrid and hot. Eating these substances together may cause the fulminant toxin of blocked wind and fire to enter the five viscera and thereby damage the person's health.

Line 24.48

猪肉共羊肝和食之，令人心闷。

Zhū ròu gòng yáng gān hé shí zhī, lìng rén xīn mèn.

Eating pork together with goat's liver causes the person [to suffer from] heart oppression.

COMMENTARY, LINE 24.48

Eating pork can have the effect of stagnating blood in the vessels, while goat liver is slimy by nature. Eating these together can therefore cause qì stagnation, and hence glomus and oppression in the heart and chest.

Line 24.49

猪肉以生胡荽同食，烂人脐。

Zhū ròu yǐ shēng hú suī tóng shí, làn rén qí.

Eating pork together with fresh cilantro putrefies the person's umbilicus.

COMMENTARY, LINE 24.49

Fresh cilantro, also called coriander, is very acrid and hot. Eating a lot of it in combination with slimy and binding pork can cause putrefaction in the stomach in persons who have constitutional heat exuberance.

Line 24.50

猪脂不可合梅子食之。

Zhū zhī bù kě hé méi zǐ shí zhī.

Pork lard must not be eaten in combination with mume.

COMMENTARY, LINE 24.50

Pork lard is slimy and lubricating, while mume is sour and astringent. Because their natures are opposite, eating them together can cause congestion in the stomach and qì turbidity in the stomach duct.

Line 24.51

猪肉合葵食之，少气。

Zhū ròu hé kuí shí zhī, shǎo qì.

Eating pork together with mallow causes shortage of qì.

COMMENTARY, LINE 24.51

Pork is slimy and stagnates qì, while mallow is cold and disinhibiting, engenders phlegm, and stirs wind. In combination, these substances can cause coursing, discharge, and downpour in the stomach and intestines, and consequently shortage of qì in the lung.

Line 24.52

鹿肉不可合蒲白作羹，食之发恶疮。

Lù ròu bù kě gě pú bái zuò gēng, shí zhī fā è chuāng.

Venison must not be combined with typha rhizome[1] to make meat broth. Eating them will cause malign sores to erupt.

TEXT NOTE, LINE 24.52

[1] Typha rhizome 蒲白 *pú bái:* Also called 蒲笋 *pú sŭn* in Chinese and cattail rhizome in English.

COMMENTARY, LINE 24.52

Venison is warm by nature. Eating cooked venison alone can cause reactions like heart vexation, insomnia, and dry mouth and tongue. Typha rhizome is acrid by nature. When these two substances are eaten together in broth, acrid hot qì can move into the interstices of the flesh and cause malign sores.

Line 24.53

麋脂及梅李子，若妊妇食之，令子青盲，男子伤精。

Mí zhī jí méi lǐ zǐ, ruò rèn fù shí zhī, lìng zǐ qīng máng, nán zǐ shāng jīng.

il eaten by a pregnant female, Elaphure [Père David's deer] fat together with plums will cause clear-eye blindness[1] in the fetus. If eaten by a male it will damage essence.

TEXT NOTE, LINE 24.53

[1] Clear-eye blindness 青盲 *qīng máng:* Blindness without visible obstruction, such as a cataract, in the eye, hence "clear-eye." The Chinese 青 *qīng* is the word for "blue-green," in this context meaning "black," the natural color of the eye free of obstructions.

COMMENTARY, LINE 24.53

Elaphure's fat (*mí zhī*) is acrid, warm, and disinhibiting, while mume and plum are clearing, cool, sour, and astringent. Eating these two substances in combination can deplete liver qì in pregnant women, therefore damaging the eyes of the fetus, and exhaust kidney essence in men, thereby damaging essential qì to the point of yáng wilting (impotence).

Line 24.54

獐肉不可合虾及生菜、梅、李果食之，皆病人。

Zhāng ròu bù kě hé xiā jí shēng cài, méi, lǐ guǒ shí zhī, jiē bìng rén.

Water deer's flesh must not be combined with prawn, raw greens, mume, and plums. Eating any of these will make the person sick.

Commentary, Line 24.54

Eating water deer's flesh stirs qì, while prawn stirs wind heat, and raw greens and plums stir phlegm. Eating these in combination can easily cause wind-phlegm hot qì disease.

Line 24.55

痼疾人不可食熊肉，令终身不愈。

Gù jí rén bù kě shí xióng ròu, lìng zhōng shēn bù yù.

People with intractable disease must not eat bear meat, or they will not recover for the rest of their life.

Commentary, Line 24.55

Bear meat is sweet and slimy and has a vacuity-supplementing effect on patients with emaciation. However, it also has the effect of lodging evil and can therefore make it difficult to eliminate the root of disease.

Line 24.56

白犬自死，不出舌者，食之害人。

Bái quǎn zì sǐ, bù chū shé zhě, shí zhī hài rén.

Eating a white dog that has died a natural death without sticking out its tongue will harm the person.

Line 24.57

食狗鼠余，令人发瘘疮。

Shí gǒu shǔ yú, lìng rén fā lòu chuāng.

Eating dogs' or rats' leftovers will make the person suffer from erupting fistulas.

COMMENTARY, LINE 24.57

Food or drink that has been touched by dogs or rats can be contaminated by their saliva. If humans eat this, the toxin can scatter into the sinews and network vessels and thereby engender fistulas.

Line 24.58

治食犬肉不消，心下坚，或腹胀，口干大渴，心急发热，妄语如狂，或洞下方

杏仁（合皮熟研用）一升

上一味，以沸汤三升，和取汁，分三服，利下肉片，大验。

Zhì shí quǎn ròu bù xiāo, xīn xià jiān, huò fù zhàng, kǒu gān dà kě, xīn jí fā rè, wàng yǔ rú kuáng, huò dòng xià fāng

Xìng rén (hé pí shú yán yòng) yī shēng

Yī fèi tāng sān shēng, huó qǔ zhī, fēn sān fú, lì xià ròu piàn, dà yàn.

A formula to treat eating dog's flesh and not being able to disperse it, with hardness below the heart or abdominal distention, dry mouth and great thirst, tension in the heart and heat effusion, mania-like reckless speech, and possibly throughflux diarrhea:

apricot kernel (杏仁 *xìng rén*, Armeniacae Semen) 1 *shēng* (cook with the peel and grind finely)

Mix the single ingredient above with three *shēng* of boiling water, take the juice, and divide into three doses. It will disinhibit and precipitate the piece of meat. Well-tested.

COMMENTARY, LINE 24.58

Eating dog's flesh strengthens the spleen and stomach and fortifies kidney yáng, but its nature is very dry and hot. Overeating it without dispersing may cause heat obstruction and food stagnation, as a result of which you will see hardness and fullness below the heart or abdominal distention.

Fire heat damaging yīn and harassing the heart results in dry mouth and great thirst, heat effusion, and manic reckless speech. If heat toxin pours downward, there is incessant throughflux diarrhea.

Dog's flesh fears apricot kernel (*xìng rén*), which is slippery and disinhibits qì. It is thus an appropriate treatment for precipitating dog's flesh accumulation.

Line 24.59

妇人妊娠，不可食兔肉、山羊肉，及鳖、鸡、鸭，令子无声音。

Fù rén rèn shēn, bù kě shí tù ròu, shān yáng ròu, jí biē, jī, yā, lìng zǐ wú shēng yīn.

During pregnancy, women may not eat the flesh of rabbit and goat, as well as soft-shelled turtle, chicken, and duck, which will make the child mute.

COMMENTARY, LINE 24.59

Rabbit meat is acrid and neutral. It supplements the center and boosts qì, cools blood, and resolves toxin. Goat meat is sweet and hot; it warms the center and expels cold, and warms and supplements qì and blood. Soft-shelled turtle meat is sweet and neutral; it enriches yīn and cools blood. Chicken meat is sweet and slightly warm, and boosts qì and supplements vacuity. Duck meat enriches yīn and supplements vacuity, disinhibits urine, and disperses swelling. To avoid harm duringuring pregnancy, you must select among these nutritious and supplementing substances in accord with the body's tendency towards yīn or yáng.

These dietary prohibitions are an important aspect of "fetal education" (胎教 *tāi jiào*), a set of dietary and behavioral guidelines and taboos that pregnant women traditionally observed during pregnancy to ensure the physical, emotional, and even moral health of the fetus. In other texts, eating rabbit during pregnancy is said to cause hare's lip, while eating tortoise causes the child to be mute or have a short neck. Chicken, goat, and duck meats are generally considered as appropriate, nourishing foods during pregnancy, and the prohibition above should be applied to over-consumption of these foods.

Line 24.60

兔肉不可合白鸡肉食之, 令人面发黄。

Tù ròu bù kě hé bái jī ròu shí zhī, lìng rén miàn fā huáng.

You may not eat rabbit meat in combination with the meat of white chickens. It will cause yellowing of the person's face.

COMMENTARY, LINE 24.60

Eating rabbit meat can stir damp-heat and thereby cause yellowing of the facial complexion.

Line 24.61

兔肉着干姜食之，成霍乱。

Tù ròu zhuó gān jiāng shí zhī, chéng huò luàn.

Eating rabbit meat that has touched dried ginger creates cholera.

COMMENTARY, LINE 24.61

Rabbit meat is sour, cold, and belongs to yīn, while dried ginger is acrid, hot, and belongs to yáng. Since these two substances are thus opposite in flavor, eating them together may cause disharmony of stomach qì and consequently cholera with vomiting and diarrhea.

Line 24.62

凡鸟自死，口不闭，翅不合者，不可食之。

Fán niǎo zì sǐ, kǒu bù bì, chì bù hé zhě, bù kě shí zhī.

Birds that have died a natural death without closing the beak and folding the wings together are inedible.

COMMENTARY, LINE 24.62

Closing the beak and folding the wings is a natural physical reaction in dying birds. If they die with the beak gaping open and the wings spread out, this indicates that their death has an abnormal cause and they are most likely contaminated by poisoning. Hence, they are inedible.

Line 24.63

诸禽肉，肝青者，食之杀人。

Zhū qín ròu, gān qīng zhě, shí zhī shā rén.

In all poultry, if the liver is green-blue, eating the meat kills the person.

COMMENTARY, LINE 24.63

In all birds and beasts, a shiny greenish-black liver indicates that the animal has died from poisoning and is therefore not fit for human consumption.

Line 24.64

鸡有六翮四距者，不可食之。
Jī yǒu liù hé sì jù zhě, bù kě shí zhī.

Chickens with six wings and four legs are inedible.

Line 24.65

乌鸡白首者，不可食之。
Wū jī bái shǒu zhě, bù kě shí zhī.

Black chickens with white heads are inedible.

Line 24.66

鸡不可共葫蒜食之，滞气。
Jī bù kě gòng hú suàn shí zhī, zhì qì.

Chicken must not be eaten together with garlic, [because] it stagnates qì.

COMMENTARY, LINE 24.66

Eating chicken meat can stir wind, while garlic can stir phlegm. In combination, they can arouse wind-phlegm, and as a result, stagnation of the qì dynamic and shortage of qì.

Line 24.67

山鸡不可合鸟兽肉食之。
Shān jī bù kě hé niǎo shòu ròu shí zhī.

Red junglefowl (*shān jī*) must not be eaten in combination with meat from [other] birds and beasts.

COMMENTARY, LINE 24.67

Because red junglefowl (*shān jī*, Gallus gallus jabouillei), a member of the pheasant family, often consume toxic substances like worms and ants or plants such as aconite (*wū tóu*) and pinellia (*bàn xià*), they can be toxic and should therefore not be eaten together with other meat.

Line 24.68

雉肉久食之，令人瘦。

Zhì ròu jiǔ shí zhī, lìng rén shòu.

Eating the flesh of ring-necked pheasants over time makes the person thin.

Line 24.69

鸭卵不可合鳖肉食之。

Yā luǎn bù kě hé biē ròu shí zhī.

Duck eggs must not be eaten together with turtle flesh.

COMMENTARY, LINE 24.69

Both duck eggs and turtle flesh are cold and can cause eruption of cold qì. Hence they should not be eaten together.

Line 24.70

妇人妊娠，食雀肉，令子淫乱无耻。

Fù rén rèn shēn, shí què ròu, lìng zǐ yín luàn wú chǐ.

If a woman during pregnancy eats sparrow's flesh, this makes the child lascivious, deranged, and without shame.

Line 24.71

雀肉不可合李子食之。

Què ròu bù kě hé lǐ zǐ shí zhī.

Sparrow's flesh must not be eaten in combination with plum.

COMMENTARY, LINE 24.71

Sparrow's flesh is hot and has the effect of invigorating yáng and boosting qì. Nevertheless, when combined with plum, which is cold, sour, and astringent, the heat does not move and may instead stagnate qì.

Line 24.72

燕肉勿食，入水为蛟龙所噉。

Yàn ròu wù shí, rù shuǐ wéi jiāo lóng suǒ dàn.

Do not eat swallow's flesh, or you will get eaten by the flood dragon when entering water.

Line 24.73

鸟兽有中毒箭死者, 其肉有毒, 解之方:

大豆

煮汁及蓝汁服之解。

Niǎo shòu yǒu zhòng dú jiàn sǐ zhě, qí ròu yǒu dú, jiě zhī fāng:

Dà dòu

Zhǔ zhī jí yán zhī fú zhī jiě.

The flesh of birds and beasts that have been killed with a poisoned arrow contains toxin. A formula for resolving it:

yellow soybean (大豆 *dà dòu*, Sojae Semen Flavum)

Boil and take the juice. Also take isatis juice. It resolves [the toxin].

COMMENTARY, LINE 24.73

Poisoned arrows are most commonly created with a preparation of wild aconite juice, which is bitter, hot, and very toxic. Juice from soybean or indigo plant seed can both be used to resolve this toxin.

Line 24.74

鱼头正白如连珠至脊上，食之杀人。

Yú tóu zhèng bái rú lián zhū zhì jǐ shàng, shí zhī shā rén.

Eating fish with pure white on the head all the way to the spine kills the person.

Line 24.75

鱼头中无腮者，不可食之，杀人。

Yú tóu zhōng wú sāi zhě, bù kě shí zhī, shā rén.

Fish that does not have cheeks in the head is inedible and kills the person.

Line 24.76

鱼无肠胆者，不可食之，三年阴不起，女子绝生。

Yú wú cháng dăn zhě, bù kě shí zhī, sān nián yīn bù qĭ, nǚ zĭ jué shēng.

Fish that lacks intestines or a gallbladder is inedible. [Eating it] causes yīn failing to rise[1] for three years, and infertility in women.

TEXT NOTE, LINE 24.76

[1] Yīn failing to rise 阴不起 *yīn bù qĭ:* Impotence. The genitals of either sex, and here specifically the penis, were often referred to as "yīn." Later, the penis came to be called "yáng."

Line 24.77

鱼头似有角者，不可食之。鱼目合者，不可食之。

Yú tóu sì yǒu jiăo zhě, bù kě shí zhī. Yú mù hé zhě, bù kě shí zhī.

Fish with horn-like [protrusions] on the head is inedible. Fish with closed eyes is inedible.

Line 24.78

六甲日，勿食鳞甲之物。

Liù jiă rì, wù shí lín jiă zhī wù.

On the six *jiă* days, do not eat things with scales or shells.

Line 24.79

鱼不可合鸡肉食之。

Yú bù kě hé jī ròu shí zhī.

Fish must not be eaten in combination with chicken.

COMMENTARY, LINE 24.79

Fish belongs to fire and likes to stir, while chicken belongs to wood and engenders wind. If these two substances are combined, wind and fire can fan each other.

Line 24.80

鱼不得合鸬鹚肉食之。

Yú bù dé hé lú cí ròu shí zhī.

Fish must not be eaten in combination with cormorant's flesh.

COMMENTARY, LINE 24.81

The cormorant is a wild bird that loves to eat fish. Hence, these two substances are opposed to each other and should not be eaten together.

Line 24.81

鲤鱼鲊，不可合小豆藿食之；其子不可合猪肝食之，害人。

Lǐ yú zhǎ, bù kě hé xiǎo dòu huò shí zhī; qí zǐ bù kě hé zhū gān shí zhī, hài rén.

Salted carp must not be eaten in combination with rice bean leaves. Its roe must not be eaten in combination with pork liver, [since] it will injure the person.

COMMENTARY, LINE 24.81

Both carp and rice bean leaves are salty, and saltiness can overcome blood. Eaten in combination, they can therefore cause dispersion-thirst.

Line 24.82

鲤鱼不可合犬肉食之。

Lǐ yú bù kě hé quǎn ròu shí zhī.

Carp must not be eaten in combination with dog's flesh.

COMMENTARY, LINE 24.82

Both carp and dog's flesh are hot. Eaten together, they may cause center dispersion and internal welling-abscess from heat toxin.

Line 24.83

鲫鱼不可合猴雉肉食之。一云不可和猪肝食。

Jì yú bù kě hé hóu zhì ròu shí zhī. Yī yún bù kě hé zhū gān shí.

Golden carp must not be eaten in combination with the flesh of monkey or ring-necked pheasant. It is also said that it must not be eaten in combination with pork liver.

COMMENTARY, LINE 24.83

Golden carp penetrates to the spleen and stomach, monkey's flesh tends to stir, and pheasant's flesh belongs to fire. Eaten together, these three substances can engender heat sores or vomiting and diarrhea, dry stomach, and intestinal bind.

Line 24.84

鳀鱼合鹿肉生食，令人筋甲缩。

Tí yú hé lù ròu shēng shí, lìng rén jīn jiă suō.

Eating raw Chinese catfish in combination with venison causes the person's sinews and nails to shrink.

COMMENTARY, LINE 24.84

Chinese catfish has the effect of treating wind-cold and cold impediment, but if combined with sour and warm venison, it can easily stir wind disease, thereby depriving the sinews and vessels of nourishment.

Line 24.85

青鱼鲊，不可合生葫荽及生葵并麦中食之。

Qīng yú zhă, bù kě hé shēng hú suī jí shēng kuí bìng mài zhōng shí zhī.

Green-blue salted fish must not be eaten together with raw coriander, raw mallow, or with grains.

Line 24.86

鳅、鳝不可合白犬血食之。

Qiū, shàn bù kě hé bái quǎn xuè shí zhī.

Loach and eel must not be eaten in combination with blood from a white dog.

Line 24.87

龟肉不可合酒果子食之。

Guī ròu bù kě hé jiǔ guǒ zǐ shí zhī.

Tortoise meat must not be eaten in combination with alcohol or fruit.

COMMENTARY, LINE 24.87

Tortoise meat can subdue yáng, and is sour and warm. Alcohol is dissipating, and fruit is sour and astringing. Because their natures differ, eating them together may cause [aversion to] cold and heat [effusion].

Line 24.88

鳖目凹陷者，及压下有王字形者，不可食之。

Biē mù āo xiàn zhě, jí yā xià yǒu wáng zì xing zhě, bù kě shí zhī.

Turtles with sunken eyes and markings below the abdomen in the shape of the character 王 are inedible.

Line 24.89

其肉不得合鸡、鸭子食之。

Qí ròu bù dé hé jī, yā zǐ shí zhī.

Their[1] flesh must not beaten in combination with chicken or duck eggs.

TEXT NOTE, LINE 24.88

[1] Their 其 *qí*: A reference to the subject of the previous line, namely turtles.

COMMENTARY, LINE 24.88

Turtle meat, when consumed in large quantities, can stagnate the spleen and lodge dampness; chicken eggs engender heat and stir wind; and duck eggs stagnate qì and lubricate the intestines.

Line 24.90

龟、鳖肉不可合苋菜食之。

Guī, biē ròu bù kě hé xiàn cài shí zhī.

The meat of tortoises and turtles must not be eaten in combination with amaranth.

COMMENTARY, LINE 24.90

Tortoise and turtle meat is astringing, while amaranth is disinhibiting. Because of their opposite nature, they should not be eaten together.

Line 24.91

虾无须，及腹下通黑，煮之反白者，不可食之。

Xiā wú xū, jí fù xià tōng hēi, zhǔ zhī fǎn bái zhě, bù kě shí zhī.

A shrimp with no beard[1] and a thoroughly black underside of the abdomen that turns white when cooked is inedible.

TEXT NOTE, LINE 24.91

[1] No beard 无须 *wú xū*: This may be a reference to missing palpus or antenna.

Line 24.92

食脍，饮乳酪，令人腹中生虫为瘕。

Shí kuài, yǐn rǔ lào, lìng rén fù zhōng shēng chóng wéi jiǎ.

Eating minced [raw] meat and drinking koumiss engenders worms in the abdomen and forms conglomerations.

Line 24.93

鲙食之，在心胸间不化，吐复不出，速下除之，久成癥病，治之方

橘皮一两　大黄二两　朴硝二两

右三味，以水一大升，煮至小升，顿服即消。

Kuài shí zhī, zài xīn xiōng jiān bù huà, tù fù bù chū, sù xià chú zhī, jiǔ chéng zhēng bìng, zhì zhī fāng

Jú pí yī liǎng; dà huáng èr liǎng; pò xiāo èr liǎng

Yòu sān wèi, yǐ shuǐ yī dà shēng, zhǔ zhì xiǎo shēng, dùn fú jí xiāo.

A formula to treat [over]consumption of minced [raw] fish such that it stays in the heart and chest region without being transformed and further cannot be expelled through vomiting. Speedily precipitate to eliminate it, because over time it can form concretions.

tangerine peel (橘皮 *jú pí*, Citri Reticulatae Pericarpium) 1 *liǎng*
rhubarb (大黄 *dà huáng*, Rhei Radix et Rhizoma) 2 *liǎng*
impure mirabilite (朴硝 *pò xiāo*, Natrii Sulfas Non-Purus) 2 *liǎng*

Boil the three above ingredients in one large *shēng* of water to get one small *shēng*. Quaff, and dispersion will ensue.

Commentary, Line 24.93

Excessive consumption of raw cold fish or meat can cause toxin to gather in the stomach duct, resulting in food accumulation and qì stagnation, and over time in concretions and conglomerations. Treatment should consist of medicinals that move qì and resolve toxin, disperse food and abduct stagnation, and offensively precipitate conglomeration lumps. In the recommended formula, tangerine peel (*jú pí*) moves qì and resolves fish toxin, while impure mirabilite (*pò xiāo*) and rhubarb (*dà huáng*) offensively precipitate concretions and disperse food accumulations. As a result, the undigested fish is eliminated by defecation.

Line 24.94

食鲙多不消，结为癥病，治之方

马鞭草

右一味，捣汁饮之。或以姜叶汁饮之一升，亦消。又可服吐药吐之。

Shí kuài duō bù xiāo, jié wéi zhēng bìng, zhì zhī fāng

Mǎ biān cǎo

Yòu yī wèi, dǎo zhī yǐn zhī. Huò yǐ jiāng yè zhī yǐn zhī yī shēng, yì xiāo. Yòu kě fú tù yào tù zhī.

A formula to treat overeating on minced [raw] fish that does not digest, binding into concretions.

verbena (马鞭草 *mǎ biān cǎo*, Verbenae Herba)

Pound the single above ingredient and drink the juice. Alternatively, use ginger leaves to make a juice and drink one *shēng* of that. It will also disperse it. Furthermore, you can take ejecting medicinals to eject it.

COMMENTARY, LINE 24.94

Verbena (*mǎ biān cǎo*) is bitter and cold, breaks blood and disperses concretions, resolves toxin, and kills worms. As an alternative treatment, ginger leaf juice resolves fish toxin, rectifies qì, and disperses accumulations.

Line 24.95

食鱼后中毒，两种烦乱，治之方
橘皮
浓煎汁服之，即解。

Shí yú hòu zhòng dú, liǎng zhǒng fán luàn, zhì zhī fāng

Jú pí

Nóng jiān zhī fú zhī, jí jiě.

A formula to treat poisoning after eating fish, with swelling in the face,[1] vexation, and derangement:

jú pí (Citri Reticulatae Pericarpium)

Decoct until concentrated. Taking the juice will resolve [the toxin].

TEXT NOTE, LINE 24.95

[1] Swelling in the face 两种 *liǎng zhǒng*: The present translation reflects the correction of the text on the basis of quotations in the *Qiān Jīn Fāng* and *Zhǒu Hòu Bèi Jí Fāng*, where 两种 is replaced with 面肿 *miàn zhǒng* (swelling of the face).

COMMENTARY, LINE 24.95

Vexation, derangement, and qì counterflow can result from food poisoning as well as from fish poisoning. Both of these are treatable with tangerine peel (*jú pí*), which has the effect of dispersing food, resolving toxin, eliminating vexation, and downbearing counterflow.

Line 24.96

食鯸鮧鱼中毒方
芦根
煮汁服之，即解。

Shí hóu yí yú zhòng dú fāng

Lú gēn

Zhǔ zhī fú zhī, jí jiě.

A formula to treat poisoning from eating globefish[1]:

phragmites (芦根 *lú gēn*, Phragmitis Rhizoma)

Boiling it and taking the juice will resolve [the toxin].

TEXT NOTE, LINE 24.96

[1] Globefish 鯸鮧 *hóu yí*: In Chinese, it is more commonly called 河豚 *hé tún* (Fugu Caro). In English, it is variously called referred to as puffer fish, blowfish, swellfish, and by the Japanese name *fugu*.

COMMENTARY, LINE 24.96

Globefish is toxic and fears phragmites (*lú gēn*), which means that the latter has the ability to resolve its toxin. This method is effective and widely used.

Line 24.97

蟹目相向，足斑目赤者，不可食之。

Xiè mù xiāng xiàng, zú bān mù chì zhě, bù kě shí zhī.

Crabs that have eyes that face each other or spotted feet and red eyes are inedible.

Line 24.98

食蟹中毒治之方

紫苏

煮汁饮之三升。紫苏子捣汁饮之，亦良。

又方:冬瓜汁饮二升，食冬瓜亦可。

Shí xiè zhòng dú zhì zhī fāng

Zǐ sū

Zhǔ zhī yǐn zhī sān shēng. Zǐ sū zǐ dǎo zhī yǐn zhī, yì liáng.

Yòu fāng: Dōng guā zhī yǐn èr shēng, shí dōng guā yì kě.

A formula to treat poisoning from eating crab:

perilla (紫苏 ***zǐ sū***, Perillae Folium, Caulis et Calyx)

Boil and drink three *shēng* of the juice. Pounding perilla (*zǐ sū zǐ*) and drinking the juice is also good.

Another formula: Drink two *shēng* of wax gourd (*dōng guā*) juice. Eating wax gourd (*dōng guā*) is also possible.

COMMENTARY, LINE 24.98

According to the *Zhū Bìng Yuán Hòu Lùn* ("The Origin and Indicators of Disease"), eating cooked crabs can cause poisoning, because crabs eat *Ranunculus japonicas* (水茛 *shuǐ gèn*, also called 毛茛 *máo gèn*), which is highly poisonous.

In the *Běn Cǎo Gāng Mù* ("Herbal Foundation Compendium"), perilla (*zǐ sū zǐ*) is said to "disinhibit the diaphragm, widen the intestines, and resolve the toxin of fish and crabs." Wax gourd (*dōng guā*) juice can resolve fish and crab toxin, as well as wine toxin, eliminating toxin by disinhibiting water.

Line 24.99

凡蟹未遇霜，多毒，其熟者乃可食之。

Fán xiè wèi yù shuāng, duō dú, qí shú zhě nǎi kě shí zhī.

Whenever crabs have not yet encountered frost, they are very toxic. But if they are cooked, you can eat them.

Commentary, Line 24.99

See the commentary for the previous line for an explanation of why crabs are poisonous. After the frost, when their diet consists of rice plants instead, their toxicity is reduced.

Line 24.100

蜘蛛落食中，有毒，勿食之。

Zhī zhū luò shí zhōng, yǒu dú, wù shí zhī.

When a spider drops on food, [the food] becomes toxic. Do not eat it.

Line 24.101

凡蜂、蝇、虫、蚁等多集食上，食之致瘘。

Fán fēng, yíng, chóng, yǐ děng duō jí shí shàng, shí zhī zhì lòu.

Whenever bees, flies, worms, or ants have gathered on top of food, eating it will cause fistulas.

Commentary, Line 24.101

Bees, flies, worms, and ants all contain toxin and can transmit all sorts of diseases, especially when gathering on food. After a person eats the contaminated food, damp-heat toxin flows into the flesh, channels, and network vessels and can therefore easily engender fistulas, as well as cholera or epidemics.

果实菜谷禁忌并治第二十五

CHAPTER 25

Fruits, Vegetables, and Grains

Contraindications and Treatments

‡ Overview

Fruits, vegetables, and grain nourish the human body with the five flavors. As stated in the *Nèi Jīng* ("The Inner Canon"), "The five grains provide nourishment, the five fruits provide assistance, and the five vegetables provide fullness." Early Chinese medicine thus already paid close attention to diet and the clinical application of food.

The present chapter discusses plant-based foods in terms of dietetic hygiene and offers methods and formulas for the prevention and treatment of food poisoning from plants. It contains 88 lines with 14 formulas, including 70 lines on dietetic hygiene with methods for identifying unclean food, adjusting a seasonal diet to disease, and dietary prohibitions during pregnancy; 5 lines on signs of poisoning from alum (*bái fán*), phytolacca (*shāng lù*), lepidii/descurainia (*tíng lì zǐ*), mercury (*shuǐ yín*), and chinaberry bark (*kǔ liàn pí*); and 13 lines on the treatment of poisoning from eating unclean plant-based foods.

Line 25.1

果子生食生疮。

Guǒ zǐ shēng shí shēng chuāng.

Eating fruit raw engenders sores.

COMMENTARY, LINE 25.1

Eating raw fruit that is not properly cleaned can allow for the transmission of disease toxin. This can engender sores and scabs, or damp-heat in the stomach and intestines, causing diarrhea.

Line 25.2

果子落地经宿，虫蚁食之者，人大忌食之。

Guǒ zǐ luò dì jīng xiǔ, chóng yǐ shí zhī zhě, rén dà jì shí zhī.

If fruit has dropped to the ground and remained there overnight, so that worms and ants have eaten [from it], it is greatly contraindicated for human consumption.

Line 25.3

生米停留多日有损处，食之伤人。

Shēng mǐ tíng liú duō rì yǒu sǔn chù, shí zhī shāng rén.

When uncooked rice has been kept in a detrimental location for several days, eating it damages the person.

COMMENTARY, LINE 25.3

Uncooked rice can be damaged during storage by contamination from insects and rodents or by spoilage due to damp-heat toxin. This will make it unfit for human consumption.

Line 25.4

桃子多食，令人热，仍不得入水浴，令人病淋沥寒热病。

Táo zǐ duō shí, lìng rén rè, réng bù dé rù shuǐ yù, lìng rén bìng lín lì hán rè bìng.

Eating too many peaches makes a person hot. Hence they may not enter water to bathe, because this will make them suffer from dripping[1] and [aversion to] cold and heat [effusion].

TEXT NOTE, LINE 25.4

[1] Dripping 淋沥 *lín lì*: This can be taken to mean strangury (淋 *lín*), but according to Wú Qiān 吴谦, it should be interpreted as 癃 *lóng*, dribbling urinary block.

COMMENTARY, LINE 25.4

Overconsumption of peaches, which are sour, sweet, and hot, can impair digestion and cause vexation and heat in the heart. If such a person is exposed to water, dampness and heat can combine and cannot be effused. The external result is aversion to cold and heat effusion, and the internal result is strangury.

Line 25.5

杏酪不熟伤人。

Xìng lào bù shú shāng rén.

If apricot paste has not matured, it damages the person.

COMMENTARY, LINE 25.5

Apricot paste (杏酪 *xìng luò*, also called 杏酥 *xìng sū*) is a product made from processed apricots. If prepared properly, it is able to moisten the five viscera, clear lung dryness, and rid phlegm panting. However, if the apricots are not processed sufficiently by soaking to remove the bitterness, they are toxic and can cause signs of poisoning, such as nausea, dizzy head and flowery vision, encumbered breathing, blue mouth and lips, and sudden clouding collapse.

Line 25.6

梅多食坏人齿。

Méi duō shí huài rén chǐ.

Eating too much mume ruins a person's teeth.

Line 25.7

李不可多食，令人胪胀。

Lǐ bù kě duō shí, lìng rén lú zhàng.

Plums must not be eaten in excess. They will cause abdominal distention.

COMMENTARY, LINE 25.7

The sour astringent nature of plums can prevent the movement of spleen qì, which would result in stagnation of the center burner.

Line 25.8

林檎不可多食，令人百脉弱。

Lìn qín bù kě duō shí, lìng rén bǎi mài ruò.

Chinese crabapple must not be eaten in excess. It makes the person's hundred vessels weak.

COMMENTARY, LINE 25.8

Chinese crabapple is sour and astringent. If eaten in excess, it can block the vessels and cause the person to sleep deeply.

Line 25.9

橘柚多食，令人口爽，不知五味。

Jú yòu duō shí, lìng rén kǒu shuǎng, bù zhī wǔ wèi.

Overconsumption of tangerine or pomelo makes a person's mouth err[1] and become unable to distinguish the five flavors.

TEXT NOTE, LINE 25.9

[1] Makes a person's mouth err (令人口爽 *lìng rén kǒu shuǎng*): Makes the palate fail in the proper detection of flavors.

COMMENTARY, LINE 25.9

Both tangerine and pomelo are cold and sour, and can engender phlegm and gather rheum. Rheum gathering above the diaphragm causes blandness in the mouth and inability to distinguish flavors.

Line 25.10

梨不可多食，令人寒中，金疮、产妇，亦不宜食。

Lí bù kě duō shí, lìng rén hán zhōng, jīn chuāng, chǎn fù, yì bù yí shí.

Pears must not be eaten in excess. They make the person cold in the center. Persons with incised wounds or women in childbed should also not eat them.

COMMENTARY, LINE 25.10

Excessive consumption of pears can cause cold-rheum patterns in persons with spleen-stomach vacuity cold. Because the coldness of pear can stagnate blood in the vessels, it is contraindicated for persons with an insufficiency of qì and blood, such as after injury or childbirth.

Line 25.11

樱桃、杏，多食伤筋骨。

Yīng táo, xìng, duō shí shāng jīn gǔ.

Eating cherries or apricots in excess damages sinew and bone.

COMMENTARY, LINE 25.11

Both cherries and apricots are sour and cold by nature. Sourness damages the sinews, and coldness damages the bones.

Line 25.12

安石榴不可多食，损人肺。

Ān shí liú bù kě duō shí, sǔn rén fèi.

Pomegranates must not be eaten in excess. They injure the person's lung.

COMMENTARY, LINE 25.12

Pomegranates are sour and astringent, and stagnate qì and engender phlegm. Lung qì must be disinhibited, not stagnant; hence pomegranates cause detriment to the lung.

Line 25.13

胡桃不可多食，令人动痰饮。

Hú táo bù kě duō shí, lìng rén dòng tán yǐn.

Walnuts must not be eaten in excess. They stir phlegm-rheum.

COMMENTARY, LINE 25.13

Walnuts are normally able to moisten the lung and disperse phlegm. Nevertheless, their hot and astringent nature can stir fire, which decocts liquid into phlegm when they are eaten in excess. Because of their astringency, they furthermore gather moisture to create dampness and rheum.

Line 25.14

生枣多食，令人热渴气胀，寒热羸弱者，弥不可食，伤人。

Shēng zǎo duō shí, lìng rén rè kě qì zhàng, hán rè léi ruò zhě, mí bù kě shí, shāng rén.

Eating raw jujubes in excess causes heat, thirst, and qì distention. Persons with [aversion to] cold and heat [effusion] or emaciation and weakness can eat them even less. They will damage such persons.

COMMENTARY, LINE 25.14

Raw jujubes are sweet, acrid, and hot. Their acrid, hot nature causes thirst; their sweetness causes qì distention. Persons with frequent aversion to cold and heat effusion or emaciation and weakness generally suffer from spleen-stomach yīn vacuity. Eating jujubes aggravates the vacuity heat and thereby damages their health.

Line 25.15

食诸果中毒治之方

猪骨（烧过）

右一味，末之，水服方寸匕。亦治马肝、漏脯等毒。

Shí zhū guǒ zhōng dú zhì zhī fāng

Zhū gǔ (shāo guò)

Yòu yī wèi, mò zhī, shuǐ fú fāng cùn bǐ. Yì zhì mǎ gān, lòu fǔ děng dú.

A formula to treat poisoning from eating the various fruits:

pig's bone (猪骨 *zhū gǔ*, Suis Os) (char excessively)

Pulverize the above single ingredient and take a square-inch-spoonful in water. It also treat poisoning from horse liver, leaked-on minced meat, etc.

Line 25.16

木耳赤色及仰生者，勿食。菌仰卷及赤色者，不可食。

Mù ěr chì sè jí yǎng shēng zhě, wù shí. Jùn yǎng juàn jí chì sè zhě, bù kě shí.

Do not eat wood ear that is red or growing facing upward. Mushrooms that are curled upward or are red are inedible.

Line 25.17

食诸菌中毒，闷乱欲死，治之方
人粪汁饮一升，土浆饮一二升，大豆浓煮汁饮之，服诸吐利药，并解。

Shí zhū jùn zhōng dú, mèn luàn yù sǐ, zhì zhī fāng

Rén fèn zhī yǐn yī shēng, tǔ jiāng yǐn yī èr shēng, dà dòu nóng zhǔ zhī yǐn zhī, fú zhū tù lì yào, bìng jiě.

A formula to treat poisoning strike from eating the various mushrooms, with resultant oppression, derangement, and impending death.

Drink one *shēng* of liquefied human excrement; drink one or two *shēng* of yellow earth water; and drink the concentrated juice from boiled soybeans. Taking these various ejecting and disinhibiting medicinals will resolve [the toxin].

COMMENTARY, LINE 25.17

Oppression, derangement, and pending death from mushroom poisoning is caused by heat toxin in the stomach. Liquefied human excrement resolves heat toxin and also hastens ejection; yellow earth water clears summerheat and resolves toxin; and soybean juice disperses swelling toxin. Alternatively, you can take other medicinals that induce ejection or vomiting, in order to disperse toxic qì above or below.

Line 25.18

食枫柱菌而哭不止，治之以前方。

Shí fēng zhù jùn ér kū bù zhǐ, zhì zhī yǐ qián fāng.

Incessant crying[1] from eating mushrooms that grow on liquidambar wood can be treated with the formula above.

TEXT NOTE, LINE 25.18

[1] Crying 哭 *kū*: Another version of this text has 笑 *xiào* ("laughing") instead.

COMMENTARY, LINE 25.18

Incessant laughing from eating mushrooms that grow in liquidambar wood indicates that toxic qì has entered the heart, which governs laughter. Treat this with the formula above in line 25.17, to resolve the toxin.

Line 25.19

误食野芋，烦毒欲死，治之以前方。

Wù shí yě yù, fán dú yù sǐ, zhì zhī yǐ qián fāng.

Vexing poisoning and pending death from mistakenly eating wild taro can be treated with the formula above.[1]

TEXT NOTE, LINE 25.19

[1] A comment included in the received text reads: "The roots of wild taro are called "*kuí* taro" (魁芋, literally, "eminent taro") by the people east of the mountains. When people plant taro and do not harvest it for three years, it also turns into wild taro and kills a person." (其野芋根，山東人名魁芋，人種芋，三年不收，亦成野芋，並殺人。)

COMMENTARY, LINE 25.19

Wild taro is cold, acrid, and toxic. When eaten, it poisons the person, causing numbness and irritation in the stomach, stomach duct, chest, and diaphragm, and when the toxin enters the lung, it causes vexation, derangement, and pending death. The formula above in line 25.17 can resolve the toxin.

Line 25.20

蜀椒闭口者有毒，误食之，戟人咽喉，气病欲绝，或吐下白沫，身体痹冷，急治之。

肉桂煎汁饮之，多饮凉水一二升，或食蒜，或饮地浆，或浓煮豉汁饮之，并解。

Shǔ jiāo bì kǒu zhě yǒu dú, wù shí zhī, jǐ rén yān hóu, qì bìng yù jué, huò tù xià bái mò, shēn tǐ bì lěng, jí zhì zhī.

Ròu guì jiān zhī yǐn zhī, duō yǐn liáng shuǐ yī èr shēng, huò shí suàn, huò yǐn dì jiāng, huò nóng zhǔ chǐ zhī yǐn zhī, bìng jiě.

Zanthoxylum with a closed mouth[1] is toxic. If eaten by mistake, it irritates the person's throat and causes qì disease verging on expiry, possibly vomiting and diarrhea of white foam, and generalized impediment and cold. Urgently treat it.

Decoct cinnamon bark and drink the juice. Repeatedly drink one or two *shēng* of cool water. Alternatively, eat garlic, drink yellow earth water, or boil fermented soybean until concentrated and drink the juice. All these resolve [the toxin].

TEXT NOTE, LINE 25.20

[1] Zanthoxylum with a closed mouth 蜀椒闭口者 *shǔ jiāo bì kǒu*: Dried zanthoxylum fruit that is not split open. This increases its toxicity.

COMMENTARY, LINE 25.20

Zanthoxylum is acrid and spicy, and its nature is hot and toxic. If the seed pod is not cracked, the toxicity is increased. In that case, its acridity can irritate the person's throat, blocking the qì dynamic in the spleen, lung, intestines, and stomach. When qì blockage obstructs construction and defense, we see generalized impediment and cold.

For treatment, resolve heat toxin with the coldness of cold water or yellow earth water, and drink concentrated fermented soybean juice to remove the toxin by ejection. Cinnamon bark and garlic are both greatly acrid and hot and therefore free blood in the vessels and repel foul evil, thus treating heat with heat.

Line 25.21

正月勿食葱，令人面生游风。

Zhèng yuè wù shí cōng, lìng rén miàn shēng yóu fēng.

In the first month, do not eat scallions. They engender wandering wind on the person's face.

COMMENTARY, LINE 25.21

In the first month, wind qì stirs. Scallions are contraindicated at this time because they are acrid and dissipating, freeing yáng qì and penetrating to the head and face. Eating raw scallion at this time thus induces wind evil to stir.

Line 25.22

二月勿食蓼，伤人肾。

Èr yuè wù shí liáo, shāng rén shèn.

In the second month, do not eat smartweed. It damages the person's kidney.

COMMENTARY, LINE 25.22

In the second month, liver-wood is effulgent. Smartweed is acrid and dissipating, and can penetrate into the kidney, which governs closure and storage. Excessive consumption of smartweed can damage kidney essence, and since water engenders wood, it can also affect the engenderment of liver-wood.

Line 25.23

三月勿食小蒜，伤人志性。

Sān yuè wù shí xiǎo suàn, shāng rén zhì xìng.

In the third month, do not eat rocambole. It damages the person's mind and nature.

COMMENTARY, LINE 25.23

Rocambole (*Allium scorodoprasum,* sand leek) is acrid, hot, malodorous, turbid, and toxic. It despoliates qì and damages the spirit. In the third month, yáng qì is exuberant. The mind is rooted in the kidney, and nature is controlled by the heart. Over-consumption of rocambole thus damages the person's kidney and mind, and heart and nature.

Line 25.24

四月、八月勿食胡荽，伤人神。

Sì yuè, bā yuè wù shí hú suī, shāng rén shén.

In the fourth and eighth months, do not eat wu shi coriander. It damages the person's spirit.

COMMENTARY, LINE 25.24

In the fourth month, heart fire is effulgent, and in the eighth month, lung qì is effulgent. Coriander is acrid and warm, and its aroma penetrates the orifices. Eating it at these times damages the spirit.

Line 25.25

五月勿食韭，令人乏气力。

Wǔ yuè wù shí jiǔ, lìng rén fá qì lì.

In the fifth month, do not eat garlic chive. It causes the person to lack qì and physical strength.

COMMENTARY, LINE 25.25

Garlic chive is fragrant in the spring, but has a strong malodor by the fifth month, and should therefore be avoided at this time. In early medicine, the spleen was said to govern the four limbs and to be averse to malodor. Hence the acrid, warm, and upbearing and effusing nature of garlic chive, when eaten in excess, can cause a lack of qì and physical strength.

Line 25.26

五月五日勿食一切生菜，发百病。

Wǔ yuè wǔ rì wù shí yī qiē shēng cài, fā bǎi bìng.

On the fifth day of the fifth month, do not eat any raw vegetables. It will cause the hundred diseases to arise.

COMMENTARY, LINE 25.26

The fifth day of the fifth month is the time of pure yáng exuberance. Raw vegetables are cold and disinhibiting; they do not boost the intestines and stomach, but discharge yáng qì. Eating them can therefore cause disease.

Line 25.27

六月、七月勿食茱萸，伤神气。

Liù yuè, qī yuè wù shí zhū yú, shāng shén qì.

In the sixth and seventh months, do not eat Japanese prickly ash. It damages spirit qì.

COMMENTARY, LINE 25.26

Japanese prickly ash (食茱萸 *shí zhū yú*), *Zanthoxylum ailanthoides*, is acrid and hot and penetrates qì. In the sixth month, yáng qì is in its prime; in the seventh month, yīn begins to constrain. Eating Japanese prickly ash at this time can damage spirit qì.

Line 25.28

八月、九月勿食姜，伤人神。

Bā yuè, jiǔ yuè wù shí jiāng, shāng rén shén.

In the eighth and ninth months, do not eat ginger. It damages the person's spirit.

COMMENTARY, LINE 25.28

The eighth and ninth months are the time when spirit qì contracts. If eaten at this time, ginger, which is acrid and dissipating, damages the spirit.

Line 25.29

十月勿食椒，损人心，伤人脉。

Shí yuè wù shí jiāo, sǔn rén xīn, shāng rén mài.

In the tenth month, do not eat zanthoxylum. It damages the person's heart and vessels.

COMMENTARY, LINE 25.29

The tenth month is the time when heart yáng is in charge of defense qì. Hot, acrid and spicy zanthoxylum (Sichuan peppercorn) penetrates qì to damage the heart. Eaten in excess, it will damage heart yáng and defense qì, and wear the heart vessels.

Line 25.30

十一月，十二月勿食薤 令人多涕唾。

Shí yī yuè, shí èr yuè wù shí xiè, lìng rén duō tì tuò.

In the eleventh and twelfth months, do not eat long-stamen onion. It causes profuse snivel and spittle.

COMMENTARY, LINE 25.30

Long-stamen onion is warm and lubricating by nature. It dissipates and discharges lung and stomach qì, and draws snivel and spittle. This effect is particularly pronounced in the eleventh and twelfth months, which is the coldest season of the year.

Line 25.31

四季勿食生葵，令人饮食不化，发百病，非但食中，药中皆不可用，深宜慎之。

Sì jì wù shí shēng kuí, lìng rén yǐn shí bù huà, fā bǎi bìng, fēi dàn shí zhōng, yào zhōng jiē bù kě yòng, shēn yí shèn zhī.

In the last months of the four seasons, do not eat raw mallow. It causes non-transformation of food and drink and eruption of the hundred diseases. This [rule] applies not only for its use in food, but you must not use it in medicines either. Pay close attention to this.

Commentary, Line 25.31

In the last month of each season, spleen-earth is effulgent. Mallow is lubricating and disinhibiting and thereby damages the spleen. It causes indigestion, from which the other diseases can arise.

Line 25.32

时病差未健，食生菜，手足必肿。

Shí bìng chài wèi jiàn, shí shēng cài, shǒu zú bì zhǒng.

Eating raw vegetables after recovering from seasonal disease, when health is not yet firmly established, invariably causes swelling of the extremities.

Commentary, Line 25.32

Seasonal disease means heat disease. After a recent recovery from heat disease, the spleen and stomach are still weak. Raw vegetables, when eaten in excess, can damage spleen yáng with their cold and thereby impair splenic movement, so that water-damp stagnates in the skin and flesh. Hence we see puffy swelling of the extremities.

Line 25.33

夜食生菜，不利人。

Yè shí shēng cài, bù lì rén.

Eating raw vegetables at night does not benefit people.

Commentary, Line 25.33

Consuming excessive amounts of raw vegetables at night can impair the movement of spleen yáng and thus inhibit digestion.

Line 25.34

十月勿食被霜生菜，令人面无光，目涩心痛，腰疼，或发心疟，疟发时，手足十指爪皆青，困萎。

Shí yuè wù shí bèi shuāng shēng cài, lìng rén miàn wú guāng, mù sè xīn tòng, yāo téng, huò fā xīn nüè, nüè fā shí, shǒu zú shí zhǐ zhǎo jiē qīng, kùn wěi.

In the tenth month, do not eat raw vegetables that have been exposed to frost, [this] will cause a dull facial complexion, dry eyes, heart and lumbar pain, and possibly malaria in the heart, green-blue nails on all the fingers and toes, and encumbrance and wilting at the time of attacks.

COMMENTARY, LINE 25.34

The tenth month is the beginning of winter, and the time when heart yáng is in charge of defense qì. The cold nature of raw vegetables is further increased after they have been exposed to frost. Eating them can thus damage heart yáng, causing the symptoms described here. When visiting cold and heart yáng struggle with each other, in extreme cases this can cause malaria.

Line 25.35

葱、韭初生芽者，食之伤人心气。

Cōng, jiǔ chū shēng yá zhě, shí zhī shāng rén xīn qì.

Eating scallion and garlic chive when they first begin to sprout damages the person's heart qì.

COMMENTARY, LINE 25.35

The heart is averse to acrid and hot scallion and garlic chive in any state, but particularly when they are just beginning to sprout, because they are not mature yet and their ability to fight depression is not developed yet. Eating them can cloud and dissipate the person's spirit light, thus damaging heart qì.

Line 25.36

饮白酒食生韭，令人病增。

Yǐn bái jiǔ shí shēng jiǔ, lìng rén bìng zēng.

Drinking white wine and eating raw long-stamen onions increases a person's diseases.

COMMENTARY, LINE 25.36

White wine is floating by nature and engenders dampness, while raw long-stamen onions are acrid and warm and stir heat. When eaten together, dampness and heat combine and can easily aggravate damp-heat conditions like panting, cough, dizziness, and surging qì.

Line 25.37

生葱不可共蜜，食之杀人。独颗蒜，弥忌。

Shēng cōng bù kě gòng mì shí zhī, shā rén. Dú kē suàn, mí jì.

Raw scallion must not be combined with honey. Eating it kills the person. Single-stalk garlic[1] is particularly forbidden.

TEXT NOTE, LINE 25.37

[1] "Single-stalk" garlic 独颗蒜 *dú kē suàn*: likely refers simply to garlic, emphasizing that it only has one flower stalk, by contrast to scallions, which have multiple flower stalks.

COMMENTARY, LINE 25.37

According to the *Qiān Jīn Fāng* ("Thousand Gold Pieces Prescriptions"), "Eating raw scallion and then honey causes diarrhea. Eating burned scallion and then honey causes death from qì congestion."

Line 25.38

枣合生葱食之，令人病。

Zǎo gě shēng cōng shí zhī, lìng rén bìng.

Eating jujube with raw scallion makes the person ill.

COMMENTARY, LINE 25.38

Raw jujube is acrid, hot, and sweet. When eaten in excess, it promotes damp-heat and causes heat thirst and inflation. In combination with acrid and warm raw scallion, it causes disharmony of the five viscera.

Line 25.39

生葱和雄鸡、雉、白犬肉食之，令人七窍经年流血。

Shēng cōng hé xióng jī, zhì, bái quǎn ròu shí zhī, lìng rén qī qiào jīng nián liú xuè.

Eating raw scallion together with the meat of roosters, ring-necked pheasants, or white dogs causes bleeding from the seven orifices for years to come.

COMMENTARY, LINE 25.39

All the substances mentioned in this line are acrid, floating, and warm or hot. Hence they engender wind and flare fire. Eaten in combination, they can cause disharmony of qì and blood, and easily stir wind-heat, which results in frequent bleeding from the seven orifices. This prohibition is particularly relevant to persons having vacuity of yīn and effulgence of yáng.

Line 25.40

食糖、蜜后四日内食生葱、韭，令人心痛。

Shí tang, mì hòu sì rì nèi shí shēng cōng, jiǔ, lìng rén xīn tòng.

Eating raw scallion or garlic chive within four days of eating sugar or honey causes heart pain.

COMMENTARY, LINE 25.40

In early texts, raw scallion and garlic chive were said to clash with sugar and honey. Hence they were not to be eaten too closely together.

Line 25.41

夜食诸姜、蒜、葱等，伤人心。

Yè shí zhū jiāng, suàn, cōng děng, shāng rén xīn.

Eating any ginger, garlic, or scallions at night damages the person's heart.

COMMENTARY, LINE 25.41

In the human body, qì moves in yáng during the day, and in yīn during the night. Eating excessive amounts of acrid hot foods like ginger, garlic, or scallion can easily damage yīn-blood, stir heart yáng, and have a stimulating effect that keeps the person from sleeping.

Line 25.42

芜菁根，多食令人气胀。

Wú jīng gēn, duō shí lìng rén qì zhàng.

Eating turnip root in excess causes qì distention.

COMMENTARY, LINE 25.42

Turnip root and leaf is bitter, warm, acrid, and sweet, and is especially delicious when eaten with goat meat. However, eaten in excess it can stir qì and congest the center, hence causing qì distention.

Line 25.43

薤不共牛肉作羹，食之成瘕病，韭亦然。

Xiè bù gòng niú ròu zuò gēng, shí zhī chéng jiǎ bìng, jiǔ yì rán.

You must not combine long-stamen onion with beef to make meat broth. Eating it creates conglomerations. The same is true for garlic chive.

Line 25.44

莼多食，动痔疾。

Chún duō shí, dòng zhì jí.

Eating water shield (*Brasenia schreberi*) in excess causes stirring and hemorrhoidal disease.

COMMENTARY, LINE 25.44

Water shield, also called 水葵 *shuǐ kuí* in Chinese, is sweet, cold, and extremely stagnating and slimy. Eaten in excess, it can easily cause qì congestion, and in severe cases vanquishing and stirring of stomach qì, abdominal cold and pain, and hemorrhoids due to blood stagnation in the intestinal vessels and to downpour of toxic qì.

Line 25.45

野苣不可同蜜食之，作内痔。

Yě jù kě tóng mì shí zhī, zuò nèi zhì.

You must not eat bitter sow thistle[1] together with honey. It will cause internal hemorrhoids.

TEXT NOTE, LINE 25.45

[1] Bitter sow thistle 野苣 *yě jù*: According to the commentary, this is identical with 苦菜 *kǔ cài*, the more common term for bitter sow thistle (*Sonchi Oleracei Herba*).

COMMENTARY, LINE 25.45

The *Shén Nóng Běn Cǎo Jīng* ("Divine Husbandman's Herbal Foundation Canon") describes bitter sow thistle as bitter, cold, and non-toxic, and able to treat hemorrhoids. By contrast, honey is sweet and warm and when eaten in excess can engender conditions of wind-damp-heat. These two substances have opposite natures, and eating them together can force heat to descend into the intestines, resulting in hemorrhoids.

Line 25.46

白苣不可共酪同食，作䘌虫。

Bái jù bù kě gòng luò tóng shí, zuò nì chóng.

Lettuce must not be eaten together with koumiss (fermented mare's milk), as it causes invisible eroding worms.[1]

TEXT NOTE, LINE 25.46

[1] Invisible eroding worms (䘌虫 *nì chóng*): In early China, skin conditions characterized by erosion and ulceration were often attributed to the action of worms that could not be seen with the naked eye.

COMMENTARY, LINE 25.46

Lettuce, also called 莴苣 *wō jù* in Chinese, is bitter and cold, while koumiss is sweet and hot. Combining cold and heat creates dampness, thereby engendering worms.

Line 25.47

黄瓜食之，发热病。

Huáng guā shí zhī, fā rè bìng.

Eating cucumber causes heat diseases to erupt.

COMMENTARY, LINE 25.47

Cucumber, also called 胡瓜 *hú guā* in Chinese, is sweet, cold, and slightly toxic. Eaten in excess, it stirs heat and cold, consumes yīn-blood, and causes counterflow ascent of vacuity heat and shortage of qì. It should be avoided particularly after heaven-current heat disease.

Line 25.48

葵心不可食，伤人；叶尤冷，黄背赤茎者，勿食之。

Kuí xīn bù kě shí, shāng rén; yè yóu lěng, huáng bèi chì jīng zhě, wù shí zhī.

Mallow heart[1] is inedible. It damages people. The leaves are exceptionally cold. Do not eat ones with a yellow back and red stalk.

Text Note, Line 25.48

[1] Mallow heart 葵心 *kuí xīn*: The tender leaves at the heart of the plant.

Commentary, Line 25.48

The tender heart of mallow leaves and leaves with a yellow back and red stalk all are toxic. Because of their bitter, cold, and lubricating nature, they can injure yáng qì in the spleen, stomach, and heart.

Line 25.49

胡荽久食之，令人多忘。

Hú suī jiǔ shí zhī, lìng rén duō wàng.

Eating coriander over a long period of time causes forgetfulness.

Commentary, Line 25.49

Coriander is acrid, warm, fuming, and malodorous. It dissipates qì and opens the orifices. Over time, it can wear on heart blood and therefore reduce a person's memory.

Line 25.50

病人不可食胡荽及黄花菜。

Bìng rén bù kě shí hú suī jí huáng huā cài.

Sick people must not eat coriander or Yúnnán day lily root.

Commentary, Line 25.49

These two substances are contraindicated because coriander wears on qì, while day lily breaks qì and wears on blood.

According to one commentary, Yúnnán day lily root (黄花菜 *huáng huā cài*) does not refer to day lily, but rather is an alternative term for cucumber leaf (黄瓜叶 *huáng guā yè*), which in the third to fifth months has yellow flowers. It is sweet, slightly bitter, slightly cold, frees bound qì, and disinhibits the intestines and stomach.

Line 25.51

芋不可多食，动病。

Yù bù kě duō shí, dòng bìng.

Taro must not be eaten in excess, as it stirs disease.[1]

TEXT NOTE, LINE 25.51

[1] Stirs disease 动病 *dòng bìng*: According to an alternate textual version, this should be read as 动气 *dòng qì* "stirs qì" instead.

COMMENTARY, LINE 25.51

Taro is stagnating and difficult to digest. When eaten in excess, it causes distention and oppression in the chest and abdomen. The *Běn Cǎo Gāng Mù* states that taro, "when eaten in excess, stirs abiding cold."

Line 25.52

妊娠食姜，令子余指。

Rèn shēn shí jiāng, lìng zǐ yú zhǐ.

Eating ginger in pregnancy can cause the child to have extra fingers.

COMMENTARY, LINE 25.52

This contraindication relates to the appearance of ginger, which has appendages that resemble fingers and was therefore believed to stimulate the growth of extra fingers in the fetus.

Line 25.53

蓼多食，发心痛。

Liáo duō shí, fā xīn tòng.

Eating water pepper fruit in excess causes heart pain to erupt.

COMMENTARY, LINE 25.53

Water pepper fruit is acrid, hot, and toxic. Eaten in excess, it can dissipate qì with its acridity, and consume blood with its dryness and heat.

Line 25.54

蓼和生鱼食之，令人夺气，阴咳疼痛。

Liáo hé shēng yú shí zhī, lìng rén duó qì, yīn ké téng tòng.

Eating water pepper fruit together with raw fish despoliates the person's qì and causes pain in the scrotum.[1]

Text Note, Line 25.54

[1] Pain in the scrotum 阴咳疼痛 *yīn ké téng tòng*: The quotation of this passage in the *Qiān Jīn Fāng* and *Yī Xīn Fāng* ("Heart of Medicine") has 核 *hé* instead of 咳 *ké*. 阴核 is a synonym for 阴囊 *yīn náng*.

Commentary, Line 25.54

Because water pepper fruit downbears qì, and raw fish is cold, eating them in combination despoliates the person's qì and causes pain in the scrotum from damp-heat pouring downward. Alternatively, we can interpret 阴咳 *yīn ké* literally as "yīn cough," which is the opposite of yáng cough or qì congestion counterflow.

Line 25.55

芥菜不可共兔肉食之，成恶邪病。

Jiè cài bù kě gòng tù ròu shí zhī, chéng wù xié bìng.

Mustard leaf must not be eaten together with rabbit's flesh. It creates malign and evil disease.

Commentary, Line 25.55

Mustard leaf is acrid and hot, and, because of its strong aroma, dissipating. Eaten in excess, it consumes the person's true original spirit qì. Rabbit's flesh is sweet, cold, and sour. These two substances are opposite by nature and should therefore not be eaten together. According to Chéng Lín 程林, "mustard leaf clouds the person's vision, and rabbit's flesh damages the person's spirit qì."

Line 25.56

小蒜多食，伤人心力。

Xiǎo suàn duō shí, shāng rén xīn lì.

Eating rocambole in excess damages the person's heart strength.

COMMENTARY, LINE 25.56

Rocambole is acrid and hot and consumes qì. A person's strength relies on qì, and when qì is consumed by eating rocambole, the heart strength is damaged.

Line 25.57

食躁或躁方

豆豉

浓煮汁饮之。

Shí zào huò zào fāng

Dòu chǐ

Nóng zhǔ zhī yǐn zhī.

A formula for agitation from eating or agitation from possible [other causes]:

fermented soybean (豆豉 *dòu chǐ*, Glycines Semen Fermentatum)

Boil into a concentrated liquid and drink..

COMMENTARY, LINE 25.57

Agitation from eating refers to vexation and agitation that arises as a result of eating toxic food. It is due to toxin entering the stomach, so that vacuity fire in the stomach floats upward into the stomach duct. Agitation from possible other sources refers to vexation and agitation that can also be due to any other cause besides food. It is a sign of yīn vacuity, and fire surging into the stomach duct and diaphragm. Fermented soybean is able to enrich yīn, resolve toxin, downbear fire, and stop vexation. Drinking the concentrated liquid is therefore a suitable treatment here.

Line 25.58

钩吻与芹菜相似，误食之杀人，解之方

荠苨八两

右一味, 水六升, 煮取二升, 分温二服。

Gōu wěn yǔ qín cài xiāng sì, wù shí zhī shā rén, jiě zhī fāng

Jì ní bā liǎng

Yòu yī wèi, shuǐ liù shēng, zhǔ qǔ èr shēng, fēn wēn èr fú.

Yellow jessamine (Gelsemii Herba) resembles mustard leaf.[1] Eating it by mistake will kill the person. A formula to resolve [the toxin]:[2]

apricot-leaved adenophora (荠苨 *jì ní*, Adenophorae Trachelioidis Radix) 8 *liǎng*

Boil the above single ingredient in six *shēng* of water to get two *shēng*. Divide into two doses and take warm.[3]

TEXT NOTES, LINE 25.58

[1] Celery 芹菜 *qín cài:* 芹 *qín*, celery, is probably a mistake for 芥 *jiè*, mustard leaf, which is the leaf of *Sinapis juncea*, since 芥 *jiè* appears in other texts, including the *Zhǒu Hòu Bèi Jí Fāng* ("Emergency Standby Remedies") quoted under the formula, and unlike celery has long leaves like yellow jessamine.

[2] A comment included in the received text reads: "The *Zhǒu Hòu Bèi Jí Fāng* ("Emergency Standby Remedies") states that it resembles ailanthus zanthoxylum and edible mustard leaf." (《肘后》云：与茱萸食芥相似). The quotation says 茱萸 *zhū yú*, which might mean the medicinals evodia (吴茱萸 *wú zhū yú*, Evodiae Fructus) or cornus (山茱萸 *shān zhū yú*, Corni Fructus). Alternatively, it may well denote Japanese prickly ash (食茱萸 *shí zhū yú*), Zanthoxylum ailanthoides, of which the fruit was eaten as food.

[3] The commentary notes: "Yellow jessamine grows on soil where no other herbs grow. Its stalk is hairy. By these signs you can differentiate it."

COMMENTARY, LINE 25.58

Yellow jessamine is acrid and warm and very toxic. As the name implies, it "hooks the corners of the mouth" when it is eaten. The main symptoms of poisoning by this plant include dizziness, numbness of the four limbs, lack of strength in the flesh, difficulty swallowing, stupor, vacuity desertion, difficulty breathing, and in severe cases paralysis. This is accompanied by scorching pain in the oral cavity and throat, abdominal pain and diarrhea, nausea and vomiting, dilated pupils, diplopia, and drooping eyelids.

Apricot-leaved adenophora is sweet and cold, and in the materia medica texts it is described as treating poisoning from yellow jessamine, as well as poisoning from the hundred herbs in general.

Line 25.59

菜中有水莨菪，叶圆而光，有毒，误食之，令人狂乱，状如中风，或吐血，治之方

甘草

煮汁服之，即解。

Cài zhōng yǒu shuǐ làng dàng, yè yuán ér guāng, yǒu dú, wù shí zhī, lìng rén kuáng luàn, zhuàng rú zhōng fēng, huò tù xuè, zhì zhī fāng

Gān cǎo

Zhǔ zhī fú zhī, jí jiě.

If among other vegetables there is water henbane (*shuǐ làng dàng*), which has round and shiny leaves and is toxic, eating it will cause manic derangement that resembles wind-stroke, possibly with blood ejection. A formula to treat this:

licorice (甘草 *gān cǎo*, Glycyrrhizae Radix)

Boil and take the juice. This will resolve [the toxin].

COMMENTARY, LINE 25.59

Mistakenly eating henbane shoots or leaves that may be hidden among other greens causes a severe eruption of heat toxin, clouding the person's spirit light and dissipating heart qì. The result is manic derangement and an appearance like wind-stroke. If the blood follows qì and gushes forth, blood ejection may be seen.

Licorice resolves toxin and clears heat; hence it is a suitable treatment for henbane poisoning.

Line 25.60

春秋二时，龙带精入芹菜中，人偶食之为病。发时手青背腹满，痛不可忍，名蛟龙病。治之方：

硬糖二三升

右一味，日两度服之，吐出如蜥蜴三五枚，差。

Chūn qiū èr shí, lóng dài jīng rù qín cài zhōng, rén ǒu shí zhī wéi bìng. Fā shí shǒu qīng fù mǎn, tòng bù kě rěn, míng jiāo lóng bìng. Zhì zhī fāng:

Yìng táng èr sān shēng

Yòu yī wèi, rì liǎng duò fú zhī, tù chū rú xī yì sān wǔ méi, chài.

During the two seasons of spring and fall, the flood dragon carries essence and enters celery. If a person happens to eat it, disease arises. Outbreaks [manifest with] greenish blackness in the hands, abdominal fullness, and unbearable pain. This is called "Flood Dragon Disease." A formula to treat it:

hard malt sugar[1] (硬糖 *yìng táng*, Maltosum Durum) 2–3 *shēng*

Take the above single ingredient twice a day. Ejecting 3–5 lizard-like [creatures] indicates recovery.

TEXT NOTE, LINE 25.60

[1] Hard malt sugar (硬糖 *yìng táng*, Maltosum Durum): This is explained as a thick, hard form of malt sugar (饴糖 *yí táng*, Maltosum).

COMMENTARY, LINE 25.60

Celery grows in moist places. According to old Chinese legend, in the spring and fall, the flood dragon, a creature related to lizards and poisonous snakes, leaves its essence on celery, which can enter humans when they consume the celery. The resulting poisoning manifests as green-blue hands, abdominal fullness, and unbearable pain. Warm, relaxing, and toxin-resolving hard malt sugar (*yìng táng*) can treat this.

Line 25.61

食苦瓠中毒治之方
黎穰
煮汁，数服之，解。

Shí kŭ hù zhōng dú zhì zhī fāng
Lí ráng
Zhŭ zhī, shù fú zhī, jiě.

A formula to treat poisoning from eating bitter calabash:

lí rang[1] 黎穰

Boil and take the juice several times to resolve [the toxin].

TEXT NOTE, LINE 25.61

[1] 黎穰 *lí ráng*: Commentators disagree on the identity of this medicinal substance. According to Lǐ Shí-Zhēn 李时珍, the character 黎 *lí* refers to broomcorn millet (黍 *shŭ*), while Gāo Xué-Shān 高学山 identifies it as sorghum (高梁 *gāo liáng*). The second character of the compound, 穰 *ráng*, means grain stalks.

COMMENTARY, LINE 25.61

Both the pulp and seeds of bitter calabash are bitter, cold, and toxic. If eaten in excess, they cause incessant vomiting and diarrhea. The stalk and roots of broomcorn millet are acrid, hot, and slightly toxic. Because its nature is feared by bitter calabash, drinking the juice of boiled broomcorn millet stalk can resolve bitter calabash toxin.

Line 25.62

扁豆，寒热者不可食之。

Biăn dòu, hán rè zhě bù kě shí zhī.

Persons with [aversion to] cold and heat [effusion] must not eat lablab.

COMMENTARY, LINE 25.62

Lablab is stagnating by nature; it is sweet and warm, and boosts qì. However, it is contraindicated in patients with aversion to cold and heat effusion, so as to avoid lodging external evil.

Line 25.63

久食小豆，令人枯燥。

Jiŭ shí xiăo dòu, lìng rén kū zào.

Eating black gram[1] for a long time causes dryness in the person.

TEXT NOTE, LINE 25.63

[1] Black gram 小豆 *xiǎo dòu*: According to one commentator, this refers to rice bean (赤小豆 *chì xiǎo dòu*).

COMMENTARY, LINE 25.63

Consumption of rice beans over a long period of time can excessively disinhibit urine and in severe cases remove oils and percolate liquid and blood, thereby emaciating the flesh and desiccating the skin.

Line 25.64

食大豆屑，忌啖猪肉。

Shí dà dòu xiè, jì dàn zhū ròu.

When eating soybean flakes, it is forbidden to [also] eat pork.

COMMENTARY, LINE 25.64

Soybean congests qì, while pork stagnates the diaphragm. Therefore eating these foods in combination is contraindicated, especially in children under 10 years of age.

Line 25.65

大麦久食，令人作癣。

Dà mài jiǔ shí, lìng rén zuò xiǎn.

Eating barley for a long time will cause lichen.

COMMENTARY, LINE 25.65

Barley is one of the five grains mentioned by Lǐ Shí-Zhēn 李时珍. The *Qiān Jīn Fāng* ("Thousand Gold Pieces Prescriptions") describes the effect of eating barley over a long period of time as "increasing strength and fortifying one's actions." Nevertheless, Chéng Lín 程林 stated that it "precipitates qì and therefore over time causes wilting, weakness, and laziness in the hands and feet." It is possible that the character 癣 *xiǎn* (literally, lichen) is here a mistake for 懈 *xiè* (sluggishness). On the other hand, the appearance of lichen as a result of eating barley can also be explained by the fact that it enters the heart and over time causes an exuberance of heart qì and internal heat, which is the cause of all itching and sores.

Line 25.66

白黍米不可同饴蜜食，亦不可合葵食之。

Bái shǔ mǐ bù kě tóng yí mì shí, yì bù kě gě kuí shí zhī.

You must not eat white broomcorn millet together with malt sugar or honey or in combination with mallow.

Commentary, Line 25.66

White broomcorn millet is sweet and warm, and when eaten over a long period of time can cause increased heat vexation. Malt sugar and honey are also sweet and cause center fullness. Thus eating these substances together will lead to abiding heat. In particular, chronically ill patients must also avoid combining white broomcorn millet with foods of the opposite nature, such as mallow, which is cold and lubricating. Otherwise a chronic condition will become even more difficult to treat.

Line 25.67

荍麦面多食之，令人发落。

Qiáo mài miàn duō shí zhī, lìng rén fǎ luò.

Eating buckwheat flour in excess causes the person's hair to fall out.

Commentary, Line 25.67

Buckwheat flour is sour and slightly cold, and difficult to digest. Eaten in excess, it stirs wind and causes dizziness. When eaten with pork or goat meat, it can cause the eyebrows and whiskers to fall out. According to Lǐ Shí-Zhēn 李时珍, "it downbears qì and thickens the intestines and is therefore able to… treat turbid discharge, diarrhea, and dysentery, and abdominal pain and qì ascent. It is suitable for patients with qì exuberance and damp-heat. [However,] if eaten by patients with spleen-stomach vacuity cold, it results in great desertion of original qì and loss of whiskers and eyebrows."

Line 25.68

盐多食，伤人肺。

Yán duō shí, shāng rén fèi.

Eating salt in excess damages the person's lung.

COMMENTARY, LINE 25.68

Eating excessive amounts of salt causes the gathering of rheum and engenders dampness. These enter the kidney, which is connected to the lung. The lung is averse to rheum and dampness. Hence salt damages the lung, causing cough, wheezing and panting, loss of color and blackened skin, and reduced physical strength. Persons with water swelling and dispersion-thirst should particularly avoid it.

Line 25.69

食冷物, 冰人齿。食热物, 勿饮冷水。

Shí lěng wù, bīng rén chǐ. Shí rè wù, wù yǐn lěng shuǐ.

Eating cold foods makes a person's teeth cold. When eating hot foods, do not drink cold water.

COMMENTARY, LINE 25.69

Eating excessively cold foods causes cold to collect on the surface of the teeth, so that they contract. This can easily damage the teeth. In addition, you should not drink cold water immediately after eating hot foods, because cold and heat contend with each other. This damages the spleen and stomach, resulting in vomiting and diarrhea, or transmuting into dampness patterns.

Line 25.70

饮酒，食生苍耳，令人心痛。

Yǐn jiǔ, shí shēng cāng ěr, lìng rén xīn tòng.

Drinking wine and eating fresh xanthium causes heart pain.

COMMENTARY, LINE 25.70

Xanthium is bitter, warm, and toxic by nature. Its bitterness enters the heart first. Drinking wine, which is pure yáng, after eating xanthium (cocklebur) will further move its poison and endanger the heart, causing heart pain.

Line 25.71

夏月大醉汗流，不得冷水洗着身，及使扇，即成病。

Xià yuè dà zuì hàn liú, bù dé lěng shuǐ xǐ zhù shēn, jí shǐ shàn, jí chéng bìng.

When a person gets greatly intoxicated in the summer months so that sweat pours out, they must not wash with cold water or fan the sweat, as this will create disease.

COMMENTARY, LINE 25.71

Getting drunk and sweating during the summer months causes the interstices to be open. Bathing in cold water or being fanned causes wind and dampness to contend, creating disease. According to the *Shén Nóng Běn Cǎo Jīng* ("Divine Husbandman's Herbal Foundation Canon"), bathing when sweating causes yellow sweat, and the *Nèi Jīng* ("The Inner Canon") warns that being struck by wind after drinking wine causes the disease of "leaking wind" and must therefore be avoided.

Line 25.72

饮酒大忌灸腹背，令人肠结。

Yǐn jiǔ dà jì jiǔ fù bèi, lìng rén cháng jié.

When drinking wine, burning moxa on the abdomen or back is greatly contraindicated. It causes intestinal bind.

COMMENTARY, LINE 25.72

The abdomen contains many alarm points and is the place where channel qì gathers. The back has many transport points and is the place where channel qì is transferred. Wine is hot by nature and disinhibits the movement of blood. Moxibustion uses moxa, which is bitter, acrid, and warm, to free the twelve channels and disinhibit qì and blood. After drinking wine, the blood is hot and moves frenetically. Hence, burning moxa at this time on the abdominal and back points can internally attack with force, in spite of the fact that the force of fire itself is small. The two yáng scorch each other, heat and dryness bind in the intestines and stomach, and thereby cause intestinal bind.

Line 25.73

醉后勿饱食，发寒热。

Zuì hòu wù bǎo shí, fā hán rè.

After becoming inebriated, do not eat to satiety. It causes [aversion to] cold and heat [effusion].

COMMENTARY, LINE 25.73

In and of itself, inebriation greatly damages liver qì. Overeating when in this condition will cause liver and gallbladder qì to move wantonly. Consequently, wood rebels against earth and damages the spleen and stomach. This affects the disinhibited movement of construction and defense, as a result of which center qì is not contained and overacts towards defense. Yáng merging with the outside results in heat effusion, and yīn interfering with the exterior results in aversion to cold.

Line 25.74

饮酒食猪肉，卧秫稻穰中，则发黄。

Yǐn jiǔ shí zhū ròu, wò shú dào ráng zhōng, zé fā huáng.

Drinking wine, eating pork, and [then] sleeping on sorghum or rice straw results in yellowing.

COMMENTARY, LINE 25.74

Drinking wine causes the interstices to be open, as a result of which damp-heat is able to enter the spleen and stomach and invade the blood aspect. Moved by depressed heat, this can then cause generalized yellowing.

Line 25.75

食饴，多饮酒大忌。

Shí yí, duō yǐn jiǔ dà jì.

Eating malt sugar and excessively drinking wine is greatly contraindicated.

COMMENTARY, LINE 25.75

When a person eats malt candy, which is very sweet, while drinking excessive amounts of alcohol, damp-heat can easily lodge in the center burner and possibly engender the various symptoms of retching, oppression, fullness, and veiling. Hence we say that "drinkers must avoid sweetness" (酒家忌甘 *jiǔ jiā jì gān*).

Line 25.76

凡水及酒, 照见人影动者, 不可饮之。

Fán shuǐ jí jiǔ, zhào jiàn rén yǐng dòng zhě, bù kě yǐn zhī.

Whenever a person's reflection in water or wine stirs, they must not drink it.

COMMENTARY, LINE 25.76

This line describes a situation where a person looking at their reflection in water or wine and perceives it as moving even though they themselves are still. This could be understood in two different ways. According to Chéng Lín 程林, the stirring water or wine indicates that a supernatural entity is involved that is moving the fluid, as a result of which the fluid should not be drunk. According to a modern commentary, the fact that a person perceives their reflection as moving indicates that the person is already overly intoxicated and must therefore not be allowed to drink any more wine.

Line 25.77

醋合酪食之，令人血瘕。

cù gě luò shí zhī, lìng rén xuè jiǎ.

Eating vinegar in combination with koumiss causes blood conglomerations.

COMMENTARY, LINE 25.77

Vinegar is sour and constraining, while koumiss (fermented mare's milk) is sticky and stagnating. Eating these substances together invariably damages the liver and inhibits the blood flow, as a result of which blood conglomerations arise.

Line 25.78

食白米粥，勿食生苍耳，成走疰。

Shí bái mǐ zhōu, wù shí shēng cāng ěr, chéng zǒu zhù.

When eating white rice gruel, do not eat raw xanthium herb. It creates wandering infixation.[1]

TEXT NOTE, LINE 25.78

[1] Wandering infixation 走疰 *zǒu zhù*: In this term, wandering refers to the fact that evil has spread into the skin and comes and goes, accompanied by pain without a fixed location.

COMMENTARY, LINE 25.78

White rice gruel is sweet, warm, and bland. It is able to percolate and disinhibit urine and to "swiftly rouse the essence in the stomach." Xanthium stalk and leaf is bitter, acrid, and slightly cold. It has the effect of tracking down wind, and if eaten raw, drying dampness and desiccating blood. These two medicinals are opposite in nature and therefore contraindicated for consumption in combination.

Line 25.79

食甜粥已，食盐即吐。

Shí tián zhōu yǐ, shí yán jí tù.

Eating salt after eating sweet gruel results in vomiting.

COMMENTARY, LINE 25.79

Eating sweet substances causes fullness in the center, and the sweetness invariably sticks to the top of the diaphragm. In this situation, consuming excessive amounts of salt will cause it to gush out.

Line 25.80

犀角筋搅饮食，沫出，及浇地坟起者，食之杀人。

Xī jiǎo jīn jiǎo yǐn shí, mò chū, jí jiāo dì fén qǐ zhě, shí zhī shā rén.

If food or drink that is stirred with chopsticks made from rhinoceros horn froths or causes veins to appear when poured on the ground, eating it kills the person.

COMMENTARY, LINE 25.80

As the *Běn Cǎo Gāng Mù* explains, rhinoceros horn is able to resolve toxin "because the rhinoceros eats the toxin of the hundred herbs and the thorns of masses of trees." For this reason, food stirred with chopsticks made from rhinoceros horn that froths when stirred or that veins when poured on the ground indicates that the rhinoceros horn is transforming the toxin. Stirring food with rhinoceros horn was therefore an ancient technique for determining the toxicity of food.

Line 25.81

饮食中毒， 烦满， 治之方

苦参三两　苦酒一升半

右二味， 煮三沸， 三上三下，服之，吐食出即差。 或以水煮亦得。

又方犀角汤亦佳。

Yǐn shí zhōng dú, fán mǎn, zhì zhī fāng

Kǔ shēn sān liǎng kǔ jiǔ yī shēng bàn

Yòu èr wèi, zhǔ sān fèi, sān shàng, sān xià fú zhī, tù shí chū jí chài. Huò yǐ shuǐ zhǔ yì dé.

Yòu fāng xī jiǎo tāng yì jiā.

A formula to treat poisoning from food or drink [that manifests] with vexation and fullness.

flavescent sophora (苦参 *kǔ shēn*, Sophorae Flavescentis Radix) 3 *liǎng*
vinegar (醋 *cù*, Acetum) 1.5 *shēng*

Bring the above two ingredients to a boil three times, letting it rise and fall three times. Take it. Ejecting the food means recovery. Alternatively, you can also boil [the flavescent sophora] in water.

Another formula: Decocted rhinoceros horn[1] is also excellent.

TEXT NOTE, LINE 25.81

[1] Rhinoceros horn is no longer used.

COMMENTARY, LINE 25.81

In poisoning that results from intake of food or drink, heat causes vexation, and toxin causes distention, oppression, and fullness. Use the bitterness of flavescent sophora and the sourness of vinegar to treat it by causing gushing discharge, resolving heat, and dispersing distention.

Line 25.82

贪食, 食多不消, 心腹坚满痛, 治之方

盐一升　水三升

右二味， 煮令盐消， 分三服， 当吐出食， 便差。

Tān shí, shí duō bù xiāo, xīn fù jiān mǎn tòng, zhì zhī fāng

Yán yī shēng shuǐ sān shēng

Yòu èr wèi, zhǔ lìng yán xiāo, fēn sān fú, dāng tù chū shí, biàn chài.

A formula to treat rapacious appetite and failure to disperse food after overeating, [which manifests] in hardness, fullness, and pain in the heart and abdomen:

salt (盐 *yán*, Sal) 1 *shēng*
water (水 *shuǐ*, Aqua) 3 *shēng*

Boil the above two ingredients until the salt is dissolved and divide into three doses. When the food is ejected, recovery ensues.

COMMENTARY, LINE 25.82

Salt is able to draw out gathering water and eject lodged food. It is therefore a suitable treatment for hardness, fullness, and pain in the heart and abdomen that is caused by overeating and non-dispersion of food.

Line 25.83

矾石生入腹，破人心肝，亦禁水。

Fán shí shēng rù fù, pò rén xīn gān, yì jìn shuǐ.

Alum that enters the abdomen raw breaks the person's heart and liver. Water is also contraindicated [after ingesting alum].

COMMENTARY, LINE 25.83

Crude (raw) alum (*bái fán*) is sour, astringent, and cold. After being ingested, its stimulating nature is very strong and therefore harmful to heart and liver qì. This action is further aggravated by drinking water, which dissolves it and thereby causes the body's fluids to be consumed. In clinic, a dosage of no more than three grams in pill form is recommended. Exceeding this amount will result in burning pain in the oral cavity and throat, retching and vomiting, and diarrhea.

Line 25.84

商陆以水服，杀人。

Shāng lù yǐ shuǐ fú, shā rén.

Taking phytolacca with water kills a person.

COMMENTARY, LINE 25.84

Phytolacca (*shāng lù*) is bitter and cold and sinking and downbearing, similar to the effect of euphorbia/knoxia (*dà jǐ*) and kansui (*gān suì*). Therefore it is contraindicated for patients with spleen vacuity water swelling. Taking an excessive amount decocted in water can cause elevated body temperature, accelerated heart beat, forced breathing, nausea and vomiting, abdominal pain and diarrhea, dizziness and clouding, lowered blood pressure, and coma or even death.

Line 25.85

葶苈子傅头疮，药成入脑，杀人。

Tíng lì zǐ chuán tóu chuāng, yào chéng rù nǎo, shā rén.

Lepidium/Descurainiae (*tíng lì zǐ*) is applied [as an external treatment for] head sores. If the qì of the medicine[1] enters the brain, this kills the person.

TEXT NOTE, LINE 25.85

[1] Qì of the medicine 药成 *yào chéng*: In accordance with alternative textual versions, this is a corruption and should be read as 药气 *yào qì* ("qì of the medicine") instead.

COMMENTARY, LINE 25.85

The bitter and cold effect of Lepidium/Descurainiae (*tíng lì zǐ*) is used to draw out the toxin in sores on the head by applying it externally. However, if it penetrates into the brain, it can endanger the patient's life and hence must be used with caution.

Line 25.86

水银入人耳，及六畜等，皆死，以金银着耳边，水银则吐。

Shuǐ yín rù rén ěr, jí liù chù děng, jiē sǐ, yǐ jīn yín zhù ěr biān, shuǐ yín zé tù.

When mercury enters a person's ears, or those of the six domestic animals, death ensues in all cases. Touching the sides of the ears with gold or silver causes the mercury to be ejected.

COMMENTARY, LINE 25.86

Mercury poisoning, which manifests with drooling, nausea and vomiting, throat pain, abdominal pain and diarrhea, hematuria, encumbered breathing, and turning blue, can result in death, Immediately attaching metal or silver to the sides of the ears, especially by using a magnetic conducting needle, may effectively draw out the mercury.

Line 25.87

苦练无子者，杀人。

Kǔ liàn wú zǐ zhě, shā rén.

Chinaberry[1] that does not have seeds kills a person.

TEXT NOTE, LINE 25.87

[1] Chinaberry 苦练 *kǔ liàn*: This is a variant form of the more common name 苦楝 *kǔ liàn*.

COMMENTARY, LINE 25.87

According to Chéng Lín 程林, chinaberry (*kǔ liàn*) has male and female plants. The male plants have no seeds, but have red roots, which are toxic, while the female plants have seeds and white roots, which are only slightly toxic and can therefore be used medicinally.

Line 25.88

凡诸毒，多是假毒以投，无知时宜煮甘草荠苨汁饮之。通除诸毒药。

Fán zhū dú, duō shì jiă dú yǐ tóu, wú zhī shí yí zhǔ gān cǎo jì ní zhī yǐn zhī. Tōng chú zhū dú yào.

The various cases of poisoning are mostly caused by [someone intentionally] adding artificial poison [to food]. If you do not know [the type of poison], boil licorice and apricot-leaved adenophora and drink the juice. This eliminates the various toxins.

COMMENTARY, LINE 25.88

Licorice and apricot-leaved adenophora are both sweet and cold. When boiled in water, they have the effect of banking up and nourishing original qì and resolving toxin.

INDEX

B

C

D

E

F

G

H

I

J

K

N

O

P

Q

R

S

T

U

V

X

Y

Z